New Insights into Intensive Care Medicine

New Insights into Intensive Care Medicine

Edited by Neil Perry

AMERICAN
MEDICAL PUBLISHERS
www.americanmedicalpublishers.com

American Medical Publishers,
41 Flatbush Avenue,
1st Floor, New York,
NY 11217, USA

Visit us on the World Wide Web at:
www.americanmedicalpublishers.com

ISBN: 978-1-63927-106-1

Cataloging-in-Publication Data

New insights into intensive care medicine / edited by Neil Perry.
p. cm.
Includes bibliographical references and index.
ISBN 978-1-63927-106-1
1. Critical care medicine. 2. Intensive care units. 3. Emergency medicine.
4. Medical emergencies. I. Perry, Neil.
RC86.7 .I58 2022
616.028--dc23

Table of Contents

Preface IX

Chapter 1 **Performance of the PEdiatric Logistic Organ Dysfunction-2 score in critically ill children requiring plasma transfusions** 1
Oliver Karam, Pierre Demaret, Alain Duhamel, Alison Shefler, Philip C. Spinella, Simon J. Stanworth, Marisa Tucci and Stéphane Leteurtre

Chapter 2 **Goal-directed fluid restriction during brain surgery** 8
Jinfeng Luo, Jing Xue, Jin Liu, Bin Liu, Li Liu and Guo Chen

Chapter 3 **Transportation of patients on extracorporeal membrane oxygenation** 15
Pedro Vitale Mendes, Cesar de Albuquerque Gallo, Bruno Adler Maccagnan Pinheiro Besen, Adriana Sayuri Hirota, Raquel de Oliveira Nardi, Edzangela Vasconcelos dos Santos, Ho Yeh Li, Daniel Joelsons, Eduardo Leite Vieira Costa, Flavia Krepel Foronda, Luciano Cesar Pontes Azevedo and Marcelo Park

Chapter 4 **Systematic review and meta-analysis of complications and mortality of veno-venous extracorporeal membrane oxygenation for refractory acute respiratory distress syndrome** 24
Sergi Vaquer, Candelaria de Haro, Paula Peruga, Joan Carles Oliva and Antonio Artigas

Chapter 5 **Intra-abdominal hypertension in patients with sellar region tumors** 37
Konstantin A Popugaev, Ivan A Savin, Andrew U Lubnin, Alexander S Goriachev, Boris A Kadashev, Pavel L Kalinin, Andrew V Oshorov, Alexander A Polupan, Ekaterina U Sokolova, Maxim A Kutin and Valeriy I Lukianov

Chapter 6 **Predictive factors of bleeding events in adults undergoing extracorporeal membrane oxygenation** 45
Cécile Aubron, Joris DePuydt, François Belon, Michael Bailey, Matthieu Schmidt, Jayne Sheldrake, Deirdre Murphy, Carlos Scheinkestel, D Jamie Cooper, Gilles Capellier, Vincent Pellegrino, David Pilcher and Zoe McQuilten

Chapter 7 **Neutrophil expression of glucocorticoid-induced leucine zipper (GILZ) anti-inflammatory protein is associated with acute respiratory distress syndrome severity** 55
Marie-Alix Espinasse, David Hajage, Philippe Montravers, Pascale Piednoir, Guillaume Dufour, Florence Tubach, Vanessa Granger, Luc de Chaisemartin, Benoît Noël, Marc Pallardy, Sylvie Chollet-Martin and Armelle Biola-Vidamment

Chapter 8 **Venovenous extracorporeal membrane oxygenation devices-related colonisations and infections** 67
Guillemette Thomas, Sami Hraiech, Nadim Cassir, Samuel Lehingue, Romain Rambaud, Sandrine Wiramus, Christophe Guervilly, Fanny Klasen, Mélanie Adda, Stéphanie Dizier, Antoine Roch, Laurent Papazian and Jean-Marie Forel

Chapter 9 **The association between FABP7 serum levels with survival and neurological complications in acetaminophen-induced acute liver failure** 77
Constantine J. Karvellas, Jaime L. Speiser, Mélanie Tremblay, William M. Lee and Christopher F. Rose

Chapter 10 **Mortality and detailed characteristics of pre-ICU qSOFA-negative patients with suspected sepsis** 88
Izumi Nakayama, Junichi Izawa, Hideyuki Mouri, Tetsuhisa Kitamura and Junji Shiotsuka

Chapter 11 **Assessment of renal hemodynamic toxicity of fluid challenge with 0.9% NaCl compared to balanced crystalloid (PlasmaLyte®) in a rat model with severe sepsis** 97
Pierre-Yves Olivier, François Beloncle, Valérie Seegers, Maher Tabka, Mathilde Renou de La Bourdonnaye, Alain Mercat, Paul Cales, Daniel Henrion, Peter Radermacher, Lise Piquilloud, Nicolas Lerolle and Pierre Asfar

Chapter 12 **Effect of HA330 resin-directed hemoadsorption on a porcine acute respiratory distress syndrome model** 105
Xuefeng Xu, Chune Jia, Sa Luo, Yanming Li, Fei Xiao, Huaping Dai and Chen Wang

Chapter 13 **Clinical features and outcome of patients with acute respiratory failure revealing anti-synthetase or anti-MDA-5 dermato-pulmonary syndrome** 122
Constance Vuillard, Marc Pineton de Chambrun, Nicolas de Prost, Claude Guérin, Matthieu Schmidt, Auguste Dargent, Jean-Pierre Quenot, Sébastien Préau, Geoffrey Ledoux, Mathilde Neuville, Guillaume Voiriot, Muriel Fartoukh, Rémi Coudroy, Guillaume Dumas, Eric Maury, Nicolas Terzi, Yacine Tandjaoui-Lambiotte, Francis Schneider, Maximilien Grall, Emmanuel Guérot, Romaric Larcher, Sylvie Ricome, Raphaël Le Mao, Gwenhaël Colin, Christophe Guitton, Lara Zafrani, Elise Morawiec, Marie Dubert, Olivier Pajot, Hervé Mentec, Gaëtan Plantefève and Damien Contou

Chapter 14 **Practical approach to diastolic dysfunction in light of the new guidelines and clinical applications in the operating room and in the intensive care** 134
F. Sanfilippo, S. Scolletta, A. Morelli and A. Vieillard-Baron

Chapter 15 **Evaluation of emotional excitation during standardized endotracheal intubation in simulated conditions** 146
Nicolas S. Marjanovic, Christelle Teiten, Nicola Pallamin and Erwan L'Her

Chapter 16 **Usefulness of video-laryngoscopy with the Airway Scope for intubation performance and learning** 154
Pierre-Louis Declercq, Michael Bubenheim, Stéphanie Gelinotte, Kévin Guernon, Jean-Baptiste Michot, Vincent Royon, Dorothée Carpentier, Gaëtan Béduneau, Fabienne Tamion and Christophe Girault

Chapter 17 **Plasma microRNAs levels are different between pulmonary and extrapulmonary ARDS patients** 167
Yi Zheng, Song-qiao Liu, Qin Sun, Jian-feng Xie, Jing-yuan Xu, Qing Li, Chun Pan, Ling Liu and Ying-zi Huang

Chapter 18 **Practice of ultrasound-guided central venous catheter technique by the French intensivists** 180
Julien Maizel, Marie-Anaïs Bastide, Jack Richecoeur, Eric Frenoy, Christian Lemaire, Bertrand Sauneuf, Hervé Dupont, Fabienne Tamion, Saad Nseir and Damien Du Cheyron

Chapter 19 **Knockout of interleukin-17A protects against sepsis-associated acute kidney injury** 188
Cong-juan Luo, Feng Luo, Li Zhang, Yan Xu, Guang-yan Cai, Bo Fu, Zhe Feng, Xue-feng Sun and Xiang-mei Chen

Chapter 20 **SAPS 3 score as a predictive factor for postoperative referral to intensive care unit** 198
João M. Silva Jr., Helder Marcus Costa Rocha, Henrique Tadashi Katayama, Leandro Ferreira Dias, Mateus Barros de Paula, Leusi Magda Romano Andraus, Jose Maria Correa Silva and Luiz Marcelo Sá Malbouisson

Chapter 21 **Outcome of in- and out-of-hospital cardiac arrest survivors with liver cirrhosis** 205
Kevin Roedl, Christian Wallmüller, Andreas Drolz, Thomas Horvatits, Karoline Rutter, Alexander Spiel, Julia Ortbauer, Peter Stratil, Pia Hubner, Christoph Weiser, Jasmin Katrin Motaabbed, Dominik Jarczak, Harald Herkner, Fritz Sterz and Valentin Fuhrmann

Chapter 22 **Carotid and femoral Doppler do not allow the assessment of passive leg raising effects** 214
Valentina Girotto, Jean-Louis Teboul, Alexandra Beurton, Laura Galarza, Thierry Guedj, Christian Richard and Xavier Monnet

Chapter 23 **Fluoroscopy-guided simultaneous distal perfusion as a preventive strategy of limb ischemia in patients undergoing extracorporeal membrane oxygenation** 222
Woo Jin Jang, Yang Hyun Cho, Taek Kyu Park, Young Bin Song, Jin-Oh Choi, Joo-Yong Hahn, Seung-Hyuk Choi, Hyeon-Cheol Gwon, Eun-Seok Jeon, Woo Jung Chun, Ju Hyeon Oh and Jeong Hoon Yang

Permissions

List of Contributors

Index

Preface

Intensive care medicine deals with the diagnosis and treatment of critically ill patients that need advanced monitoring and life saving support. Its diagnosis and treatment are carried out in special intensive care units within the hospital. Some of the equipment used in such units are ventricular assist devices, hemodynamic and cardiac monitoring systems, intra-aortic balloon pumps, extracorporeal membrane oxygenation circuits, continuous renal replacement equipment, etc. These equipment help in hemofiltration, mechanical ventilation, and invasive monitoring. There are many drugs that are used under intensive care. These include inotropes, sedatives, antibiotics and analgesics. This book explores all the important aspects of intensive care medicine in the present day scenario. It also unravels the recent studies in this field. This book is a vital tool for all researching and studying this field.

This book is the end result of constructive efforts and intensive research done by experts in this field. The aim of this book is to enlighten the readers with recent information in this area of research. The information provided in this profound book would serve as a valuable reference to students and researchers in this field.

At the end, I would like to thank all the authors for devoting their precious time and providing their valuable contribution to this book. I would also like to express my gratitude to my fellow colleagues who encouraged me throughout the process.

Editor

Performance of the PEdiatric Logistic Organ Dysfunction-2 score in critically ill children requiring plasma transfusions

Oliver Karam[1,2*], Pierre Demaret[2,3], Alain Duhamel[2,4], Alison Shefler[5], Philip C. Spinella[6], Simon J. Stanworth[7], Marisa Tucci[8], Stéphane Leteurtre[2,9] and for the PlasmaTV investigators

Abstract

Background: Organ dysfunction scores, based on physiological parameters, have been created to describe organ failure. In a general pediatric intensive care unit (PICU) population, the PEdiatric Logistic Organ Dysfunction-2 score (PELOD-2) score had both a good discrimination and calibration, allowing to describe the clinical outcome of critically ill children throughout their stay. This score is increasingly used in clinical trials in specific subpopulation. Our objective was to assess the performance of the PELOD-2 score in a subpopulation of critically ill children requiring plasma transfusions.

Methods: This was an ancillary study of a prospective observational study on plasma transfusions over a 6-week period, in 101 PICUs in 21 countries. All critically ill children who received at least one plasma transfusion during the observation period were included. PELOD-2 scores were measured on days 1, 2, 5, 8, and 12 after plasma transfusion. Performance of the score was assessed by the determination of the discrimination (area under the ROC curve: AUC) and the calibration (Hosmer–Lemeshow test).

Results: Four hundred and forty-three patients were enrolled in the study (median age and weight: 1 year and 9.1 kg, respectively). Observed mortality rate was 26.9 % (119/443). For PELOD-2 on day 1, the AUC was 0.76 (95 % CI 0.71–0.81) and the Hosmer–Lemeshow test was $p = 0.76$. The serial evaluation of the changes in the daily PELOD-2 scores from day 1 demonstrated a significant association with death, adjusted for the PELOD-2 score on day 1.

Conclusions: In a subpopulation of critically ill children requiring plasma transfusion, the PELOD-2 score has a lower but acceptable discrimination than in an entire population. This score should therefore be used cautiously in this specific subpopulation.

Keywords: Plasma transfusion, Critical care, Children, Outcome, Multiple organ failure, Score

Background

Mortality is a frequent outcome in clinical trials in critically ill adults [1–5]. However, as mortality is lower in pediatric intensive care unit (PICU) patients [6–8], other outcome measures have been developed. Multiple organ dysfunction syndrome (MODS), frequently observed in PICU, is a good candidate marker of severity of illness because MODS is the main cause of death in adult ICU [9] and in PICU patients [7]. MODS scores can be used to assess the presence and severity of organ dysfunction on admission and throughout the stay [9].

In a general PICU population, the PEdiatric Logistic Organ Dysfunction-2 score (PELOD-2) and the daily PELOD-2 scores had both a good discrimination and calibration, allowing to describe the clinical outcome of critically ill children throughout their stay [8, 10].

Little is known regarding plasma use in children. Our recent international observational study shows that non-bleeding patients represent more than half of the critically

*Correspondence: oliver.karam@hcuge.ch
[1] Pediatric Intensive Care Unit, Geneva University Hospital, Geneva, Switzerland
Full list of author information is available at the end of the article

ill children receiving plasma transfusions [11]. This marked heterogeneity in plasma transfusion patterns might be due to the absence of randomized controlled trials (RCTs) that could guide plasma transfusion strategies [12].

The first version of the PELOD score [7] has been used over the last few years as an outcome measure in studies in specific subpopulations, such as sepsis [13], hematopoietic stem cell transplant [14], acute respiratory dysfunction syndrome [15], extracorporeal life support [16], drowning [17], or seizure [18]. However, some authors have voiced their concern regarding using organ dysfunction scores in specific subpopulations [9].

Our hypothesis was that the PELOD-2 score would have the same performance in the subpopulation of patients receiving at least one plasma transfusion, validating its use as a surrogate outcome in a future RCT.

Our objective was to assess the performance of the PELOD-2 score in a subset of critically ill children requiring plasma transfusions [11] during their PICU stay.

Methods

Study sites and population

This is an ancillary study of a large point-prevalence study conducted in 101 PICUs in 21 countries. The complete methods have already been published elsewhere [11].

In brief, six 1-week periods were randomly predefined over six consecutive months (April to September 2014) for each study site. All critically ill children aged 3 days to 16 years old admitted to a participating PICU on one of the study days were considered eligible. Any eligible patient for whom at least one plasma transfusion was administered on any study day was included unless one of the exclusion criteria (i.e., plasmapheresis and gestational age less than 37 weeks at the time of PICU admission) was present. If a patient was readmitted within 24 h of PICU discharge, this was considered part of the same admission.

Variable of interest

The primary variable of interest of this analysis is the daily PELOD-2 scores [8, 10]. This score evaluates five organ functions using ten items: neurologic (Glasgow coma score and pupillary reaction), cardiovascular (lactatemia, mean arterial pressure), renal (creatinine), respiratory (PaO_2/FiO_2 ratio, $PaCO_2$, invasive ventilation), and hematologic (white blood cell count and platelets). Data were collected on days 1 (i.e., the day of first transfusion), 2, 5, 8, and 12. These time points were previously identified as the first optimal time points to estimate the daily PELOD-2 scores [8, 10].

As for previously published severity and MODS scores, the most abnormal value of each variable observed during each of these time points was considered to calculate the PELOD-2 score. No laboratory tests were performed solely to meet the needs of this research; as recommended, a non-collected value was considered normal [8].

We also collected demographic data and PICU mortality, our primary outcome, which was censored 28 days after the end of the enrollment period.

Ethics approval

Ethics committees or boards at all 101 sites approved this study.

Statistical analysis

Descriptive statistics are reported as mean ± standard deviation (SD), median and interquartile range (IQR), or proportions with their 95 % CI.

The association between PELOD-2 score and death was assessed by comparing the PELOD-2 score between survivors and non-survivors with a Mann–Whitney test. We also tested this association, adjusting for the baseline risk (PELOD-2 score at day 1) and the daily change in PELOD-2 score using a logistic regression model [10].

Discrimination refers to the ability of the score to separate non-survivors from survivors across the whole group [19]. We calculated the area under the receiver operating characteristic curve (AUC) of the PELOD-2 scores with its 95 % CI, for each time point. It is usually considered that an AUC of 1, 0.90–0.99, 0.80–0.89, 0.70–0.79, 0.60–0.69, and <0.60 is considered to be perfect, excellent, very good, good, moderate, and poor, respectively [20].

The *calibration* was assessed by directly comparing the observed and customized predicted mortality across subcategories of risk. We employed the Hosmer–Lemeshow goodness-of-fit test, where a p value >0.05 indicates acceptable calibration [20].

All tests were two sided, with an alpha level of 0.05. All statistical analyses were performed with SPSS version 20 for Mac (SPSS, Chicago, IL, USA).

Results

Population

Over the 30 study days, 13,192 patients were admitted and hence eligible and 443 (3.4 %) critically ill children receiving at least one plasma transfusion were included. The center which included the largest number of patients contributed to 11.1 % (49/443) of the results. Two hundred and fifty-three patients were from Europe, 134 from North America, and 56 from other continents.

The median age and weight were 1 year (IQR 0.2–6.4) and 9.1 kg (IQR 4.0–21.0), respectively. Forty-three percent were males. The main reasons for admission to PICU were respiratory (32 %), cardiac surgery with bypass (30 %), elective surgery (24 %), septic shock

(15 %), emergency surgery (13 %), cardiac non-surgical (11 %), renal failure (10 %), and hepatic failure (10 %). Forty-eight patients (11 %) were on extracorporeal life support, and 35 patients (8 %) were on continuous renal replacement therapy. The full demographic description is available elsewhere [11].

The primary indication for plasma transfusion was critical bleeding in 22 % of patients, minor bleeding in 21 %, planned surgery or procedure in 12 %, and high risk of postoperative bleeding in 11 %. No bleeding or planned procedures were reported in 34 % of patients.

Median length of mechanical ventilation was 5 days (IQR 1–16), and median PICU length of stay was 10 days (IQR 4–24). The median time to death was 6 days (IQR 1;17).

PELOD-2 score

PELOD-2 score was collected in all patients on day 1 and in all surviving patients still in the PICU at posttransfusion days 2, 5, 8, and 12. There were no missing data.

Median PELOD-2 scores were statistically different between survivors and non-survivors: 7 (5;9) versus 10 (7;15) on transfusion day 1 ($p < 0.001$), as well as on the other days (Table 1; Fig. 1).

The PELOD-2 score on day 1 was a significant prognostic factor: The odds ratio for death was 1.30 (95 % CI 1.22–1.39) for each PELOD-2 point. Similarly, the serial evaluation of the changes in the daily PELOD-2 scores from day 1, adjusted for baseline value (PELOD-2 at day 1), demonstrated a significant association with death, for each of the observation days (Table 2).

Discrimination

The AUC was 0.76 (95 % CI 0.71–0.81, Fig. 2) for day 1 and 0.78, 0.74, 0.74, and 0.77, for days 2, 5, 8, and 12, respectively (Table 3). Adding the INR to the PELOD-2 score resulted in an AUC of 0.77 (95 % CI 0.71–0.83). The AUC on day 1 according to plasma transfusion indication and according to the reason for admission is presented in Tables 4 and 5, respectively.

Table 1 PELOD-2 score in survivors and non-survivors

Day	Survivors		Non-survivors		*p*
	Mean	Median (IQR)	Mean	Median (IQR)	
Day 1	6.7	7 (5;9)	11.2	10 (7;15)	<0.001
Day 2	6.5	7 (4;9)	11.0	11 (8;13)	<0.001
Day 5	6.1	6 (3;9)	9.2	9 (8;11)	<0.001
Day 8	5.6	5 (3;8)	8.8	9 (7;11)	<0.001
Day 12	5.1	5 (2;7)	8.5	9 (6;11)	<0.001

PELOD-2 score PEdiatric Logistic Organ Dysfunction-2 score, *IQR* interquartile range

Calibration

The Hosmer–Lemeshow Chi-square value was 5.02 ($p = 0.76$) for PELOD-2 score on day 1. The results for the other time points, according to plasma transfusion indication, and according to the reason for admission are given in Tables 3, 4, and 5, respectively.

Adding the INR to the PELOD-2 score resulted in Hosmer–Lemeshow Chi-square value of 10.6 ($p = 0.23$).

Discussion

Our results indicate that in a subpopulation of critically ill children requiring plasma transfusions, the PELOD-2 score has an acceptable performance. These results of performance of the PELOD-2 scores are observed with the performance both according to the indications to plasma transfusion (Table 4) and according to the 5 days of the PELOD-2 scores (Tables 2, 3).

The PELOD-2 score seems to have a lower, although acceptable discrimination power compared to a general PICU population, where it had an excellent discrimination power, based on an AUC of 0.93. As the PELOD-2 score has been advocated to be "used as a surrogate outcome measure in randomized clinical trials" [7, 8], many recent trials have used these scores to assess patients [13–18]. As these studies enrolled only specific PICU subpopulations, their results should be interpreted cautiously, in light of our findings. Similar caveats have been made for adult organ dysfunction scores regarding their use in specific subpopulations [9].

The lower discrimination of the PELOD-2 score in a subset of critically ill children transfused with plasma might be explained by different observations. First, our population was sicker than the initial PELOD-2 study, with a mortality rate of 26.9 versus 6.0 %. The PICU length of stay was also longer (10 vs. 2 days), as the case-mix was different: In our population compared to the PELOD-2 population, the reasons for admission were less frequently respiratory (32 vs. 47 %, $p < 0.001$) and more frequently cardiovascular (64 vs. 19 %, $p < 0.001$) or hepatic (10 vs. 1 %, $p < 0.001$) [8]. Moreover, in the study of Pollack et al. (10,078 patients from U.S. PICUs), the mortality rate was 2.7 %, with a median age of 3.7 years and a median hospital length of stay of 4.9 days (PICU length of stay was not provided) [21]. The fact that all patients received plasma transfusions might also explain

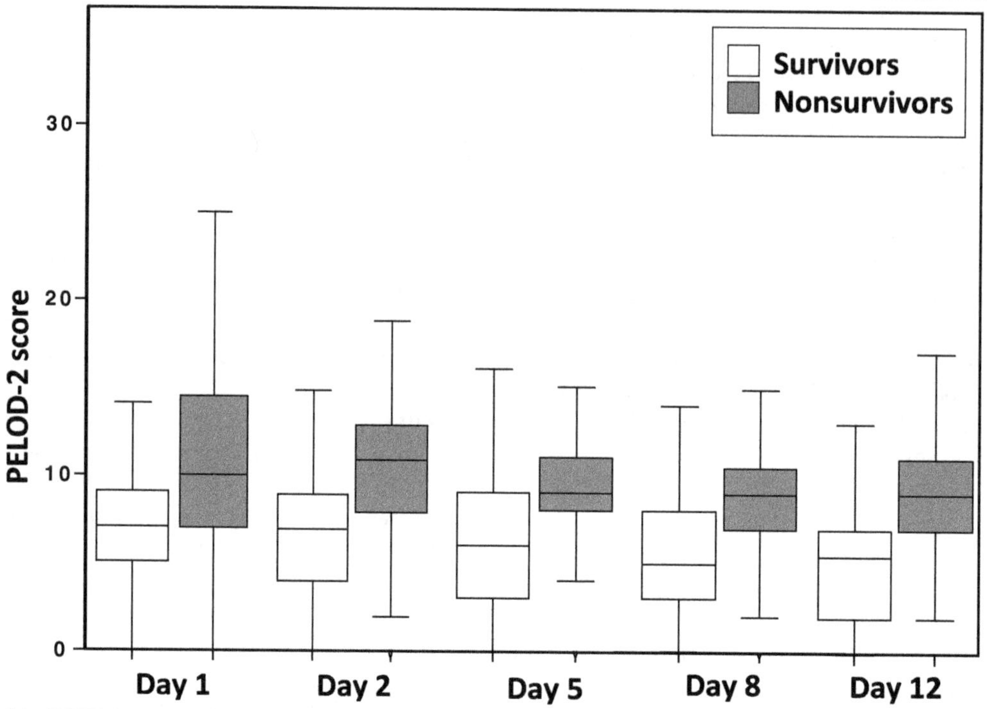

Fig. 1 Boxplot of the PELOD-2 score on days 1, 2, 5, 8, and 12, among survivors (*white*) and non-survivors (*gray*). On each study day, PELOD-2 scores were significantly different between survivors and non-survivors

Table 2 Serial evaluation of the change in the daily PELOD-2 score from day 1, adjusted for baseline value (PELOD-2 score on day 1)

Variable	Odds ratio	95 % CI	*p* value
PELOD-2 score on day 1	1.30	1.22–1.39	<0.0001
Change in PELOD-2 score			
Day 1–day 2	1.33	1.21–1.47	<0.0001
Day 1–day 5	1.26	1.15–1.39	<0.0001
Day 1–day 8	1.28	1.15–1.43	<0.0001
Day 1–day 12	1.38	1.20–1.58	<0.0001

Odds ratio (OR) for death is provided with a 95 % CI. The cumulative OR of death can be calculated as follows: (OR of PELOD-2 score on day 1)$^{\text{PELOD-2 score on day 1}}$ × (OR of change in score from day 1 to specific day)$^{\text{PELOD-2 score on specific day} - \text{PELOD-2 score on day 1}}$. For example, for a child whose score is 10 on day 1 and 6 on day 12 (change in score −4), the OR for death would be $1.30^{10} \times 1.38^{-4} = 3.80$

PELOD-2 score PEdiatric Logistic Organ Dysfunction-2 score, *OR* odds ratio

this lower discrimination, as observational studies have suggested that plasma transfusions were independently associated with increased risk of morbidity and mortality [9, 22–24], but neither coagulopathy nor plasma transfusions are items of the PELOD-2 score. Third, except for mechanical ventilation, PELOD-2 score does not take into account the support that can be offered for each organ, such as vasoactive drugs, continuous renal replacement therapies, or extracorporeal life support (ECLS). Given that the mortality rate associated with ECLS is close to 50 % [25, 26], one could hypothesize that a lower discrimination may be due at least partly to the fact that PELOD-2 score does not take this variable into account. Similarly, the PELOD-2 score does not incorporate coagulopathy, which might be associated with increased risk of bleeding or disseminated intravascular

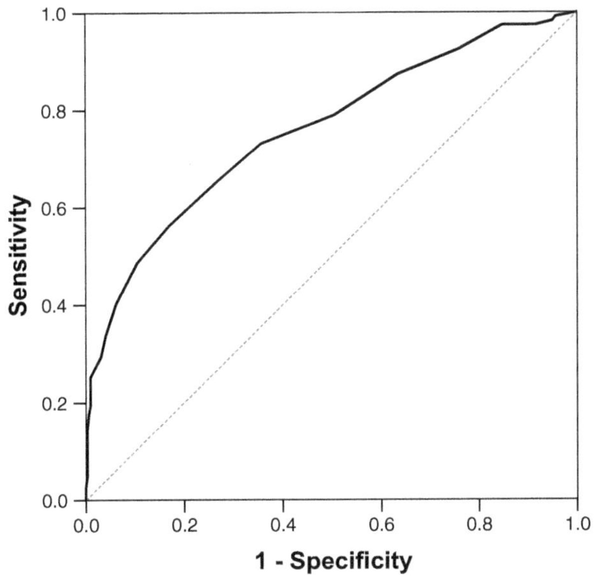

Fig. 2 Receiver operating characteristic (ROC) curve of the PELOD-2 score on day 1. The area under the curve was 0.76 (95 % CI 0.71–0.81). The *dashed line* represents the reference line

coagulopathy, which are also known to be associated with increased mortality [27].

As observed in the validation study, severity of illness is a major component to evaluate the performance of the daily PELOD-2 scores [10]. Therefore, in this study, the serial evaluation of the change in the daily PELOD-2 score has to be adjusted to the baseline value (PELOD-2 score on day 1). Our results indicate that changes in the PELOD-2 score over time are also associated with changes in the probability of death. These are important findings, as they validate the use of sequential measuring of the PELOD-2 score to assess clinical outcome. These results also highlight the relationship between organ failure and death.

Some limitations must be recognized. First, our results are only applicable to critically ill children requiring plasma transfusions and not to other PICU subpopulations. Second, our study days were not days after admission but days after plasma transfusion. It is of note, however, that the median length of PICU stay before the first plasma transfusion was 1 day. Third, although scores have classically been evaluated by their association with mortality, they might still adequately describe the clinical situation related to organ failure, as it has solid physiological basis and is clinically meaningful. Therefore, the ability of the PELOD-2 score to describe organ failure and its change over time might be more important that its ability to predict death. Fourth, additional variables to the PELOD-2 score could have been evaluated. Unfortunately, some interesting variables, such as platelet count, were not available in our database. However, adding the INR to the PELOD-2 score did not improve its performance.

Table 3 Performance of the PELOD-2 score according to study days

	Day 1	Day 2	Day 5	Day 8	Day 12
Number of patients	443	411	295	231	165
Mortality rate	119 (27 %)	98 (24 %)	67 (23 %)	51 (22 %)	41 (25 %)
PELOD-2 (median, IQR)	7 (5;10)	7 (5;10)	7 (4;9)	6 (3;9)	6 (3;9)
AUC (95 % CI)	0.76 (0.71–0.81)	0.78 (0.73–0.84)	0.74 (0.67–0.81)	0.74 (0.66–0.82)	0.77 (0.68–0.85)
Hosmer–Lemeshow test	$p = 0.76$	$p = 0.63$	$p = 0.09$	$p = 0.30$	$p = 0.77$

PELOD-2 score PEdiatric Logistic Organ Dysfunction-2 score, *IQR* interquartile range, *AUC* area under receiver the operating characteristic curve

Table 4 Performance of the PELOD-2 score on day 1, according to indications to plasma transfusion

	Critical bleeding	Minor Bleeding	Preparation[a]	Post-op risk of bleeding	No bleeding
Number of patients	99	94	52	47	151
Mortality rate	34 (35 %)	14 (16 %)	16 (32 %)	9 (19 %)	46 (31 %)
PELOD-2 (median, IQR)	8 (6–11)	7 (5–8)	7 (4–11)	7 (5–9)	7 (5–10)
AUC (95 % CI)	0.81 (0.72–0.91)	0.83 (0.70–0.96)	0.60 (0.44–0.76)	0.88 (0.74–1.00)	0.71 (0.62–0.80)
Hosmer–Lemeshow test	$p = 0.42$	$p = 0.34$	$p = 0.26$	$p = 0.54$	$p = 0.58$

PELOD-2 score PEdiatric Logistic Organ Dysfunction-2 score, *IQR* interquartile range, *AUC* area under receiver the operating characteristic curve

[a] Preparation refers to preparation for surgery or procedure

Table 5 Performance of the PELOD-2 score on day 1, according to patients' reason for admission

	Respiratory	Cardiac surgery with bypass	Elective surgery	Septic shock	Renal failure
Number of patients[a]	143	133	107	65	45
Mortality rate	54 (38 %)	19 (14 %)	9 (8 %)	21 (32 %)	19 (42 %)
PELOD-2 (median, IQR)	8 (6–11)	7 (5–9)	6 (5–8)	8 (6–12)	8 (6–10)
AUC (95 % CI)	0.76 (0.68–0.85)	0.75 (0.62–0.88)	0.80 (0.62–0.97)	0.77 (0.66–0.89)	0.69 (0.53–0.85)
Hosmer–Lemeshow test	$p = 0.99$	$p = 0.23$	$p = 0.17$	$p = 0.27$	$p = 0.39$

PELOD-2 score PEdiatric Logistic Organ Dysfunction-2 score, *IQR* interquartile range, *AUC* area under receiver the operating characteristic curve

[a] Patients could be categorized into more than one reason of admission

Conclusions

In a subpopulation of critically ill children requiring plasma transfusion, the PELOD-2 score has a lower but acceptable discrimination than in an entire population. Although using this score as an outcome in a RCT seems reasonable, it should be interpreted cautiously.

Abbreviations

AUC: area under the receiver operating characteristic curve; CI: confidence interval; ECLS: extracorporeal life support; FiO_2: inspired fraction of oxygen; IQR: interquartile range; MODS: multiple organ dysfunction syndrome; OR: odds ratio; SD: standard deviation; PaO_2: partial pressure of arterial oxygen; $PaCO_2$: partial pressure of arterial carbon dioxide; PELOD-2: PEdiatric Logistic Organ Dysfunction-2 score; PICU: pediatric intensive care unit.

Authors' contributions

All authors participated in the initial PlasmaTV study. OK and SL designed this ancillary study. OK, AD, and SL analyzed the data. OK and SL drafted the manuscript, and all authors participated in the final version of the manuscript. All authors read and approved the final manuscript.

Author details

[1] Pediatric Intensive Care Unit, Geneva University Hospital, Geneva, Switzerland. [2] Univ. Lille, EA 2694 - Santé Publique: épidémiologie et qualité des soins, 59000 Lille, France. [3] Pediatric Intensive Care Unit, CHC Liège, Liège, Belgium. [4] Department of Biostatistics, CHU Lille, 59000 Lille, France. [5] Pediatric Intensive Care Unit, Oxford University Hospitals, Oxford, UK. [6] Division of Critical Care, Department of Pediatrics, Washington University in St. Louis, St. Louis, MO, USA. [7] NHS Blood and Transplant, John Radcliffe Hospital, Oxford, UK. [8] Pediatric Intensive Care Unit, CHU Sainte-Justine, Montreal, Canada. [9] Pediatric Intensive Care Unit, CHU Lille, 59000 Lille, France.

Acknowledgements

We would like to thank all of the PlasmaTV investigators for their tremendous work. We would also like to thank the Plateforme de Recherche Clinique of the Department of Pediatrics, Geneva University Hospital, for their help with this study.

Competing interests

Dr. Spinella reports personal fees from Octapharma and personal fees from Entegrion. The authors declare that they have no competing interests.

Funding

This study was funded by the Groupe Francophone de Réanimation et Urgences Pédiatriques (GFRUP) and the Marisa Sophie Research Foundation for Critically Ill Children.

PlasmaTV investigators

Australia: Warwick Butt, Carmel Delzoppo, Kym Bain (Royal Children's Hospital, Melbourne); Simon Erickson, Nathan Smalley (Princess Margaret Hospital for Children, Perth; Tavey Dorofaeff, Debbie Long (Royal Children's Hospital, Brisbane); Nathan Smalley, Greg Wiseman (Townsville Hospital, Townsville). Belgium: Stéphan Clénent de Cléty, Caroline Berghe (Cliniquesuniversitaires Saint-Luc, Brussels); Annick de Jaeger (Princess Elisabeth Children's University Hospital, Ghent); Pierre Demaret, Marc Trippaerts (CHC-CHR, Liège); Ariane Willems, ShancyRooze (Hôpitaluniversitaire des enfantsReine Fabiola, Brussels); Jozef De Dooy (Antwerp University Hospital, Edegem). Canada: Elaine Gilfoyle, Lynette Wohlgemuth (Alberta Children's Hospital, Calgary, AB); Marisa Tucci, Mariana Dumitrascu (CHU Sainte-Justine, Montréal, QC); Davinia Withington, Julia Hickey (Montreal Children's Hospital, Montreal, QC); Karen Choong, Lois Sanders (McMaster Children's Hospital, Hamilton, ON); Gavin Morrison (IWK Health Centre, Halifax, NS); Janice Tijssen (Children's Hospital, London Health Sciences Centre, London, ON); David Wensley, Gordon Krahn (British Columbia Children's Hospital, Vancouver, BC); Marc-Andre Dugas, Louise Gosselin (Centre Mère Enfant Soleil, CHU de Québec, Québec, QC); Miriam Santschi (CHUS, Sherbrooke, QC). Chile: Bettina Von Dessauer, Nadia Ordenes (Hospital De Niños Roberto Del Río, Santiago). Denmark: Arash Afshari, Lasse Hoegh Andersen, Jens Christian Nilsson, Mathias Johansen, Anne-Mette Baek Jensen (Rigshospitalet, University of Copenhagen, Copenhagen). Ecuador: Santiago Campos Mino, Michelle Grunauer (Hospital de los Valles, Universidad San Francisco de Quito, Quito. France: Nicolas Joram (Hôpital mère enfant, Nantes); Nicolas Roullet-Renoleau (Hôpital Gatien de Clocheville, CHU Tours, Tours); Etienne Javouhey, Fleur Cour-Andlauer, Aurélie Portefaix (Hôpital Femme Mère Enfant, Hospices Civils de Lyon, Lyon); Olivier Brissaud, Julie Guichoux (Hôpital des Enfants, Bordeaux); Valérie Payen (CHU Grenoble, Grenoble); Pierre-Louis Léger (Hôpital Armand-Trousseau, Paris); Mickael Afanetti (Hopitaux Pédiatriques CHU Lenval, Nice); Guillaume Mortamet (Hopital Necker, Paris); Matthieu Maria (Hôpital d'Enfants CHRU de Nancy, Nancy); Audrey Breining (Hopitaux Universitaires de Strasbourg, Strasbourg); Pierre Tissieres (Hôpital Kremlin-Bicêtre, Paris); Aimée Dorkenoo (CHU Lille, Lille); Anna Deho (Hopital Robert Debré, Paris). Germany: Harry Steinherr (MedizinischeHochschule Hannover, Hannover). Greece: Filippia Nikolaou (Athens Children Hospital P&A Kyriakou, Athens). Italy: Anna Camporesi (Children Hospital VittoreBuzzi, Milano); Federica Mario (Department of Women's and Children's Health, Padua). Japan: Tatsuya Kawasaki, Shinya Miura (Shizuoka Children's Hospital, Shizuoka City). New Zealand: John Beca, Miriam Rea, Claire Sherring, Tracey Bushell (Starship Children's Hospital, Auckland). Norway: Gunnar Bentsen (Oslo University Hospital—Rikshospitalet, Oslo). Portugal: Alexandra Dinis (Hospital Pediátrico—CHUC, Coimbra); Gabriela Pereira (UCIP Hospital Dona Estefânia, Lisbon); Marisa Vieira (Hospital de Santa Maria, Lisbon); Marta Moniz (Hospital Prof. Dr Fernando Fonseca, Amadora). Saudi Arabia: Saleh Alshehri (King Saud Medical City, Riyadh); Manal Alasnag, Ahmad Rajab (King Fahd Armed Forces Hospital, Jeddah). Slovakia: Maria Pisarcikova (DFN Kosice, Kosice). Spain: Iolanda Jordan (Hospital Sant Joan de Déu, Barcelona); Joan Balcells (Hospital Valld'Hebron,

Barcelona); Antonio Perez-Ferrer, Jesús de Vicente Sánchez, Marta Vazquez Moyano (La Paz University Hospital, Madrid); Antonio Morales Martinez (Malaga Regional University Hospital, Malaga); Jesus Lopez-Herce, Maria Jose Solana (Hospital General Universitario Gregorio Marañón, Madrid); Jose Carlos Flores González (Puerta del Mar University Hospital, Cadiz); Maria Teresa Alonso (Hospital Virgen del Rocío, Sevilla); Manuel Nieto Faza (Hospital Universitario Cruces, Bilbao). Switzerland: Marie-Hélène Perez, Vivianne Amiet (CHUV, Lausanne); Carsten Doell (Kinderspital Zürich, Zürich); Alice Bordessoule (Geneva University Hospital, Geneva). The Netherlands: Suzan Cochius-den Otter, Berber Kapitein (Erasmus MC—Sophia Children's Hospital, Rotterdam); Martin Kneyber (Beatrix Children's Hospital, Groningen). United Kingdom: Joe Brierley, Vanessa Rea, Stephen McKeever (Great Ormond Street, London); Andrea Kelleher (Royal Brompton Hospital, London); Barney Scholefield, Anke Top, Nicola Kelly, SatnamVirdee (Birmingham Children's Hospital, Birmingham); Peter Davis, Susan George (Bristol Royal Hospital for Children, Bristol); Kay C. Hawkins, Katie McCall, Victoria Brown (Royal Manchester Children's Hospital, Manchester); Kim Sykes (University Hospital Southampton, Southampton); Richard Levin, Isobel MacLeod (Yorkhill Children's Hospital, Glasgow); Marie Horan, PetrJirasek (Alder Hey Children's hospital, Liverpool); David Inwald, Amina Abdulla, Sophie Raghunanan (Imperial College Healthcare, London); Bob Taylor (Royal Belfast Hospital for Sick Children, Belfast); Alison Shefler, Hannah Sparkes (Oxford University Hospitals, Oxford). USA: Sheila Hanson, Katherine Woods, David Triscari, Kathy Murkowski (Children's Hospital of Wisconsin, Milwaukee, WI); Caroline Ozment (Duke University, Durham, NC); Marie Steiner, Dan Nerheim, Amanda Galster (University of Minneapolis, Minneapolis, MN); Renee Higgerson, LeeAnn Christie (Dell Children's Medical Center, Austin, TX); Philip C. Spinella, Daniel Martin, Liz Rourke (Washington University in St. Louis, Saint Louis, MO); Jennifer Muszynski, Lisa Steele, (Nationwide Children's Hospital, Columbus, OH); Samuel Ajizian, Michael C. McCrory (Wake Forest School of Medicine, Winston-Salem, NC); Kevin O'Brien, Christopher Babbitt, Erin Felkel, Glenn Levine (Miller Children's Hospital Long Beach, Long Beach, CA); Edward J. Truemper, Machelle Zink (Children's Hospital and Medical Center, Omaha, NE); Marianne Nellis (NYPH—Weill Cornell Medical College, New York, NY); Neal J. Thomas, Debbie Spear (Penn State Hershey Children's Hospital, Hershey, PA); Barry Markovitz, Jeff Terry, Rica Morzov (Children's Hospital Los Angeles, Los Angeles, CA); Vicki Montgomery, Andrew Michael, Melissa Thomas (University of Louisville and Kosair Children's Hospital, Louisville, KY); Marcy Singleton, Dean Jarvis, Sholeen Nett (Dartmouth Hitchcock Medical Center, Lebanon, NH); Douglas Willson, Michelle Hoot (Virginia Commonwealth University, Richmond, VA); Melania Bembea, Alvin Yiu (Johns Hopkins University, Baltimore, MD); David McKinley, Elizabeth Scarlett, Jennifer Sankey, Minal Parikh (Geisinger, Danville, PA); E. Vincent S. Faustino (Yale School of Medicine, New Haven, CT); Kelly Michelson, Jay Rilinger, Laura Campbell (Ann & Robert H. Lurie Children's Hospital of Chicago, Chicago, IL); Shira Gertz (Hackensack University Medical Center, Hackensack, NJ); Jill M. Cholette (University of Rochester, Rochester, NY); Asumthia Jeyapalan (Holtz Children's Hospital-Jackson Memorial Hospital, Miami, FL); Margaret Parker (Stony Brook University, Stony Brook, NY); Scot Bateman, Amanda Johnson (UMass Memorial Children's Medical Center, Worcester, MA).

References

1. Rivers E, Nguyen B, Havstad S, Ressler J, Muzzin A, Knoblich B, et al. Early goal-directed therapy in the treatment of severe sepsis and septic shock. N Engl J Med. 2001;345(19):1368–77.
2. Ferguson ND, Cook DJ, Guyatt GH, Mehta S, Hand L, Austin P, et al. High-frequency oscillation in early acute respiratory distress syndrome. N Engl J Med. 2013;368(9):795–805.
3. Young D, Lamb SE, Shah S, MacKenzie I, Tunnicliffe W, Lall R, et al. High-frequency oscillation for acute respiratory distress syndrome. N Engl J Med. 2013;368(9):806–13.
4. Asfar P, Meziani F, Hamel JF, Grelon F, Megarbane B, Anguel N, et al. High versus low blood-pressure target in patients with septic shock. N Engl J Med. 2014;370(17):1583–93.
5. Lacroix J, Hebert PC, Fergusson DA, Tinmouth A, Cook DJ, Marshall JC, et al. Age of transfused blood in critically ill adults. N Engl J Med. 2015;372(15):1410–8.
6. Pollack MM, Patel KM, Ruttimann UE. PRISM III: an updated pediatric risk of mortality score. Crit Care Med. 1996;24(5):743–52.
7. Leteurtre S, Martinot A, Duhamel A, Proulx F, Grandbastien B, Cotting J, et al. Validation of the paediatric logistic organ dysfunction (PELOD) score: prospective, observational, multicentre study. Lancet. 2003;362(9379):192–7.
8. Leteurtre S, Duhamel A, Salleron J, Grandbastien B, Lacroix J, Leclerc F, et al. PELOD-2: an update of the PEdiatric logistic organ dysfunction score. Crit Care Med. 2013;41(7):1761–73.
9. Vincent JL, Bruzzi de Carvalho F. Severity of illness. Semin Respir Crit Care Med. 2010;31(1):31–8.
10. Leteurtre S, Duhamel A, Deken V, Lacroix J, Leclerc F, Groupe Francophone de Reanimation et Urgences Pediatriques. Daily estimation of the severity of organ dysfunctions in critically ill children by using the PELOD-2 score. Crit Care. 2015;19(1):324.
11. Karam O, Demaret P, Shefler A, Leteurtre S, Spinella PC, Stanworth SJ, et al. Indications and effects of plasma transfusions in critically ill children. Am J Respir Crit Care Med. 2015;191(12):1395–402.
12. Karam O, Tucci M, Combescure C, Lacroix J, Rimensberger PC. Plasma transfusion strategies for critically ill patients. Cochrane Database Syst Rev. 2013; (12):CD010654.doi:10.1002/14651858.CD010654.pub2.
13. Raj S, Killinger JS, Gonzalez JA, Lopez L. Myocardial dysfunction in pediatric septic shock. J Pediatr. 2014;164(1):72–7.e2.
14. Duncan CN, Lehmann LE, Cheifetz IM, Greathouse K, Haight AE, Hall MW, et al. Clinical outcomes of children receiving intensive cardiopulmonary support during hematopoietic stem cell transplant. Pediatr Crit Care Med. 2013;14(3):261–7.
15. Orwoll BE, Spicer AC, Zinter MS, Alkhouli MF, Khemani RG, Flori HR, et al. Elevated soluble thrombomodulin is associated with organ failure and mortality in children with acute respiratory distress syndrome (ARDS): a prospective observational cohort study. Crit Care. 2015;19:435.
16. Rambaud J, Guellec I, Leger PL, Renolleau S, Guilbert J. Venoarterial extracorporeal membrane oxygenation support for neonatal and pediatric refractory septic shock. Indian J Crit Care Med. 2015;19(10):600–5.
17. Mtaweh H, Kochanek PM, Carcillo JA, Bell MJ, Fink EL. Patterns of multiorgan dysfunction after pediatric drowning. Resuscitation. 2015;90:91–6.
18. Payne ET, Zhao XY, Frndova H, McBain K, Sharma R, Hutchison JS, et al. Seizure burden is independently associated with short term outcome in critically ill children. Brain. 2014;137(Pt 5):1429–38.
19. Shann F. Are we doing a good job: PRISM, PIM and all that. Intensive Care Med. 2002;28(2):105–7.
20. Keegan MT, Gajic O, Afessa B. Severity of illness scoring systems in the intensive care unit. Crit Care Med. 2011;39(1):163–9.
21. Pollack MM, Holubkov R, Funai T, Dean JM, Berger JT, Wessel DL, et al. The pediatric risk of mortality score: update 2015. Pediatr Crit Care Med. 2016;17(1):2–9.
22. Karam O, Lacroix J, Robitaille N, Rimensberger PC, Tucci M. Association between plasma transfusions and clinical outcome in critically ill children: a prospective observational study. Vox Sang. 2013;104(4):342–9.
23. Khan H, Belsher J, Yilmaz M, Afessa B, Winters JL, Moore SB, et al. Fresh-frozen plasma and platelet transfusions are associated with development of acute lung injury in critically ill medical patients. Chest. 2007;131(5):1308–14.
24. Sarani B, Dunkman WJ, Dean L, Sonnad S, Rohrbach JI, Gracias VH. Transfusion of fresh frozen plasma in critically ill surgical patients is associated with an increased risk of infection. Crit Care Med. 2008;36(4):1114–8.
25. Barbaro RP, Odetola FO, Kidwell KM, Paden ML, Bartlett RH, Davis MM, et al. Association of hospital-level volume of extracorporeal membrane oxygenation cases and mortality. Analysis of the extracorporeal life support organization registry. Am J Respir Crit Care Med. 2015;191(8):894–901.
26. Bokman CL, Tashiro J, Perez EA, Lasko DS, Sola JE. Determinants of survival and resource utilization for pediatric extracorporeal membrane oxygenation in the United States 1997–2009. J Pediatr Surg. 2015;50(5):809–14.
27. Levi M, Ten Cate H. Disseminated intravascular coagulation. N Engl J Med. 1999;341(8):586–92.

2

Goal-directed fluid restriction during brain surgery

Jinfeng Luo, Jing Xue, Jin Liu, Bin Liu, Li Liu and Guo Chen*

Abstract

Background: The value of goal-directed fluid therapy in neurosurgical patients, where brain swelling is a major concern, is unknown. The aim of our study was to evaluate the effect of an intraoperative goal-directed fluid restriction (GDFR) strategy on the postoperative outcome of high-risk patients undergoing brain surgery.

Methods: High-risk patients undergoing brain surgery were randomly assigned to a usual care group (control group) or a GDFR group. In the GDFR group, (1) fluid maintenance was restricted to 3 ml/kg/h of a crystalloid solution and (2) colloid boluses were allowed only in case of hypotension associated with a low cardiac index and a high stroke volume variation. The primary outcome variable was ICU length of stay, and secondary outcomes were lactates at the end of surgery, postoperative complications, hospital length of stay, mortality at day 30, and costs.

Results: A total of 73 patients from the GDFR group were compared with 72 patients from the control group. Before surgery, the two groups were comparable. During surgery, the GDFR group received less colloid (1.9 ± 1.1 vs. 3.9 ± 1.6 ml/kg/h, $p = 0.021$) and less crystalloid (3 ± 0 vs. 5.0 ± 2.8 ml/kg/h, $p < 0.001$) than the control group. ICU length of stay was shorter (3 days [1–5] vs. 6 days [3–11], $p = 0.001$) and ICU costs were lower in the GDFR group. The total number of complications (46 vs. 99, $p = 0.043$) and the proportion of patients who developed one or more complications (19.2 vs. 34.7%, $p = 0.034$) were smaller in the GDFR group. Hospital length of stay and costs, as well as mortality at 30 day, were not significantly reduced.

Conclusion: In high-risk patients undergoing brain surgery, intraoperative GDFR was associated with a reduction in ICU length of stay and costs, and a decrease in postoperative morbidity.

Trial registration Chinese Clinical Trial Registry ChiCTR-TRC-13003583, Registered 20 Aug, 2013

Keywords: Fluid management, Goal-directed therapy, Goal-directed fluid restriction, Brain surgery, Postoperative complications, ICU length of stay

Background

Perioperative fluid administration has been shown to be a major determinant of postoperative outcome [1]. The amount of fluid administered during the perioperative period depends on multiple factors such as preoperative hydration, intraoperative blood loss, hemodynamic stability, as well as habits and believes of anesthesiologists and surgeons [2]. Fluid needs may be highly variable from one patient to the other and are hardly predictable from classical physiological parameters such as heart rate, blood pressure, and central venous pressure. Fluid titration based on the measurements of advanced hemodynamic parameters, such as cardiac output and dynamic predictors of fluid responsiveness, has been shown to be useful to improve the outcome of patients undergoing major abdominal, vascular, and orthopedic procedures [3–6].

Whether such strategies may also be useful in patients undergoing brain surgery is unknown. In this specific context, the temptation is to keep patients as dry as

*Correspondence: grace_chenguo@hotmail.com
Department of Anesthesiology and Translational Neuroscience Center, West China Hospital, Sichuan University, No. 37 Guoxue Xiang, Wuhou District, Chengdu 610041, Sichuan, People's Republic of China
Jinfeng Luo and Jing Xue are co-first authors

possible to prevent brain swelling. However, blinded or uncontrolled fluid restriction may expose patients to hypovolemia-related complications [1]. We hypothesized that advanced hemodynamic measurements may be useful to objectively balance the risks of fluid restriction (hypovolemia, hypotension, and cerebral ischemia) with the risk of inducing or worsening cerebral edema [7, 8]. In line with this concept, we designed an intraoperative fluid management protocol where minimal fluid maintenance with a crystalloid solution (fluid restriction) was combined with the administration of fluid boluses in case of severe and documented hypovolemia.

The goal of the present study was therefore to assess the effects of an intraoperative goal-directed fluid restriction (GDFR) strategy on the postoperative outcome of high-risk patients undergoing brain surgery.

Methods

Patient selection

Adult patients undergoing elective craniotomy for brain tumor resection, brain abscess, or intracranial aneurysm were considered for enrollment. Inclusion criteria were age >18, ASA score III or IV, and expected duration of surgery >2 h. Patients with a body weight <40 kg or >100 kg were excluded, as well as patients with cardiac arrhythmia (well-known limitation to the use of the stroke volume variation as an indicator of fluid responsiveness) [9]. The study was approved by the Ethical Committee of the West China Hospital from Sichuan University (No. 2012-104). After obtaining written informed consent, patients were randomly assigned to a standard fluid management group (Control) or to a GDFR group. A random number table was used to generate the random number sequence. All random numbers were concealed in sealed envelopes and assigned to a patient when entering the operating room.

Intraoperative monitoring and management

In addition to pulse oximetry, capnography, and heart rate monitoring, all patients had a radial arterial line in place for continuous blood pressure monitoring and a BIS sensor in place to monitor depth of anesthesia. Tidal volume was set at 8 ml/kg and respiratory frequency was adapted to maintain end-tidal CO_2 between 30 and 35 mmHg. Anesthesia induction was done with propofol (2 mg/kg) and rocuronium (1 mg/kg), and then propofol and remifentanil were used to maintain depth of anesthesia (BIS in the range 40–60). Body temperature was maintained close to normal using warmed solutions and insulation blankets. Per our neurosurgical policy, all patients received mannitol the day before surgery (250 ml), at the beginning of the surgical procedure (250 ml), and the day after surgery (125 ml).

In the control group, no recommendation was given for fluid and hemodynamic management during and after surgery, and therapeutic decisions were left at the discretion of the attending anesthesiologist and intensivist. In the GDFR group and during surgery, fluid maintenance was set at 3 ml/kg/h of normal saline with an infusion pump, and additional colloid (gelatins or hydroxyethyl starches) boluses (200 ml) were allowed only in case of systemic hypotension (MAP < 65 mmHg) with a cardiac index (CI) <2.5 l/min/m^2 and a stroke volume variation (SVV) >15%. In case of hypotension with a CI >2.5, the recommendation was to give a vasopressor. If CI was <2.5 and SVV <15%, the recommendation was to give an inotrope. The FloTrac/Vigileo system (Edwards Lifesciences, Irvine, CA) was used to continuously monitor CI and SVV.

Outcome variables

The primary outcome variable was ICU length of stay. Secondary outcome variables were lactates at the end of surgery, postoperative complications at day 30, postoperative morbidity (the proportion of patients who developed one or more complications) at day 30, mortality at day 30, hospital length of stay, and costs.

Statistical analysis

Median ICU length of stay was 5 ± 1.6 days in our institution, and we assumed that GDFR may decrease it by 1 day or 20%. A study sample size of 60 patients in each group was calculated for two-sided tests with type I error of 5% and power of 90%. Owing to an anticipated loss of several patients entering the study, we planned to include 75 patients in each group. For a test of normal distribution, the Kolmogorov–Smirnov test was used. Continuous data with normal distribution were tested with paired or unpaired t tests, non-normally distributed data using Mann–Whitney U test and Wilcoxon rank-sum test for unpaired and paired results, respectively. Changes in lactate over time were tested using analysis of variance (ANOVA) on repeated measurements. Categorical data were tested using Chi-square test and Chi-square test for trend. Data are presented as mean ± standard deviation when normally distributed and as median [interquartile ranges] in case of abnormal distribution. A $p < 0.05$ was considered statistically significant for all tests. All calculations were done with MedCalc® version 10.4.8.0 (MedCalc Software, Mariakerke, Belgium).

Results

A total of 150 patients were randomized (75 in each group). Despite preoperative approval, five patients refused to participate in the study after surgery and had to be excluded from the analysis. Thus, 73 patients from the GDFR group were compared to 72 patients from the control group.

Baseline and surgical characteristics

Reasons for surgery were brain tumor (n = 87), intracranial aneurysm (n = 55), or brain abscess (n = 3) and were well balanced between the two groups (Table 1). The GDFR group and the control group were comparable in terms of age, comorbidities, ASA score, and POSSUM score (Table 1). Surgery duration was comparable in both groups as well as intraoperative estimated blood loss (Table 2). During surgery, the GDFR group received significantly less colloid and crystalloid than the control group (Table 2).

Outcome variables

The ICU length of stay was significantly shorter in the GDFR group (3 days [1–5] vs. 6 days [3–11], $p = 0.001$) (Fig. 1). At the end of the surgical procedure, lactates were lower in the GDFR group (1.79 ± 0.85 vs. 2.23 ± 1.36 mmol/l, $p = 0.003$). The total number of complications and the proportion of patients who developed one or more postoperative complications were lower in the GDFR group, as well as ICU costs (Table 3). Median hospital length of stay was decreased by 2 days, but the difference did not reach statistical significance (Table 3). No differences were found in heart rate, mean arterial pressure, $P_{ET}CO_2$, natremia, and urine output during the surgery between the two groups (Table 4).

Table 1 Preoperative characteristics of the study population

	GDFR group (n = 73)	Control group (n = 72)	*p* value
Male/female	30:43	32:40	0.738
Age	61 ± 13	62 ± 13	0.693
Age ≥ 70 years	20	24	0.474
Weight (kg)	59 ± 11	60 ± 12	0.417
Height (cm)	160 ± 8	162 ± 7	0.105
POSSUM (physiology score)	21 ± 7	23 ± 6	0.151
POSSUM (operative score)	13 ± 4	13 ± 3	0.394
ASA (3:4)	70:3	70:2	1.000
Comorbidities			
Coronary artery disease	5	7	0.563
Hypertension	45	37	0.243
Peripheral artery disease	0	0	1.000
COPD	11	18	0.151
Other pulmonary pathology	4	5	0.745
Cerebrovascular disease	26	29	0.610
Diabetes mellitus	10	11	0.818
Chronic kidney disease	1	1	0.992
Malignancy	33	30	0.738
Diagnosis			
Intracranial aneurysm	26	29	0.610
Intracranial mass	46	41	0.500
Brain abscess	1	2	0.620

Values are presented as mean ± standard deviation

POSSUM physiological and operative severity score for the enumeration of mortality and morbidity, *COPD* chronic obstructive pulmonary disease

Discussion

In high-risk patients undergoing brain surgery, our study shows that the use of GDFR was associated with a decrease in fluid volumes, less postoperative complications, and a shorter ICU length of stay.

Many studies have investigated the value of goal-directed fluid therapy in patients undergoing major abdominal, vascular, and orthopedic surgeries [3–6]. Conflicting results have been reported, but recent meta-analysis [3–6] has suggested an overall reduction in postoperative morbidity around 25–50%, associated with a 1–2-day reduction in hospital length of stay. As far as we know, this is the first study investigating the effects of a goal-directed fluid strategy in patients undergoing brain surgery. The main objective of goal-directed strategies is to rationalize the way fluid is administered during the perioperative period [10]. A U-shaped relationship has been described between the perioperative fluid volume and postoperative complications [1]. Patients who do not receive enough fluid may develop complications related to hypovolemia, such as acute renal failure, myocardial injury, and cerebral ischemia. On the other hand, patients receiving too much fluid may develop complications associated with fluid overload, such as tissue edema, which may be responsible for prolonged mechanical ventilation and delayed wound healing [11].

For specific surgical procedures, such as pneumonectomy, liver resection, and neurosurgery, the temptation has always been to keep patients as dry as possible to prevent pulmonary edema, surgical bleeding, and brain swelling, respectively. However, blinded or uncontrolled fluid restriction may expose patients to hypovolemia-related complications [1, 12]. We hypothesized that advanced hemodynamic measurements may be useful to prevent both insufficient and excessive fluid management and improve postoperative outcome. We therefore designed an intraoperative fluid management protocol where minimal fluid maintenance with a crystalloid solution (fluid restriction) was combined with the administration of fluid boluses only in case of severe hypovolemia defined by the association of a low cardiac index with a high SVV. The SVV has been shown to be useful to predict fluid responsiveness in many different settings [13]. Pending limitations are respected [9]; SVV >10–13%

Table 2 Patient characteristics during and 24 h after surgery

	GDFR group (n = 73)	Control group (n = 72)	*p* value
Patient position			
Supine position (n)	41	45	0.500
Left-lateral position (n)	18	14	0.549
Right-lateral position (n)	12	10	0.818
Prone position (n)	2	3	0.679
Beginning of surgery			
CI (ml/min/m^2)	3 ± 1.2	NA	NA
SVV (%)	12 ± 5	NA	NA
During surgery			
Crystalloids (ml/kg/h)	3 ± 0	5.0 ± 2.8	<0.001
Colloids (ml/kg/h)	1.9 ± 1.1	3.9 ± 1.6	0.021
Colloids (ml)	563 ± 550	1050 ± 548	<0.001
Colloids (nb of bolus per patient)	3 ± 3	5 ± 3	<0.001
Autologous blood transfusion (ml)	n = 5, 280 ± 109	n = 14, 375 ± 198	0.224
Red blood cell (ml)	n = 3, 400 ± 200	n = 2, 400 ± 282	0.089
Fresh frozen plasma (ml)	0	0	1
Estimated blood loss (ml)	287 ± 179	305 ± 273	0.535
Metaraminol (no. of patients)	39	18	<0.001
Ephedrine (no. of patients)	40	21	<0.001
Dopamine (no. of patients)	5	3	0.479
Dobutamine (no. of patients)	1	0	0.319
Norepinephrine (no. of patients)	3	3	0.981
End of surgery			
CI (ml/min/m^2)	3.6 ± 0.7	NA	NA
SVV (%)	7 ± 2	NA	NA
Length of surgery (min)	274 ± 72	276 ± 66	0.864
Dopamine (n)	1	0	0.319
Norepinephrine (n)	0	1	0.312
24 h after surgery			
Crystalloids (ml/kg/h)	2.6 ± 1.3	2.6 ± 0.8	0.881
Colloids (ml/kg/h)	0.2 ± 0.3	0.2 ± 0.3	0.868
Blood (ml/kg/h)	0	0	0.746
Fresh frozen plasma (ml)	0	0	0.744
Estimated blood loss (ml)	98 ± 65	115 ± 99	0.206
Norepinephrine (n)	3	3	0.981
Dopamine (n)	5	3	0.479
Vasodilatation therapy (n)	5	11	0.105
Diuretic support (n)	45	38	0.281

Values are presented as mean ± standard deviation

CI cardiac index, *HR* heart rate, *MAP* mean arterial pressure, *N/A* not applicable, *SVV* stroke volume variation

identifies fluid responder patients with high sensitivity and specificity [13]. We decided to use a higher cut-off value to keep our patients on the "dry" side, but we also decided to allow fluid boluses when SVV was >15% to prevent excessive fluid restriction and hypovolemia-related complications. Goal-directed fluid strategies have the advantage to rationalize the way patients are treated [10]. However, we believe that fluid management protocols must be adapted to clinical and surgical situations. The use of high SVV target values (around 18–20%) has recently been proposed in patients undergoing liver resection to limit surgical bleeding as much as possible [14]. We thought it might be wise to adopt a similar strategy in neurosurgical patients to minimize cerebral edema. With our GDFR protocol, patients received less crystalloid and colloid than the control group, but did not

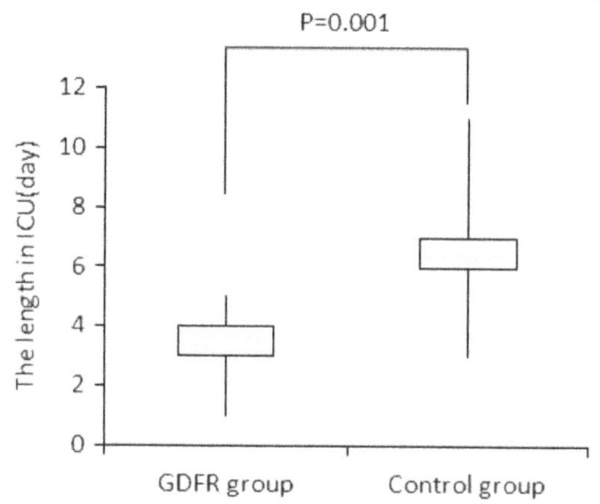

Fig. 1 Length of stay in the intensive care unit (ICU) in the goal-directed fluid restriction (GDFR) and in the control groups

develop more often hypovolemia-related complications such as acute kidney and myocardial injury.

Our study also showed a significant reduction in ICU costs with GDFR, which is logical when considering the observed reduction in ICU length of stay, likely related to the lower number of patients who developed complications (Table 3). Sadique et al. [15] recently reported the financial results of the large UK Optimise trial and showed that patients treated with goal-directed fluid therapy were on average £400 less expensive to treat than control patients. In patients undergoing head and neck surgery in the USA, in whom ICU length of stay was significantly reduced when using goal-directed fluid therapy, Hand et al. [16] recently reported savings exceeding $3000 per patient. Surgical and anesthesia costs in China are not comparable to those observed in the UK or in the USA. However, as suggested by previous studies [17, 18] our financial findings confirm that the improvement in postoperative outcome may offset the costs associated with the implementation of goal-directed fluid therapy.

Our study has several limitations. First, this is a single-center study where we compared a GDFR strategy to standard hemodynamic management at West China Hospital in Chengdu, Sichuan. We also focused on high-risk patients (ASA III & IV). Thus, our results may not be extrapolated to other institutions having different anesthesia and surgical practices, as well as to low-risk (ASA I & II) neurosurgical patients. Three patients had a brain abscess and did not require emergency surgery. Thus, they were considered as elective patients and enrolled in our study. We acknowledge their specificity but confirm that similar results were observed after excluding them from the analysis. Although based on physiological rational, the 15% cutoff value used for SVV was arbitrary and other studies would be useful to investigate whether better results could be observed when using lower (e.g., 13%) or higher (e.g., 18%) cutoff values. Also, we cannot draw any conclusion regarding the superiority of

Table 3 Postoperative outcome

Parameters	GDFR group (n = 73)	Control group (n = 72)	*p* value
ICU length of stay (days)	3 (1–5)	6 (3–11)	0.001
Mortality (n/%)	4/5.5	9/12.5	0.158
Hospital length of stay (days)	15 (7–23)	17 (9–27)	0.069
Complications (day 30)			
Total (n)	46	99	0.043
Patients with one or more complications (n/%)	14/19.2	25/34.7	0.034
Vomiting (n/%)	2/2.7	2/2.8	0.989
Coma (n/%)	3/4.1	2/2.8	0.660
Seizure (n/%)	1/1.4	3/4.2	0.304
Encephaledema (CT/MRI) (n/%)	9/12.3	16/22.2	0.115
Pneumonia (n/%)	9/12.3	20/27.8	0.020
Sepsis (n/%)	0/0	2/2.8	0.152
Ventilator support (n/%)	6/8.2	12/16.7	0.123
New onset of ventilator support (n/%)	3/4.1	8/11.1	0.111
AKI (without dialysis) (n/%)	3/4.1	5/6.9	0.455
Renal failure with dialysis (n/%)	0/0	1/1.4	0.312
Stroke (including TIA) (n/%)	1/1.4	0/0	0.319
Deep vein thrombosis (n/%)	0/0	4/5.6	0.041
Graft thrombosis (n/%)	0/0	1/1.4	0.312
Wound infection/dehiscence (n/%)	0/0	0/0	1
Skin lesions (n/%)	8/11.0	16/22.2	0.068
Arrhythmias (non-life threatening) (n/%)	1/1.4	2/2.8	0.552
Arrhythmias (life threatening) (n/%)	0/0	1/1.4	0.312
Heart failure/pulmonary edema (n/%)	0/0	4/5.6	0.041
Acute myocardial infarction (n/%)	0/0	0/0	1
Pulmonary embolism (n/%)	0/0	0/0	1
Costs			
Hospital costs ($)	9218 ± 2890	10,249 ± 3175	0.482
ICU costs ($)	1776 ± 459	3080 ± 700	0.037

Values are presented as mean ± standard deviation

ICU intensive care unit, *AKI* acute kidney injury

Table 4 Patient characteristics during surgery

Variable	Beginning of surgery	1 h	2 h	3 h	4 h	End of surgery
Number						
GDFR group	73 (100%)	73 (100%)	73 (100%)	36 (49%)	25 (34%)	73 (100%)
Control group	72 (100%)	72 (100%)	72 (100%)	37 (51%)	24 (33%)	72 (100%)
p value	1.00	1.00	1.00	0.80	0.92	1.00
MAP (mmHg)						
GDFR group	83 ± 14	75 ± 9	77 ± 10	77 ± 11	73 ± 9	82 ± 11
Control group	80 ± 15	78 ± 11	80 ± 14	76 ± 11	82 ± 11	78 ± 11
p value	0.17	0.09	0.16	0.93	0.12	0.07
$P_{ET}CO_2$ (mmHg)						
GDFR group	29 ± 3	29 ± 4	29 ± 3	29 ± 3	29 ± 3	31 ± 4
Control group	30 ± 3	29 ± 3	29 ± 3	30 ± 3	32 ± 4	28 ± 3
p value	0.20	0.68	0.69	0.44	0.06	0.79
Sodium (mmol/l)						
GDFR group	137.8 ± 4.8	134.5 ± 5.7	135.9 ± 4.7	136.8 ± 5.5	136.2 ± 3.3	137.3 ± 4.5
Control group	136.0 ± 5.5	134.3 ± 5.8	136.1 ± 5.2	137.4 ± 5.3	139.0 ± 6.7	137.5 ± 5.1
p value	0.03	0.81	0.86	0.64	0.07	0.84
Diuresis (ml/kg/h)						
GDFR group	0	5.58 ± 1.74	5.19 ± 1.37	4.97 ± 1.85	4.41 ± 1.73	4.12 ± 1.39
Control group	0	5.76 ± 1.50	5.52 ± 1.77	5.03 ± 1.63	5.01 ± 1.45	4.12 ± 1.39
p value	1	0.52	0.18	0.92	0.26	0.80

Values are presented as mean ± standard deviation

MAP mean arterial pressure, $P_{ET}CO_2$ peak end-tidal CO_2

our original GDFR strategy over a more classical goal-directed fluid strategy (e.g., stroke volume optimization) or over fluid restriction alone. The reliability of the FloTrac/Vigileo system to measure cardiac output has been questioned when compared to clinical reference techniques such as pulmonary thermodilution and echocardiography [19]. Of note, most limitations have been described in patients with septic shock receiving vasopressors, or during liver transplantation [20]. Recent meta-analysis of validation studies suggests that both accuracy and precision are comparable to those observed with other continuous cardiac output monitoring techniques currently available on the market [21]. And many studies have demonstrated that FloTrac-derived SVV is an accurate predictor of fluid responsiveness; pending limitations are respected [20].

Conclusion

In high-risk patients undergoing brain surgery, our intraoperative GDFR strategy was associated with a significant decrease in ICU length of stay, costs, and postoperative complications. Larger studies are needed to confirm our findings and assess the impact on hospital length of stay and hospital finances.

Abbreviations

GDFR: goal-directed fluid restriction; ICU: intensive care unit; ASA: American Society of Anesthesiologists; CI: cardiac index; SVV: stroke volume variation; HR: heart rate; MAP: mean arterial pressure; N/A: not applicable; POSSUM: physiological and operative severity score for the enumeration of mortality and morbidity.

Authors' contributions

GC, JL, and BL participated in study design and manuscript preparation. JL, JX, and GC participated in patient selection, intraoperative monitoring and management, data collection, analysis, and manuscript preparation. LL contributed to data collection. All authors read and approved the final manuscript.

Acknowledgements

We thank Dr Frederic Michard, Lausanne, Switzerland, for helping us to design the study and to review the manuscript.

Competing interests

The authors declare that they have no competing interests.

Funding

This study was supported by the Science and Technology Department of Sichuan Province support program (No. 2013SZ0030).

References

1. Bellamy MC. Wet, dry or something else? Br J Anaesth. 2006;97:808–16.
2. Lilot M, Ehrenfeld JM, Lee C, Harrington B, Cannesson M, Rinehart J. Variability in practice and factors predictive of total crystalloid administration during abdominal surgery: retrospective two-centre analysis. Br J Anaesth. 2015;114:767–76.
3. Hamilton MA, Cecconi M, Rhodes A. A systematic review and meta-analysis on the use of preemptive hemodynamic intervention to improve postoperative outcomes in moderate and high-risk surgical patients. Anesth Analg. 2011;112:1392–402.
4. Grocott MP, Dushianthan A, Hamilton MA, Mythen MG, Harrison D, Rowan K. Perioperative increase in global blood flow to explicit defined goals and outcomes after surgery: a Cochrane Systematic Review. Br J Anaesth. 2013;111:535–48.
5. Pearse RM, Harrison DA, MacDonald N, Gillies MA, Blunt M, Ackland G, et al. Effect of a perioperative, cardiac output-guided hemodynamic therapy algorithm on outcomes following major gastrointestinal surgery: a randomized clinical trial and systematic review. JAMA. 2014;311:2181–90.
6. Benes J, Giglio M, Brienza N, Michard F. The effects of goal-directed fluid therapy based on dynamic parameters on post-surgical outcome: a meta-analysis of randomized controlled trials. Crit Care. 2014;18:584.
7. Tummala RP, Sheth RN, Heros RC. Hemodilution and fluid management in neurosurgery. Clin Neurosurg. 2006;53:238–51.
8. Tommasino C. Fluids and the neurosurgical patient. Anesthesiol Clin North Am. 2002;20:329–46.
9. Michard F, Chemla D, Teboul JL. Applicability of pulse pressure variation: how many shades of grey? Crit Care. 2015;19:144.
10. Michard F, Biais M. Rational fluid management: dissecting facts from fiction. Br J Anaesth. 2012;108:369–71.
11. Holte K, Sharrock NE, Kehlet H. Pathophysiology and clinical implications of perioperative fluid excess. Br J Anaesth. 2002;89:622–32.
12. Thacker JK, Mountford WK, Ernst FR, Krukas MR, Mythen MM. Perioperative fluid utilization variability and association with outcomes: considerations for enhanced recovery efforts in sample US surgical populations. Ann Surg. 2016;263:502–10.
13. Yang X, Du B. Does pulse pressure variation predicts fluid responsiveness in critically ill patients: a critical review and meta-analysis. Crit Care. 2014;18:650.
14. Dunki-Jacobs EM, Philips P, Scoggins CR, McMasters KM, Martin RC. Stroke volume variation in hepatic resection: a replacement for standard central venous pressure monitoring. Ann Surg Oncol. 2014;21:473–8.
15. Sadique Z, Harrison DA, Grieve R, Rowan KM, Pearse RM, OPTIMISE study group. Cost-effectiveness of a cardiac output-guided haemodynamic therapy algorithm in high-risk patients undergoing major gastrointestinal surgery. Perioper Med (Lond). 2015;4:13.
16. Hand WR, Stoll WD, McEvoy MD, McSwain JR, Sealy CD, Skoner JM, et al. Intraoperative goal-directed hemodynamic management in free tissue transfer for head and neck cancer. Head Neck. 2016;38:1974–80.
17. Manecke GR, Asemota A, Michard F. Tackling the economic burden of post-surgical complications: would perioperative goal directed fluid therapy help? Crit Care. 2014;18:566.
18. Ebm C, Cecconi M, Sutton L, Rhodes A. A cost-effectiveness analysis of postoperative goal-directed therapy for high-risk surgical patients. Crit Care Med. 2014;42:1194–203.
19. Camporota L, Beale R. Pitfalls in haemodynamic monitoring based on the arterial pressure waveform. Crit Care. 2010;14:124.
20. Slagt C, Malagon I, Groeneveld J. Systematic review of uncalibrated arterial pressure waveform analysis to determine cardiac output and stroke volume variation. Br J Anaesth. 2014;112:626–37.
21. Peyton PJ, Chong SW. Minimally invasive measurement of cardiac output during surgery and critical care: a meta-analysis of accuracy and precision. Anesthesiology. 2010;113:1220–35.

Transportation of patients on extracorporeal membrane oxygenation

Pedro Vitale Mendes[1,2*], Cesar de Albuquerque Gallo[2], Bruno Adler Maccagnan Pinheiro Besen[2], Adriana Sayuri Hirota[2], Raquel de Oliveira Nardi[2], Edzangela Vasconcelos dos Santos[2], Ho Yeh Li[2], Daniel Joelsons[2], Eduardo Leite Vieira Costa[1,2], Flavia Krepel Foronda[2], Luciano Cesar Pontes Azevedo[1,2] and Marcelo Park[2]

Abstract

Background: Utilization of extracorporeal membrane oxygenation (ECMO) has increased worldwide, but its use remains restricted to severely ill patients, and few referral centers are properly structured to offer this support. Inter-hospital transfer of patients on ECMO support can be life-threatening. In this study, we report a single-center experience and a systematic review of the available published data on complications and mortality associated with ECMO transportation.

Methods: We reported single-center data regarding complications and mortality associated with the transportation of patients on ECMO support. Additionally, we searched multiple databases for case series, observational studies, and randomized controlled trials regarding mortality of patients transferred on ECMO support. Results were analyzed independently for pediatric (under 12 years old) and adult populations. We pooled mortality rates using a random-effects model. Complications and transportation data were also described.

Results: A total of 38 manuscripts, including our series, were included in the final analysis, totaling 1481 patients transported on ECMO support. A total of 951 patients survived to hospital discharge. The pooled survival rates for adult and pediatric patients were 62% (95% CI 57–68) and 68% (95% CI 60–75), respectively. Two deaths occurred during patient transportation. No other complication resulting in adverse outcome was reported.

Conclusion: Using the available pooled data, we found that patient transfer to a referral institution while on ECMO support seems to be safe and adds no significant risk of mortality to ECMO patients.

Keywords: Acute respiratory failure, Extracorporeal membrane oxygenation, Transport, Rescue work

Introduction

Extracorporeal membrane oxygenation (ECMO) respiratory support is a potentially lifesaving strategy that has been shown to be cost-effective in high-income countries [1–3] and in a middle-income country [4]. Although its use remains restricted to cases of severe respiratory failure refractory to mechanical ventilation [5–8], further acute and chronic organ failures are very common and increase mortality and morbidity in these patients [9, 10]. Consequently, ECMO respiratory support is lifesaving only in highly select cases—namely, early after the onset of severe respiratory failure, and only in patients without

*Correspondence: pemendes@hotmail.com
[1] Intensive Care Unit, Hospital das Clinicas, University of São Paulo School of Medicine, Rua Dr. Enéas Carvalho de Aguiar, 255, Sala 5023, São Paulo, SP 05403000, Brazil
Full list of author information is available at the end of the article

severe acute or chronic organ dysfunctions [3, 5–7, 11, 12].

Facing the paucity of such cases, and the high level of expertise needed to implement ECMO support, a proper referral system becomes necessary and has been shown to be effective [7]. In the CESAR trial, the cost-effectiveness of ECMO respiratory support was demonstrated with 81% (73 out of 90) of ECMO-supported patients being transported to only one UK ECMO referral center [3]. However, the severity of those patients' respiratory insufficiency makes transportation without ECMO support unsafe. Therefore, many referral centers transfer patients under ECMO respiratory support [13, 14] and, so far, there are no data regarding the safety of those inter-hospital ECMO transportations.

Considering the recent global increase in ECMO support, and the consequent increase in ECMO patient transportation, our objectives were the following: (a) to describe a Brazilian tertiary medical center's experience with ECMO transportation of patients with severe respiratory failure, and (b) to describe the current literature by providing pooled results of mortality and complications associated with transportation on venovenous and venoarterial ECMO support.

Background

Patients of the Brazilian tertiary medical center

Patients' data were retrieved from a prospectively collected REDCap database from the Hospital das Clínicas da Universidade de São Paulo [15]. From 2010 to 2014, physicians from various institutions directly contacted the Hospital das Clínicas ECMO team in cases of refractory hypoxemia. Initial evaluation was done through telephone contact together with a REDCap-based online form based on patients' clinical and laboratory data [15]. The decision of whether or not to undertake the rescue was based on predefined inclusion and exclusion criteria. In cases of uncertainty, we required the consultation and approval of two other members of the ECMO team. The inclusion and exclusion criteria, as well as the clinical approach to support and ECMO initiation, were standardized and already published elsewhere [11, 16].

In all cases, cannulation was performed at bedside by the ECMO team at the consultant hospital. The femoral-to-internal jugular venovenous configuration was used. Bidimensional ultrasonography was used to guide the vascular puncture, guidewire insertion and cannulae positioning. A centrifugal magnetic pump with a Permanent Life Support (PLS) system using a polymethylpentene oxygenator (Rotaflow/Jostra Quadrox - D, Maquet CardiopulmonaryAG, Hirrlingen, Germany) was employed in all cases. Approximately 1 h after ECMO initiation, patients were transported in extracorporeal support to the Hospital das Clínicas da Universidade de São Paulo through ground ambulance or helicopter. The ECMO team for patient transportation consisted of 2 ICU physicians, 1 ICU nurse and 1 ICU respiratory therapist.

Systematic review of the literature

Registration

This systematic review, including its search protocol, was registered on the PROSPERO database (registration number CRD42015024710).

Search strategy

We searched PUBMED (1966 until November 2012), EMBASE (January 1990 until November 2012), LILACS, and SCIELO to identify studies describing transportation of severely ill patients on ECMO support. Venovenous and venoarterial ECMO descriptions for respiratory support were included to better describe the population submitted to transportation while on ECMO. We relied upon observational studies, as no randomized studies comparing inter-hospital transportation of ECMO-supported patients have been published to date.

In order to enhance the sensitivity of our search, the terms were separated into two blocks for PUBMED, using medical subject headings [MeSH] and [All field] terms. The MeSH terms used in PUBMED were organized as follows: ("extracorporeal membrane oxygenation" or "extracorporeal oxygenation" or "extracorporeal life support" or ECMO) and ("transport" or "rescue work"). In the PUBMED, EMBASE, LILACS and SCIELO searches, the terms were inserted as [All fields] and were organized as follows: ("extracorporeal membrane oxygenation" or "extracorporeal oxygenation" or "extracorporeal life support" or ECMO) and ("transport" or "rescue work" or "rescue" or "retrieval").

The resulting outputs were then combined. Duplicated results were excluded. The remaining articles were independently evaluated by 3 investigators (PVM, CAG and MP) for eligibility. Only manuscripts with the agreement of a least two investigators were included. We also searched personal records and the references of the retrieved articles for other potential studies.

Study evaluation and data extraction

Manuscripts were included only if data on patients' transportation on ECMO support and hospital survival were available. Manuscripts involving animal data, case reports describing less than four subjects, language other than English, French, Spanish, or Portuguese and review articles were excluded. When available, the following data were also extracted: patients' demographic features (including illness severity), mechanical ventilation information, complications during ECMO transportation, ECMO support data, and intensive care unit (ICU) and hospital lengths of stay. Retrieved data were also analyzed separately for pediatric patients and adult patients. When additional information was needed, an e-mail was sent to the main author requesting the data.

Quality assessment

Though there is no proper scoring system for evaluating case series of patients on ECMO support, we developed a predetermined system for all included studies based on previously published reports [17], and on commonly expected measures of quality for ECMO support and ECMO transportation. Each study was scored and a final grade was calculated to estimate data quality (Additional file). The studies' final scores were classified by quality into three tertiles and mortality rate was assessed independently for each one of these groups.

Statistical analysis

Variables are shown as mean ± standard deviation if normally distributed, and median plus the 25th and 75th percentiles if otherwise. For descriptive data, a confidence interval was generated for each manuscript in accordance with the recommendations of the Association of Public Health Observatories (APHO) of England [18]. Some manuscripts did not present means and standard deviations for quantitative data. In these cases, means and standard deviations were estimated from the sample size, median, range or 25th and 75th percentiles, according to the Wan method [19]. Heterogeneity between and within studies was assessed using Cochran's Q statistic and Higgin's I^2. Either a $P < 0.10$ or an $I^2 > 50\%$ was considered suggestive of significant heterogeneity. We a priori expected that studies would present high heterogeneity. Therefore, we performed a random-effects meta-analysis using the DerSimonian and Laird method for all pooled characteristics and effects. The analyses were done using the metafor package from R open-source software [20].

Results

Brazilian medical center

During the studied period, our group was called on for consultation for a total of 12 patients. Seven patients fulfilled the predefined criteria and were supported by ECMO. All patients had received at least one rescue maneuver for refractory hypoxemia before ECMO initiation, as described in Table 1. In all cases, patients were cannulated at the remote institution and transferred under ECMO support to Hospital das Clínicas. Data on respiratory failure etiology, laboratory data, and ECMO settings are described in Table 1. Five patients were successfully weaned from ECMO support. One patient died 21 days after ECMO removal due to septic shock. Median time on ECMO support was 5 days [2, 10]. ICU and Hospital length of stay were 13 [2, 20] and 20 days [2, 60], respectively. Four patients survived to hospital discharge and were still alive after 90 days, with a survival rate of 57%.

Table 1 General characteristics, ICU support and diagnosis of the patients

General characteristics	All patients ($n = 7$)
Age (yo)	28 [14,48]
Male [n(%)]	3 [43]
SAPS 3	84 [57,118]
SOFA	13 [7,18]
Lung injury score	4 [3,4]
Acute respiratory failure etiology	
Pneumonia [n(%)]	4 [57]
Syncytial respiratory virus [n (%)]	1 [14]
Influenza A virus (H_3N_2) [n (%)]	1 [14]
Varicella zoster virus [n (%)]	1 [14]
Nosocomial pneumonia [n (%)]	2 [28]
Alveolar hemorrhage [n (%)]	1 [14]
Pre-ECMO initiation hospital data	
Hospital LOS (days)	8 [3,30]
Days on mechanical ventilation	8 [1,19]
Pre-ECMO rescue maneuvers	
Alveolar recruitment [n (%)]	7 (100)
Nitric oxide [n (%)]	1 [14]
Neuromuscular blockers [n (%)]	4 [57]
Corticosteroids [n (%)]	3 [43]
Tracheal gas insufflation [n (%)]	1 [14]
Clinical outcomes	
ECMO weaning [n (%)]	5 (71)
Time on ECMO support (days)	5 [2, 10]
Hospital discharge	4 (57)
90-day survival [n (%)]	4 (57)

Ventilatory settings	Pre-ECMO initiation	After ECMO initiation
Ventilatory mode (n)	6 PCV/1 VCV	7 PCV
Tidal volume (mL/kg)	310 [180, 500]	100 [12, 220]
Plateau pressure (cmH_2O)	35 [31, 46]	20 [20, 25]
PEEP (cmH_2O)	18 [13, 25]	10 [10, 20]
Resp. rate (insp./min.)	26 [25, 35]	10 [10, 10]
FiO_2	1.0 [1.0, 1.0]	0.3 [0.21, 1.0]

Quantitative data are expressed as median [minimum, maximum]

ECMO extracorporeal membrane oxygenation, *ICU* intensive care unit, *SAPS 3* simplified acute physiological score, *SOFA* sequential organ failure assessment; the lung injury score is the Murray's score; and the two patients in the puerperal period were, respectively, in the 1st and 10th day after delivery; *LOS* length of stay, *SBE* standard base excess, *PCV* pressure-controlled ventilation, *VCV* volume-controlled ventilation, *PEEP* positive end-expiratory pressure

Individual characteristics of the Brazilian patients transported on ECMO support are described in Additional file 1: Table 1S. The median transfer distance was 31 km [1,163] with an average rescue mission time of 345 min [270,960]. In one case, an electrical failure of the pump battery caused an unexpected pump arrest and the need for manual rotation of the hand crank during ground ambulance transportation. No deaths or any severe ECMO complications occurred during transport to our institution.

Systematic review

Study inclusion

Our literature search yielded 610 publications for possible inclusion. Of these, 46 were excluded for duplicity. Of the remaining 564, 512 did not have data for hospital survival. Five studies required author contact for data clarification. Four authors responded to our solicitation and were included in the dataset. In the end, a total of 37 manuscripts were included for analysis (Additional file 2: Fig. 1S) [13, 14, 21–55]. Three studies were considered to be low quality, and 34 were considered moderate to high quality by our scoring system (Additional file 3: Table 3S). Our case series was included in the final analysis, resulting in a total of 38 manuscripts.

Outcomes

Mortality was assessed in all included studies for a total of 1481 patients. Of these, 1025 were adults, and 456 were pediatric. A total of 951 patients survived to hospital discharge after ECMO support in a crude analysis. The pooled survival rates for adult and pediatric patients were 62% (95% CI 57–68) and 68% (95% CI 60–75), respectively (Figs. 1, 2). After stratifying studies into tertiles of quality, we found a lower mortality rate in high-quality studies and a progressive increase in mortality for intermediary and lower tertiles. Mortality rates were 69% (95% CI 52–85%), 65% (95% CI 60–71%) and 61% (95% CI 46–76%) for the first, second and third tertiles, respectively. Total number of patients transported in each country is shown in Additional file 4: Figure 2s

General characteristics, pre-ECMO status, diagnosis and ECMO support data of the entire cohort are reported in Table 2. Most studies did not report any scoring system for hospital survival. Mean time on mechanical ventilation before ECMO initiation was 4.6 days (95% CI 3.7–5.5). Acute Respiratory Distress Syndrome was the most prevalent diagnosis reported for adult patients, while meconium aspiration syndrome was the diagnosis most frequently reported for the pediatric population. ECMO support duration, ICU length of stay and hospital length of stay were 9.8 (95% CI 8.6–10.9), 22 (95% CI 15–30) and 32 (95% CI 25–28) days, respectively.

At least one complication was reported in 12 of the 38 manuscripts analyzed, totaling 80 occurrences in 1481 patients transported (Additional file 5: Table 2S). The most common complication was sudden fall in tidal volume during transportation. We found two reports of deaths during patient transportation to the referral institution. Rescue mission characteristics and adverse events are described in Table 3.

Discussion

ECMO remains a high-cost therapy with lifesaving potential in a select group of critically ill patients [3]. Given the level of expertise needed for daily care of these patients, it is preferable that ECMO candidates be transferred to a specialized referral center. Because of the severe respiratory failure, patient transfer without ECMO is usually deemed to be too risky. Conversely, there are no data regarding the safety of inter-hospital ECMO transportations. Herein, we report a case series of patients transported under ECMO support to a referral hospital in Brazil with a survival rate of 57% and no major complications or deaths during transportation. Additionally, our systematic review of the literature showed a pooled survival rate for adult and pediatric patients of nearly two-thirds—with just 2 deaths reported in this cohort of 1481 patients—and without any other major adverse events resulting from the transportation itself.

Our data are compatible with the overall mortality reported in the latest publication by the Extracorporeal Life Support Organization (ELSO), in which the expected survival rate for adult venovenous extracorporeal support was 58% [56]. Similarly, using the available published data, we found a survival rate of 62% for adult patients transported while on ECMO. For the pediatric population, our pooled analysis retrieved a survival rate of 68%, in comparison with the 57% reported in ELSO guidelines [56]. Therefore, in this case series and in our overall analysis, we found no increase in mortality for ECMO support despite the need for patient transfer to a referral institution.

Concerns regarding the safety of transport of critically ill patients in need of extracorporeal support are an important question to be solved considering the recent global increase in ECMO support [5, 56, 57]. In the Cesar trial, patients who were randomized for the ECMO group were transferred to the referral center only after transport was considered safe by the ECMO Team, therefore delaying the initiation of support. As reported in the text, patients were not transported while on ECMO and, despite precautions, two deaths were reported during patient transfer [3]. Similarly, in a previous publication of 158 infants accepted for ECMO initiation, Boedy et al. reported 18 (39.1%) deaths associated with

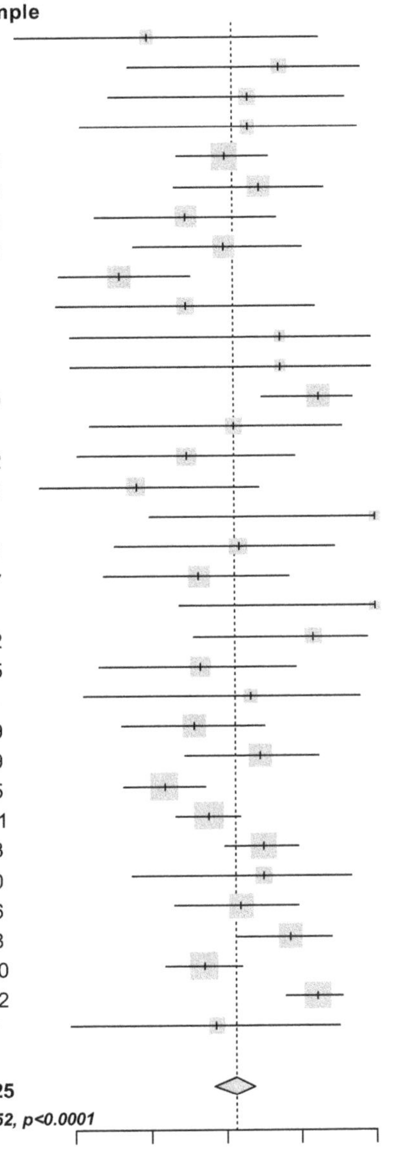

Author - year	Survivals	Sample	Percentage	CI - 95%	Weight
Bennett - 1994	2	5	40	[5; 85]	1.4%
Rossaint - 1997	6	8	75	[35; 97]	1.6%
Linden - 2001	6	9	67	[30; 93]	2.0%
Bulpa - 2002	4	6	67	[22; 96]	1.5%
Foley - 2002	41	68	60	[48; 72]	5.2%
Wagner - 2008	16	23	70	[47; 87]	3.4%
Haneya - 2009	9	18	50	[26; 74]	3.3%
Arlt - 2009	12	20	60	[36; 81]	3.4%
Clement - 2010	10	31	32	[17; 51]	3.9%
Bessereau - 2010	4	8	50	[16; 84]	2.0%
Forrest - 2011	3	4	75	[19; 99]	0.9%
Ciapetti - 2011	3	4	75	[19; 99]	0.9%
Forrest - 2011	34	40	85	[70; 94]	3.5%
DAncona - 2011	5	8	62	[24; 91]	1.9%
Isgro - 2011	6	12	50	[21; 79]	2.6%
Chenaitia - 2011	4	11	36	[11; 69]	2.3%
Cianchi - 2011	4	4	100	[40; 100]	0.6%
Diaz - 2011	7	11	64	[31; 89]	2.3%
Javidfar - 2011	9	17	53	[28; 77]	3.2%
Bein - 2012	5	5	100	[48; 100]	0.6%
Lebreton - 2012	10	12	83	[52; 98]	1.8%
Haneya - 2012	8	15	53	[27; 79]	3.0%
Roncon - 2012	4	6	67	[22; 96]	1.5%
Desebbe - 2013	15	29	52	[33; 71]	4.0%
Lucchini - 2014	20	29	69	[49; 85]	3.8%
Roch - 2014	37	85	44	[33; 55]	5.4%
Bryner - 2014	78	141	55	[47; 64]	5.9%
Broman - 2015	65	93	70	[60; 79]	5.4%
Delnoij - 2015	7	10	70	[35; 93]	2.1%
Raspé - 2015	23	36	64	[46; 79]	4.3%
Sherren - 2015	37	48	77	[63; 88]	4.3%
Biscotti - 2015	54	100	54	[44; 64]	5.6%
Vaja - 2015	86	102	84	[76; 91]	4.9%
Mendes - 2016	4	7	57	[18; 90]	1.8%
Total number of patients	**638**	**1025**	**62**	**[57; 68]**	**100%**

Heterogeneity: I-squared=57.2%, tau-squared=0.2152, p<0.0001

Fig. 1 Forest plot of the adult case series of inter-hospital transportation on ECMO respiratory support, showing the weighted mean of hospital survival

transport. Five infants died waiting for ECMO initiation and 13 died either during transport without ECMO assistance or, after arriving moribund, before ECMO could be started. Considering all these deaths occurred before ECMO initiation, the authors concluded that there may be a hidden mortality associated with ECMO transportation that is generally excluded when we look exclusively at ECMO-supported patients [58]. Therefore, a strategy of rapid ECMO initiation and patient transport while on ECMO support may be safer than the use of conventional mechanical ventilation during transfer to the referral center.

However, it is important to highlight that the presence of complications is common, and nearly a third of the analyzed studies reported at least one complication during transport. Sudden fall in tidal volume was the most common complication reported. Power failure, circuit rupture and other more severe complications were also reported, but no deaths or any adverse outcomes related to these complications during transport were described.

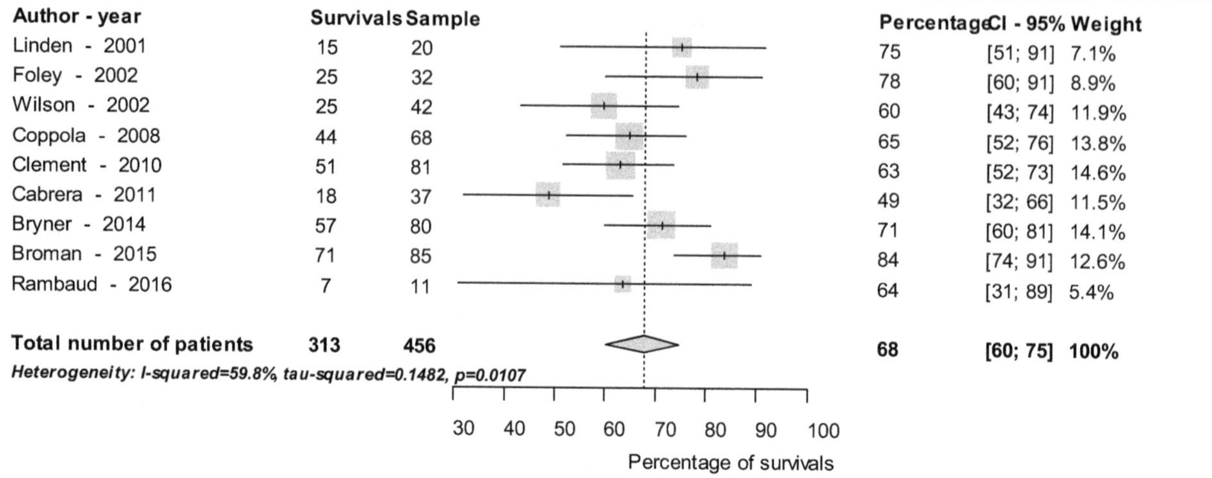

Fig. 2 Forest plot of the pediatric case series of inter-hospital transportation on ECMO respiratory support showing the weighted mean of hospital survival

Table 2 General characteristics, pre-ECMO status, diagnosis and ECMO support data of the patients

Characteristic	≥12 years old		<12 years old	
	Patients analyzed Total $N = 682$	Mean (CI 95%)	Patients analyzed Total $N = 365$	Mean (CI 95%)
Age (yo)	627	38 (35–41)	114	3.1 (1.4–4.8)
Male gender (%)	482	61 (45–77)	365	17 (13–21)
Weight (kg)	119	74 (67–82)	37	23.6 (17.6–29.6)
Pre-ECMO status				
Time on MV (days)	246	4.6 (3.7–5.5)	–	–
pH	242	7.24 (7.19–7.28)	32	7.26 (7.23–7.29)
P/F ratio (mmHg)	373	59 (40–78)	–	–
PCO_2 (mmHg)	306	71 (63–78)	–	–
APACHE II	53	22 (21–23)	–	–
SAPS 2	128	46 (40–52)	–	–
SAPS 3	10	86 (80–92)	–	–
Diagnosis				
ARDS (%)	682	30 (26–34)	365	14 (11–18)
Bacterial pneumonia (%)	682	27 (23–31)	365	6 (4–9)
Viral pneumonia (%)	682	22 (19–25)	365	5 (3–7)
Respiratory and right ventricle failure (%)	682	19 (12–26)	365	17 (13–21)
Trauma (%)	682	4 (3–6)	365	0
Aspiration syndromes (%)	682	3 (1–4)	365	1.0 (0.1–2.5)
Meconium aspiration syndrome (%)	682	0	365	19 (15–23)
Congenital diaphragmatic hernia (%)	682	0	365	8 (5–11)
Persistent newborn pulmonary hypertension (%)	682	0	365	8 (5–10)
ECMO support and outcome data				
ECMO support duration (days)	458	9.8 (8.6–10.9)	7.5	–
Venovenous configuration (%)	682	62 (59–66)	365	42 (35–50)
Venoarterial configuration (%)	682	16 (13–19)	365	58 (50–65)
ICU LOS (days)	64	22 (15–30)	–	–
Hospital LOS (days)	119	32 (25–38)	–	–

ECMO extracorporeal membrane oxygenation, *CI* confidence interval, *BMI* body mass index, *MV* mechanical ventilation, *APACHE* Acute Physiological and Chronic Health Evaluation score, *SAPS* Simplified Physiological Score, *ARDS* acute respiratory distress syndrome, *ICU* intensive care unit, *LOS* length of stay

Table 3 Rescue mission characteristics and adverse events

	Patients analyzed (Total *N* = 1481)	Mean (CI 95%)
Rescue mission		
Distance of transportation (km)	444	486 (68–904)
Rescue time lasting (hours)	318	17 (9–27)
Ambulance (%)	1481	53 (50–56)
Fixed wing (%)	1481	27 (25–31)
Helicopter (%)	1481	22 (19–24)
International transportation (%)	1481	7 (5–8)
Adverse events on the rescue mission		
Death during transport (%)	1481	2 deaths (0.1%)
Tidal volume fall (%)	1481	4 (3–5)
System rupture (%)	1481	1.0 (0.4–1.6)
Any bleeding (%)	1481	0.9 (0.3–1.4)
Power failure (%)	1481	0.5 (0.1–0.9)
Hypotension (%)	1481	0.4 (0.1–0.8)
Cannulae dislodgement (%)	1481	0.2 (0.1–0.7)
Others (%)	1481	0.9 (0.3–1.4)
Absence of complications (%)	1481	92 (91–94)

It is interesting to note that the majority of complications (74%) were reported in one single study [43] (Additional file 5: Table 2s), suggesting that most reports on ECMO transportation did not focus on looking for adverse events. Certainly, the definition of complications during patient transportation varied between studies, making it difficult to understand the real size of this problem. It is very likely that the incidence of adverse events is much higher than described in this manuscript.

Our study has several limitations: (1) The absence of any scoring system in most of the studies makes it difficult to correlate expected mortality with final results. However, as previously described, overall mortality rate was compatible with the expected mortality previously published in the ELSO guidelines for ECMO-supported patients. (2) A publication bias may have affected our results. As observed in our analysis, low-quality studies were associated with a high mortality rate and, possibly, even higher mortality rates may be found in unpublished data. (3) No randomized clinical trial has directly evaluated the safety of transporting ECMO patients. Our data were extracted mainly from case series, and the results are limited by the inherent flaws of such studies. (4) The studies included in this manuscript span several years of ECMO transportation worldwide. Therefore, clinical and technical development, which may have influenced the presence of complications and death in ECMO patients throughout the years, are not addressed in this manuscript.

Conclusions

ECMO support is a high-cost therapy restricted to highly specialized referral centers. The analysis of pooled data from available literature suggests that patient transfer to a referral institution while on ECMO support seems to be safe and to not increase mortality in ECMO-supported patients. This modality should possibly be preferred over transport of such patients under conventional ventilation exclusively.

Abbreviations

ECMO: extracorporeal membrane oxygenation; ICU: intensive care unit.

Authors' contributions

PVM, CAG and MP performed the statistical analysis, interpretation of data and drafted the manuscript. ASH, RON, EVS, HYL and DJ contributed to the conception of the work, interpretation of data and drafted the manuscript. BAMPB, ELVC and LCPA contributed to the conception of the work, interpretation of data and final critical review of the manuscript. All authors read and approved the final manuscript.

Author details

[1] Intensive Care Unit, Hospital das Clinicas, University of São Paulo School of Medicine, Rua Dr. Enéas Carvalho de Aguiar, 255, Sala 5023, São Paulo, SP 05403000, Brazil. [2] Research and Education Institute, Hospital Sírio-Libanês, São Paulo, Brazil.

Acknowledgements

We are indebted to Dr. Alberto Lucchini, Dr. Roberto Roncon-Albuquerque Jr., Dr. Alain Morris and Dr. Richard T. Fizer for providing additional data regarding their previously published manuscripts.

Competing interests

The authors declare that they have no competing interests.

References

1. Petrou S, Edwards L. Cost effectiveness analysis of neonatal extracorporeal membrane oxygenation based on four year results from the UK Collaborative ECMO Trial. ArchDisChild Fetal Neonatal Ed. 2004;89(3):F263–8.
2. Schumacher RE, Roloff DW, Chapman R, Snedecor S, Bartlett RH. Extracorporeal membrane oxygenation in term newborns.A prospective cost-benefit analysis. ASAIO J. 1993;39(4):873–9.
3. Peek GJ, Mugford M, Tiruvoipati R, Wilson A, Allen E, Thalanany MM, et al. Efficacy and economic assessment of conventional ventilatory support versus extracorporeal membrane oxygenation for severe adult respiratory failure (CESAR): a multicentre randomised controlled trial. Lancet. 2009;374(9698):1351–63.
4. Park M, Mendes PV, Zampieri FG, Azevedo LC, Costa EL, Antoniali F, et al. The economic effect of extracorporeal membrane oxygenation to support adults with severe respiratory failure in Brazil: a hypothetical analysis. Rev Bras Ter Intensiva. 2014;26(3):253–62.
5. Davies A, Jones D, Bailey M, Beca J, Bellomo R, Blackwell N, et al. Extracorporeal membrane oxygenation for 2009 influenza A(H1N1) acute respiratory distress syndrome. JAMA. 2009;302(17):1888–95.

6. Pham T, Combes A, Rozé H, Chevret S, Mercat A, Roch A, et al. Extracorporeal membrane oxygenation for pandemic influenza A(H1N1) induced acute respiratory distress syndrome. A cohort study and propensity-matched analysis. Am J Respir Crit Care Med. 2012;187(3):276–85.
7. Noah MA, Peek GJ, Finney SJ, Griffiths MJ, Harrison DA, Grieve R, et al. Referral to an extracorporeal membrane oxygenation center and mortality among patients with severe 2009 influenza A(H1N1). JAMA. 2011;306(15):1659–68.
8. Brogan TV, Thiagarajan RR, Rycus PT, Bartlett RH, Bratton SL. Extracorporeal membrane oxygenation in adults with severe respiratory failure: a multi-center database. Intensive Care Med. 2009;35(12):2105–14.
9. Schmidt M, Zogheib E, Rozé H, Repesse X, Lebreton G, Luyt CE, et al. The PRESERVE mortality risk score and analysis of long-term outcomes after extracorporeal membrane oxygenation for severe acute respiratory distress syndrome. Intensive Care Med. 2013;39(10):1704–13.
10. Schmidt M, Bailey M, Sheldrake J, Hodgson C, Aubron C, Rycus PT, et al. Predicting survival after extracorporeal membrane oxygenation for severe acute respiratory failure. The respiratory extracorporeal membrane oxygenation survival prediction (RESP) score. Am J Respir Crit Care Med. 2014;189(11):1374–82.
11. Park M, Azevedo LC, Mendes PV, Carvalho CR, Amato MB, Schettino GP, et al. First-year experience of a Brazilian tertiary medical center in supporting severely ill patients using extracorporeal membrane oxygenation. Clinics (Sao Paulo). 2012;67(10):1157–63.
12. Wetsch WA, Spöhr FA, Hinkelbein J, Padosch SA. Emergency extracorporeal membrane oxygenation to treat massive aspiration during anaesthesia induction. A case report. Acta Anaesthesiol Scand. 2012;56(6):797–800.
13. Forrest P, Cheong JY, Vallely MP, Torzillo PJ, Hendel PN, Wilson MK, et al. International retrieval of adults on extracorporeal membrane oxygenation support. Anaesth Intensive Care. 2011;39(6):1082–5.
14. Forrest P, Ratchford J, Burns B, Herkes R, Jackson A, Plunkett B, et al. Retrieval of critically ill adults using extracorporeal membrane oxygenation: an Australian experience. Intensive Care Med. 2011;37(5):824–30.
15. Harris PA, Taylor R, Thielke R, Payne J, Gonzalez N, Conde JG. Research electronic data capture (REDCap)—a metadata-driven methodology and workflow process for providing translational research informatics support. J Biomed Inform. 2009;42(2):377–81.
16. Azevedo LC, Park M, Costa EL, Santos EV, Hirota A, Taniguchi LU, et al. Extracorporeal membrane oxygenation in severe hypoxemia: time for reappraisal? J Bras Pneumol. 2012;38(1):7–12.
17. Quality Assessment Tool for Case Series Studies 2014 [Available from: https://www.nhlbi.nih.gov/health-pro/guidelines/in-develop/cardiovascular-risk-reduction/tools/case_series.
18. Cunningham A, Fryers P, Abbas J, Flowers J, Stockton D. Technical Briefing 3: Commonly Used Public Health Statistics and their Confidence Intervals Public Health England Webpage2008 [Available from: http://www.apho.org.uk/resource/item.aspx?RID=48457].
19. Wan X, Wang W, Liu J, Tong T. Estimating the sample mean and standard deviation from the sample size, median, range and/or interquartile range. BMC Med Res Methodol. 2014;14:135.
20. Team RDC. R: a language and environment for statistical computing. R Foundation for Statistical Computing. 2009. https://www.R-project.org/.
21. Bennett JB, Hill JG, Long WB, Bruhn PS, Haun MM, Parsons JA. Interhospital transport of the patient on extracorporeal cardiopulmonary support. Ann Thorac Surg. 1994;57(1):107–11.
22. Rossaint R, Pappert D, Gerlach H, Lewandowski K, Keh D, Falke K. Extracorporeal membrane oxygenation for transport of hypoxaemic patients with severe ARDS. Br J Anaesth. 1997;78(3):241–6.
23. Bulpa P, Evrard P, Dive A, Pranger D, Gonzales M, Installe E. Inter-hospital transportation of patients with severe acute respiratory failure on extracorporeal membrane oxygenation. Intensive Care Med. 2002;28(6):802.
24. Foley DS, Pranikoff T, Younger JG, Swaniker F, Hemmila MR, Remenapp RA, et al. A review of 100 patients transported on extracorporeal life support. ASAIO J. 2002;48(6):612–9.
25. Wagner K, Sangolt GK, Risnes I, Karlsen HM, Nilsen JE, Strand T, et al. Transportation of critically ill patients on extracorporeal membrane oxygenation. Perfusion. 2008;23(2):101–6.
26. Haneya A, Philipp A, Foltan M, Mueller T, Camboni D, Rupprecht L, et al. Extracorporeal circulatory systems in the interhospital transfer of critically ill patients: experience of a single institution. Ann Saudi Med. 2009;29(2):110–4.
27. Arlt M, Philipp A, Zimmermann M, Voelkel S, Amann M, Bein T, et al. Emergency use of extracorporeal membrane oxygenation in cardiopulmonary failure. Artif Organs. 2009;33(9):696–703.
28. Bessereau J, Chenaitia H, Michelet P, Roch A, Gariboldi V. Acute respiratory distress syndrome following 2009 H1N1 virus pandemic: when ECMO come to the patient bedside. Ann Fr Anesth Reanim. 2010;29(2):165–6.
29. Ciapetti M, Cianchi G, Zagli G, Greco C, Pasquini A, Spina R, et al. Feasibility of inter-hospital transportation using extra-corporeal membrane oxygenation (ECMO) support of patients affected by severe swine-flu(H1N1)-related ARDS. Scand J Trauma Resusc Emerg Med. 2011;19:32.
30. D'Ancona G, Capitanio G, Chiaramonte G, Serretta R, Turrisi M, Pilato M, et al. Extracorporeal membrane oxygenator rescue and airborne transportation of patients with influenza A (H1N1) acute respiratory distress syndrome in a Mediterranean underserved area. Interact CardioVasc Thorac Surg. 2011;12(6):935–7.
31. Isgrò S, Patroniti N, Bombino M, Marcolin R, Zanella A, Milan M, et al. Extracorporeal membrane oxygenation for interhospital transfer of severe acute respiratory distress syndrome patients: 5-year experience. Int J Artif Organs. 2011;34(11):1052–60.
32. Chenaitia H, Massa H, Toesca R, Michelet P, Auffray JP, Gariboldi V. Mobile cardio-respiratory support in prehospital emergency medicine. Eur J Emerg Med. 2011;18(2):99–101.
33. Cianchi G, Bonizzoli M, Pasquini A, Bonacchi M, Zagli G, Ciapetti M, et al. Ventilatory and ECMO treatment of H1N1-induced severe respiratory failure: results of an Italian referral ECMO center. BMC Pulm Med. 2011;11:2.
34. Diaz Rodrigo. ECMO y ECMO mobile. Soporte Cardio Respiratorio Avanzado. 2011;22(3):377–87.
35. Javidfar J, Brodie D, Takayama H, Mongero L, Zwischenberger J, Sonett J, et al. Safe transport of critically ill adult patients on extracorporeal membrane oxygenation support to a regional extracorporeal membrane oxygenation center. ASAIO J. 2011;57(5):421–5.
36. Bein T, Zonies D, Philipp A, Zimmermann M, Osborn EC, Allan PF, et al. Transportable extracorporeal lung support for rescue of severe respiratory failure in combat casualties. J Trauma Acute Care Surg. 2012;73(6):1450–6.
37. Lebreton G, Sanchez B, Hennequin JL, Resière D, Hommel D, Léonard C, et al. The French airbridge for circulatory support in the Carribean. Interact CardioVasc Thorac Surg. 2012;15(3):420–5.
38. Haneya A, Philipp A, Foltan M, Camboni D, Müeller T, Bein T, et al. First experience with the new portable extracorporeal membrane oxygenation system Cardiohelp for severe respiratory failure in adults. Perfusion. 2012;27(2):150–5.
39. Roncon-Albuquerque R, Basílio C, Figueiredo P, Silva S, Mergulhão P, Alves C, et al. Portable miniaturized extracorporeal membrane oxygenation systems for H1N1-related severe acute respiratory distress syndrome: a case series. J Crit Care. 2012;27(5):454–63.
40. Desebbe O, Rosamel P, Henaine R, Vergnat M, Farhat F, Dubien PY, et al. Interhospital transport with extracorporeal life support: results and perspectives after 5 years experience. Ann Fr Anesth Reanim. 2013;32(4):225–30.
41. Lucchini A, De Felippis C, Elli S, Gariboldi R, Vimercati S, Tundo P, et al. Mobile ECMO team for inter-hospital transportation of patients with ARDS: a retrospective case series. Heart Lung Vessel. 2014;6(4):262–73.
42. Roch A, Hraiech S, Masson E, Grisoli D, Forel JM, Boucekine M, et al. Outcome of acute respiratory distress syndrome patients treated with extracorporeal membrane oxygenation and brought to a referral center. Intensive Care Med. 2014;40(1):74–83.
43. Broman LM, Holzgraefe B, Palmér K, Frenckner B. The Stockholm experience: interhospital transports on extracorporeal membrane oxygenation. Crit Care. 2015;19:278.
44. Delnoij TS, Veldhuijzen G, Strauch U, Van Mook WN, Bergmans DC, Bouman EA, et al. Mobile respiratory rescue support by off-centre initiation of extracorporeal membrane oxygenation. Perfusion. 2015;30(3):255–9.
45. Raspé C, Rückert F, Metz D, Hofmann B, Neitzel T, Stiller M, et al. Inter-hospital transfer of ECMO-assisted patients with a portable miniaturized ECMO device: 4 years of experience. Perfusion. 2015;30(1):52–9.

46. Sherren PB, Shepherd SJ, Glover GW, Meadows CI, Langrish C, Ioannou N, et al. Capabilities of a mobile extracorporeal membrane oxygenation service for severe respiratory failure delivered by intensive care specialists. Anaesthesia. 2015;70(6):707–14.
47. Lindén V, Palmér K, Reinhard J, Westman R, Ehrén H, Granholm T, et al. Inter-hospital transportation of patients with severe acute respiratory failure on extracorporeal membrane oxygenation—national and international experience. Intensive Care Med. 2001;27(10):1643–8.
48. Wilson BJ, Heiman HS, Butler TJ, Negaard KA, DiGeronimo R. A 16-year neonatal/pediatric extracorporeal membrane oxygenation transport experience. Pediatrics. 2002;109(2):189–93.
49. Coppola CP, Tyree M, Larry K, DiGeronimo R. A 22-year experience in global transport extracorporeal membrane oxygenation. J Pediatr Surg. 2008;43(1):46–52 **(discussion)**.
50. Clement KC, Fiser RT, Fiser WP, Chipman CW, Taylor BJ, Heulitt MJ, et al. Single-institution experience with interhospital extracorporeal membrane oxygenation transport: a descriptive study. Pediatr Crit Care Med. 2010;11(4):509–13.
51. Cabrera AG, Prodhan P, Cleves MA, Fiser RT, Schmitz M, Fontenot E, et al. Interhospital transport of children requiring extracorporeal membrane oxygenation support for cardiac dysfunction. Congenit Heart Dis. 2011;6(3):202–8.
52. Vaja R, Chauhan I, Joshi V, Salmasi Y, Porter R, Faulkner G, et al. Five-year experience with mobile adult extracorporeal membrane oxygenation in a tertiary referral center. J Crit Care. 2015;30(6):1195–8.
53. Rambaud J, Léger PL, Larroquet M, Amblard A, Lodé N, Guilbert J, et al. Transportation of children on extracorporeal membrane oxygenation: one-year experience of the first neonatal and paediatric mobile ECMO team in the north of France. Intensive Care Med. 2016;42(5):940–1.
54. Biscotti M, Agerstrand C, Abrams D, Ginsburg M, Sonett J, Mongero L, et al. One hundred transports on extracorporeal support to an extracorporeal membrane oxygenation center. Ann Thorac Surg. 2015;100(1):34–9 **(discussion 9–40)**.
55. Bryner B, Cooley E, Copenhaver W, Brierley K, Teman N, Landis D, et al. Two decades' experience with interfacility transport on extracorporeal membrane oxygenation. Ann Thorac Surg. 2014;98(4):1363–70.
56. Extracorporeal Life Suport Organization—ECLS Registry Report 2016. Available from: http://www.elso.org/Registry/Statistics/InternationalSummary.aspx.
57. Hinkelbein J, Spelten O, Mey C. High-quality logistical concept for interhospital transport is crucial. Dtsch Arztebl Int. 2013;110(27–28):485–6.
58. Boedy RF, Howell CG, Kanto WP. Hidden mortality rate associated with extracorporeal membrane oxygenation. J Pediatr. 1990;117(3):462–4.

4

Systematic review and meta-analysis of complications and mortality of veno-venous extracorporeal membrane oxygenation for refractory acute respiratory distress syndrome

Sergi Vaquer[1*], Candelaria de Haro[1], Paula Peruga[1], Joan Carles Oliva[2] and Antonio Artigas[1]

Abstract

Veno-venous extracorporeal membrane oxygenation (ECMO) for refractory acute respiratory distress syndrome (ARDS) is a rapidly expanding technique. We performed a systematic review and meta-analysis of the most recent literature to analyse complications and hospital mortality associated with this technique. Using the PRISMA guidelines for systematic reviews and meta-analysis, MEDLINE and EMBASE were systematically searched for studies reporting complications and hospital mortality of adult patients receiving veno-venous ECMO for severe and refractory ARDS. Studies were screened for low bias risk and assessed for study size effect. Meta-analytic pooled estimation of study variables was performed using a weighted random effects model for study size. Models with potential moderators were explored using random effects meta-regression. Twelve studies fulfilled inclusion criteria, representing a population of 1042 patients with refractory ARDS. Pooled mortality at hospital discharge was 37.7% (CI 95% = 31.8–44.1; $I^2 = 74.2\%$). Adjusted mortality including one imputable missing study was 39.3% (CI 95% = 33.1–45.9). Meta-regression model combining patient age, year of study realization, mechanical ventilation (MV) days and prone positioning before veno-venous ECMO was associated with hospital mortality ($p < 0.001$; $R^2 = 0.80$). Patient age ($b = 0.053$; $p = 0.01$) and maximum cannula size during treatment ($b = -0.075$; $p = 0.008$) were also independently associated with mortality. Studies reporting H1N1 patients presented inferior hospital mortality (24.8 vs 40.6%; $p = 0.027$). Complication rate was 40.2% (CI 95% = 25.8–56.5), being bleeding the most frequent 29.3% (CI 95% = 20.8–39.6). Mortality due to complications was 6.9% (CI 95% = 4.1–11.2). Mechanical complications were present in 10.9% of cases (CI 95% = 4.7–23.5), being oxygenator failure the most prevalent (12.8%; CI 95% = 7.1–21.7). Despite initial severity, significant portion of patients treated with veno-venous ECMO survive hospital discharge. Patient age, H1N1-ARDS and cannula size are independently associated with hospital mortality. Combined effect of patient age, year of study realization, MV days and prone positioning before veno-venous ECMO influence patient outcome, and although medical complications are frequent, their impact on mortality is limited.

Keywords: Extracorporeal life support (ECLS), Extracorporeal CO_2 removal ($ECCO_2R$), Acute respiratory failure (ARF), Mechanical ventilation, H1N1, Extracorporeal bypass

*Correspondence: sergivaquer@gmail.com
[1] Critical Care Center, CIBER de Enfermedades Respiratorias, Corporació Sanitària Universitària Parc Taulí, Autonomous University of Barcelona, Parc Taulí 1, 08208 Sabadell, Spain
Full list of author information is available at the end of the article

Background

Despite extensive research and improved clinical management, mortality of severe forms of acute respiratory distress syndrome (ARDS) remains high [1–3]. However, in most cases, no specific treatment exists but to provide supportive therapy while the initial decompensating factor is treated. In this context, mechanical ventilation (MV) is cornerstone; however, ventilator-induced lung injury (VILI) remains a principal problem, with an impact on patient outcome [4]. Furthermore, despite best evidence-based respiratory care, a percentage of patients still die from refractory ARDS [5]. Therefore, in patients presenting with severe ARDS who become unresponsive to conventional treatment, the use of extracorporeal membrane oxygenation (ECMO), able to temporary replace pulmonary function, can represent a life-saving alternative, while time is gained for resolving the underlying cause [6].

ECMO can be used as a rescue therapy to avoid injurious effects of mechanical ventilation and to rescue from extreme gasometrical alterations [6]. These objectives can be attained by means of veno-venous ECMO circuits and can be used in patients with a large spectrum of underlying pathologies leading to refractory ARDS. New technologies with easier and more reliable equipment and procedures have allowed the expansion of veno-venous ECMO to many intensive care units (ICU) worldwide [7], and recent evidence suggested a potential positive effect of the use of these systems in refractory ARDS [8] as compared with initial experiences [9, 10]. However, despite the increasing number of reports, an adequate estimation of the effects of veno-venous ECMO use on complication rate and patient outcome using a meta-analytical approach is still lacking. Available studies provide either a general overview of a large historical database without pooled analysis [11], included high percentage of patients requiring cardiovascular support [12], are based on a specific population of patients [13] or were based on a low number of reports representing a small population of patients [14]. Therefore, we performed a systematic review and meta-analysis of the latest available peer-reviewed published literature to adequately estimate complication rate and hospital mortality associated with veno-venous ECMO in patients presenting refractory ARDS.

Methods

The MEDLINE database from the National Library of Medicine (USA) and EMBASE were systematically searched to find articles reporting the utilization of veno-venous ECMO for treating any form of severe and refractory ARDS. Studies were included if they reported medical or technical complications in adult patients (>18 years old) from 1972 to December 2015. The search string was comprised of the following MESH terms and Booleans: (("Extracorporeal Membrane Oxygenation"[Mesh] OR "Oxygenators, Membrane"[Mesh]) AND ("Respiratory Distress Syndrome, Adult"[Mesh] OR "Respiratory Insufficiency"[Mesh])) OR (("Extracorporeal Membrane Oxygenation"[Mesh] OR "Oxygenators, Membrane"[Mesh]) AND "Respiratory Insufficiency"[Mesh] AND ("Carbon Dioxide"[Mesh] OR "Hypercapnia"[Mesh])) AND "humans"[MeSH Terms] AND ("adolescent"[MeSH Terms] OR "adult"[MeSH Terms]). The term "Oxygenators, Membrane" was added to include older articles classified before 1988. The term "adolescent" was included to permit allocation of studies reporting patients ageing 18 years old (PubMed search engine identifies an "adult" as a 19 years or more subject). This implied the inclusion of a number of paediatric cases ageing >16 years, who had to be later excluded from the analysis. Additional articles were allocated by reviewing article reference lists, textbooks and grey literature.

Articles retrieved were included or rejected based on information obtained from the title, abstract or main text. Only studies reporting the use of veno-venous ECMO techniques were included. In studies reporting a combination of veno-venous ECMO and veno-arterial ECMO, only patients who received VV-ECMO were included if information about patient outcome and technique complications could be differentiated for each technique. In all other cases, studies were included if the percentage of VA-ECMO utilization was below 10%. This percentage was arbitrarily selected on the basis of its expected negligible effect on the statistical analysis and to account for the reduced percentage of patients that present associated cardiac failure to refractory ARDS. Meta-analysis and systematic reviews were excluded to avoid overlapping of results with original articles. Articles reporting analysis from the international ELSO—Extracorporeal Life Support Organization—were also excluded to avoid overlapping of patients with those presented in articles published by the original submitting centre. Only articles written in English were included in this systematic review.

A minimum number of 50 veno-venous ECMO cases per report were arbitrarily established as an initial threshold to minimize publication bias. Risk of bias of studies was further assessed using a scoring system for evaluating selection, attrition and reporting biases for randomized controlled trials (max. 3 points) [15] and the Ottawa–Newcastle scale for non-randomized studies (max. 9 points) [16]. Studies were identified to have high risk of bias and were excluded if their scoring results were below 3 and 5 points, respectively, or if information on patient outcome and complications was not provided.

Additionally, small study effect was evaluated by means of visual evaluation of funnel plots and the Egger's test of the intercept, using mortality at discharge from hospital as the main outcome variable and a random effects model analysis, with significant threshold at one-tailed $p < 10\%$ as originally described [17]. Duval and Tweedie's Trim and Fill method [18] was used to impute potentially missing studies on both sides of the plot using a random effects model and to compute corrected mean point estimates if required.

Three investigators reviewed all articles, performed data extraction and complied the database using equal digital templates (VS, dHC, PP). Results were compared, and discrepancies were solved by agreement. A fourth investigator approved the final database and decided upon remaining conflictive data (AA). In case of suspected unreliable information due to insufficient clarity in data presentation, the article was excluded from the analysis. Any other source of conflict was solved by consensus of the research team (VS, dHC, PP, OJ, AA). The process followed the PRISMA guidelines for systematic reviews and meta-analyses [19] and the Cochrane guidelines for systematic review of interventions [20].

Once appropriate articles were allocated, the following general study and technical information were collected: type of study, centre and country of realization, year of study start and year of finalization, number and cause of veno-venous ECMO (ARDS, lung transplant, trauma, hypoventilation, mixed), patient age, pre-ECMO PO_2/FiO_2 ratio (P/F), positive end-expiratory pressure and plateau pressure (Pplat), Sequential Organ Failure Assessment Score (SOFA) [21] if available, MV days before ECMO initiation, Lung Injury Score (LIS) [22], centre experience (determined by the number of veno-venous ECMO cases per year), veno-venous ECMO duration, cannulation site (jugulo-femoral or J-F, femoro-jugular or F-J, femoro-femoral or F-F, J double, F double or mixed), maximum cannula size used (in French), membrane type (silicone—spiral, polymethylpentene/polypropylene—hollow fibre), pump type (rotary, centrifugal), mean measured or targeted coagulation time ratio during ECMO treatment, total number of complications, mortality attributable to complications and mortality at hospital discharge. Patient deceases were considered to be attributable to complications of veno-venous ECMO whenever authors of the original article clearly identified a direct relation between the occurrence of the complication and the fatal outcome. Such complication must have occurred during the course of veno-venous ECMO treatment or immediately after its discontinuation. The presented average coagulation time during ECMO in each article was divided by the standard laboratory time of the specific test if provided, or by 107 s for activated coagulation time (ACT), 35 s for partial thromboplastin time (PTT) and 22 s for thrombin time (TT) to obtain a comparable coagulation ratio across studies. Studies were sorted according to their finalization and start year to allow evaluation of the impact of study realization time on study variables. If such information was not available, one year before acceptance for publication was arbitrarily selected as the study finalization year.

The following medical complications were recorded: total bleeding events, significant bleeding events (defined as major/severe bleeding by the authors of the original article due to relevant impact on patient status, bleeding requiring surgical control or haemoderivate transfusion and bleeding events leading to fatal outcome), number of specific site bleeding events (surgical site, respiratory system, gastrointestinal, cannulation site, intracerebral, haemothorax and other), pneumothorax (if related to cannulation only), limb ischaemia, diffuse intravascular coagulopathy, heparin-induced thrombocytopenia, haemolysis, deep venous thrombosis, pulmonary embolism, severe arrhythmia, hypothermia, confirmed bloodstream infection after veno-venous ECMO initiation, veno-venous ECMO catheter infection, tamponade or direct cardiac injury. The total number of haemoderivates administered was also recorded (packed red blood cell units—RBC; platelet + fresh frozen plasma concentrates—PL/FFP).

The following equipment complications were recorded: oxygenator failure (oedema, coagulation or rupture), cannulas failure (disconnection, coagulation or rupture), decannulation events, pump failure (coagulation or rupture) and tubing malfunction (rupture, leak or coagulation).

Statistical evaluation was performed using SPSS version 22 statistical software (International Business Machines. Armonk, NY, USA), Comprehensive Meta-Analysis version 3 (Biostat Inc. Englewood, NJ, USA) and OpenMetaAnalyst version 10.10 [23]. Meta-analytic pooled estimation of mortality at hospital discharge, complications and mortality due to veno-venous ECMO complications was performed using a weighted random effects model for study size. Results are presented as overall average point estimate (in %) with 95% CI and usual statistics (mean, median, CI 95% and IQR). Heterogeneity values (I^2) are provided when appropriate. Meta-regression using a random effects model analysis was employed to explore the potential effect of moderators on study variables. The following variables were evaluated as potential independent moderators: percentage of prone positioning before extracorporeal support, patient age, P/F ratio, PEEP, Pplat, driving pressure, MV duration, LIS and SOFA before veno-venous ECMO, cause of ARDS, extracorporeal support duration, centre experience, realization year, targeted/measured coagulation ratio during treatment, maximum cannula size used and membrane and pump type used. Combinations of moderator variables were evaluated by means of a stepwise meta-regression analysis in a random effects model. Variables included in the model were selected to maximize study inclusion in the analysis according to completeness of the database.

Results

The systematic search performed returned a total of 1423 studies. The complete list of studies can be found as Additional file 1: Study Database. One thousand four hundred eleven studies were excluded from the analysis based on exclusion criteria established for this systematic review and meta-analysis (Fig. 1). Main excluded studies are presented in Table 1. The study performed by Schmidt et al. [24] provided data from patients treated in three different centres from two nationalities. Since detailed information was provided for each of them, they were considered as independent studies and included separately to enhance statistical power of the analysis. The reports by Schmid et al. [25] and Camboni et al. [26] were excluded from the analysis to minimize the chance of patient overlap among studies performed in the same institution (University Medical Center, Regensburg, Germany). Main features of the final 12 included studies are presented in Table 2. All included studies were performed in the last fifteen years and used veno-venous ECMO for supporting patients under severe and refractory ARDS. Using hospital mortality as the main variable, included studies were evaluated for study size effect. The generated funnel plot presented no clear asymmetry upon visual inspection (Fig. 2), and the Egger's test of the intercept did not identify any significant association between study size and hospital mortality ($t = 1.23$; df $= 10$; $p = 0.12$). Pooled mortality at hospital discharge was 37.7% ($z = -3.73$; CI 95% = 31.8–44.1%; $p < 0.001$) with a heterogeneity of $I^2 = 74.2\%$ ($Q = 42.66$; $Tau^2 = 0.153$; $p < 0.001$) (Fig. 3). One imputable missing study was found using Duval and Tweedie's Trim and Fill method on the right side of the funnel plot (Fig. 2). Corrected hospital mortality including the calculated missing study was 39.3% (CI 95% = 33.1–45.9%). The following moderator variables were found to be independently associated with hospital mortality: patient age ($b = 0.053$; $Q = 6.6$; $n = 12$; $p = 0.01$), maximum cannula size used during treatment ($b = -0.075$; $Q = 7.04$; $n = 4$; $p = 0.008$) and cause of ARDS (H1N1 = 24.8 vs other = 40.6%; $Q = 4.894$; $p = 0.027$). The meta-regression model combining patient age ($b = 0.192$; $p < 0.001$), year of study realization ($b = -0.176$; $p = 0.003$), MV days before veno-venous ECLS ($b = 0.209$; $p = 0.003$) and prone position before extracorporeal support ($b = -2.383$; $p = 0.01$) was associated with the observed hospital mortality ($Q = 19.48$; $n = 11$; $p < 0.001$; $R^2 = 0.80$). No additional moderator variables were associated with hospital

Table 1 Main excluded studies

Study	Year	Patients	Reason for exclusion
Lehle et al. [42]	2014	317	No complications reported
Cheng et al. [43]	2013	216	Unable to identify data associated with veno-venous ECMO
Schmid et al. [44]	2012	176	Risk of patient overlap (duplicate)
Hemmila et al. [28]	2004	168	>10% veno-arterial ECMO
Bartlett et al. [45]	2000	146	>10% veno-arterial ECMO
Camboni et al. [26]	2011	127	Risk of patient overlap (duplicate)
Lindskov et al. [46]	2013	124	>10% veno-arterial ECMO
Pham et al. [35]	2013	123	>10% veno-arterial ECMO
Pranikoff et al. [47]	1999	94	Risk of bias
Bein et al. [48]	2006	90	Arterio-venous CO_2 removal
Nehra et al. [49]	2009	81	Reports patients <18 years
Rubino et al. [50]	2014	72	Risk of bias
Liebold et al. [51]	2002	70	Reports patients <18 years
Chiu et al. [52]	2015	65	No complications reported
Pappalardo et al. [53]	2013	60	ELSO database
Ma et al. [54]	2012	56	Risk of bias
Chimot et al. [55]	2013	52	Risk of bias
Pranikoff et al. [56]	1994	51	>10% veno-arterial ECMO
Zimmermann et al. [57]	2009	51	Arterio-venous CO_2 removal
Peek et al. [58]	1997	50	Reports patients <18 years

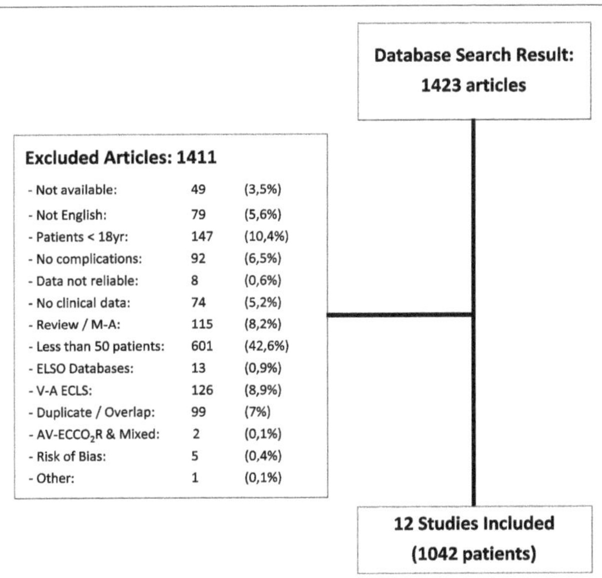

Fig. 1 Consort chart of included/excluded studies

Table 2 List of included studies

Study	Year	Centre	Type	Patients	Population	P/F ratio	MV (days)	Prone (%)	LIS	Age (years)	Heparin coating	Membrane type	Pump type	Coagulation ratio[b]	Max cannula size (French)	Cannulation	ECMO duration (days)
Mols et al. [59]	2000	University of Freiburg, Freiburg, Germany	CP	62	Mixed	64	10	81	3.2	35	Y	n/a	R	1.26	25	F-J	14.5
Davies et al. [36]	2009	Multi-centre, Australia	CR	68	H1N1	56	2	18	3.2	34[a]	Y	HF-PMP	C	n/a	n/a	Mixed	10[a]
Mueller et al. [60]	2009	University Medical Center, Regensburg, Germany	CR	60	Mixed	64	1	n/a	3.6	53[a]	Y	HF-PMP	C	1.50	23	F-J	9[a]
Peek et al. [8]	2010	The Glenfield Hospital, Leicester, UK	RCT	68	Mixed	70[a]	1.5[a]	47	3.5[a]	40	n/a	HF-PP	R	1.58	n/a	n/a	9[a]
Noah et al. [61]	2011	Multicentre, UK	CC	69	H1N1	55[a]	4[a]	39	3.5[a]	36	n/a	n/a	n/a	n/a	23	n/a	9[a]
Patroniti et al. [62]	2011	Multicentre, Italy	CP	60	ARDS	63[a]	2	27	3.6	41	Y	HF-PMP	C	1.6	n/a	Mixed	9[a]
Schmidt et al. [27]	2013	Multi-centre, France	CR	140	Mixed	53	5	61	n/a	44[a]	Y	HF mixed	C	1.357	n/a	Mixed	15[a]
Roch et al. [63]	2014	Marseille North Hospital, France	CP	85	Mixed	60	2	20	3.5	47	Y	HF mixed	C	1.28	25	F-J	9
Haneya et al. [64]	2015	University Medical Center, Regensburg, Germany	CR	262	Mixed	64	1	n/a	3.3	49	Y	HF mixed	C	1.57	31	Mixed	9
Schmidt et al. [24] (Melbourne)	2015	Alfred Hospital, Australia	CR	52	Mixed	75	1	2	n/a	37	n/a	n/a	n/a	n/a	n/a	Mixed	10

Table 2 continued

Study	Year	Centre	Type	Patients	Population	P/F ratio	MV (days)	Prone (%)	LIS	Age (years)	Heparin coating	Membrane type	Pump type	Coagulation ratio[b]	Max cannula size (French)	Cannulation	ECMO duration (days)
Schmidt et al. [24] (Paris)	2015	Pitié-Salpètrière Hospital, France	CR	57	Mixed	61	4	20	n/a	46	n/a	n/a	n/a	n/a	n/a	Mixed	10
Schmidt et al. [24] (Sydney)	2015	Royal Prince Alfred Hospital, Australia	CR	59	Mixed	66	2	54	n/a	40	n/a	n/a	n/a	n/a	n/a	Mixed	9

CP cohort prospective, *CR* cohort retrospective, *CC* case–control, *RCT* randomized controlled trial, *P/F* ratio: PO_2/FiO_2 ratio, *MV* mechanical ventilation before ECMO initiation, *LIS* Lung Injury Score, *HF* hollow fibre, *PP* polypropylene, *PMP* polymethylpentene, *C* centrifugal, *R* rotatory, *F-J* femoro-jugular. Mean values are presented unless indicated

[a] Median values

[b] Normalized coagulation ratio, see "Methods" section for explanation

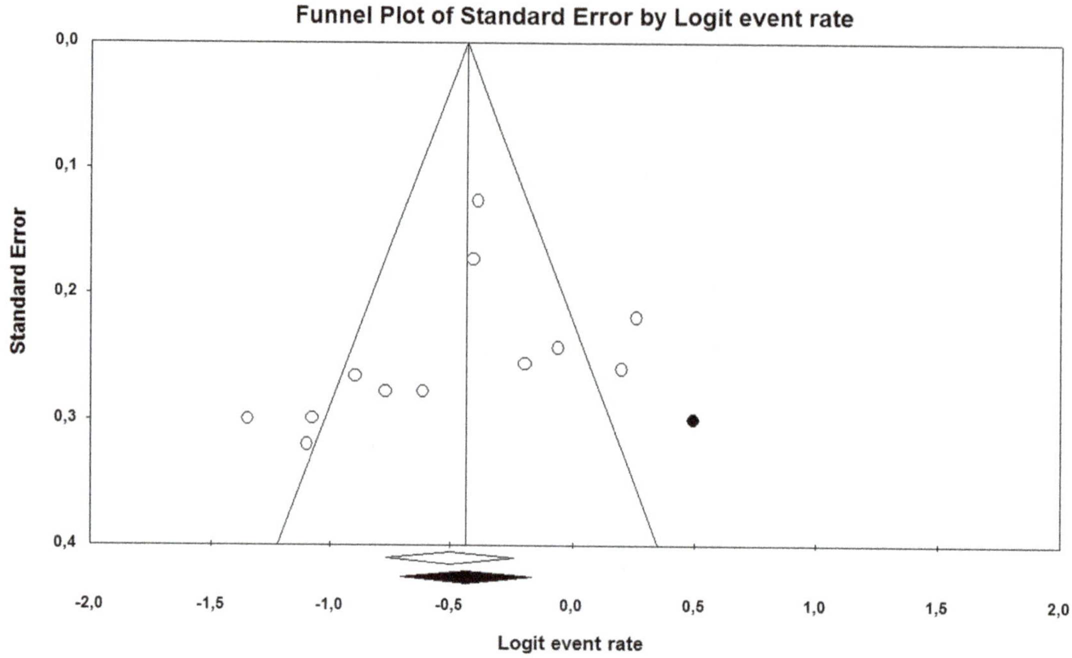

Fig. 2 *Funnel plot* of included studies. *White circles* represent observed studies. Mean point was computed using a random effects model and is presented as white rhomboid. Using the Trim and Fill method, one additional imputable study was identified. The estimated corrected mean point with confidence interval is presented as a *black rhomboid*

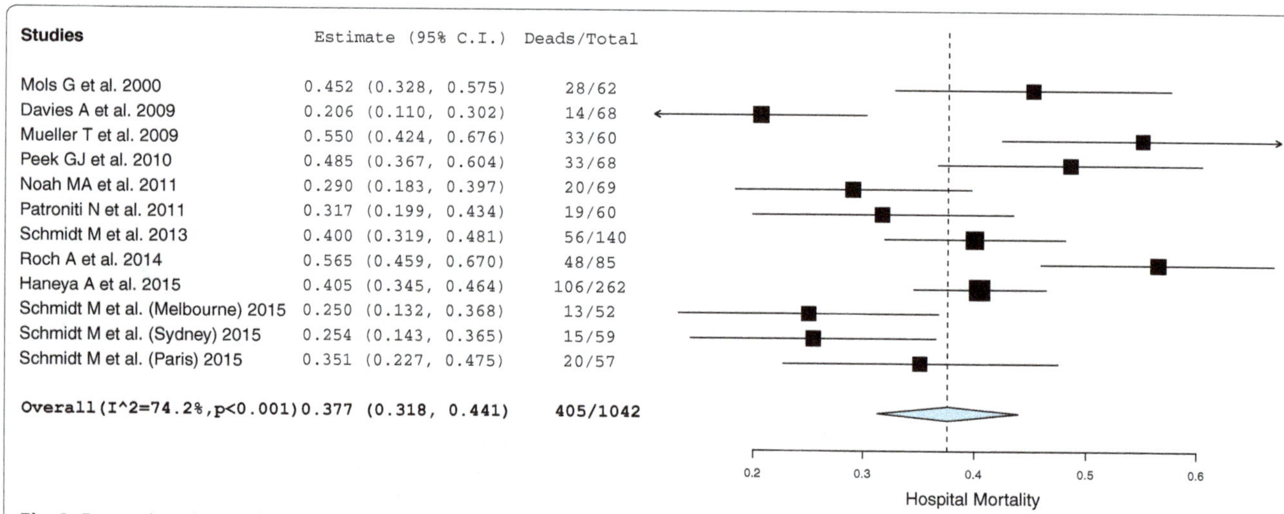

Fig. 3 Forest plot—hospital mortality

mortality. Medical complications occurred in 40.2% of patients, being bleeding the most frequent (29.3%). Mechanical complications affected 11% of patients, with 12.8% of them requiring oxygenator replacement for malfunction. However, mortality caused by complications accounted for only 7% of deceases (Table 3).

Discussion

Results of the present meta-analysis indicate that more than 60% of the patients with refractory ARDS who receive veno-venous ECMO survive hospital discharge despite initial high illness severity. These results are unexpected, given the observed mortality ratios in

Table 3 Patient outcome and complication rate

	Number of studies reporting data	Average point estimate (CI 95%)
Hospital mortality	12	37.7% (31.8–44.1)
Mortality due to complications	8	6.9% (4.1–11.2)
Mortality due to bleeding	7	3.3% (2–5.4)
Medical complications	12	40.2% (25.8–56.5)
Bleeding	12	29.3% (20.8–39.6)
Significant bleeding	9	10.4% (5.6–18.7)
Cannula bleeding	8	9.3% (5.3–15.6)
ICH	5	5.4% (2.7–10.3)
Pulmonary bleeding	5	6.4% (3.2–12.4)
Other bleeding	6	9.3% (4.9–16.9)
DVT/PE	3	4.6% (2.2–9.2)
Pneumothorax	3	5.7% (1.1–24.2)
Cannula infections	3	9.9% (4.2–21.5)
Mechanical complications	4	10.9% (4.7–23.5)
Oxygenator failure	2	12.8% (7.1–21.7)
Cannula failure	3	4.5% (2.5–8.1)

ICH intracerebral haemorrhage, *DVT/PE* deep venous thrombosis/pulmonary embolism

severe forms of ARDS [1–3]. Interestingly, Zampieri et al. [14] had already identified a potential beneficial effect of veno-venous ECMO on survival [14] in a meta-analysis of three studies including patients with severe and refractory ARDS (1 RCT and 2 case–control studies). However, reduction of hospital mortality could only be found if alternative severity-pairing method in two of the three included studies was used (OR = 0, 52; CI 95% = 0.35–0.76; $p < 0.001$). The low number of studies included representing a limited population of refractory ARDS patients may explain these results. Conversely, data from the present meta-analysis are supported by a larger number of studies, more recently published and by a larger population size of refractory ARDS patients receiving veno-venous ECMO. Moreover, thanks to the larger population being studied, details on technique-associated complications, their effect on patient outcome and the effect of potential moderator variables could be evaluated. Results of the present report are also consistent with those published in studies based on the Extracorporeal Life Support Organization (ELSO) database. The ELSO is an international association of ECMO-providing centres, which maintains a registry of ECMO cases and provides annual ECMO survival information and centre-based performance reports [7]. In the study by Paden et al., based on a large cohort of refractory ARDS patients receiving veno-venous ECMO, mortality rates oscillated between 36 and 49% depending on the condition leading to ARDS [7]. However, these results may be not completely representative of the true reality of ECMO use in ICUs worldwide. Selection and notification bias may affect studies based on the ELSO database, for that inclusion of patients into the registry is voluntary and only selected centres can be members of the network. Interestingly, two of the three studies included in the above-mentioned meta-analysis by Zampieri et al. were based on the ELSO database [14]. In this sense, the present report provides more reliable information by excluding studies from the ELSO database, which avoids above-mentioned biases and ensures minimum overlapping of patients and duplication of results. Finally, it also allowed us to gather more detailed information about procedural and centre characteristics not included in more general studies.

To explain the observed levels of hospital mortality found in the present meta-analysis and its associated heterogeneity, we explored the effect of potential moderator variables independently and in combination in a logistic meta-regression model. Patient age at study inclusion was independently associated with hospital mortality in our results, which confirm previous observations [27, 28] and is supportive of the validity of the database and the analysis performed. Such association was also found in the combined meta-regression model which suggests the principal role of this moderator variable. Indeed, patient age is a strong determinant of patient outcome that must be taken into account when ECMO treatment is indicated. Nevertheless, it is challenging to find a proper comparable population of patients with severe ARDS without ECMO to compare the specific effect of age on outcome. In the study by Guérin et al. [29], patients in the prone group had an average age of 58 years (compared to the present 42 years of ECMO patients determined in this meta-analysis) and presented inferior mortality rates (16 vs 39.3%). However, such patients probably had less severe lung injuries, not yet refractory to conventional treatment, including prone positioning. In the study by Guérin et al. [29], P/F ratio was substantially higher in the prone group than in patients included in the present meta-analysis (100 vs 62), and PEEP, Pplat and driving pressure values were higher in ECMO patients (14.2 vs 10; 32.6 vs 23; 7.6 vs 4 cmH_2O, respectively). These findings indicate the need for higher ventilator loads to maintain minimum oxygenation, which would be caused by a more severe and established lung injury in veno-venous ECMO patients. Conversely, according to other reports published by Villar et al. [2] and Bellani et al. [3], higher mortality ratios in older patients with severe ARDS can be identified (58.1% and 46% vs 39.3%). It is therefore paramount that multiple factors are taken into account when trying to compare ECMO and non-ECMO patients, such as patient comorbidities and patient typology. In fact, the inclusion of an undetermined number of H1N1 patients in the present meta-analysis could have contributed to the observed association between mortality and patient age, given the younger average age of these patients. Other factors, such as immunocompromised status and malignancies, have the potential for significantly influencing outcome and are discussed later in this section.

Present results also suggest that cannula size used during veno-venous ECMO is also a determinant factor for patient outcome. Insufficient cannula size implies limited oxygenation capabilities of the extracorporeal system and consequently impossibilities the reduction of mechanical ventilation loads exerted on the patient during veno-venous ECMO treatment. As recently demonstrated, driving pressure is associated with patient outcome [30] and inability to reduce it during veno-venous ECMO has a negative influence on patient evolution [31]. Although insufficient information on driving pressure during extracorporeal support could be found to be included in the general meta-regression evaluation, the identified inverse association between cannula size and mortality could be indicative of the risks of insufficient extracorporeal support due to smaller-than-necessary cannula use. However, these results need to be evaluated cautiously, given the limited number of studies that reported the size of the used cannulas.

We were also able to find a statistically significant difference in hospital mortality in studies reporting predominantly H1N1 patients when compared to those in which veno-venous ECMO was initiated for a combination of causes leading to ARDS. This finding is also in accordance with previous observations, in which patients with viral pneumonia receiving ECMO presented inferior levels of mortality [7, 13]. These results are also not unexpected given the inferior mortality rates of H1N1 patients when compared with general ARDS population [32–34]. In another meta-analysis by Zangrillo et al. on mortality of H1N1 patients receiving veno-venous ECMO, authors estimated 28% (CI 95% = 18–37%) of pooled hospital mortality [13], which is similar to what has been observed in our results. However, high variability can be observed in results of studies evaluating the use of ECMO for severe and refractory ARDS induced by H1N1 infection. These oscillate between 17% in Schmidt et al. [27], 36% in Pham et al. [35] and 35% in Davies et al. [36]. Such variability could be caused by several factors ranging from pre-existing comorbidities to centre experience and patient management differences. As discussed below, the use of prone positioning before veno-venous ECMO is associated with improved outcomes. In the above-mentioned studies, the highest percentage of prone positioning can be observed in the study with the lowest mortality ratios (Schmidt et al. = 59%, Pham et al. = 45%, Davies et al. = 22%). In addition, the use of veno-arterial ECMO for concomitant cardiovascular failure in these studies was the lowest in the study with the lowest mortality ratios (5, 7.3 and 13%, respectively). As it will also be discussed later in this section, the use of veno-arterial ECMO implies exposure to a different pattern of associated complications, which have the potential for exerting an impact on patient outcome. Higher use of veno-arterial ECMO could also illustrate higher severity of patients, with added cardiovascular dysfunction, which would worsen prognosis and explain the different mortality rates.

Another variable, study realization time, was also associated with hospital mortality in the evaluated meta-regression model. Increasing centre ECMO experience during the studied time frame could be a factor explaining such association. Interestingly, centre experience has already been associated with improved outcomes in previous reports [37] but could not be identified as a moderator variable in the model used in the present analysis. Nevertheless, it is important to highlight that the used estimator of centre experience in our study does not take into account other forms of extracorporeal life support, which share technical and operational characteristics with veno-venous ECMO and could have been performed in the reporting centres during the same study time frame. Such additional extracorporeal support experience could not be incorporated into our analysis. Furthermore, other patient types that received veno-venous ECMO simultaneously but presented other pathologies not matching the objectives of the included studies were also not incorporated in the estimation of experience. This would be especially true for studies reporting only H1N1 patients. The effect of such underestimation of centre experience may be the cause of the observed lack of association with hospital mortality. Furthermore, the impossibility to ascertain centre experience in multicentre studies also limited the use of this variable in the combined meta-regression evaluation due to excessive missing information. On another side, progressive technological evolution of veno-venous ECMO equipment, with improved biocompatibility and reduced complication rates, could have had a potential positive impact on patient evolution [38]. Interestingly, previous reports have identified the opposite effect of study realization time in other forms of ECMO for cardiovascular support, in which mortality increased with publication year [12].

Mortality of refractory ARDS patients treated with veno-venous ECMO was also associated with MV days before extracorporeal support initiation in the combined meta-regression model. It has already been well established that a delayed instauration of ECMO and a prolonged MV before treatment (>7 days) have deleterious effects on outcome [28, 39]. Despite the fact that in most of the included studies veno-venous ECMO was initiated without much delay (median = 2, IQR = 1.1–4), we were able to identify an association of MV duration before extracorporeal support and mortality. This corroborates previous observations and justifies the initiation of veno-venous ECMO in refractory ARDS patients within the first days after admission, before irreversible lung injury is established.

Implementation of prone position before ECMO was also evaluated in the present report. Despite the already demonstrated beneficial effect of prone positioning in moderate–severe ARDS patients [29], prone positioning before veno-venous ECMO was only used in 40% of the included patients in the present systematic review and meta-analysis and presented high variability (range 2–73%). As recently published, prone position use is also very variable in patients with severe ARDS in ICUs worldwide [3]. In our results, prone positioning before veno-venous ECMO initiation was identified as a cofactor associated with positive outcomes. These results are also in accordance with those in previous studies [27]. In spite of the fact that in all included studies veno-venous ECMO was used in patients considered refractory to conventional treatment and followed pre-established protocols, which aimed at optimizing patients before treatment initiation, present results indicate that prone positioning was used insufficiently before veno-venous ECMO initiation. We were unable to ascertain whether such findings were due to excessive severity and instability of patients, or because other rescue therapies had been used instead of prone positioning. Limited information was available in this regard in the original studies included.

Finally, adequate patient selection of veno-venous ECMO treatment instauration also has the potential for influencing outcome [27, 28, 39] and may have also influenced results. Outcomes of ECMO treatment are highly dependent on the underlying cause of ARDS and patient comorbidities. In addition to already mentioned differences according to the cause of ARDS (H1N1 vs. other causes), patients with haematological malignancies and ARDS present markedly higher mortality ratios than those observed in present results (haematological = 50% present other = 40.6%, present H1N1 = 24.8%) [40]. Furthermore, patient immunocompromised status has already been identified as a prognostic factor in patients receiving veno-venous ECMO [27]. However, we were unable to allocate information on immune status or malignancy prevalence in the included studies to confirm previous observations.

Marked differences can be found in studies evaluating patients receiving ECMO for cardiovascular support when compared to ECMO for respiratory support. Veno-arterial ECMO has been associated with mortality rates that vary from 57%, in highly experienced centres [37], to 66% according to the ELSO database [7]. In these reports, patients received extracorporeal support for isolated cardiovascular failure mainly. Indeed, veno-arterial ECMO for cardiovascular failure must be differentiated from veno-venous ECMO for respiratory patients, for that it uses a different cannulation technique in which blood is directly reinjected into the arterial mainstream. This technique is also applied to a different type of patient with specific underlying pathology. Zangrillo et al. performed another meta-analysis to evaluate mortality rates and complications associated with ECMO use [12]. Studies included were developed in high case volume centres (>100 patients per study) and included patients who received support with veno-arterial ECMO for cardiac failure predominantly (92%). When such results are compared with present observations, marked differences in mortality at hospital discharge can be observed (39 vs 54%). Interestingly, Zangrillo et al. also identified a significant reduction in mortality rates in the subgroup of patients who only received veno-venous ECMO ($b = -0.203$; CI 95% = −0.412 to 0.005; $p = 0.005$). These results support that veno-arterial and veno-venous ECMO represent different techniques with different outcome rates. This important conceptual differentiation is of high relevance when designing a national ECMO programme for respiratory support, since both hospital resources and required professional expertise differ for both techniques. This also has a significant impact in cost estimation [8] and should be taken into account by healthcare administrators.

Data from our meta-analysis also indicate that, like in veno-arterial ECMO, medical complications associated with veno-venous ECMO are common. However, despite their high incidence during the treatment course, medical complications associated with ECMO support have a small impact in overall mortality, accounting only for 7% of fatal outcome cases. Additionally, although bleeding has been historically considered the most feared complication during ECMO, present results suggest that while bleeding episodes are rather frequent, their attributable mortality in veno-venous ECMO is reduced. Similarly, although catastrophic, ICH affects a limited number of patients. When present data are compared with results from the previous meta-analysis by Zangrillo et al., in which high rates of patients treated with veno-arterial ECMO were included [12], meaningful differences between the two techniques are once again noticeable. Bleeding episodes were inferior in the present report (33 vs 29%), so was the occurrence of intracerebral haemorrhage (8 vs 5.4%). Interestingly, limb ischaemia events were not reported in the included studies of the present meta-analysis. These findings illustrate the key differential features of veno-venous and veno-arterial ECMO circuits. The lack of arterial catheterization implies minimum risk of arterial ischaemia and also reduces the risk of arterial emboli and central nervous system complications. Furthermore, bleeding has been reported to be commonly observed in the cannula insertion site and in recent surgical wounds in either form of ECMO [7]. However, in the present report, surgical bleeding was reported only in a limited number of included studies. Since the likelihood of veno-arterial ECMO being performed close to cardiac surgery is higher, more frequent surgical site bleeding events should be expected in patients receiving this type of therapy. Also, the fact that cannulas are placed in a pressurized vessel may also predispose to increased bleeding. On the other side observed coagulation ratios in included studies with veno-venous ECMO were inferior to those attained in previously reported veno-arterial ECMO patients (mean = 1.45 vs 1.64) [12]; however, no association between coagulation ratio and increased bleeding rates could be observed in our results with veno-venous ECMO patients. It is necessary to comment that this lack of association may be caused by the insufficient validity of an average/target coagulation point that does not represent the true course of anticoagulation therapy. Oscillations of anticoagulation values not illustrated by mean values can occur during treatment and may have an impact on bleeding occurrence. Nevertheless, the possible benefits of veno-venous ECMO must be gauged to the lethality of the above-mentioned complications. This is specially true in case of ICH and other similar complications, which can have a significant impact on patient morbi-mortality and long-term effects on patient's quality of life. Despite low attributable mortality to medical complications, emphasis must be put in adequate patient selection and experienced management of ECMO to further minimize their occurrence and impact on patient outcome.

Mechanical complications were present in 11% of patients. These findings contrast with historical reports in which high number of both oxygenator and pump failures were observed. However, two recent evaluations of complications associated with ECMO use in ARDS found that acute replacements of the ECMO system were required in 14.4 and 16.1% of cases [7, 41]. These results fall within the observed range of failures found in our meta-analysis. Nevertheless, the reduced number of studies reporting on technical and mechanical complications included in the present meta-analysis makes the interpretation of the above-mentioned results difficult and should be evaluated cautiously. Further and more technically oriented evaluations are required to provide a definitive answer on the technical improvement of veno-venous ECMO systems.

In addition to the already mentioned limitations of this study, some further aspects which may limit the interpretation of present results must be discussed. The highest statistical quality of systematic reviews and meta-analysis is obtained when randomized controlled trials (RCT) are used to estimate pooled outcomes [20]. Indeed, this minimizes the risk of multiple biases and enhances the quality of information obtained from the analysis. However, in the present report, the only recent RCT available on the use of ECMO for respiratory failure [8] was combined with non-randomized studies. In order to reduce bias in our results, strict inclusion criteria were implemented and careful care was taken to minimize the impact of confounding factors. In addition, specific statistical methods to identify publication bias and to quantify the impact of study size on results were implemented in the present report. None of the implemented evaluations suggested unreliability of present analyses, and results were adjusted to include potentially missing reports. Nevertheless, as new RCT become available, new meta-analyses should be performed to include newest data and improve reliability of present estimations. Another limitation of the present report is that not all studies provided information in all variables. While the main study variables were widely covered by most of the reports included, information on certain medical and technical complications was only provided in a few studies. Thus, the pooled point estimate for certain variables needs to be interpreted cautiously. Future studies will also be beneficial to provide better estimations of these variables. The present report is also limited by the fact that only articles written in English were included, which could represent a source of bias. However, the impact of such idiomatic bias was estimated to be negligible given the low number of reports written in other languages (5.6%). Finally, the high heterogeneity levels observed for hospital mortality rates implied increased variance among the included studies. Although we were able to identify one model that could explain a high proportion of the observed variance, additional unexplored factors can be present. The inclusion of data from upcoming RCTs, with more homogeneous patient characteristics, objectives and methodologies, may help in minimizing heterogeneity and yield more reliable and definitive results.

Conclusion

Results suggest that despite high initial severity, patients treated with veno-venous ECMO for refractory ARDS present reduced mortality ratios. Patient age, H1N1-related ARDS and cannula size are independently associated with hospital mortality, and the combined effect of patient age, year of study realization, MV days and prone positioning before extracorporeal support are also associated with better outcomes. Medical complications are commonly present in veno-venous ECMO but have limited impact on patient outcome. When compared with veno-arterial ECMO for cardiovascular support, veno-venous ECMO presents a different pattern of complications and outcomes, probably due to differences in technical and patient characteristics.

In conclusion, veno-venous ECMO has evolved substantially and has become a widespread technique with progressively improving outcomes in recent years. Appropriate patient selection, timing and use of validated treatment options, including prone positioning before initiation of extracorporeal support, are key to treatment success. Despite the still relevant number of complications associated with veno-venous ECMO, attributable mortality is limited.

Abbreviations

ARDS: acute respiratory distress syndrome; MV: mechanical ventilation; VILI: ventilation-induced lung injury; ECMO: extracorporeal membrane oxygenation; $ECCO_2R$: extracorporeal CO_2 removal; ICU: intensive care unit; ELSO: Extracorporeal Life Support Organization; P/F: PO_2/FiO_2 ratio; SOFA: Sequential Organ Failure Assessment Score; LIS: Lung Injury Score; J-F: jugulo-femoral; F-J: femoro-jugular; F-F: femoro-femoral; ACT: activated coagulation time; PTT: partial thromboplastin time; TT: thrombin time; RBC: red blood cell unit; PL/FFP: platelet + fresh frozen plasma concentrate; ICH: intracerebral haemorrhage; DVT/PE: deep venous thrombosis/pulmonary embolism.

Authors' contributions

VS designed the project, performed data search, selected appropriate studies, extracted information, compiled the database, analysed results, drafted the manuscript and approved the final text; dHC performed data search, selected appropriate studies, extracted information, compiled the database, analysed results, drafted the manuscript and approved the final text; PP performed data search, selected appropriate studies, extracted information, compiled the database and approved the final text; OJ analysed results and approved the final text; AA compiled the database and approved the final text. All authors read and approved the final manuscript.

Author details

[1] Critical Care Center, CIBER de Enfermedades Respiratorias, Corporació Sanitària Universitària Parc Taulí, Autonomous University of Barcelona, Parc Taulí 1, 08208 Sabadell, Spain. [2] Fundació Parc Taulí, Parc Taulí University Institute, Parc Taulí 1, 08208 Sabadell, Spain.

Acknowledgements

We express our gratitude to Dr. Haneya H and col. for providing information to complete our database.

Competing interests

The authors declare that they have no competing interests.

References

1. Ranieri VM, Rubenfeld GD, Thompson BT, et al. Acute respiratory distress syndrome: the Berlin Definition. JAMA. 2012;307:2526–33.
2. Villar J, Pérez-Méndez L, Blanco J, et al. A universal definition of ARDS: the PaO2/FiO2 ratio under a standard ventilatory setting—a prospective, multicenter validation study. Intensive Care Med. 2013;39:583–92.
3. Bellani G, Laffey JG, Pham T, et al. Epidemiology, patterns of care, and mortality for patients with acute respiratory distress syndrome in intensive care units in 50 countries. JAMA. 2016;315:788–800.
4. Terragni PP, Rosboch G, Tealdi A, et al. Tidal hyperinflation during low tidal volume ventilation in acute respiratory distress syndrome. Am J Respir Crit Care Med. 2007;175:160–6.
5. Stapleton RD, Wang BM, Hudson LD, et al. Causes and timing of death in patients with ARDS. Chest. 2005;128:525–32.
6. Del Sorbo L, Cypel M, Fan E. Extracorporeal life support for adults with severe acute respiratory failure. Lancet Respir Med. 2014;2:154–64.
7. Paden ML, Conrad SA, Rycus PT, et al. Extracorporeal life support organization registry report 2012. ASAIO J. 2013;59:202–10.
8. Peek GJ, Mugford M, Tiruvoipati R, et al. Efficacy and economic assessment of conventional ventilatory support versus extracorporeal membrane oxygenation for severe adult respiratory failure (CESAR): a multicentre randomised controlled trial. Lancet. 2009;374:1351–63.
9. Zapol WM, Snider MT, Hill JD, et al. Extracorporeal membrane oxygenation in severe acute respiratory failure. A randomized prospective study. JAMA. 1979;242:2193–6.
10. Morris AH, Wallace CJ, Menlove RL, et al. Randomized clinical trial of pressure-controlled inverse ratio ventilation and extracorporeal CO_2 removal for adult respiratory distress syndrome. Am J Respir Crit Care Med. 1994;149:295–305.
11. Schmidt M, Hodgson C, Combes A. Extracorporeal gas exchange for acute respiratory failure in adult patients: a systematic review. Crit Care. 2015;19:99.
12. Zangrillo A, Landoni G, Biondi-Zoccai G, et al. A meta-analysis of complications and mortality of extracorporeal membrane oxygenation. Crit Care Resusc. 2013;15:172–8.
13. Zangrillo A, Biondi-Zoccai G, Landoni G, et al. Extracorporeal membrane oxygenation (ECMO) in patients with H1N1 influenza infection: a systematic review and meta-analysis including 8 studies and 266 patients receiving ECMO. Crit Care. 2013;17:R30.
14. Zampieri FG, Mendes PV, Ranzani OT, et al. Extracorporeal membrane oxygenation for severe respiratory failure in adult patients: a systematic review and meta-analysis of current evidence. J Crit Care. 2013;28:998–1005.
15. Wu S-C, Chen WT-L, Lin H-H, et al. Use of extracorporeal membrane oxygenation in severe traumatic lung injury with respiratory failure. Am J Emerg Med. 2015;33:658–62.
16. GA Wells, B Shea, D O'Connell, J Peterson, V Welch, M Losos PT, Wells GA, Shea B, O'Connell D, Peterson J, Welch V, Losos M, Tugwell P. The Newcastle-Ottawa Scale (NOS) for assessing the quality of nonrandomised studies in meta-analyses. http://www.ohri.ca/programs/clinical_epidemiology/oxford.html.
17. Egger M, Davey Smith G, Schneider M, et al. Bias in meta-analysis detected by a simple, graphical test. BMJ. 1997;315:629–34.
18. Duval S, Tweedie R. Trim and fill: a simple funnel-plot-based method of testing and adjusting for publication bias in meta-analysis. Biometrics. 2000;56:455–63.
19. Liberati A, Altman DG, Tetzlaff J, et al. The PRISMA statement for reporting systematic reviews and meta-analyses of studies that evaluate health care interventions: explanation and elaboration. J Clin Epidemiol. 2009;62:e1–34.
20. Higgins J, Green S: Cochrane handbook for systematic reviews of interventions. Cochrane Collaboration 2011; Version 5. pp 1–639.
21. Vincent JL, de Mendonça A, Cantraine F, et al. Use of the SOFA score to assess the incidence of organ dysfunction/failure in intensive care units: results of a multicenter, prospective study. Working group on "sepsis-related problems" of the European Society of Intensive Care Medicine. Crit Care Med. 1998;26:1793–800.
22. Murray JF, Matthay MA, Luce JM, et al. An expanded definition of the adult respiratory distress syndrome. Am Rev Respir Dis. 1988;138:720–3.
23. Wallace BC, Dahabreh IJ, Trikalinos TA, et al. Closing the gap between methodologists and end-users: R as a computational back-end. J Stat Softw. 2012;49:1–15.

24. Schmidt M, Stewart C, Bailey M, et al. Mechanical ventilation management during extracorporeal membrane oxygenation for acute respiratory distress syndrome: a retrospective international multicenter study. Crit Care Med. 2015;43:654–64.
25. Schmid C, Philipp A, Hilker M, et al. Venovenous extracorporeal membrane oxygenation for acute lung failure in adults. J Hear Lung Transplant. 2012;31:9–15.
26. Camboni D, Philipp A, Lubnow M, et al. Support time-dependent outcome analysis for veno-venous extracorporeal membrane oxygenation. Eur J Cardiothorac Surg. 2011;40:1341–7.
27. Schmidt M, Zogheib E, Rozé H, et al. The PRESERVE mortality risk score and analysis of long-term outcomes after extracorporeal membrane oxygenation for severe acute respiratory distress syndrome. Intensive Care Med. 2013;39:1704–13.
28. Hemmila MR, Rowe SA, Boules TN, et al. Extracorporeal life support for severe acute respiratory distress syndrome in adults. Ann Surg. 2004;240:595–607.
29. Guérin C, Reignier J, Richard J-C, et al. Prone positioning in severe acute respiratory distress syndrome. N Engl J Med. 2013;368:2159–68.
30. Amato MBP, Meade MO, Slutsky AS, et al. Driving pressure and survival in the acute respiratory distress syndrome. N Engl J Med. 2015;372:747–55.
31. Chiu L-C, Hu H-C, Hung C-Y, et al. Dynamic driving pressure associated mortality in acute respiratory distress syndrome with extracorporeal membrane oxygenation. Ann Intensive Care. 2017;7:12.
32. Duggal A, Pinto R, Rubenfeld G, et al. Global variability in reported mortality for critical illness during the 2009–10 influenza A (H1N1) pandemic: a systematic review and meta-regression to guide reporting of outcomes during disease outbreaks. PLoS ONE. 2016;11:e0155044.
33. Máca J, Jor O, Holub M, et al. Past and present ARDS mortality rates: a systematic review. Respir Care. 2016;62(1):113–22.
34. Noah MA, Peek GJ, Finney SJ, et al. Referral to an extracorporeal membrane oxygenation center and mortality among patients with severe 2009 influenza A (H1N1). JAMA. 2011;306:1659–68.
35. Pham T, Combes A, Rozé H, et al. Extracorporeal membrane oxygenation for pandemic influenza A (H1N1)-induced acute respiratory distress syndrome: a cohort study and propensity-matched analysis. Am J Respir Crit Care Med. 2013;187:276–85.
36. Davies A, Jones D, Bailey M, et al. Extracorporeal membrane oxygenation for 2009 influenza A (H1N1) acute respiratory distress syndrome. JAMA. 2009;302:1888–95.
37. Barbaro RP, Odetola FO, Kidwell KM, et al. Association of hospital-level volume of extracorporeal membrane oxygenation cases and mortality. Analysis of the extracorporeal life support organization registry. Am J Respir Crit Care Med. 2015;191:894–901.
38. Combes A, Bacchetta M, Brodie D, et al. Extracorporeal membrane oxygenation for respiratory failure in adults. Curr Opin Crit Care. 2012;18:99–104.
39. Brogan TV, Thiagarajan RR, Rycus PT, et al. Extracorporeal membrane oxygenation in adults with severe respiratory failure: a multi-center database. Intensive Care Med. 2009;35:2105–14.
40. Wohlfarth P, Ullrich R, Staudinger T, et al. Extracorporeal membrane oxygenation in adult patients with hematologic malignancies and severe acute respiratory failure. Crit Care 2014;18(1):R20
41. Lubnow M, Philipp A, Foltan M, et al. Technical complications during veno-venous extracorporeal membrane oxygenation and their relevance predicting a system-exchange–retrospective analysis of 265 cases. PLoS ONE. 2014;9:e112316.
42. Lehle K, Philipp A, Hiller K-A, et al. Efficiency of gas transfer in venovenous extracorporeal membrane oxygenation: analysis of 317 cases with four different ECMO systems. Intensive Care Med. 2014;40:1870–7.
43. Cheng A, Sun H-Y, Lee C-W, et al. Survival of septic adults compared with nonseptic adults receiving extracorporeal membrane oxygenation for cardiopulmonary failure: A propensity-matched analysis. J Crit Care. 2013;28:532-e1–10.
44. Schmid C, Philipp A, Hilker M, et al. Venovenous extracorporeal membrane oxygenation for acute lung failure in adults. J Heart Lung Transplant. 2012;31:9–15.
45. Bartlett RH, Roloff DW, Custer JR, et al. Extracorporeal life support: the University of Michigan experience. JAMA. 2000;283:904–8.
46. Lindskov C, Jensen RH, Sprogoe P, et al. Extracorporeal membrane oxygenation in adult patients with severe acute respiratory failure. Acta Anaesthesiol Scand. 2013;57:303–11.
47. Pranikoff T, Hirschl RB, Remenapp R, et al. Venovenous extracorporeal life support via percutaneous cannulation in 94 patients. Chest. 1999;115:818–22.
48. Bein T, Weber F, Philipp A, et al. A new pumpless extracorporeal interventional lung assist in critical hypoxemia/hypercapnia. Crit Care Med. 2006;34:1372–7.
49. Nehra D, Goldstein AM, Doody DP, et al. Extracorporeal membrane oxygenation for nonneonatal acute respiratory failure: the Massachusetts General Hospital experience from 1990 to 2008. Arch Surg. 2009;144:427–32 **(discussion 432)**.
50. Rubino A, Vuylsteke A, Jenkins DP, et al. Direct complications of the Avalon bicaval dual-lumen cannula in respiratory extracorporeal membrane oxygenation (ECMO): single-center experience. Int J Artif Organs. 2014;37:741–7.
51. Liebold A, Philipp A, Kaiser M, et al. Pumpless extracorporeal lung assist using an arterio-venous shunt. Applications and limitations. Minerva Anestesiol. 2002;68:387–91.
52. Chiu L-C, Tsai F-C, Hu H-C, et al. Survival predictors in acute respiratory distress syndrome with extracorporeal membrane oxygenation. Ann Thorac Surg. 2015;99:243–50.
53. Pappalardo F, Pieri M, Greco T, et al. Predicting mortality risk in patients undergoing venovenous ECMO for ARDS due to influenza A (H1N1) pneumonia: the ECMOnet score. Intensive Care Med. 2013;39:275–81.
54. Ma DS, Kim JB, Jung S-H, et al. Outcomes of venovenous extracorporeal membrane oxygenation support for acute respiratory distress syndrome in adults. Korean J Thorac Cardiovasc Surg. 2012;45:91–4.
55. Chimot L, Marque S, Gros A, et al. Avalon(copyright) bicaval dual-lumen cannula for venovenous extracorporeal membrane oxygenation: survey of cannula use in France. ASAIO J. 2013;59:157–61.
56. Pranikoff T, Hirschl RB, Steimle CN, et al.: Efficacy of extracorporeal life support in the setting of adult cardiorespiratory failure. *ASAIO* J 1994;40:M339–43
57. Zimmermann M, Bein T, Arlt M, et al. Pumpless extracorporeal interventional lung assist in patients with acute respiratory distress syndrome: a prospective pilot study. Crit Care. 2009;13:R10.
58. Peek GJ, Moore HM, Moore N, et al. Extracorporeal membrane oxygenation for adult respiratory failure. Chest. 1997;112:759–64.
59. Mols G, Loop T, Geiger K, et al. Extracorporeal membrane oxygenation: a ten-year experience. Am J Surg. 2000;180:144–54.
60. Müller T, Philipp A, Luchner A, et al. A new miniaturized system for extracorporeal membrane oxygenation in adult respiratory failure. Crit Care. 2009;13:R205.
61. Noah MA, Peek GJ, Finney SJ, et al. Referral to an extracorporeal membrane oxygenation center and mortality among patients with severe 2009 influenza A(H1N1). JAMA. 2011;306:1659–68.
62. Patroniti N, Zangrillo A, Pappalardo F, et al. The Italian ECMO network experience during the 2009 influenza A(H1N1) pandemic: preparation for severe respiratory emergency outbreaks. Intensive Care Med. 2011;37:1447–57.
63. Roch A, Hraiech S, Masson E, et al. Outcome of acute respiratory distress syndrome patients treated with extracorporeal membrane oxygenation and brought to a referral center. Intensive Care Med. 2014;40:74–83.
64. Haneya A, Diez C, Philipp A, et al. Impact of acute kidney injury on outcome in patients with severe acute respiratory failure receiving extracorporeal membrane oxygenation. Crit Care Med. 2015;43:1898–906.

5

Intra-abdominal hypertension in patients with sellar region tumors

Konstantin A Popugaev*, Ivan A Savin, Andrew U Lubnin, Alexander S Goriachev, Boris A Kadashev, Pavel L Kalinin, Andrew V Oshorov, Alexander A Polupan, Ekaterina U Sokolova, Maxim A Kutin, Valeriy I Lukianov

Abstract

Background: Data on intra-abdominal hypertension [IAH] and secondary abdominal compartment syndrome [ACS] due to neurological insults are limited.

Methods: This was a prospective observational study conducted between January 2010 and January 2011 in the neurological ICU [NICU]. Forty-one consecutive patients with sellar region tumors [SRT] were enrolled into the study. If conservative therapy was ineffective in patients with ACS, thoracic epidural anesthesia [EA] was performed. Primary endpoint was defined as the efficacy of conservative treatment and EA in patients with IAH and ACS; secondary endpoint, the influence of IAH and ACS on outcomes.

Results: Of the 41 patients, 13 (31.7%) had normal intra-abdominal pressure and 28 (68.3%) developed IAH, of whom 9 (22%) had ACS (group II). On average, IAH developed on the second postoperative day, while ACS, between the third and the fifth day. Multiple organ dysfunction developed in 3 (23.1%) patients of group I and in 23 (82%) patients of group II ($p = 0.0003$). Ileus due to gastrointestinal dysmotility was present in 6 (46.2%) patients of group I and in all patients of group II ($p = 0.0001$). Significant risk factors for ileus were diencephalon dysfunction (whole group - in 33 patients (80.5%); group I - in 6 patients (46.2%); group II - in 27 patients (96.4%), $p = 0.0002$) and sepsis (whole group - in 8 patients (19.5%); group I - no cases; group II - in 8 patients (28.6%), $p = 0.03$). Conservative treatment was effective in the majority of patients (78.9%) with IAH and only in 3 (33%) patients with ACS. Thoracic EA was performed in four patients with ACS with success. Length of stay in the NICU was 6.5 ± 4.6 days in group I and 24.1 ± 25.7 ($p = 0.02$) days in group II. Five out of nine (55.6%) patients with ACS died. None of these patients received EA. All patients with EA had favorable outcomes.

Conclusion: The development of IAH is common after SRT surgery. If conservative treatment is ineffective, EA can be considered in patients with secondary ACS. Further studies are warranted.

Introduction

Intra-abdominal hypertension [IAH] is associated with increased morbidity and mortality in critically ill patients [1-3]. Abdominal compartment syndrome [ACS] leads to multiple organ dysfunction [MOD] and carries a high mortality [4,5]. Ileus is considered as a contributing factor leading to IAH [1]. Patients with recent removal of sellar region tumors [SRT] represent a special neurocritical care population because they have an increased risk of postoperative ileus [4].

* Correspondence: Stan.Popugaev@yahoo.com
Department of Neurological Intensive Care Unit (NICU), Burdenko Neurosurgical Research Institute, 16 4th Tverskaya-Yamskaya, Moscow, 125047, Russia

The ideal management for secondary ACS has not yet been well defined [6,7]. The evidence-based therapeutic options are scarce [5,8]. The consensus conference on IAH and ACS recommends to maintain an abdominal perfusion pressure [APP] above 50 to 60 mmHg (grade 1C), to use a brief trial of neuromuscular blockage (grade 2C), to avoid elevation of the head of the bed above 30° (grade 2C), and to use hypertonic crystalloid and colloid-based resuscitation fluids (grade 1C) [5]. The benefit of analgesia/sedation, prokinetic motility agents, and naso-gastric/colonic decompression is unclear [5]. Intra-abdominal pressure [IAP] should be decreased before it reaches the threshold that will lead to the development of irreversible MOD. Urgent abdominal decompression is recommended in patients in whom medical treatment for

ACS has failed [9]. In spite of the relative safety and absolute efficacy of abdominal decompression, this operation has inherent risks and morbidity [8]. Prolonged thoracic epidural anesthesia [EA] has been shown to be effective in the reduction of IAP in patients with primary ACS [10]. To date, there are no data on the efficacy of EA in patients with secondary ACS. The purpose of the study was (1) to investigate the incidence of raised IAP in the postoperative period in SRT patients, (2) to evaluate the efficacy of conservative treatment in IAH and (3) to evaluate the efficacy of EA as a treatment option for ACS.

Methods

Study patients and definitions

Between January 2010 and January 2011, a prospective observational study was conducted in the 38-bed neurological intensive care unit [NICU] of Burdenko Neurosurgical Research Institute, Moscow, Russia. Inclusion criteria were: (1) adult patients, (2) SRT, and (3) a complicated postoperative period. Exclusion criteria were: (1) deep coma, (2) phimosis or contraindication for bladder pressure measurement, and (3) a contracted bladder. Patients were selected consecutively. All consecutive patients who met the inclusion criteria were included into the study. The study was conducted in accordance with the study protocol, the Declaration of Helsinki, and applicable regulatory requirements. The institutional review board and the local institutional ethics committee approved the protocol. Informed consent was obtained from each patient before inclusion.

A complicated postoperative period was recognized if the patient had an unstable neurological status or a new organ dysfunction. The clinical picture in SRT patients is typically a combination of altered level of consciousness, water and electrolyte disturbances (fluid balance dysregulation with hyper- or hyponatremia in the absence of iatrogenic causes, such as inadequate use of desmopressin, vaptans (V_2-receptor antagonists), or hyperosmotic solutions), and at least one new organ dysfunction/failure as defined by a sequential organ failure assessment [SOFA] subscore equal to or above 3 [4]. This entity has been defined previously as diencephalon dysfunction [DD].

IAH is defined as a sustained elevation of IAP equal to or above 12 mmHg, and ACS is defined as a sustained increase in IAP over 20 mmHg that is associated with a new organ dysfunction/failure [2]. The APP is calculated as mean arterial pressure minus IAP.

One of the causes of IAH and secondary ACS is gastrointestinal dysmotility resulting in ascites and ileus. Ileus has been classified into three forms: (1) impaired gastric emptying, (2) impaired intestinal/colonic emptying, (3) or both. Impaired gastric emptying is defined as a gastric residual volume above 400 ml per day (gastrostasis) with preserved intestinal peristalsis and defecation. Impaired intestinal/colonic emptying is defined as preserved gastric emptying with depressed intestinal peristalsis and constipation. Gastrostasis, depressed intestinal peristalsis, and constipation comprise the combined form of ileus. Outcomes were evaluated with the Glasgow Outcome Scale [GOS] (Table 1).

Patient management

Severity scores (acute physiology and chronic health evaluation [APACHE]-II and SOFA) were recorded in all patients admitted to NICU. Routine CT imaging of the brain was performed immediately postsurgery. Most patients were ventilated, and crystalloids or colloids and sympathomimetics were started early when indicated and to maintain perfusion pressure [4].

All patients received polyhormonal replacement therapy with glucocorticoids (hydrocortisone 150 to 200 mg/day which gradually decrease to 30 mg/day, orally) and thyroid hormones (L-thyroxin 1 to 3 μg/kg/day, orally or IV). Central diabetes insipidus was corrected with desmopressin.

All physiological, clinical, and biochemical data were collected. All patients were assessed with APACHE-II and SOFA scores.

IAP, APP measurement, and IAH management

IAP was measured every 6 h from the second postoperative day and during ICU stay, or until the 28th postoperative day. Measurements were carried out via the bladder with an installation volume of 25 ml sterile saline. Urinary catheter was connected to a Philips MP60 (Eindhoven, The Netherlands) monitor via a standard pressure transducer [11]. The APP was registered simultaneously.

All the patients underwent ultrasound investigation in order to rule out ascites. Patients were screened for IAH risk factors according to an international consensus [2]. Risk factors for ileus were considered to be either independent or related to the presence of DD. Independent risk factors are the use of narcotic analgetics, sympathomimetics, positive fluid balance, sepsis, and hypokalemia.

Conservative treatment of IAH was started immediately in accordance to the IAH/ACS medical management algorithm [5,12]. If conservative treatment was ineffective in patients with ACS for longer than a 24-h period, thoracic EA was performed via an 18-gauge epidural catheter that was inserted at the level of T8 to T9 through a Touhy needle and advanced up to 5 to 6 cm in a cephalad direction. After confirmation of catheter position, a 0.25% bupivacaine infusion at 7 to 8 ml/h was initiated and titrated. The EA remained in place for 3 days. Sepsis was a contraindication for EA. According to our department protocol, treatment of IAH was considered effective

Table 1 Glasgow Outcome Scale

GOS	Outcome	Functional outcome
1	Dead	Unfavorable
2	Vegetative state	
3	Severely disabled (conscious but requires others for daily support)	
4	Moderately disabled (independent but disabled)	Favorable
5	Good recovery (resumed most normal activity)	

if IAP normalized within 72 h; and treatment of ACS was considered effective if IAP normalized within 24 h.

Statistical methods

The primary endpoint was defined as the efficacy of conservative treatment and EA to lower IAP in patients with IAH and ACS. The secondary endpoint was defined as the influence of IAP and ACS on the outcome. Descriptive analyses were performed for all study variables. Data are presented as mean and standard deviation. We used variance analysis, χ^2 (Pearson's and maximum likelihood chi-square), and Fisher's exact test in the analysis of contingency tables. We also calculated the relative risk when appropriate. A p value of < 0.05 was defined as a significant difference. For this purpose, we used program Statistica v6 (StatSoft Inc., Tulsa, OK, USA).

Results

Patient characteristics and patient groups

Five hundred and seventy-eight SRT patients underwent tumor removal during the study period. Five hundred and thirty-four patients were excluded because they had a normal postoperative period; another three patients were excluded because they developed deep coma on the second postoperative day. The remaining 41 patients were enrolled. The IAP was normal in 13 patients (group I). IAH developed in 28 patients (group II, Figure 1). Baseline APACHE-II and SOFA scores for group II patients indicate that their condition was more severe at the time of NICU admission (Table 2).

IAP and APP

The majority of patients were admitted to NICU without IAH. In group I, IAP was significantly lower than in group II, 6.5 ± 3.1 mmHg versus 10.6 ± 3.9 mmHg (p = 0.003, Table 2). In group I, the duration of IAP monitoring was 5.6 ± 4.8 days; in group II, it was 14.9 ± 8.5 days. The IAP was significantly higher in group II from the second to the sixth postoperative day. Maximal IAP was 8.9 ± 2.3 mmHg in group I and 18.6 ± 5.6 mmHg in group II. In group II, maximal IAP developed on 2.5 ± 0.9 postoperative day; in group I, significantly later - on 6.2 ± 0.9 postoperative day (p = 0.01). ACS developed in nine patients. On average, IAH developed on the second postoperative day, while ACS, between the third and the

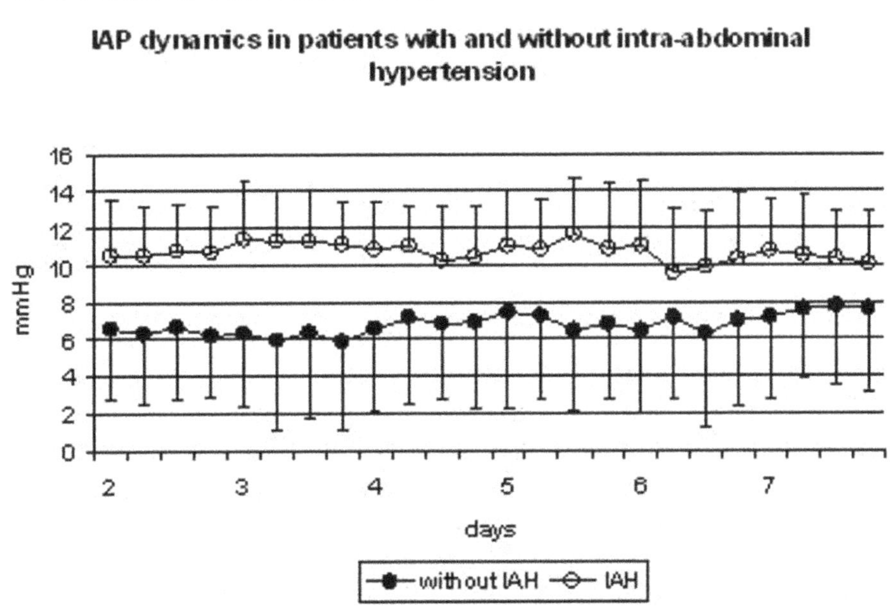

Figure 1 Mean IAP in groups I and II during the first seven days of postoperative period.

Table 2 Characteristics of group I and group II

	Whole group	Group I (no IAH)	Group II (IAH)	*p* Value (significance of difference between groups I and II)
Number (patients)	41	13	28	
Sex (male/female)	19:22	8:5	11:17	0.2
Age (mean ± SD)	48.3 ± 15	46.3 ± 17.7	49.3 ± 13.8	0.8
APACHE-II (mean ± SD)	13 ± 5.6	9.1 ± 6.1	14.9 ± 4.4	0.0004*
SOFA score (mean ± SD)	2.5 ± 1.8	1.9 ± 2.3	2.7 ± 1.6	0.2
Neurosurgical pathology (patients)				
Pituitary adenoma	18	6	12	0.8
Craniopharyngioma	11	1	10	0.06
Sellar region meningioma	8	3	5	0.7
III ventricular glioma	3	2	1	0.2
III ventricular ganglioma	1	1	0	0.1
Admission value of IAP (mmHg, mean ± SD)	9.2 ± 4.0	6.5 ± 3.1	10.6 ± 3.9	0.003*
Mean value of IAP mmHg (mean ± SD)	9.3 ± 3.1	6.4 ± 2.0	10.7 ± 2.5	0.000003*
Maximal value of IAP (mmHg, mean ± SD)	15.2 ± 6.2	8.9 ± 2.3	18.6 ± 5.6	0.002*
Minimal value of APP (mmHg, mean ± SD)	79.0 ± 9.0	86.5 ± 5.8	75.6 ± 8.2	0.0001*
Risk factors for IAH (patients (%))				
Positive fluid balance	7 (17.1)	1 (7.7)	6 (21.4)	0.3
Acidosis	2 (4.9	0 (0)	2 (7.1)	0.3
Hypothermia	4 (9.8)	1 (7.7)	3 (10.7)	0.7
Coagulopathy	6 (14.6)	1 (7.7)	5 (17.9)	0.4
MOD	26 (63.4)	3 (23.1)	23 (82)	0.0003*
MV	24 (58.5)	6 (46.2)	18 (64.3)	0.3
Ileus	34 (82.9)	6 (46.2)	28 (100)	0.0001*
Type of ileus (patients (%))				
Impaired gastric emptying	-	-	-	
Impaired intestinal and colonic emptying	21 (51.2)	4 (30.8)	17 (60.7)	0.07
Combined form	13 (31.7)	2 (15.4)	11 (39.3)	0.1
Onset time of ileus (postoperative day)	2.3 ± 1.4	1.7 ± 0.5	2.4 ± 1.5	0.17
Duration of ileus (days)	10.6 ± 7.6	4.3 ± 1.0	11.9 ± 7.7	0.01*
Risk factors of ileus (patients (%))				
DD	33 (80.5)	6 (46.2)	27 (96.4)	0.0002*
Independent risk factors (patients (%))				
Narcotics	2 (4.9)	0 (0)	2 (7.1)	0.3
Sympathomimetics	7 (17.1)	5 (38.5)	2 (7.1)	0.01*
Positive fluid balance	7 (17.1)	1 (7.7)	6 (21.4)	0.3
Sepsis	8 (19.5)	0 (0)	8 (28.6)	0.03*
Hypokalemia, hypomagnesaemia	28 (68.3)	8 (61.5)	20 (71.4)	0.5
LOS (days, mean ± SD)	18.5 ± 22.8	6.5 ± 4.6	24.1 ± 25.7	0.02*
Outcome (patients (%))				
Favorable outcome GOS 4	26 (63.4)	11 (85)	15 (54)	0.06
Unfavorable outcome	15 (36.6)	2 (15)	13 (46)	0.06
GOS 2,3	4 (9.8)	0 (0)	4 (14)	
GOS 1	11 (26.8)	2 (15)	9 (32)	

*Significant difference. IAH, intra-abdominal hypertension; SD, standard deviation; APACHE-II, acute physiology and chronic health evaluation, and SOFA, sequential organ failure assessment, scores on ICU admission; IAP, intra-abdominal pressure; APP, abdominal perfusion pressure; MOD, multiple organ dysfunction; MV, mechanical ventilation; GOS, Glasgow Outcome Scale; LOS, length of stay.

fifth day. Minimal APP was normal in both groups, however, it was significantly higher in group I - 86.5 ± 5.8 mmHg versus 75.6 ± 8.2 mmHg in group II (p = 0.0001).

Causes of IAH and types of ileus

None of the patients developed ascites. Ileus was the most common risk factor for IAH in both groups, 46.2% and 100%, respectively. MOD and the need for mechanical ventilation [MV] for more than 24 h occurred also more frequently in group II (Table 2). Ileus developed within the first two postoperative days, and its onset time did not differ between groups (p = 0.17). Duration of ileus was significantly longer in group II (p = 0.01). There were no cases with isolated impaired gastric emptying. The impaired intestinal and colonic emptying was diagnosed in 4 patients of group I and in 17 patients of group II (p = 0.07). An interesting observation was that ileus developed prior to IAH, but it lasted longer.

A major cause of ileus was DD. DD developed in 46.2% cases of group I and in 96.4% cases of group II. Among the list of independent risk factors, electrolyte disorders and sympathomimetics were common in both groups (Table 2).

Diencephalon dysfunction

DD significantly increased the risk for IAH development (relative risk 6.56, 95% confidence interval 1.04 to 16.46).

Therapy of IAH and ACS

Conservative treatment was effective in 15 patients out of 19 (79%) with IAH, but without ACS and in 3 patients out of 9 (33%) with ACS. EA was performed in four cases with ACS. In all these cases, EA effectively normalized IAP rapidly after bupivacaine infusion. No complications were associated with EA. In three ACS cases, conservative treatment was effective, and in two patients with sepsis and ACS, EA was contraindicated.

Outcomes

Eleven patients (85%) of group I had a favorable outcome, and only two patients (15%) died due to brain edema and herniation early in the postoperative period. In group II, a favorable outcome was observed in 15 patients (54%), while 4 patients (14%) had severe disability, and 9 patients died (32%). Causes of death were: sepsis (n = 3), meningitis (n = 1), combination of sepsis and meningitis (n = 2), brain edema and herniation (n = 1), acromegalic cardiomyopathy (n = 1), and pulmonary thromboembolism (n = 1). An absolute risk of having a poorer neurologic recovery (any other below GOS 5) in patients with IAH was 0.89, with a 95% confidence interval of 0.77 to 1.0. The length of stay [LOS] in the NICU was significantly longer in patients with IAH (p = 0.02, Table 2).

IAH developed in 19 (63.3%) survivors and in 9 (81.8%) non-survivors (p = 0.3). ACS developed in 13.3% of survivors and in 45.5% of non-survivors (p = 0.03) (Table 3). The evolution of IAP in survivors and non-survivors during the first seven days of the postoperative period is shown in Figure 2.

In survivors, isolated impairment of intestinal/colonic emptying developed in 66.7% of patients; the combination of impaired gastric emptying and impaired intestinal/colonic emptying was revealed in 33.3% of patients. In non-survivors, isolated impairment of intestinal/colonic emptying developed in 9.1% of patients; the combination of impaired gastric emptying and impaired intestinal/colonic emptying was revealed in 90.9% of patients. Therefore, isolated impairment of intestinal/colonic emptying was observed significantly more frequently in group I (p = 0.01), whereas the combination of impaired gastric emptying and impaired intestinal/colonic emptying was observed significantly more frequently in group II (p = 0.01). Independent risk factors such as positive fluid balance, sympathomimetics, administration of narcotics, and sympathomimetics were revealed significantly more frequently in non-survivors than in survivors. Ileus persisted significantly longer in non-survivors than in survivors, 15.3 ± 8.5 versus 8.5 ± 6.6 days (p = 0.01).

All four patients with ACS, who had received EA, survived with favorable outcomes. Three patients with ACS and effective conservative therapy died due to causes independent of IAH (thromboembolism, cardiomyopathy, and sepsis). The other two patients with ACS, who had not received EA, died due to sepsis and meningitis.

Discussion

A complicated postoperative period developed in 7% of patients with SRT. Two thirds of this neurocritical care population has IAH, which developed on the second postoperative day. IAH correlated with worse APACHE-II and SOFA scores, and it occurred more frequently in non-survivors. Patients with normal IAP had better outcomes. However, the cause-and-effect relationship between IAP and severity of the patients' condition remains unclear. Severe injury to the hypothalamo-pituitary axis can lead to MOD [4]. On the other hand, our patients had high maximal IAP values, and IAH can also be considered as a cause of MOD [5,12]. Our data show the importance of IAP monitoring in these neurocritical care patients since early recognition and timely medical management can affect outcome.

Ileus was a leading cause of IAH in our cohort. Theoretically, capillary leak syndrome and fluid accumulation can also cause IAH [1,3,5]. This syndrome can be due to decompensated hypothyroidism [13] in patients with SRT and can lead to polyserositis with ascites, hydrothorax, and/or hydropericardium [6,14]. In our population, severe

Table 3 Characteristics of survivors and non-survivors

	Survivors	Non-survivors	*p* Value
Number (patients)	30	11	
Sex (male/female)	12:18	7:4	0.17
Age (mean ± SD)	46.6 ± 15.9	53.0 ± 11.3	0.8
APACHE-II (mean ± SD)	11.0 ± 4.5	18.6 ± 4.6	0.05
SOFA score (mean ± SD)	1.9 ± 1.4	4.1 ± 2.1	0.04*
Admission value of IAP (mmHg, mean ± SD)	9.1 ± 3.9	9.6 ± 4.6	0.8
Normal IAP (patients (%))	11 (36.7)	2 (18.2)	0.3
Maximal value of IAP (mmHg, mean ± SD)	14.1 ± 5.6	18.2 ± 6.9	0.06
Minimal value of APP (mmHg, mean ± SD)	80.9 ± 8.8	74.9 ± 7.7	0.05
IAH (patients (%))	19 (63.3)	9 (81.8)	0.3
ACS (patients)	4 (13.3)	5 (45.5)	0.03*
Ileus	23 (76.7)	11 (100)	0.08
Type of ileus (patients (%))			
Impaired gastric emptying	0	0	
Impaired intestinal and colonic emptying	20 (66.7)	1 (9.1)	0.01*
Combined form	10 (33.3)	10 (90.9)	0.01*
Onset time of ileus (postoperative day)	2.6 ± 1.6	1.6 ± 0.7	0.06
Duration of ileus (days)	8.5 ± 6.6	15.3 ± 8.5	0.01*
Risk factors of ileus (patients (%))			
DD	25 (83.3)	8 (72.7)	0.4
Independent risk factors (patients (%))			
Narcotics	0	2 (18.2)	0.02*
Sympathomimetics	12 (40)	9 (81.8)	0.02*
Positive fluid balance	1 (3.3)	6 (54.5)	0.0001*
Sepsis	2 (6.7)	6 (54.5)	0.0006*
Hypokalemia, hypomagnesaemia	19 (63.3)	9 (81.8)	0.3

*Significant difference. SD, standard deviation; APACHE-II, acute physiology and chronic health evaluation, and SOFA, sequential organ failure assessment, scores on ICU admission; IAP, intra-abdominal pressure; APP, abdominal perfusion pressure; IAH, intra-abdominal hypertension; ACS, abdominal compartment syndrome; DD, diencephalon dysfunction.

hypothyroidism was ruled out because all the patients received postoperative polyhormonal therapy, and the levels of thyroid hormones in plasma were routinely controlled. Also, there were no patients with ascites in our study population.

Different types of ileus were observed: impaired intestinal and colonic emptying and a combined form. The leading cause of ileus was DD, and this can be explained by the surgery site. Hypothalamic nuclei directly regulate gastrointestinal motility [7,15]. Furthermore, a normal thyroid status is necessary for an adequate function of the gastrointestinal tract [13]. Independent risk factors had minor importance for the ileus development in our patients, especially narcotics, sympathomimetics, or positive fluid balance. The last is insignificant for SRT patients because central diabetes insipidus is a common postoperative complication. Sepsis was an important risk factor for ACS. Our results are in concordance with previous literature data [16-18]. Hypokalemia and hypomagnesaemia developed frequently due to glucocorticoid therapy [19].

Conservative treatment was effective in the majority of patients with IAH, but without ACS. In ACS, on the other hand, conservative treatment was ineffective in two thirds of the patients. Guidelines recommend urgent laparotomy if conservative therapy fails [5,8,20]. There are no publications on the timing and efficacy of urgent laparotomy in patients with secondary ACS due to neurosurgical pathology. Thoracic EA, used before laparotomy, should therefore be considered as a safe and effective therapeutic option.

The use of EA is generally accepted in the ICU and has been previously described [10,21,22]. The pathophysiological basis of thoracic EA for the treatment of ACS is: (1) sympathetic block and accordingly, prevalence of parasympathetic tonus in the innervation of the gastrointestinal tract, (2) strong analgetic effect, (3) abdominal wall

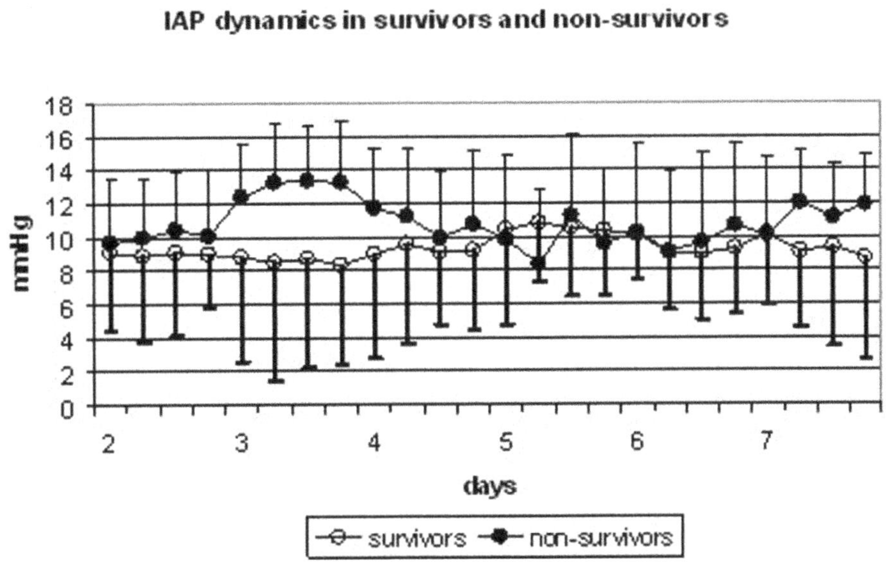

Figure 2 Mean IAP in survivors and non-survivors during the first seven days of postoperative period.

muscle relaxation, (4) increase of gastrointestinal blood flow, gastric mucosal perfusion, improvement of tissue oxygenation, and (5) prevention of bacterial translocation [22-25]. These mechanisms can interrupt the deleterious pathological processes caused by ACS. We showed that the use of EA can be effective in a selected group of patients. In these patients, the IAP normalized within several hours, and signs of MOD regressed within 1 to 2 days. The duration of IAH in patients with EA was significantly shorter than that in patients without EA. We could not perform EA in two septic patients with ineffective conservative treatment for ACS. Traditionally, sepsis is a contraindication for EA due to an increased risk of infectious complications [21,26]. All patients with ACS, who did not receive EA, died, irrespective of the duration of ACS. These data allow us to conclude the following: (1) early thoracic EA can be an effective treatment option for secondary ACS in neurosurgical patients; and (2) if the main cause of ACS in neurosurgical patients is sepsis, the only effective method of ACS treatment would probably be urgent laparotomy.

To our knowledge, this is the first study to investigate secondary ACS in patients with SRT. Our study has several serious limitations. First, 41 patients are still a small number for a meaningful statistical analysis, especially concerning the calculation of the risk of unfavorable outcomes and death in patients with IAH. Second, it is a single-center study. Third, we only performed intermittent measurements of IAP, not continuous monitoring, which could have changed the therapeutic approach and accordingly, the results. Fourth, four patients with EA are a small number for decision-making about the significance of EA for ACS treatment.

Conclusions

The development of IAH is common in patients after SRT surgery during a complicated postoperative period. If conservative treatment is ineffective, EA can be attempted in patients with secondary ACS when it is not contraindicated. Further studies are warranted.

Abbreviations

ACS: abdominal compartment syndrome; DD: diencephalon dysfunction; EA: epidural anesthesia; GOS: Glasgow Outcome Scale; IAP: intra-abdominal pressure; IAH: intra-abdominal hypertension; LOS: length of stay; MOD: multiple organ dysfunction; MV: mechanical ventilation; NICU: neurosurgical intensive care unit; SRT: sellar region tumors.

Acknowledgements

This article has been published as part of *Annals of Intensive Care* Volume 2 Supplement 1, 2012: Diagnosis and management of intra-abdominal hypertension and abdominal compartment syndrome. The full contents of the supplement are available online at http://www.annalsofintensivecare.com/supplements/2/S1

We are grateful to Professor Manu Malbrain and our peers for their great support in the preparation of our manuscript and for their advice and encouragement. Also, we deeply appreciate the assistance in the manuscript preparation of Dr. Andy Eynon and Dr. Leonid Krivskiy from the University Hospital Southampton. Also, we would like to express our sincere gratitude to the nurses of our department for their scrupulous measurement of IAP and their excellent care of severely ill patients.

Authors' contributions

PLK, IAS, and AUL contributed to the conception and design of the study. ASG, BAK, and KAP did the acquisition of funding, systematic search, and drafting of the manuscript. AVO, AAP, and EUS did the interpretation of data and drafting of the manuscript. MAK and VIL contributed substantially to the interpretation of data and critically revised the manuscript. All authors read and approved the final manuscript for publication.

Competing interests

The authors declare that they have no competing interests.

References

1. Cheatham ML: **Intra-abdominal hypertension and abdominal compartment syndrome.** *New Horiz* 1999, **7**:96-115.
2. Malbrain ML, Cheatham ML, Kirkpatrick A, Sugrue M, Parr M, De Waele J, Balogh Z, Leppäniemi A, Olvera C, Ivatury R, D'Amours S, Wendon J, Hillman K, Wilmer A: **Results from the International Conference of Experts on Intra-abdominal Hypertension and Abdominal Compartment Syndrome. I. Definitions.** *Intensive Care Med* 2006, **32**:1722-1732.
3. Malbrain ML, Chiumello D, Pelosi P, Wilmer A, Brienza N, Malcangi V, Bihari D, Innes R, Cohen J, Singer P, Japiassu A, Kurtop E, De Keulenaer BL, Daelemans R, Del Turco M, Cosimini P, Ranieri M, Jacquet L, Laterre PF, Gattinoni L: **Prevalence of intra-abdominal hypertension in critically ill patients: a multicentre epidemiological study.** *Intensive Care Med* 2004, **30**:822-829.
4. Popugaev KA, Savin IA, Goriachev AS, Kadashev BA: **Hypothalamic injury as a cause of refractory hypotension after sellar region tumor surgery.** *Neurocrit Care* 2008, **8**:366-373.
5. Malbrain ML, Cheatham ML, Kirkpatrick A, Sugrue M, Parr M, De Waele J, Balogh Z, Leppäniemi A, Olvera C, Ivatury R, D'Amours S, Wendon J, Hillman K, Wilmer A: **Results from the International Conference of Experts on Intra-abdominal Hypertension and Abdominal Compartment Syndrome. II. Recommendations.** *Intensive Care Med* 2007, **33**:951-962.
6. de Azevedo AM, D Goldberg Tabak: **Life-threatening capillary leak syndrome after G-CSF mobilization and collection of peripheral blood progenitor calls for allogenic transplantation.** *Bone Marrow Transplant* 2001, **28**:311-312.
7. Akmayev IG, Vikhreva OV, Konovalova LK: **The origin of the hypothalamic-vagal descending pathway: an experimental ultrastructural study.** *Brain Res* 1981, **230**:342-345.
8. Balogh Z, Moore FA, Goettler CE, Rotondo MF, Schwab WC, Kaplan MJ: **Surgical management of abdominal compartment syndrome.** In *Abdominal Compartment Syndrome.* Texas: Landes Bioscience;Ivatury RR, Cheatham ML, Malbrain M, Sugrue M 2006:266-270.
9. De Waele JJ, Hoste EA, Malbrain ML: **Decompressive laparotomy for abdominal compartment syndrome-a critical analysis.** *Crit Care* 2006, **10**: R51.
10. Hakobyan RV, Mkhoyan GG: **Epidural analgesia decreases intraabdominal pressure in postoperative patients with primary intra-abdominal hypertension.** *Acta Clin Belg* 2008, **63**:86-92.
11. Malbrain ML: **Different techniques to measure intra-abdominal pressure (IAP): time for a critical re-appraisal.** *Intensive Care Med* 2004, **30**:357-371.
12. Cheatham ML: **Abdominal compartment syndrome.** *Curr Opin Crit Care* 2009, **15**:154-62.
13. Ji JS, Chae HS, Cho YS, Kim HK, Kim SS, Kim CW, Lee CD, Lee BI, Choi H, Lee KM, Lee HK, Choi KY: **Myxedema ascites: case report and literature review.** *J Korean Med Sci* 2006, **21**:761-764.
14. Garces S, Araujo F, Rego F, Soares JL, Carlos AG: **Capillary leakage syndrome: a case report and a review.** *Allerg Immunol (Paris)* 2002, **34**:361-364.
15. Blessing WW, Jaeger CB, Ruggiero DA, Reis DJ: **Hypothalamic projections of medullary catecholamine neurons in the rabbit: a combined catecholamine fluorescence and HRP transport study.** *Brain Res Bull* 1982, **9**:279-286.
16. Fruhwald , Holzer P, Metzler H: **Intestinal motility disturbances in intensive care patients pathogenesis and clinical impact.** *Intensive Care Med* 2007, **33**:36-44.
17. Overhaus M, Tögel S, Pezzone MA, Bauer AJ: **Mechanisms of polymicrobial sepsis-induced ileus.** *Am J Physiol Gastrointest Liver Physiol* 2004, **287**: G685-694.
18. Bauer AJ, Schwarz NT, Moore BA, Türler A, Kalff JC: **Ileus in critical illness: mechanisms and management.** *Curr Opin Crit Care* 2002, **8**:152-157.
19. Arzel-Hezode M, McGoey S, Stenberg D, Vicart S, Eymard B, Fontaine B: **Glucocorticoids may trigger attacks in several types of periodic paralysis.** *Neuromuscul Disord* 2009, **19**:217-219.
20. De Laet IE, Ravyts M, Vidts W, Valk J, De Waele JJ, Malbrain ML: **Current insights in intra-abdominal hypertension and abdominal compartment syndrome: open the abdomen and keep it open!** *Langenbecks Arch Surg* 2008, **393**:833-847.
21. Sielenkamper AW, Van Aken H: **Epidural analgesia in sepsis: too early to judge a new concept.** *Intensive Care Med* 2004, **30**:1987-1989.
22. Steinbrook RA: **Epidural anesthesia and gastrointestinal motility.** *Anesth Analg* 1998, **86**:837-844.
23. Kapral S, Collmann G, Bachmann D, Prohaska B, Likar R, Jandrasits O, Weinstabl C, Lehofer F: **The effect of thoracic epidural anesthesia on intraoperative visceral perfusion and metabolism.** *Anesth Analg* 1999, **88**:402-406.
24. Buggy DJ, Doherty WL, Hart EM: **Postoperative wound oxygen tension with epidural or intravenous analgesia: a prospective, randomized, single-blind clinical trial.** *Anesthesiology* 2002, **97**:952-958.
25. Spackman DR, McLeod AD, Prineas SN, Leach RM, Reynolds F: **Effect of epidural blockage on indicators of splanchnic perfusion and gut function in critically ill patients with peritonitis: a randomized comparison of epidural bupivacaine and systemic morphine.** *Intensive Care Med* 2000, **26**:1638-1645.
26. Adolphs J, Schmidt DK, Korsukewitz I, Kamin B, Habazettl H, Schäfer M, Welte M: **Effects of thoracic epidural anesthesia on intestinal microvascular perfusion during normotensive endotoxemia in rats.** *Intensive Care Med* 2004, **30**:2094-2101.

6

Predictive factors of bleeding events in adults undergoing extracorporeal membrane oxygenation

Cécile Aubron[1,2,7,8*], Joris DePuydt[3,4], François Belon[5], Michael Bailey[1], Matthieu Schmidt[1,9], Jayne Sheldrake[3], Deirdre Murphy[3,6], Carlos Scheinkestel[3,6], D Jamie Cooper[1,3], Gilles Capellier[5], Vincent Pellegrino[3,6], David Pilcher[1,3] and Zoe McQuilten[1,2]

Abstract

Background: Bleeding is the most frequent complication associated with extracorporeal membrane oxygenation (ECMO) support in critically ill patients. Nonetheless, risk factors for bleeding have been poorly described especially those associated with coagulation anomalies and anticoagulant therapy during ECMO support. The aim of this study is to describe bleeding complications in critically ill patients undergoing ECMO and to identify risk factors for bleeding events.

Methods: We retrospectively analysed ICU charts of adults who received either veno-venous (VV) or veno-arterial (VA) ECMO support in two participating ICUs between 2010 and 2013. Characteristics of patients with and without bleeding complications, as per the Extracorporeal Life Support Organisation (ELSO) definition, were compared, and the impact of bleeding complications on patient outcomes was assessed using survival analysis. Variables that were independently associated with bleeding, including daily clinical and biological variables during ECMO courses, were modelled.

Results: Of the 149 ECMO episodes (111 VA ECMO and 38 VV ECMO) performed in 147 adults, 89 episodes (60 %) were complicated by at least one bleeding event. The most common bleeding sources were: ECMO cannula (37 %), haemothorax or cardiac tamponade (17 %) and ear–nose and throat (16 %). Intra-cranial haemorrhage occurred in five (2.2 %) patients. Bleeding complications were independently associated with worse survival [adjusted hazard ratio (HR) 2.17, 95 % confidence interval (CI) 1.07–4.41, $P = 0.03$]. Higher activated partial thromboplastin time (aPTT) [adjusted odds ratio (OR) 3.00, 95 % CI 1.64–5.47, $P < 0.01$], APACHE III score [adjusted OR 1.01, 95 % CI 1.01–1.02, $P = 0.01$] and ECMO following surgery [adjusted OR 3.04, 95 % CI 1.62–5.69, $P < 0.01$] were independently associated with greater risk of bleeding occurrence. A similar association between bleeding and higher aPTT was found when non-post-surgical VA ECMO was considered separately.

Conclusions: Bleeding events based on the ELSO bleeding definition occurred in more than 60 % of ECMO episodes and were associated with hospital mortality. We identified higher aPTT prior bleeding as an independent risk factor for bleeding event, suggesting that better control of the aPTT (through a better control of either coagulopathy or anticoagulation) may improve patients' outcome.

Keywords: Extra corporeal membrane oxygenation, Critically ill patients, Haemorrhage, Bleeding, Anticoagulation, Coagulopathy, Thromboembolic events

*Correspondence: Cecile.aubron@chu-brest.fr; cecile.aubron@monash.edu
[7] Medical Intensive Care Unit, Centre Hospitalier Régional et Universitaire de Brest, site La Cavale Blanche, Bvd Tanguy Prigent, 29609 Brest Cedex, France
Full list of author information is available at the end of the article

Background

Bleeding is one of the most frequent complications occurring in patients undergoing extracorporeal membrane oxygenation (ECMO), occurring in approximately 30 % of patients receiving ECMO therapy [1–4]. Bleeding events independently impact on patient prognosis, including mortality [1, 2]. This association may be explained by the site of bleeding, with intra-cranial haemorrhage (ICH) identified in more than 40 % of non-survivors in patients treated with ECMO during the H1N1 flu outbreak [5].

Many factors that may place patients undergoing ECMO at higher risk of bleeding have been identified [6], and these can be classified into patient, treatment and circuit related. The systemic inflammatory response syndrome (SIRS) and contact between the patient's blood with the ECMO circuit lead to activation of the coagulation cascade, with effects on fibrinolysis, thrombin formation and platelet function [6–8]. The results of these changes to haemostatic balance may be difficult to predict, with the coexistence of both thrombotic and haemorrhagic risks. Although use of bioline surface-heparinised extracorporeal perfusion circuits reduces the risk of thrombosis, with decreases in inflammation, coagulation activation and platelet consumption, anticoagulation remains standard practice in patients undergoing ECMO to offset circuit-associated thrombotic risks [9, 10]. Indeed, thrombotic events might complicate ECMO therapy with significant morbidity and mortality. Thrombotic events have been identified in approximately 15 % of ECMO courses [11], but they are likely to be underdiagnosed and underreported [12].

A better knowledge of characteristics of bleeding during ECMO is essential to improve management and outcomes of patients undergoing ECMO. Studies on risk factors for haemorrhagic complications have predominantly been performed in paediatric patients or suffer limitations, including lack of standard bleeding definition and the timing of the study with many advances in ECMO circuit and care over the past decades [13, 14].

Therefore, we aimed to study bleeding complications in critically ill patients undergoing ECMO to define incidence, consequences on patient prognosis and factors associated with increased bleeding risk.

Patients and methods

Study design

We conducted a retrospective study in two centres, the Alfred Hospital (Melbourne, Australia) and the Hospital of Besançon (France). The Alfred Hospital is a teaching hospital affiliated to Monash University, which provides heart and lung transplantation services for the states of Victoria, South Australia and Tasmania. It has an intensive care unit (ICU) with a 45-bed capacity and is the referral centre for adult trauma and ECMO in Victoria. The Hospital of Besançon is a teaching hospital affiliated to the University of Franche-Comté; its 21-bed medical ICU has long-standing experience in ECMO support.

All adults admitted to ICU between January 2010 and June 2013 at the Alfred Hospital and between January 2013 and December 2013 at the Hospital of Besançon and who underwent ECMO were included.

The study was approved by the Alfred Health Human Research Ethics Committee (202/11) and by the Ethics Committee of Besançon Hospital.

ECMO haemostatic practice

Both hospitals had anticoagulation protocols and local guidelines for haemostatic management for patients undergoing ECMO, and these protocols were similar for VV and VA ECMO. In both centres, systemic anticoagulation with a heparin infusion targeting an activated partial thromboplastin time (aPTT) between 50 and 70 s was standard practice, unless patients were bleeding or at increased risk of bleeding (usually related to peri-operative and traumatic injuries). Red blood cell (RBC) transfusion was given to maintain a haemoglobin (Hb) concentration above 8 g/dL. Prophylactic blood products were not routinely given for coagulation abnormalities, with the exception of severe thrombocytopenia ($<$50,000 platelets/mm^3). In the case of bleeding, platelets were administered to maintain a platelet count $\geq$80,000/mm^3, fresh frozen plasma (FFP) to maintain the international normalised ratio (INR) $\leq$1.5 or prothrombin (PT) $>$70 %, and cryoprecipitate or fibrinogen concentrate to maintain fibrinogen plasma concentration $\geq$1.5 g/L. Coagulation factor concentrates, antifibrinolytic agents (tranexamic acid), antithrombin III and protamine were administered when deemed appropriate by the intensivist in charge. Heparin was the anticoagulant of choice; however, alternatives (warfarin, lepirudin) were used if necessary. ECMO circuits were phosphorylcholine and heparin bonded in both centres. Circuit membrane was changed at the Alfred Hospital if there was evidence of systemic fibrinolysis presumed to be due to circuit or clot in the oxygenator and at both sites in cases of poor oxygenator function and increases in trans-oxygenator pressure. Proton pump inhibitors were routinely administered to ECMO patients. At the Alfred Hospital, both cannulae of VA and VV ECMO were percutaneously inserted, while at Hospital of Besançon cannula of VA ECMO was surgically inserted.

Clinical and biological data

Medical history and clinical charts were retrospectively reviewed, and the following data were collected: demographics, comorbidities, ICU and hospital admission and discharge dates, diagnosis and Acute Physiology and Chronic Health Evaluation (APACHE III) score at admission. Treatment with aspirin, clopidogrel or vitamin K antagonist, surgery or cardiopulmonary resuscitation prior to ECMO initiation was recorded. The Sequential Organ Failure Assessment (SOFA) scores prior to ECMO initiation and on the third day of ECMO were calculated. Requirement for renal replacement therapy (RRT), mechanical ventilation (MV) or intra-aortic balloon pump while on ECMO were also collected. The daily highest and lowest values of the following biological data were recorded for each day on ECMO: Hb on formal full blood examination, platelet count, aPTT, INR, PT and fibrinogen level. The lowest temperature, the lowest value of arterial pH and ionised calcium, the highest D-dimer, urea, bilirubin and free Hb were also collected for each day on ECMO.

ECMO data

ECMO data included the commencement and cessation date, whether the ECMO was initiated in another hospital, the main indication for ECMO and the type of ECMO [veno-venous (VV) or veno-arterial (VA) including central and peripheral VA ECMO]. The following data were also recorded: outcomes of ECMO, status at ICU and hospital discharge and location of hospital discharge.

Bleeding events and thromboembolic events

Daily information on blood product and haemostatic agent use, including type and dose of anticoagulant, was collected for the duration of ECMO.

Bleeding events were defined according to the Extracorporeal Life Support Organisation (ELSO) definition [15]: we defined a bleeding event if there was clinically overt bleeding recorded in the medical and/or nursing charts associated with either administration of 2 or more RBC units in 24 h or a drop in haemoglobin greater than 2 g/L over 24 h, or if there was a haemothorax, central nervous system or retroperitoneal bleeding, or if bleeding required an intervention. If there were consecutive days with the same primary source of bleeding as preceding days, these were considered the same bleeding event. When a patient had more than one bleeding source on the same day, this was also recorded.

Thromboembolic complications, including deep venous thrombosis, ischaemic stroke, intra-cardiac thrombus, pulmonary embolism and membrane circuit clotting requiring membrane change, were collected from the medical record.

Statistical analysis

All analyses were performed using Stata 12.0 (College Station, Texas). Descriptive statistics are reported as mean (standard deviation) or median (inter-quartile range, IQR) according to data distribution. Hypothesis testing for patient level data was performed using Chi-square for categorical variables, Student's *t* test for normally distributed data and Wilcoxon's rank sum for non-normally distributed data. For comparisons between ECMO days with and without bleeding, to account for the repeated measures per patient (with bleeding recorded on each day of ECMO treatment), a repeated measures mixed model was performed for continuous variables and random effects logistic model for binomial variables. Mean and 95 % confidence interval (CI) are reported adjusted for repeated measures.

Survival curves were plotted using the Kaplan–Meier method, and groups were compared using the log-rank test. Multivariable analysis for predictors of survival was performed using a Cox proportional hazard regression model, including those variables that were associated with the outcome with a $P < 0.2$. As the relationship between bleeding and survival was time dependent (with bleeding occurring at different times during the course of ECMO treatment), bleeding variables were treated as time-varying covariates in the Cox proportional hazard models. The final models were assessed for proportionality using the proportional hazards assumption test.

To investigate predictors of bleeding, multiple logistic regression modelling was performed. Initially, a backward stepwise logistic model was performed, which only included variables recorded prior to the day of bleeding (e.g. highest aPTT on the day prior to the bleeding event, anticoagulation on the day prior to the bleeding event, etc.). aPTT was categorised into quartiles for the multivariable analysis. To account for the repeated measures per patient, variables that were found to be independently associated with the bleeding outcomes in the stepwise logistic model were then included in a multi-level logistic regression model, with each patient now modelled as a random effect. Subgroup analyses were performed in patients undergoing non-post-surgical VA ECMO.

Results

Over the study period, 149 episodes of ECMO support, 38 VV and 111 VA ECMO, were conducted in both hospitals (Alfred, $n = 125$, and Besançon, $n = 24$). The median duration of support was 8 days (first and third quartiles: 5–14) for the VV ECMO and 6 days (first and third quartiles: 4–10) for the VA ECMO. Characteristics of study cohort are given in Table 1.

Bleeding events

Overall there were 128 bleeding events (with a bleeding event defined as consecutive days meeting the bleeding definition with the same source of bleeding) over 203

Table 1 Comparison of ECMO episodes with and without bleeding events

Variable	All episodes ($n = 149$)	No bleeding ($n = 60$)	Bleeding ($n = 89$)	P
Age (year ± SD)	46.5 ± 14.9	44.5 ± 15.1	47.8 ± 14.7	0.18
Male sex	92 (62 %)	38 (63 %)	54 (61 %)	0.74
Weight (kg ± SD)	80.7 ± 22	80.7 ± 22	80.7 ± 22	1.00
APACHE III score ± SD	77.3 ± 33.6	70.1 ± 30	82.1 ± 35.2	0.03
Comorbidities				
Immunosuppressed	34 (23 %)	8 (14 %)	26 (29 %)	0.027
Hepatic failure	3 (2 %)	2 (3 %)	1 (1 %)	0.34
Cirrhosis liver disease	2 (1.3 %)	0 (0 %)	2 (2 %)	0.25
Insulin dependent diabetes	7 (5 %)	3 (5 %)	4 (5 %)	0.87
Chronic respiratory failure	23 (16 %)	4 (7 %)	19 (21 %)	0.018
Chronic cardiovascular disease	38 (26 %)	14 (24 %)	24 (27 %)	0.66
Chronic renal failure	2 (1.3 %)	0 (0 %)	2 (2 %)	0.25
Indications for ECMO				
Acute cardiomyopathy	20 (13 %)	12 (20 %)	8 (9 %)	0.05
AMI	28 (19 %)	9 (15 %)	19 (21 %)	0.33
Chronic cardiomyopathy	14 (9 %)	8 (13 %)	6 (7 %)	0.18
Heart transplant	16 (11 %)	4 (7 %)	12 (13 %)	0.19
Lung transplant	15 (10 %)	3 (5 %)	12 (13 %)	0.09
Pneumonia	27 (18 %)	16 (27 %)	11 (12 %)	0.03
Post CAGS or valve surgery	9 (6 %)	1 (2 %)	8 (9 %)	0.07
Other	20 (13 %)	7 (12 %)	13 (15 %)	0.61
Post-surgical ECMO	39 (26 %)	4 (7 %)	35 (39 %)	<0.001
Transplantation prior	33 (22 %)	8 (13 %)	25 (28 %)	0.033
Cardiac arrest before	39 (26 %)	14 (23 %)	25 (28 %)	0.52
Medication prior ECMO				
Aspirin	35 (24 %)	13 (22 %)	22 (26 %)	0.59
Clopidogrel	17 (12 %)	5 (8 %)	12 (14 %)	0.32
Warfarin	16 (11 %)	4 (7 %)	12 (14 %)	0.16
ECMO started in another hospital	40 (27 %)	20 (33 %)	20 (22 %)	0.14
ECMO type				
VA ECMO	111 (74 %)	40 (67 %)	71 (80 %)	0.07
VV ECMO	38 (26 %)	20 (33 %)	18 (20 %)	0.07
Days on support, median [IQR]	7 [5–11]	6 [5–10]	8 [5–12]	0.09
Centre Alfred Hospital	128 (86 %)	52 (87 %)	76 (85 %)	0.83
RRT at any time	60 (43 %)	18 (31 %)	42 (51 %)	0.02
MV at any time	145 (97 %)	57 (95 %)	88 (99 %)	0.15
SOFA score prior ECMO median [IQR]				
Total	10 [7–13]	9 [7–12]	11 [9–14]	0.01
SOFA respiratory	3 [2–4]	3 [2– 4]	3 [1–4]	0.95
SOFA coagulation	0 [0–1]	0 [0–1]	1 [0–2]	0.17
SOFA liver	0 [0–2]	0 [0–1]	1 [0–2]	0.02
SOFA cardiovascular	4 [4–4]	4 [3–4]	4 [4–4]	0.02
SOFA neurology	1 [0–2]	0 [0–1]	1 [0–3]	0.02
SOFA renal	1 [0–3]	1 [0– 2]	1 [0–3]	0.21
Blood product use during ECMO				
Median RBC unit (IQR)	6 [2–14]	2 [0.5–4]	12 [6–19]	<0.01
Median PLT doses (IQR)	1 [0–3]	0 [0–1]	2 [0–5]	<0.01
Median FFP unit (IQR)	2 [0–6]	0 [0–1]	5 [1–10]	<0.01
Median cryoprecipitate (IQR)	0 [0–0]	0 [0–0]	0 [0–1]	<0.01

Table 1 continued

Variable	All episodes ($n = 149$)	No bleeding ($n = 60$)	Bleeding ($n = 89$)	*P*
Other adverse events				
Ischaemic stroke	4 (2.7 %)	1 (2 %)	3 (3 %)	0.53
Membrane change	16 (11 %)	6 (10 %)	10 (11 %)	0.81
Limb ischaemia any stage	11 (7 %)	2 (3 %)	9 (10 %)	0.12
Outcomes				
Weaned off ECMO	95 (64 %)	42 (70 %)	53 (60 %)	0.19
Never weaned	36 (24 %)	10 (17 %)	26 (29 %)	0.08
Bridge to other assistance	18 (12 %)	8 (13 %)	10 (11 %)	0.70
Median (IQR) ICU LOS (days)	17 [9–28]	13.5 [8–23]	16 [9–28]	0.18
Median (IQR) hospital LOS (days)	36.5 [15–56]	27.5 [13.5–36.5]	36.5 [15–56]	0.04
ICU status, alive	101 (68 %)	45 (75 %)	56 (63 %)	0.12
Hospital status, alive	99 (66 %)	45 (75 %)	54 (61 %)	0.07
Discharge home	65 (66 %)	33 (55 %)	32 (36 %)	0.02

Data presented as *n* (%) categorical variables and median (interquartile range) for nonparametric variables

"Post-surgical ECMO" includes any surgery (CAGS and other)

ECMO extracorporeal membrane oxygenation, *APACHE III* score Acute Physiology and Chronic Health Evaluation III score, *AMI* acute myocardial infarction, *CAGS* coronary artery graft surgery, *VA ECMO* veno-arterial ECMO, *VV ECMO* veno-venous ECMO, *RRT* renal replacement therapy, *MV* mechanical ventilation, *SOFA* Sequential Organ Failure Assessment, *RBC* red blood cell unit, *FFP* fresh frozen plasma, *PLT* platelets bag, *ICU* intensive care unit, *LOS* length of stay

ECMO days with 224 bleeding sources identified. Of the 149 ECMO episodes, 58 (39 %) had one, 14 (9 %) had two, 9 (6 %) had three, 5 (3 %) had four and 3 (2 %) had five bleeding events during the ECMO course. The median time to the first bleeding event from starting ECMO was 4 days (first and third quartiles: 0–8 days). Of the 224 sources of bleeding identified, the three most frequent were ECMO cannula, post-cardiothoracic surgical haemothorax or tamponade, and ear–nose and throat (ENT) haemorrhage (Fig. 1). Intra-cranial haemorrhage (ICH) occurred in 5 patients (2.2 %) and was fatal in all cases. There were 67 specific haemostatic interventions for bleeding in 43 ECMO episodes that included surgical intervention ($n = 56$), angiography ($n = 5$), gastroscopy ($n = 4$) and bronchoscopy ($n = 2$). Tranexamic acid was administered in 15 bleeding events, activated recombinant factor VII in 3 events and prothrombin complex concentrate and fibrinogen concentrate in 5 and 2 bleeding events, respectively.

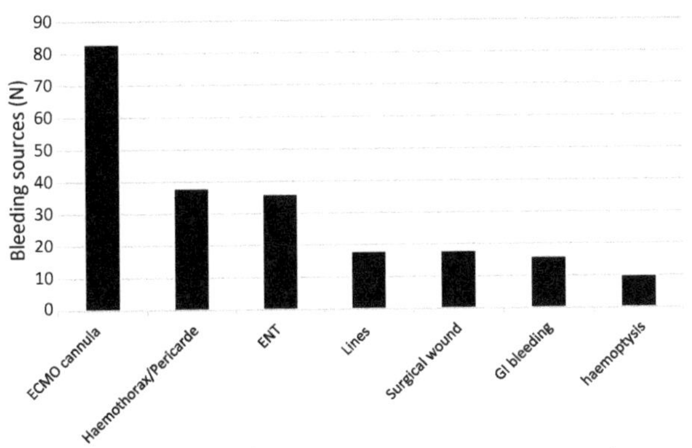

Fig. 1 Bleeding sources. Results are expressed as absolute values (*n*). There were 224 sources identified in 128 haemorrhage events. *Lines* include central venous catheter; *ENT* ear–nose and throat, *GI* gastrointestinal

Eighty-nine ECMO episodes (60 %) were complicated by at least one bleeding event. There were no differences in patient demographics and comorbidities between those who experienced bleeding complications and those who did not (Table 1). When haemorrhagic complications occurred during ECMO, patients were more likely to have surgery prior to ECMO (39 vs. 7 %, $P < 0.001$), had greater illness severity at ECMO initiation with a median SOFA score of 11 (first and third quartiles: 9–14) vs. 9 (first and third quartiles: 7–12) ($P = 0.01$) and more often required RRT (64 vs. 35 %; $P < 0.01$). Antiplatelet therapy or warfarin prior to ECMO was not associated with bleeding events in univariate analysis, nor was the duration of ECMO.

When considering the days on ECMO individually, 1144 days on ECMO were free of bleeding while 203 met the ELSO definition of bleeding. Lower Hb [mean 87 g/L (95 % CI 84–89) vs. 93 g/L (95 % CI 90–95); $P < 0.01$], lower arterial pH [mean 7.30 (95 % CI 7.28–7.32) vs. 7.35 (95 % CI 7.33–7.36); $P < 0.01$], lower ionised calcium [mean 1.02 mmol/L (95 % CI 1.01–1.05) vs. 1.09 mmol/L (95 % CI 1.07–1.10); $P < 0.01$] and higher aPTT [mean 90 s (95 % CI 81–98) vs. 71 s (95 % CI 67–76); $P < 0.01$] recorded on the day prior to bleeding were associated with bleeding occurrence when considering all patients with and without heparin (Table 2). A lower proportion of patients with bleeding had received heparin on the previous day compared to those without bleeding; however, those who did receive it and who were bleeding had higher aPTT compared to the non-bleeding patients [mean 86 s (95 % CI 76–95) vs. 69 s (95 % CI 64–73); $P < 0.01$]. Intra-aortic balloon pump was present in 4 % ($n = 6$) of days with bleeding compared with 1 % ($n = 12$) of days without bleeding. Type of ECMO was also associated with bleeding (Table 2).

Four patients had an ischaemic stroke (2.7 %), limb ischaemia occurred in 11 patients (7.4 %), and membrane was changed for 16 circuits. There was no difference in thrombotic events between bleeding and non-bleeding patients. None of the patients who received tranexamic acid or activated factor VII were diagnosed with thrombotic complications.

Factors associated with bleeding

After adjusting for repeated measures in the same patient, factors that were significantly associated with increased risk of bleeding were: higher aPTT on the day prior, with a significant association for the highest quartile compared to the lowest quartile, higher APACHE III score and post-surgical ECMO. Variables associated with lower risk of bleeding were anticoagulation on the day prior to the event (Table 3). ECMO type was not associated with the risk of bleeding in the adjusted model. When considering only the 75 non-post-surgical VA ECMO episodes, higher aPTT on the day prior remained associated with bleeding [adjusted OR 3.24 (95 % CI 1.11–9.44); $P = 0.03$] (Table 4). In this subgroup analysis, the daily lowest temperature was also associated with bleeding occurrence.

Independent predictors for survival

Bleeding was associated with worse survival [HR 3.04 (95 % CI 1.58–5.89); $P < 0.01$] on univariate analysis. When adjusting for other variables predictive of survival, bleeding was associated with worse survival [HR 2.17 (95 % CI 1.07–4.41); $P = 0.03$] as given in Table 5. The other variables associated with worse survival were SOFA score at ECMO initiation [HR 1.10 (95 % CI 1.01–1.20); $P = 0.03$] and indication for ECMO (Table 5). When considering only patient undergoing non-post-surgical VA ECMO, bleeding was also associated with worse survival [HR 3.05 (95 % CI 1.11–8.38); $P = 0.03$] (Table 6).

Table 2 Comparison of biological and transfusion characteristics of days on ECMO with and without bleeding events

Variable[a]	ECMO days without bleeding ($n = 1144$)	ECMO days with bleeding ($n = 203$)	P
Lowest Hb (g/dL)[b]	93 (90–95)	87 (84–89)	<0.01
Lowest platelet count ($\times 10^9$ cells/L)[b]	125 (115–134)	131 (122–141)	0.15
Highest INR[b]	1.6 (1.5–2.0)	1.9 (1.7–2.0)	0.14
Lowest Fg (g/L)[b]	4.0 (3.8–4.3)	3.9 (3.7–4.2)	0.59
Highest aPTT (s)[b]	71 (67–76)	90 (81–98)	<0.01
Lowest arterial pH[b]	7.35 (7.33–7.36)	7.30 (7.28–7.32)	<0.01
Lowest temperature (°C)[b]	36.1 (35.9–36.2)	36.1 (35.9–36.2)	0.85
Highest urea (mmol/L)[b]	11.1 (10.4–11.7)	11.4 (10.6–12.2)	0.40
Lowest corrected calcium (mmol/L)[b]	1.09 (1.07–1.10)	1.02 (1.01–1.05)	<0.01
Highest free haemoglobin[b]	0.07 (0.06–0.08)	0.07 (0.05–0.10)	0.65
RRT[b]	461 (40 %)	76 (37 %)	0.43
Bilirubin[b]	22.6 (19.6–26.0)	22.1 (20.0–24.4)	0.67
Anticoagulation			
Heparin infusion[b]	816 (71 %)	106 (52 %)	<0.01
Hours on heparin per day[b]	22 (19–24)	18 (15–20)	0.04
Highest aPTT if receiving heparin (s)[b]	69 (64–73)	86 (76–95)	<0.01
Daily dose heparin if receiving heparin (unit)[b]	19,256 (17,292–21,219)	21,400 (19,187–23,614)	0.06
Centre Alfred Hospital	1085 (95 %)	181 (89 %)	0.10
Max membrane gradient (mmHg)	21 (19–23)	20 (17–22)	0.55
VA ECMO	737 (64 %)	164 (81 %)	<0.01
Type of access if VA ECMO, peripheral	697 (94 %)	146 (89 %)	0.04

Hb haemoglobin, *INR* international normalised ratio, *Fg* fibrinogen, *aPTT* activated partial thromboplastin time, *RRT* renal replacement therapy, *IABP* intra-aortic balloon pump, *VA* ECMO veno-arterial ECMO

[a] Mean (95 % CI) adjusted for repeated measures presented for continuous variables and number (%) for categorical variables. *P* values are adjusted for repeated measures

[b] Values are for day prior to bleeding event when considering ECMO days with bleeding

Table 3 Factors independently associated with bleeding in multivariable analysis

Variable	Adjusted odds ratio	95 % confidence interval	P
Previous-day aPTT[a]			
≥46 and ≤55 s	1.35	0.73–2.49	0.33
≥56 and ≤69 s	1.45	0.75–2.82	0.26
≥70 s	3.00	1.64–5.47	<0.01
Previous-day anticoagulation	0.40	0.24–0.66	<0.01
APACHE III score	1.01	1.01–1.02	0.01
Post-surgical ECMO	3.04	1.62–5.69	<0.01

Analysis includes 1125 days with complete data

aPTT activated partial thromboplastin time, *APACHE III* score Acute Physiology and Chronic Health Evaluation III score

[a] aPTT < 46 s is the reference

Table 4 Factors independently associated with bleeding in non-post-surgical VA ECMO (*N* = 75) (adjusted for ECMO indication and severity)

Variables	Adjusted odds ratio	95 % confidence interval	P
Previous-day aPTT[a]			
≥46 and ≤55 s	2.03	0.68–6.10	0.30
≥56 and ≤69 s	1.32	0.41–4.27	0.47
≥70 s	3.24	1.11–9.44	0.03
Previous-day anticoagulation	0.21	0.06–0.52	<0.01
Daily lowest corporeal temperature	1.79	1.20–2.66	<0.01
APACHE III score	1.03	1.01–1.04	<0.01

aPTT activated partial thromboplastin time, *APACHE III* score Acute Physiology and Chronic Health Evaluation III score

[a] aPTT < 46 s is the reference

Table 5 Factors independently associated with reduced survival

Variables	Adjusted hazard ratio	95 % confidence interval	P
Bleeding on one or more days	2.17	1.07–4.41	0.03
Hospital	2.14	0.92–4.94	0.08
APACHE III score	0.99	0.98–1.01	0.39
SOFA score prior to ECMO	1.10	1.01–1.20	0.03
Indication for ECMO (lung transplant reference)			
AMI	15.40	1.89–125	0.01
Acute cardiomyopathy	2.05	0.18–23.18	0.56
Chronic cardiomyopathy	1.38	0.08–25.06	0.83
Heart transplant	7.26	0.96–55.23	0.06
Cardiac surgery	9.07	1.06–77.28	0.04
Pneumonia	3.68	0.45–30.12	0.22
Other	12.11	1.73–84.41	0.01

aPTT activated partial thromboplastin time, *APACHE III* score Acute Physiology and Chronic Health Evaluation III score, *SOFA* Sequential Organ Failure Assessment, *AMI* acute myocardial infarction

Discussion

Bleeding complications, as defined by ELSO, occurred in more than half of critically ill patients undergoing ECMO and were strongly and independently associated with hospital mortality. The most frequent bleeding sources identified in our study included ECMO cannula, post-cardiothoracic surgery site and ENT. We found that illness severity and higher aPTT on the day prior to bleeding onset were independently associated with bleeding, while anticoagulant administration on the day prior was associated with a lower risk of bleeding. Our results emphasise the importance of further studies on coagulation abnormalities in this population.

Comparison with available literature

We found that 60 % of ECMO courses were complicated by bleeding, which is higher than previously reported bleeding rates. This difference may be due to differences in bleeding definitions [3, 11]. Bleeding events in ECMO patients, when reported in the literature, are either not clearly defined or reported on the basis of organ site involved, death due to bleeding, requirement for surgical intervention or using only RBC transfusion as a surrogate of bleeding [2, 11, 13]. Extracorporeal Life Support Organization (ELSO) guidelines recently provided definition criteria for bleeding complications [15]. Although this definition has not commonly been used in studies related to bleeding in ECMO, it may allow and facilitate comparison between findings of ours and future studies.

We found that post-surgical bleeding and ECMO cannula were the most common sources of bleeding in patients undergoing ECMO, as previously reported [1, 11, 16]. However, ENT has not commonly been reported as a source of bleeding in this patient population. Severity of ENT bleeding may be difficult to estimate, and its

Table 6 Factors independently associated with reduced survival in the sub group of patients undergoing non-post-surgical VA ECMO (*N* = 75)

Variables	Adjusted hazard ratio	95 % confidence interval	*P*
Bleeding on one or more days	3.05	1.11–8.38	0.03
Hospital	1.41	0.47–3.62	0.47
SOFA score prior to ECMO	1.11	0.98–1.26	0.11
ECMO indication (AMI reference)			
Acute cardiomyopathy	0.16	0.03–0.77	0.02
Chronic cardiomyopathy	0.34	0.07–1.71	0.19
Heart transplant	0.86	0.16–4.69	0.86
Other	0.51	0.19–1.42	0.20

aPTT activated partial thromboplastin time, *SOFA* Sequential Organ Failure Assessment, *AMI* acute myocardial infarction

haemodynamic consequences may be less acute than other bleeding sites. Nonetheless, ENT bleeding is important to diagnose because it may require specific investigation for primary haemostatic disorders, such as platelet function abnormalities and von Willebrand disease, and specific treatment including local haemostatic packing [17]. In our study, ICH complicated ECMO in 2.2 % of cases. This figure is comparable to those reported by Paden et al. but lower than those found in other cohorts [5, 11]. ICH may also be underestimated in our study, as CT brain scans and post-mortem examination were not routinely performed.

Risk factors for bleeding previously studied include parameters available at ECMO initiation (i.e. demographics, ECMO characteristics, patient characteristics at ECMO initiation). There are few reports evaluating bleeding risk factors measured during ECMO treatment. A few decades ago, Kasirajan et al. reported an association between ICH and platelet count [14]. In our study, we did not find an independent association between thrombocytopenia and haemorrhage, possibly because the median platelet count remained relatively high and possibly because of the low rate of the ICH. The same authors reported an association between ICH and heparin therapy. However, information about heparin regimen and coagulation results were not provided [14]. In our study, the fact that a lower proportion of patients with bleeding had received heparin on the previous day compared to those without bleeding may be explained if the onset of bleeding was prior to when the patients met the ELSO bleeding definition, resulting in clinicians ceasing heparin infusion. It could also be explained by physicians selecting patients at lower risk of bleeding for therapeutic anticoagulation, and that patients who remain on heparin have proven their tolerance to anticoagulation without bleeding. However, we also found that the intensity of anticoagulation (as measured by aPTT) was associated with increased bleeding risk (with increasing OR with increasing aPTT categories), suggesting that high aPTT in anticoagulated patients are deleterious. This supports the need for further research on anticoagulation and risk of bleeding in this population. In a recent prospective observational study using thromboelastography (TEG) to evaluate anticoagulation profile during 32 VV ECMO episodes, heparin therapy and aPTT were associated with a reaction time of >90 min ("flat-line" profile); these results also emphasise the need for optimisation of anticoagulation management in this population [18]. Both ECMO and cardiac surgery lead to decrease in fibrinogen level [7, 19]. Association between low fibrinogen level and bleeding events has been recently reported in paediatrics ECMO and in surgical setting [20, 21]. The key role of coagulation abnormalities has been suggested indirectly in other studies, in which a benefit of carefully monitoring and treating coagulopathy in ECMO patients was found [19, 22].

Patients who undergo VA ECMO have different comorbidities, underlying diseases and anticoagulant requirement compared to patients who undergo VV ECMO. While VA ECMO was associated with more bleeding days in the univariate analysis, this association did not remain in the adjusted analysis; however, we may have been underpowered to detect a difference if one did exist. Likewise, there were some differences in bleeding risk according to diagnosis; however, this did not remain associated in the adjusted analysis. Finally, with a high incidence of post-surgical VA ECMO (32 %), we may have missed an association between type of ECMO and bleeding risk despite the absence of colinearity between these post-surgical ECMO and ECMO type.

Implications of study findings and future research

This risk of bleeding should be taken into consideration in clinical management, including invasive procedures in this population. Although this is a retrospective study with the limitations secondary to this design, our findings on the association between coagulation abnormalities and bleeding in adults on ECMO highlight the importance of closely monitoring coagulation and bleeding in this population. Having local haemostatic guidelines to manage bleeding and non-bleeding patients undergoing ECMO should be a priority for ECMO centres.

Prospective studies evaluating optimal haemostatic treatment, including blood components, intensity of anticoagulation, use of tranexamic acid, concentrate of coagulation factors and antithrombin III with their effects on bleeding and thromboembolic complications are warranted. Beside coagulation monitoring by thromboelastography might also be beneficial in this high-risk population [18, 23].

It would also be meaningful to perform a larger prospective study considering separately fatal bleeding as an outcome.

Strengths and limitations

Our work addresses an important issue in the management of patients on ECMO, as bleeding complications remain common and associated with poor prognosis. It studies clinical, biological and therapeutic parameters that may be risk factors for bleeding complications. We used a clear definition of bleeding events, thereby ensuring accuracy of our outcome measure and allowing comparisons with other studies. Inclusion of patients from two ECMO centres provides external validity to our results. Time-dependent survival analysis enables identification of parameters not only at ECMO initiation but also during the ECMO course.

Our study does, however, suffer several limitations. Due to the retrospective study design, we could only explore associations between risk factors and bleeding outcomes and cannot make any conclusions regarding causation. We also cannot exclude the possibility of confounding by unmeasured factors, for example cannulation method. The retrospective design may also lead to misclassification of bleeding events. However, the definition of bleeding that we used relies on transfusion volumes, bleeding at specific sites and/or requirement for intervention, all of which could be objectively measured from electronic laboratory data and medical records. As it was not possible to identify the time at which bleeding started, we analysed association between variables collected on the preceding day. Furthermore, we could not perform relevant statistical analysis considering subgroups of either patients undergoing VV ECMO only or post-surgical ECMO because of their small sample size. Finally, thrombosis complications are likely to be underreported because of the retrospective design.

Conclusions

In conclusion, our study shows that bleeding events as defined by the ELSO remain a common and serious complication in patients undergoing ECMO, with 60 % of ECMO courses complicated by at least one bleeding complication. Bleeding while on ECMO is independently associated with hospital mortality. Among identified risk factors for bleeding event, besides patient severity, coagulation anomalies are the only identified which may be targeted with interventions. These findings highlight the importance of further research to determine the safest haemostatic management in this population.

Authors' contributions

All authors have contributed substantially to the submitted work. CA, DP, MD, JS, MS and VP have designed the study. CA, JD and FB have collected the data. MB and ZM have performed the statistical analysis. CA, DP, VP and ZM have analysed the results. CA and ZM have written the first draft of the manuscript that has been substantially reviewed by all authors. All authors read and approved the final manuscript.

Author details

[1] The Australian and New Zealand Intensive Care Research Centre, Department of Epidemiology and Preventive Medicine, Monash University, Melbourne, Australia. [2] The Transfusion Research Unit, Department of Epidemiology and Preventive Medicine, Monash University, Melbourne, Australia. [3] The Intensive Care Unit, The Alfred Hospital, Melbourne, Australia. [4] University Hospital of Antwerp, 2000 Antwerp, Belgium. [5] The Intensive Care Unit, Jean Minjoz Hospital, 25030 Besançon, France. [6] School of Public Health and Preventive Medicine, Monash University, Melbourne, Australia. [7] Medical Intensive Care Unit, Centre Hospitalier Régional et Universitaire de Brest, site La Cavale Blanche, Bvd Tanguy Prigent, 29609 Brest Cedex, France. [8] LUBEM, EA 3882 - Université de Bretagne Occidentale, 29 200 Brest, France. [9] Medical Intensive Care Unit, iCAN, Institute of Cardiometabolism and Nutrition, Hôpital de la Pitié–Salpetrière, Assistance Publique–Hôpitaux de Paris, Paris, France.

Acknowledgements

This work is part of a research programme "Centre of Research Excellence for Patient Blood Management in Critical Illness and Trauma", which is funded by the Australian National Health and Medical Research Council.

Competing interests

The authors declare that they have no competing interests.

References

1. Brogan TV, Thiagarajan RR, Rycus PT, Bartlett RH, Bratton SL. Extracorporeal membrane oxygenation in adults with severe respiratory failure: a multi-center database. Intensive Care Med. 2009;35(12):2105–14.
2. Aubron C, Cheng AC, Pilcher D, Leong T, Magrin G, Cooper DJ, et al. Factors associated with outcomes of patients on extracorporeal membrane oxygenation support: a 5-year cohort study. Crit Care. 2013;17(2):R73.
3. Zangrillo A, Landoni G, Biondi-Zoccai G, Greco M, Greco T, Frati G, et al. A meta-analysis of complications and mortality of extracorporeal membrane oxygenation. Crit Care Resusc J Aust Acad Crit Care Med. 2013;15(3):172–8.
4. Combes A, Leprince P, Luyt CE, Bonnet N, Trouillet JL, Leger P, et al. Outcomes and long-term quality-of-life of patients supported by extracorporeal membrane oxygenation for refractory cardiogenic shock. Crit Care Med. 2008;36(5):1404–11.
5. Davies A, Jones D, Bailey M, Beca J, Bellomo R, Blackwell N, et al. Extracorporeal membrane oxygenation for 2009 influenza A (H1N1) acute respiratory distress syndrome. JAMA. 2009;302(17):1888–95.
6 Murphy DA, Hockings LE, Andrews RK, Aubron C, Gardiner EE, Pellegrino VA, et al. Extracorporeal membrane oxygenation-hemostatic complications. Transfus Med Rev. 2015;29(2):90–101.
7 Hunt BJ, Parratt RN, Segal HC, Sheikh S, Kallis P, Yacoub M. Activation of coagulation and fibrinolysis during cardiothoracic operations. Ann Thorac Surg. 1998;65(3):712–8.
8 Heilmann C, Geisen U, Beyersdorf F, Nakamura L, Benk C, Trummer G, et al. Acquired von Willebrand syndrome in patients with extracorporeal life support (ECLS). Intensive Care Med. 2012;38(1):62–8.

9 Palatianos GM, Foroulis CN, Vassili MI, Astras G, Triantafillou K, Papadakis E, et al. A prospective, double-blind study on the efficacy of the bioline surface-heparinized extracorporeal perfusion circuit. Ann Thorac Surg. 2003;76(1):129–35.
10 Bembea MM, Annich G, Rycus P, Oldenburg G, Berkowitz I, Pronovost P. Variability in anticoagulation management of patients on extracorporeal membrane oxygenation: an international survey. Pediatr Crit Care Med J Soc Crit Care Med World Fed Pediatr Intensive Crit Care Soc. 2013;14(2):e77–84.
11 Paden ML, Conrad SA, Rycus PT, Thiagarajan RR. Extracorporeal life support organization registry report 2012. ASAIO J. 2013;59(3):202–10.
12 Rastan AJ, Lachmann N, Walther T, Doll N, Gradistanac T, Gommert JF, et al. Autopsy findings in patients on postcardiotomy extracorporeal membrane oxygenation (ECMO). Int J Artif Organs. 2006;29(12):1121–31.
13 Werho DK, Pasquali SK, Yu S, Donohue J, Annich GM, Thiagarajan RR, et al. Hemorrhagic complications in pediatric cardiac patients on extracorporeal membrane oxygenation: an analysis of the Extracorporeal Life Support Organization Registry. Pediatr Crit Care Med J Soc Crit Care Med World Fed Pediatr Intensive Crit Care Soc. 2015;16(3):276–88.
14 Kasirajan V, Smedira NG, McCarthy JF, Casselman F, Boparai N, McCarthy PM. Risk factors for intracranial hemorrhage in adults on extracorporeal membrane oxygenation. Eur J Cardio Thorac Surg. 1999;15(4):508–14.
15 Extracorporeal Life Support Organization. ELSO Anticoagulation guideline. Ann Arbor, MI USA 2014. p. 17. Available on https://www.elso.org/Portals/0/Files/elsoanticoagulationguideline8-2014-table-contents.pdf.
16 Marasco SF, Lukas G, McDonald M, McMillan J, Ihle B. Review of ECMO (extra corporeal membrane oxygenation) support in critically ill adult patients. Heart Lung Circ. 2008;17(Suppl 4):S41–7.
17 Kalbhenn J, Schmidt R, Nakamura L, Schelling J, Rosenfelder S, Zieger B. Early diagnosis of acquired von Willebrand Syndrome (AVWS) is elementary for clinical practice in patients treated with ECMO therapy. J Atheroscler Thromb. 2015;22(3):265–71.
18 Panigada M, Iapichino G, L'Acqua C, Protti A, Cressoni M, Consonni D, et al. Prevalence of "Flat-Line" thromboelastography during extracorporeal membrane oxygenation for respiratory failure in adults. ASAIO J. 2016;62(3):302–9.
19 Kalbhenn J, Wittau N, Schmutz A, Zieger B, Schmidt R. Identification of acquired coagulation disorders and effects of target-controlled coagulation factor substitution on the incidence and severity of spontaneous intracranial bleeding during veno-venous ECMO therapy. Perfusion. 2015.
20 Doymaz S, Zinger M, Sweberg T. Risk factors associated with intracranial hemorrhage in neonates with persistent pulmonary hypertension on ECMO. J Intensive Care. 2015;3(1):6.
21 Montan C, Johansson F, Hedin U, Wahlgren CM. Preoperative hypofibrinogenemia is associated with increased intraoperative bleeding in ruptured abdominal aortic aneurysms. Thromb Res. 2015;135(3):443–8.
22 Northrop MS, Sidonio RF, Phillips SE, Smith AH, Daphne HC, Pietsch JB, et al. The use of an extracorporeal membrane oxygenation anticoagulation laboratory protocol is associated with decreased blood product use, decreased hemorrhagic complications, and increased circuit life. Pediatr Crit Care Med J Soc Crit Care Med World Fed Pediatr Intensive Crit Care Soc. 2015;16(1):66–74.
23 Davis MC, Andersen NE, Johansson P, Andersen LW. Use of thromboelastograph and factor VII for the treatment of postoperative bleeding in a pediatric patient on ECMO after cardiac surgery. J Extra Corpor Technol. 2006;38(2):165–7.

7

Neutrophil expression of glucocorticoid-induced leucine zipper (GILZ) anti-inflammatory protein is associated with acute respiratory distress syndrome severity

Marie-Alix Espinasse[1], David Hajage[4], Philippe Montravers[2,3], Pascale Piednoir[2,3], Guillaume Dufour[2,3], Florence Tubach[4], Vanessa Granger[1,5], Luc de Chaisemartin[1,5], Benoît Noël[1], Marc Pallardy[1], Sylvie Chollet-Martin[1,5†] and Armelle Biola-Vidamment[1*†]

Abstract

Background: Glucocorticoid-induced leucine zipper (GILZ) is a potent anti-inflammatory protein involved in neutrophil apoptosis and the resolution of inflammation. Given the numerous pathophysiologic roles of neutrophils in the acute respiratory distress syndrome (ARDS), we postulated that neutrophil GILZ expression might be induced during ARDS, to modulate the inflammatory process and participate in lung repair.

Methods: This single-center, prospective, observational cohort study took place in the surgical intensive care unit of Bichat Hospital (Paris, France) and involved 17 ARDS patients meeting the Berlin criteria at inclusion, and 14 ventilated controls without ARDS. Serial blood samples were obtained every 2 days until extubation or death (from 1 to 9 samples per patient). GILZ protein and gene expression was quantified in blood neutrophils, along with markers of inflammation (CRP, extracellular DNA) or its resolution (Annexin A1).

Results: Neutrophil GILZ expression was detected at the transcriptional and/or translational level in 9/17 ARDS patients (in particular 7/10 severe ARDS) and in 2/14 ventilated controls. The highest mRNA levels were observed in the most severely ill patients ($p < 0.028$). GILZ was expressed in about ¾ of the corticosteroid-treated patients and its expression could also occur independently of corticosteroids, suggesting that inflammatory signals may also induce neutrophil GILZ expression in vivo.

Conclusions: In this pilot study, we show for the first time that blood neutrophils from patients with ARDS can express GILZ, in keeping with an anti-inflammatory and regulatory endogenous role of GILZ in humans. Contrary to some markers of inflammation or its resolution, the levels of *gilz* gene expression were related to ARDS severity.

Keywords: Neutrophils, Glucocorticoid-induced leucine zipper (GILZ), ARDS, Extracellular DNA, Annexin A1

Background

The acute respiratory distress syndrome (ARDS) is one of the most severe forms of acute respiratory failure [1] characterized by diffuse alveolar damage. High alveolar concentrations of inflammatory mediators trigger excessive neutrophil influx and activation, leading to the release of reactive oxygen species (ROS), proteases, cytokines and neutrophil extracellular traps (NETs), all of which can contribute to alveolar injury [2]. Both circulating and alveolar neutrophils exhibit delayed apoptosis in this setting, and this is associated with lung injury, impaired resolution of inflammation, clinical severity, and poor outcome [3, 4].

*Correspondence: armelle.biola-vidamment@u-psud.fr
†Sylvie Chollet-Martin and Armelle Biola-Vidamment have contributed equally to this work
[1] INSERM UMR-996 - Inflammation, Chemokines and Immunopathology, Univ Paris-Sud, Faculté de pharmacie, Université Paris-Saclay, 5 rue JB Clément, 92296 Châtenay-Malabry Cedex, France
Full list of author information is available at the end of the article

Despite significant research, ARDS management still consists mainly of supportive care, based on optimized ventilation and extracorporeal membrane oxygenation (ECMO) [5]. New therapeutic strategies based on modulation of inflammation, using mesenchymal stromal cells, miRNA, or regulatory T cells, have recently been proposed [6–8]. Steroids have controversial effects when used early during the course of ARDS [9], but have been shown to reduce fibroblast proliferation and cytokine release when used in the late phase, thereby improving recovery [10]. Another effect of steroid therapy might be the induction of glucocorticoid-induced leucine zipper (GILZ).

GILZ is an immunomodulatory protein belonging to the transforming growth factor-β-stimulating clone 22 domain (TSC-22D) family [11]. GILZ can also be induced in vitro by TGF-β and IL-10 [12], and has been detected both in a murine model of arthritis and in the joints of patients with rheumatoid arthritis [13]. These recent in vivo findings suggest that, in some inflammatory conditions, GILZ may be induced independent from exogenous corticosteroid administration.

In vitro, GILZ regulates major inflammatory signal transduction pathways such as activator protein 1 (AP-1), nuclear factor-kappa B (NF-κB), and forkhead box O (FOXO) [11, 14]. GILZ has also been implicated in the control of apoptosis and cell survival in various cell types [11, 15, 16]. We recently showed that GILZ expression by human neutrophils in vitro promotes their apoptosis [17]. These results were confirmed in vivo by Vago et al. [18] who found that preventive or therapeutic administration of the cell-permeable TAT-GILZ fusion protein improved resolution in a mouse model of LPS-induced pleurisy. GILZ thus appears to be an important regulator of neutrophil apoptosis in vitro and in vivo, contributing to the resolution of inflammation. The mechanisms of GILZ action involve the well-described anti-inflammatory and pro-resolving factor Annexin A1 [18, 19]. Indeed, endogenous Annexin A1 induces neutrophils to undergo apoptosis and promotes their efferocytosis by macrophages, as demonstrated in vivo in the mouse model of LPS-induced pleurisy [20].

We postulated that neutrophil GILZ expression might be induced during ARDS, to modulate the inflammatory process and participate in lung repair. The aim of this pilot study was thus to analyze the kinetics of blood neutrophil GILZ expression at the protein and mRNA levels in ventilated septic patients with and without ARDS, and treated or not by corticosteroids. The levels of *gilz* mRNA were then analyzed according to ARDS severity, in comparison with some markers of inflammation (circulating CRP and extracellular DNA) or its resolution (Annexin A1), to assess whether GILZ might be included in a new biological signature of ARDS severity.

Methods

Study setting and population

We conducted a single-center, prospective, pilot, observational cohort study of ARDS patients hospitalized in the intensive care unit (ICU) of Bichat Hospital (Paris, France) from January 2012 to March 2013. Patients with HIV infection, hepatitis, transplantation, end-stage cancer, age below 18 years, or ongoing pregnancy were excluded. The protocol was approved by the ethics committee of Paris-Bichat Hospital (CEERB, comité d'évaluation de l'éthique des projets de recherche biomédicale, No. 12-028, Paris, France), and informed consent was obtained from the patients' legally authorized relatives. Patients mechanically ventilated with a positive end-expiratory pressure above 5 cm H_2O were prospectively included and classified into two groups: patients with ARDS ($n = 17$) and ARDS-free ventilated controls ($n = 14$), according to the Berlin definition of ARDS (acute hypoxemia, ratio of partial pressure of arterial oxygen (PaO_2)/ fraction of inspired oxygen (FiO_2) of 300 mmHg or less, and bilateral infiltrates on chest X-ray) [1]. The control group consisted mainly of postoperative care or trauma patients receiving mechanical ventilation for respiratory failure without ARDS criteria. Blood samples were obtained prospectively during routine care, the first within 24 h after ARDS diagnosis or ICU hospitalization and then every 2 days until extubation or death. The following clinical parameters were collected at inclusion: age, sex, reason for ICU admission, CRP plasma level (Dimension Vista®1500, Siemens Healthcare diagnostics, $n < 6$ mg/L), ARDS etiology, Simplified Acute Physiology Score II (SAPS II) [21], Sequential Organ Failure Assessment Score (SOFA) [22], Lung Injury Score (LIS) [23], ventilation parameters (PaO_2/FiO_2 ratio), and use of extracorporeal membrane oxygenation (ECMO) and other treatments (steroids and vasoactive agents) as recommended by the standard of care of patients with ARDS [24]. ECMO was used as rescue therapy if hypoxemia persisted despite optimal mechanical ventilation, neuromuscular blocking agent administration, and nitric oxide inhalation. Intravenous hydrocortisone hemisuccinate (200 mg/day) was administered in case of severe septic shock with an inadequate response to vascular filling and cardiovascular treatment [25]. Vital status was recorded 28 days after inclusion.

Blood neutrophil isolation

Neutrophils were isolated immediately after blood sampling by sedimentation on a separating medium containing 5% Dextran T500® (Pharmacia, Uppsala, Sweden) in 0.9% saline and centrifugation on a Ficoll gradient

(Eurobio, Les Ulis, France) as previously described [26, 27]. Erythrocytes were removed by hypotonic lysis.

Immunoblotting of neutrophil-derived GILZ protein

Neutrophils were lysed in cold Laemmli buffer (5% Tris pH 6.8 1.25 M, 10% glycerol, 10% SDS, 1 mM PMSF, 1 mM Na_3VO_4, 25 mM β-glycerophosphate, 10 µg/ml aprotinin, 10 µg/ml leupeptin, and 10 µg/ml pepstatin), then boiled, and sonicated. The total protein concentration was measured by bicinchoninic acid assay, and equal amounts of denatured protein were loaded on 12% SDS-PAGE gels and transferred to PVDF membranes. The membranes were incubated with a polyclonal rabbit antibody raised against human GILZ that was developed in our laboratory [15], stripped, and reprobed with an antibody against p38 MAP Kinase (Cell signaling, Danvers, USA, ref 9212) as a loading control.

Real-time PCR analysis of the neutrophil *gilz* and annexin A1 genes

Neutrophils were lysed in RLT buffer (Qiagen, Courtaboeuf, France) and stored after homogenization of the lysate through a QIAshreder column. Total RNA was isolated with the Qiagen Mini Plus Kit according to the manufacturer's protocol. RNA integrity was evaluated by capillary electrophoresis using RNA 6000 Nano chips and the Bioanalyzer 2100 (Agilent Technologies). Reverse transcription was carried out as previously described [28]. Real-time PCR analysis was performed using SYBR Green technology on a Biorad CFX96 system with Sso Fast EvaGreen Supermix (Bio-Rad, Marnes la Coquette, France) and appropriate primers for *gilz* [5′-TCTGCTTGGAGGGGATGTGG-3′ and 5′-ACTTGTGGGGATTCGGGAGC-3′] [29], *gapdh* [5′-CAGCCTCAAGATCATCAGC A-3′ and 5′-TGTGGTCATGAGTCCTTCCA-3′], *b2m* (beta-2-microglobulin) [5′-ACCCCCACTGAAAAAGATGA-3′ and 5′-ATCTTCAAACCTCCATGATG-3′], and *annexin A1* (Qiagen QuantiTect primer assay QT00078197), as previously described [28]. The cDNA was amplified with 500-nM final concentrations of each primer, in duplicate 10-µl reactions, by 45 two-step cycles (95 °C 5 s; 60 °C 30 s). "No RT" controls were amplified on all genes to control for genomic DNA contamination, and melting curve analysis was performed to assess the purity of the PCR products. Serial dilutions of a pool of cDNA samples were used to construct linear standard curves, from which PCR efficiencies (E) were calculated for each gene. GeNorm in qBase Plus tool [29] was used to select *b2m* and *gapdh* as reference genes for normalization of mRNA expression results. The normalized relative expression of target genes in samples was determined using the $\Delta\Delta Cq$ method with correction for PCR efficiencies, where $\text{NRQ} = E_{\text{Target}}{}^{-\Delta Cq\ \text{Target}}/E_{\text{Ref}}{}^{-\Delta Cq\ \text{Reference}}$ and $\Delta Cq = Cq_{\text{sample}} - Cq_{\text{calibrator}}$ [30, 31]. Final results were expressed as the *n*-fold differences in target gene expression in a given ARDS patient vs one arbitrarily chosen control patient.

Circulating extracellular DNA quantification

Circulating DNA was extracted from plasma by using the QiAmp Ultrasens Kit (Qiagen) and stored at −20 °C until use. Cell-free DNA was quantified by fluorimetry in the Quanti-iT™ Picogreen dsDNA assay (Molecular Probes, Eugene, USA) according to the manufacturer's instructions. The fluorescence signal was recorded on a plate reader (TECAN Infinite® M200, Männedorf, Switzerland).

Statistical analysis

Demographic data were expressed as the median corrected by the interquartile range (IQR). Fisher's exact test or the Chi-square test was used to assess the comparability of the study cohort with the control group. Nonparametric variables were compared by using the Mann–Whitney *U* test or the Kruskal–Wallis test for multiple comparisons.

Neutrophil expression of *gilz* and *annexin A1* mRNA and plasma levels of extracellular DNA and CRP were compared between mild/moderate ARDS patients, severe ARDS patients, and controls. A linear mixed-effects regression model was used to take into account the repeated nature of the data and the different times of measurement, and to compensate for data attrition.

In the mixed-effects models, we considered the *gilz* mRNA expression logarithm in order to improve data normality. The 95% confidence interval and corresponding (two-tailed) *p* value were estimated by boostrapping with 1000 replications. A p value < 0.05 was considered statistically significant.

We defined an arbitrary positivity threshold for *gilz* mRNA expression as the mean plus twice the standard deviation of the controls' *gilz* mRNA levels in at least one of the first two serial samples; this value was 2.8 arbitrary units. We used only the first two samples in order to compensate for data attrition, allowing us to analyze an equivalent number of data for each group. Consequently, a "*gilz*-positive" patient had a *gilz* expression level above the threshold in at least one of his/her first two samples. We then analyzed several features of "*gilz*-positive" patients by using the Chi-square test.

All analyses were done using GraphPad software (San Diego, CA, USA) and R version 3.0.2 (R Foundation for Statistical Computing, Vienna, Austria) implemented in the lme4 package version 1.0-4.

The sample size was not calculated in this pilot study because this is the first study to report the *gilz* expression levels in neutrophils from patients with ARDS, and no evidence could be referenced for statistical power analysis. Instead, the sample size was determined by our previous experience.

Results

Characteristics of the patients

A total of 17 ARDS patients and 14 controls were consecutively enrolled. Their main characteristics are shown in Table 1. The ARDS and controls had similar general severity scores (SAPS II and SOFA). The reasons for ICU admissions were similar (mainly sepsis, postoperative care, or trauma). The ARDS patients stayed longer in the ICU than the controls, allowing serial blood sampling for GILZ analysis.

The *gilz* gene is transiently expressed by blood neutrophils from ARDS patients, which depends on corticosteroids but not on vasoactive agent administration

Neutrophil *gilz* expression was transiently detected in several ARDS patients (9/17) but only in few controls (2/14). Figure 1a shows the time course of *gilz* mRNA expression in two representative controls and two representative ARDS patients. Depending on the patients, 1–9 mRNA samples could be obtained during the ICU stay and analyzed. Neutrophil *gilz* mRNA relative quantity was significantly increased in patients with steroid therapy as compared with patients without corticosteroids ($p < 0.05$) (4.2 ± 6.7 and 1.7 ± 3.2 arbitrary units) (Fig. 1b), but was also evidenced in the absence of corticotherapy (Fig. 1a, b). Vasoactive agents were administered to 65% of the 31 patients; *gilz* expression was similar in patients who did and did not receive vasoactive agents (2.2 ± 4.3 and 2.6 ± 5.0 arbitrary units) (Fig. 1c).

GILZ protein is transiently expressed by blood neutrophils from ARDS patients

GILZ was detected in neutrophil homogenates from 7 upon the 8 ARDS patients that could be studied (good quality protein samples for 47% of the ARDS patients) and was almost undetectable in the 6 controls studied (Fig. 2).

Depending on the patients, 1–5 protein samples could be obtained during the ICU stay and analyzed. GILZ protein was transiently expressed during ARDS, as described above for *gilz* gene expression (Fig. 2).

Neutrophil *gilz* mRNA levels are related to ARDS severity

We then wanted to compare neutrophil *gilz* mRNA levels in controls, mild/moderate ARDS patients, and severe ARDS patients. We first analyzed the highest value of *gilz* expression for each patient and found that it tended to be higher in ARDS patients than in controls, particularly when only severe ARDS patients were considered (Fig. 3). We then used a linear mixed-effects regression model to refine this comparison and to compensate for data attrition linked to differences in the numbers of serial samples analyzed for each patient ($n = 1–9$). This allowed us to calculate predicted *gilz* mRNA levels based on available measured values. As shown in Fig. 4a, predicted *gilz* mRNA levels did not differ between mild/moderate ARDS patients and controls ($p = 0.665$). However, predicted *gilz* mRNA levels were higher in severe ARDS patients than in controls ($p = 0.035$) and mild/moderate ARDS patients ($p = 0.028$) (Fig. 4a). Although *gilz* mRNA expression appeared variable in time, no linear interaction or association with time was found. We then examined whether *gilz* expression was related to the PaO_2/FiO_2 ratio and found that the correlation between *gilz* expression and a PaO_2/FiO_2 below 100 was very close to statistical significance ($p = 0.054$) (data not shown). Interestingly, *gilz* expression was significantly higher in ARDS patients receiving ECMO than in other ARDS patients ($p < 0.005$) (Fig. 4b).

To evaluate GILZ as a possible new marker of ARDS severity, we used the same linear mixed-effects regression model to analyze three other parameters related to inflammation (CRP, extracellular DNA) or its regulation (Annexin A1). We found that predicted circulating CRP levels did not differ across the three patient groups (Fig. 5a) and that *gilz* gene expression did not correlate with CRP levels (data not shown). As extracellular DNA levels have been linked to organ injury in some forms of acute lung injury and sepsis, we measured extracellular DNA in the same samples and found no difference across the three groups of patients (Fig. 5b), confirming that this parameter is not specific for ARDS. Finally, we analyzed neutrophil-derived Annexin A1, as this glucocorticoid-inducible pro-resolving protein can cooperate with GILZ to dampen inflammation. We found that predicted *annexin A1* mRNA levels did not differ across the three groups of patients (Fig. 5c), suggesting that *annexin A1* regulation may occur at a different level than *gilz* regulation.

Together, these results show that GILZ can be expressed by neutrophils during the course of ARDS, at both the protein and gene level, and that its expression level is associated with clinical severity, more specifically than other markers of inflammation or its resolution.

Clinical definition of "*gilz*-positive" ARDS patients

We then analyzed several features of "*gilz*-positive" patients (see above), including clinical parameters (ARDS, septic shock at inclusion, and pneumonia at inclusion [32]), treatment, and mortality. Using the

Table 1 Characteristics of the patients

Patients	Ventilated controls ($n = 14$)	Mild ($n = 1$) and moderate ($n = 6$) ARDS	Severe ARDS ($n = 10$)	p value
Age (years, median ± IQR)	56 ± 19	52 ± 24	59 ± 6	0.82
Male/female (number)	9/5	6/1	7/3	0.78
Comorbidities				
Smoking (number, percentage)	4 (29%)	5 (71%)	2 (20%)	0.07
Obstructive airway diseases (number, percentage)	5 (36%)	5 (71%)	4 (40%)	0.27
Cardiovascular disease (number, percentage)	1 (7%)	1 (14%)	–	0.49
Diabetes (number, percentage)	2 (14%)	1 (14%)	–	0.45
Malignancy (number, percentage)	–	1 (14%)	1 (10%)	0.39
Reasons for ICU admission				
Sepsis (number, percentage)	7 (50%)	6 (86%)	8 (80%)	0.15
Pneumonia (number, percentage)	5 (36%)	5 (71%)	5 (50%)	0.30
Postoperative care (number, percentage)	11 (79%)	7 (100%)	9 (90%)	0.36
Congestive heart failure (number, percentage)	2 (14%)	1 (14%)	–	0.45
Hemorrhagic shock (number, percentage)	1 (14%)	2 (29%)	–	0.13
Trauma (number, percentage)	4 (29%)	1 (14%)	3 (30%)	0.73
SAPS II (median ± IQR)	39.0 ± 13.5	45.0 ± 21.0	43.5 ± 20.5	0.67
SOFA at inclusion (median ± IQR)	6 ± 4	7 ± 2	7.5 ± 3.5	0.06
CRP at inclusion (mg/L, median ± IQR)	217 ± 325	211 ± 195	273 ± 313	0.80
Number of samples per patient (range)	1–5	1–5	1–9	–
Cause of lung injury				
Pneumonia at inclusion (number, percentage)	5 (36%)	5 (71%)	8 (80%)	0.081
Aspiration (number, percentage)	1 (7%)	2 (29%)	3 (30%)	0.29
Septic shock at inclusion (number, percentage)	5 (36%)	6 (86%)	8 (80%)	0.043
Extra pulmonary cause (number, percentage)	–	3 (43%)	2 (20%)	0.038
Steroid therapy[a] (number, percentage)	1 (7%)	1 (14%)	5 (50%)	0.051
Vasoactive agent therapy[a] (number, percentage)	7 (50%)	7 (100%)	6 (60%)	0.065
Lung injury score at inclusion (median ± IQR)	0.67 ± 0.91	2.33 ± 0.66	3.00 ± 0.72	<0.0001
Respiratory variables				
Positive end-expiratory pressure, cmH20 (median ± IQR)	5 ± 0.5	8 ± 1	9 ± 2	0.001
PaO_2/FiO_2 at inclusion mmHg (median ± IQR)	253 ± 85	210 ± 49	67 ± 29	<0.0001
$PaCO_2$ at inclusion mmHg (median ± IQR)	41 ± 5	43 ± 4	43 ± 4	0.72
ECMO[a] (number, percentage)	–	–	6 (60%)	0.0004
Mortality at day 28 (number, percentage)	4 (28%)	2 (29%)	6 (60%)	0.26

ARDS acute respiratory distress syndrome, *LIS* Lung Injury Score [23], *SOFA* Sequential Organ Failure Assessment, *SAPS II* Simplified Acute Physiology Score II [21], *ECMO* Extracorporeal membrane oxygenation, *CRP* C-reactive protein, *IQR* interquartile range

p values: determined by Kruskal–Wallis test or Fisher's exact test for continuous and categorical variables, respectively

[a] During the ICU stay

Chi-square test to assess whether or not two variables were independent, we found that neutrophil *gilz* gene expression was associated with ARDS ($p < 0.05$) but not with septic shock or pneumonia (Table 2). The percentage of "*gilz*-positive" patients was higher in the severe ARDS group (70%) than in the mild/moderate ARDS group (29%) and than in the ventilated controls (14%). Corticosteroid therapy might play a role in *gilz* induction as neutrophils from steroid-treated patients expressed *gilz* in 71% of cases (Table 2). However, these results also suggest that steroid therapy was not required for *gilz* expression and that other inducers could be active. This model also confirmed that neutrophil *gilz* expression was not linked to administration of vasoactive agents (Table 2). Finally, *gilz* positivity was not linked to day-28 mortality among ARDS patients (Table 2).

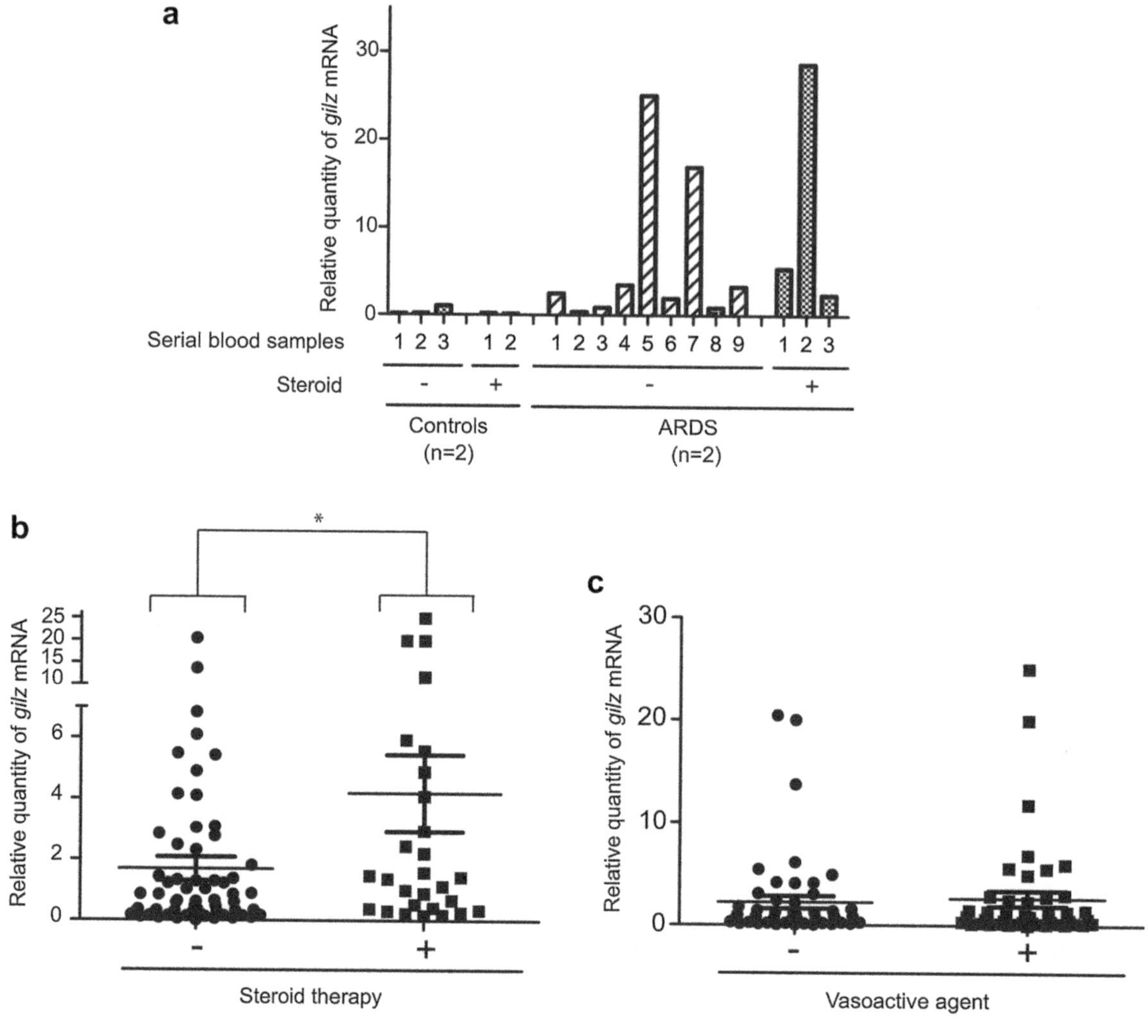

Fig. 1 **a** Kinetics of *gilz* mRNA expression in neutrophils from 2 representative controls and 2 representative ARDS patients. The number of serial blood samples obtained (every 2 days until extubation or death) is indicated ($n = 2$–9 per patient, depending on the patient). Some patients received hydrocortisone hemisuccinate (200 mg/day; steroid). Relative quantity of *gilz* mRNA was expressed as *gilz* expression level divided by the mean of *gapdh* and *b2m* levels. **b** Implication of corticoid therapy in *gilz* mRNA expression in all samples studied. Results are expressed as the relative quantity of *gilz* mRNA (mean ± standard error of the mean). *$p < 0.05$, Mann–Whitney test. **c** Implication of vasoactive agent administration in all samples studied. Results are expressed as the relative quantity of *gilz* mRNA (mean ± standard error of the mean). *ARDS* acute respiratory distress syndrome, *GILZ* glucocorticoid-induced leucine zipper

Discussion

The main findings of this pilot study are that GILZ, a potent regulator of inflammation, can be induced in ARDS patients' blood neutrophils, that its expression is transient, and that mRNA levels are related to ARDS severity. Therapeutic GILZ upregulation might thus constitute a potential beneficial approach in ARDS.

During ARDS, lung edema and endothelial/epithelial cell damage promote the recruitment and activation of neutrophils in interstitial and bronchoalveolar spaces. The overwhelming inflammatory response associated with ARDS not only targets the lung but also causes persistent elevation of circulating protease and cytokine levels, and primed or hyperactivated neutrophil numbers, leading to extrapulmonary organ dysfunction [2, 33]. The mechanisms that regulate this acute, severe inflammatory response are poorly understood. Neutrophils themselves might help to dampen this inflammation, by releasing IL-1RA or TGF-β, by adopting an immunosuppressive phenotype (CD16^{bright} CD62-L^{dim}) or by engaging in crosstalk with other immune cells [34, 35]. Indeed, we have previously shown that neutrophil-derived extracellular traps (NETs) can downregulate dendritic cell activation in vitro, thereby inducing Th2 T

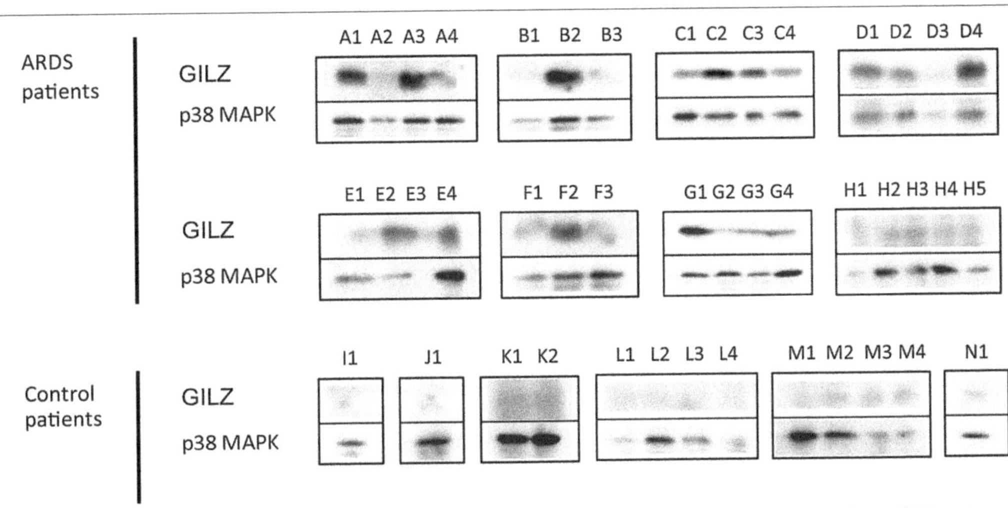

Fig. 2 Kinetics of GILZ protein expression in ARDS patients and controls. Representative serial Western blot data for 8 ARDS patients (A to H) and 6 controls (I to N) performed every 2 days. p38 MAPK expression served as control. *A1* sample 1 of patient A, *A2* sample 2 of patient A

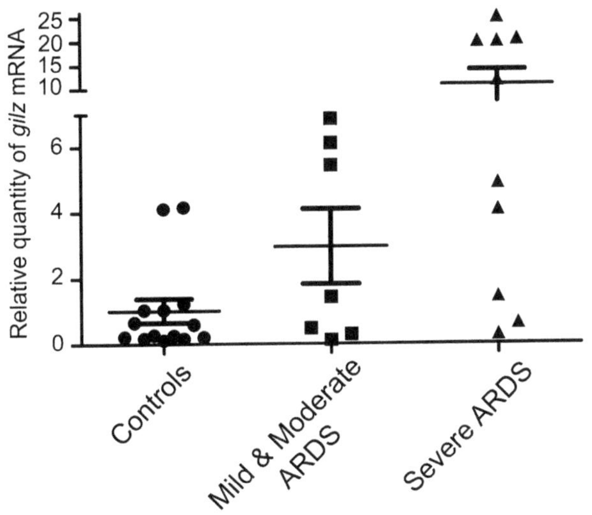

Fig. 3 *gilz* mRNA expression in the neutrophils of ARDS and controls (highest point of *gilz* expression for each patient). Results are expressed as the mean ± standard error of the mean. Relative quantity of *gilz* mRNA was expressed as *gilz* expression level divided by the mean of *gapdh* and *b2m* levels. *ARDS* acute respiratory distress syndrome, *GILZ* glucocorticoid-induced leucine zipper

lymphocyte polarization [27]. Moreover, a new neutrophil-related gene signature has been described in patients with early sepsis-induced ARDS, based on two anti-inflammatory genes: *OLFM4* (encoding olfactomedin 4) and *LCN2* (encoding lipocalin 2) [36]. The main objective of the present study was to determine whether GILZ, an anti-inflammatory protein that we recently found to be expressed by human neutrophils in particular stimulatory conditions in vitro [17], is modulated during ARDS.

We show for the first time that *gilz* is expressed by blood neutrophils of most severe ARDS patients but in only a minority of mild/moderate ARDS patients or ARDS-free ventilated controls. Interestingly, GILZ expression during ARDS was transient. The very short half-life of *gilz* transcripts, of around 2 h in murine lymphocytes [16] and macrophages [37], would explain, at least in part, this transient expression. Our study provides new insights into the neutrophil-related events, adding a new gene in the recently described signature [36].

Neutrophil *gilz* mRNA levels were related to ARDS severity, being significantly higher in severe ARDS patients (reaching levels of 7–9 times the threshold value) than in mild/moderate ARDS patients and in ventilated controls. Moreover, patients receiving ECMO had higher *gilz* expression than patients without ECMO. This rescue therapy is used in severe ARDS when conventional mechanical ventilation fails [5, 38]. As ECMO has been shown to have pro-inflammatory effects in vivo [39, 40], it is conceivable that GILZ induction was aimed at compensating for these effects.

In order to better document the clinical relevance of *gilz* expression in this setting, we used the linear mixed-effects regression model to compare circulating levels of two classical markers of inflammation (CRP and extracellular DNA) in the three patient groups. CRP levels did not differ across the three groups and did not correlate with the neutrophil *gilz* expression level, suggesting that GILZ expression is not only induced by inflammatory signals. Extracellular DNA levels are a marker of NET release. NETs are decondensed DNA fibers that bear histones and several proteins from the granular and

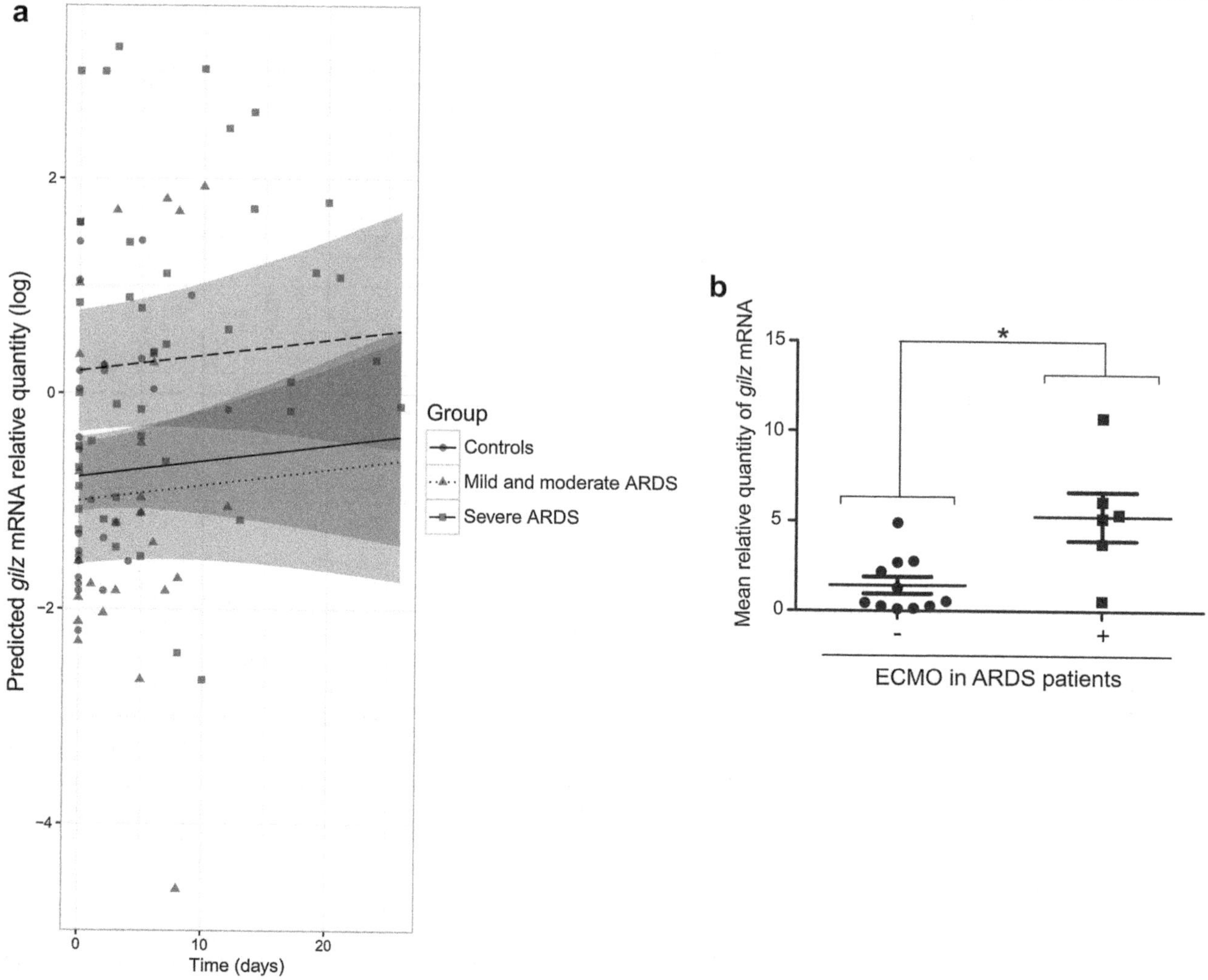

Fig. 4 *gilz* gene expression in relation to ARDS severity. **a** *gilz* expression levels predicted by a linear mixed model. Controls (full line), mild/moderate ARDS patients (*small dotted line*), and severe ARDS patients (*large dotted line*) are represented. For each prediction, the confidence interval is represented by the *gray region*. Fixed effects of the model are: − 0.773 − 0.222 × mild/moderate ARDS + 0.984 × severe ARDS + 0.014 × time. All values are represented on the graph: *circles* for controls, *triangles* for mild/moderate ARDS patients, and *squares* for severe ARDS patients. **b** Mean *gilz* mRNA expression in neutrophils from ARDS patients with ($n = 6$) and without extracorporeal membrane oxygenation ($n = 11$). Results are expressed as the mean ± standard error of the mean *gilz* mRNA value. (*$p < 0.05$, Mann–Whitney test)

cytoplasmic compartments, which can induce lung damage [41]. We found that circulating extracellular DNA levels were similarly elevated in the three patient groups, independently of clinical severity. This concurs with the results of Yildiz et al. [42] who found that mechanical ventilation induced netosis in an animal model of sepsis, but that netosis had no major pathogenic effect. However, netosis intensity has been linked to severity in two models of sterile ARDS: acid-aspiration-induced ARDS [43] and transfusion-related acute lung injury [44]. *Gilz* expression might thus be a more specific marker of ARDS severity than other markers such as CRP and NETs.

The stimuli leading to neutrophil *gilz* expression in vivo are probably multiple in ARDS. Even if steroid therapy did not appear to be a prerequisite for *gilz* expression, it was observed in almost ¾ of corticosteroid-treated patients. We found a near-significant negative correlation between *gilz* levels and the PaO_2/FiO_2 ratio, suggesting that hypoxia could play a role. Consistent with our results, GILZ expression was recently reported to be induced by hypoxia in vitro, in both murine macrophages [45] and human epithelial cells [46]. The presence of areas of hypoxia being a prominent feature of inflamed tissues, GILZ expression could be induced not

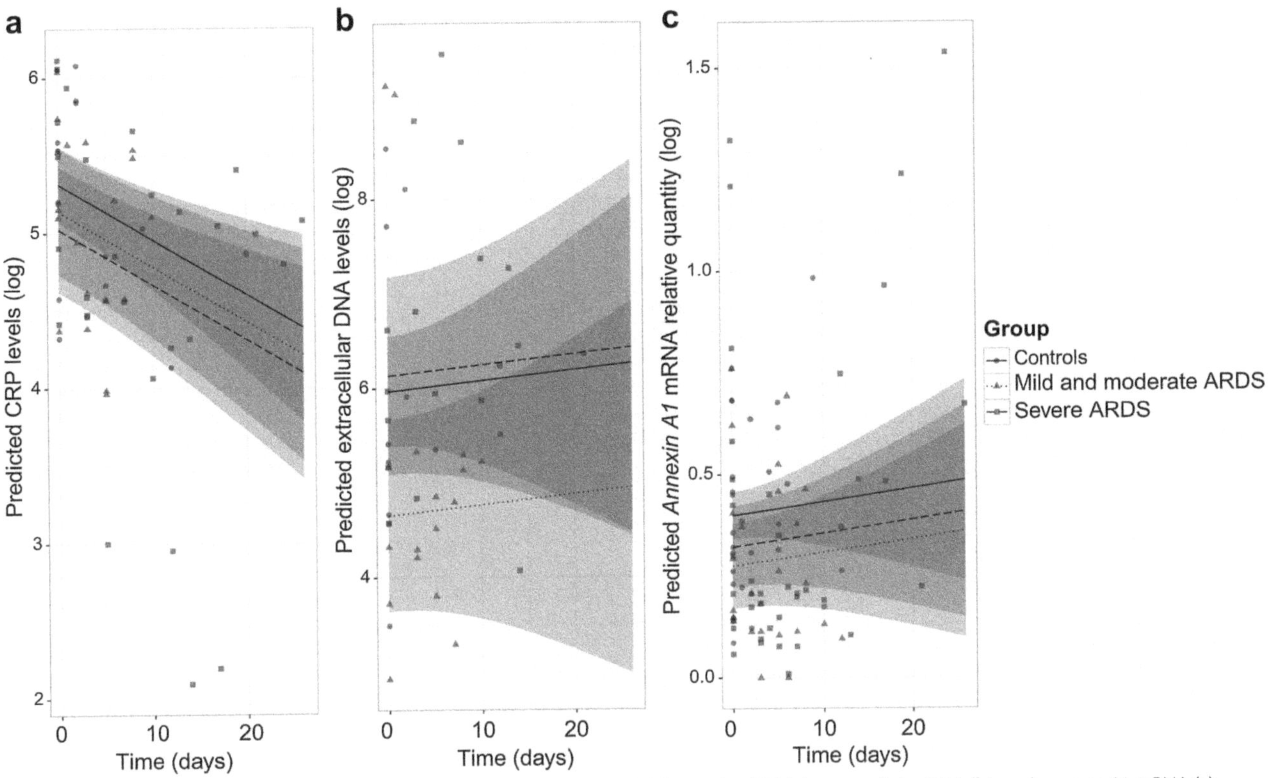

Fig. 5 CRP, extracellular DNA and *annexin A1* mRNA levels in relation to ARDS severity. CRP (**a**), extracellular DNA (**b**), and *annexin A1* mRNA (**c**) levels predicted by a linear mixed model. controls (*full line*), mild/moderate ARDS patients (*small dotted line*), and severe ARDS patients (*large dotted line*) are represented. For each prediction, the confidence interval is represented by the *gray region*. All values are represented on the graph: *circles* for controls, *triangles* for mild/moderate ARDS patients, and squares for severe ARDS patients. Fixed effects of the model with the CRP are: 5.314 − 0.175 × mild/moderate ARDS − 0.291 × severe ARDS − 0.036 × time. Fixed effects of the model with DNA are: 5.969 − 1.311 × mild/moderate ARDS + 0.167 × severe ARDS − 0.011 × time. Fixed effects of the model with *annexin A1* are: 0.400 − 0.125 × mild/moderate ARDS − 0.077 × severe ARDS + 0.003 × time

only by anti-inflammatory signals such as glucocorticoids (GCs), but also by the inflammatory context as previously hypothesized in arthritis [13].

We recently demonstrated that the induction of neutrophil *gilz* expression promotes apoptosis [17]. Moreover, the combination of GCs and hypoxia has also been recently reported to induce neutrophil apoptosis in vitro [47]. Taken together, we could postulate that the induction of neutrophil *gilz* expression by GCs, hypoxia, and/or other inflammatory signals could contribute to neutrophil apoptosis, necessary for lung repair.

Neutrophil *gilz* expression may thus help to resolve inflammation. There is growing interest in the possible role of two GC-induced proteins (Annexin A1 and GILZ) in the anti-inflammatory effects of GCs in vivo. Annexin A1 is upregulated during natural resolution of acute inflammation and has been shown to have pro-resolving and immunosuppressive properties both in vitro [48, 49] and in vivo at the site of inflammation [18]. It was also recently demonstrated that Annexin A1 can control GILZ expression [19], revealing close cooperation between the two proteins in the resolution of inflammation. Here, we found that blood neutrophil *annexin A1* mRNA levels were not linked to ARDS severity, suggesting that *annexin A1* is rather a general marker of inflammation resolution.

An anti-inflammatory role of endogenous GILZ in humans was first suggested by Beaulieu et al. [13] in rheumatoid arthritis. More recently, Vago et al. [18] demonstrated that GILZ administration accelerated and improved resolution of inflammation in a mouse model of acute lung injury (ALI). Interestingly, in a mouse model of LPS-induced ALI, we have found that GILZ is expressed in alveolar neutrophils and peaks when pulmonary inflammation is maximal (Espinasse et al., unpublished observations). GILZ might thus participate in the regulation of inflammation in vivo.

This prospective observational pilot study has several limitations. First, we had no access to alveolar neutrophils. Second, the cohort size was modest and not

Table 2 Characteristics of "*gilz*-positive" patients

Overall patients $n = 31$	ARDS		Steroids[a]		Vasoactive agents[a]		Pneumonia at inclusion		Septic shock at inclusion		Vital status on day 28	
	No $n = 14$	Yes $n = 17$	No $n = 24$	Yes $n = 7$	No $n = 10$	Yes $n = 21$	No $n = 13$	Yes $n = 18$	No $n = 12$	Yes $n = 19$	Dead $n = 12$	Alive $n = 19$
gilz-positive patients	2/14 (14%)	9/17 (53%)	6/24 (25%)	5/7 (71%)	3/10 (30%)	8/21 (38%)	3/13 (23%)	8/18 (44%)	3/12 (25%)	8/19 (42%)	4/12 (33%)	7/19 (37%)
p value	0.025		0.024		0.660		0.220		0.332		0.842	

"*gilz*-positive" patients had *gilz* mRNA levels above the threshold in at least one of the first two serial samples

p values: determined by the Chi-square test

[a] At least one injection

sufficiently large for biomarker exploration. Third, we did not perform a power analysis because no reference data are available in this setting. Finally, because blood samples were obtained prospectively during usual care of patients until death or extubation, the number of samples is different for each patient and some patients may have a longer follow-up than others. This data attrition can be viewed as a missing data issue, and mixed effect modeling that we used in this study has been found robust in this setting [50], as they implicitly impute outcome trajectories beyond the time of death or extubation. More complex modeling techniques could have been considered in this situation [51], but they were not applicable because of the relatively small sample size of this pilot study.

Conclusions

We show for the first time that GILZ, a potent regulator of inflammation and an inducer of apoptosis, can be expressed by blood neutrophils of ARDS patients at both the gene and protein level. GILZ expression was transient and could occur without steroid therapy. Interestingly, the highest neutrophil *gilz* expression levels were observed in patients with severe ARDS, and these levels correlated with the PaO_2/FiO_2 ratio; neutrophil GILZ may prove to be a potential biomarker for ARDS severity in a larger study. These data also suggest that blood neutrophil activation during ARDS might not only contribute to lung injury but also participate in endogenous inflammation regulation.

Abbreviations

ARDS: acute respiratory distress syndrome; ALI: acute lung injury; CRP: C-reactive protein; ECMO: extracorporeal membrane oxygenation; FiO_2: fraction of inspired oxygen; ICU: intensive care unit; GCs: glucocorticoids; GILZ: glucocorticoid-induced leucine zipper; NETs: neutrophil extracellular traps; PaO_2: partial pressure of arterial oxygen; PEEP: positive end-expiratory pressure; ROS: reactive oxygen species; SAPS II: Simplified Acute Physiology Score II; SOFA: Sequential Organ Failure Assessment Score; SS: septic shock.

Authors' contributions

MAE and BN carried out quantitative PCR and Western blot. VG and LdC performed extracellular DNA analysis. PP, GD, and PM conducted patient inclusions. DH performed the statistical analysis. MAE, FT, SCM, PM, and MP participated in the design of the study and in the interpretation of the results. ABV conceived the study and participated in its design and coordination. MAE, SCM, and ABV wrote the manuscript. All authors read and approved the final manuscript.

Author details

[1]

INSERM UMR-996 - Inflammation, Chemokines and Immunopathology, Univ Paris-Sud, Faculté de pharmacie, Université Paris-Saclay, 5 rue JB Clément, 92296 Châtenay-Malabry Cedex, France. [2] Département d'Anesthésie-Réanimation, Hôpital Bichat-Claude Bernard, AP-HP, Paris, France. [3] Université Paris Diderot, Sorbonne Paris Cité, Paris, France. [4] Département d'Epidémiologie et Recherche Clinique, Assistance Publique-Hôpitaux de Paris Hôpital Bichat, INSERM, CIE 801, Université Paris Diderot, Sorbonne Paris Cité, Paris, France. [5] Laboratoire d'immunologie, «Autoimmunité et hypersensibilités», Hôpital Bichat-Claude Bernard, AP-HP, Paris, France.

Acknowledgements

The authors particularly thank Pr Jean Mantz (Department of Anesthesia, Critical Care and Pain Medicine, European Georges Pompidou Hospital, Paris Descartes University) for his critical reading of the manuscript. The authors thank Cécile Joie, Inès Mallet, Elsa Le Bonhomme, and Raed Daher for their scientific and technical support. The authors acknowledge Claudine Deloménie from IPSIT, Trans-Prot facility, for her support in transcriptomic analysis and the Region Ile de France for financial support to this facility. We also thank Dr. Jérémie Botton (INSERM UMR-S 1018) for help with statistical analysis. Marie-Alix Espinasse is a fellow of La Fondation du Souffle et du Fonds de Dotation de Recherche en Santé Respiratoire.

Competing interests

The authors declare that they have no competing interests.

Funding

The study was funded by INSERM institutional grants.

References

1. Ranieri VM, Rubenfeld GD, Thompson BT, Ferguson ND, Caldwell E, Fan E, et al. Acute respiratory distress syndrome: the Berlin Definition. JAMA. 2012;307(23):2526–33.
2. Williams AE, Chambers RC. The mercurial nature of neutrophils: Still an enigma in ARDS? Am J Physiol Lung Cell Mol Physiol. 2014;306(3):L217–30.
3. Fialkow L, Fochesatto Filho L, Bozzetti MC, Milani AR, Rodrigues Filho EM, Ladniuk RM, et al. Neutrophil apoptosis: a marker of disease severity in sepsis and sepsis-induced acute respiratory distress syndrome. Crit Care. 2006;10(6):R155.
4. Chopra M, Reuben JS, Sharma AC. Acute lung injury: apoptosis and signaling mechanisms. Exp Biol Med (Maywood). 2009;234(4):361–71.
5. Klinzing S, Wenger U, Steiger P, Starck CT, Wilhelm M, Schuepbach RA, et al. External validation of scores proposed for estimation of survival probability of patients with severe adult respiratory distress syndrome undergoing extracorporeal membrane oxygenation therapy: a retrospective study. Crit Care. 2015;19:142.
6. Monsel A, Zhu YG, Gennai S, Hao Q, Hu S, Rouby JJ, et al. Therapeutic effects of human mesenchymal stem cell-derived microvesicles in severe pneumonia in mice. Am J Respir Crit Care Med. 2015;192(3):324–36.
7. Cardinal-Fernandez P, Ferruelo A, Esteban A, Lorente JA. Characteristics of micro RNAs and their potential relevance for the diagnosis and therapy of the acute respiratory distress syndrome: from bench to bedside. Transl Res. 2016;169:102–11.
8. Yu ZX, Ji MS, Yan J, Cai Y, Liu J, Yang HF, et al. The ratio of Th17/Treg cells as a risk indicator in early acute respiratory distress syndrome. Crit Care. 2015;19:82.
9. Horita N, Hashimoto S, Miyazawa N, Fujita H, Kojima R, Inoue M, et al. Impact of corticosteroids on mortality in patients with acute respiratory distress syndrome: a systematic review and meta-analysis. Intern Med. 2015;54(12):1473–9.
10. Meduri GU, Bridges L, Shih MC, Marik PE, Siemieniuk RA, Kocak M. Prolonged glucocorticoid treatment is associated with improved ARDS outcomes: analysis of individual patients' data from four randomized trials and trial-level meta-analysis of the updated literature. Intensive Care Med. 2016;42:829–40.
11. Ayroldi E, Riccardi C. Glucocorticoid-induced leucine zipper (GILZ): a new important mediator of glucocorticoid action. Faseb J. 2009;23(11):3649–58.

12. Beaulieu E, Morand EF. Role of GILZ in immune regulation, glucocorticoid actions and rheumatoid arthritis. Nat Rev. 2011;7(6):340–8.
13. Beaulieu E, Ngo D, Santos L, Yang YH, Smith M, Jorgensen C, et al. Glucocorticoid-induced leucine zipper is an endogenous antiinflammatory mediator in arthritis. Arthritis Rheum. 2010;62(9):2651–61.
14. Latre de Late P, Pepin A, Assaf-Vandecasteele H, Espinasse C, Nicolas V, Asselin-Labat ML, et al. Glucocorticoid-induced leucine zipper (GILZ) promotes the nuclear exclusion of FOXO3 in a Crm1-dependent manner. J Biol Chem. 2010;285(8):5594–605.
15. Asselin-Labat ML, David M, Biola-Vidamment A, Lecoeuche D, Zennaro MC, Bertoglio J, et al. GILZ, a new target for the transcription factor FoxO3, protects T lymphocytes from interleukin-2 withdrawal-induced apoptosis. Blood. 2004;104(1):215–23.
16. Pepin A, Espinasse MA, Latre de Late P, Szely N, Pallardy M, Biola-Vidamment A. TSC-22 promotes interleukin-2-deprivation induced apoptosis in T-lymphocytes. J Cell Biochem. 2016;117(8):1855–68.
17. Espinasse MA, Pepin A, Virault-Rocroy P, Szely N, Chollet-Martin S, Pallardy M, et al. Glucocorticoid-induced leucine zipper is expressed in human neutrophils and promotes apoptosis through Mcl-1 down-regulation. J Innate Immun. 2016;8(1):81–96.
18. Vago JP, Tavares LP, Garcia CC, Lima KM, Perucci LO, Vieira EL, et al. The role and effects of glucocorticoid-induced leucine zipper in the context of inflammation resolution. J Immunol. 2015;194(10):4940–50.
19. Yang YH, Aeberli D, Dacumos A, Xue JR, Morand EF. Annexin-1 regulates macrophage IL-6 and TNF via glucocorticoid-induced leucine zipper. J Immunol. 2009;183(2):1435–45.
20. Vago JP, Nogueira CR, Tavares LP, Soriani FM, Lopes F, Russo RC, et al. Annexin A1 modulates natural and glucocorticoid-induced resolution of inflammation by enhancing neutrophil apoptosis. J Leukoc Biol. 2012;92(2):249–58.
21. Le Gall JR, Lemeshow S, Saulnier F. A new simplified acute physiology score (SAPS II) based on a European/North American multicenter study. JAMA. 1993;270(24):2957–63.
22. Vincent JL, Moreno R, Takala J, Willatts S, De Mendonca A, Bruining H, et al. The SOFA (Sepsis-related Organ Failure Assessment) score to describe organ dysfunction/failure. On behalf of the Working Group on Sepsis-Related Problems of the European Society of Intensive Care Medicine. Intensive Care Med. 1996;22(7):707–10.
23. Murray JF, Matthay MA, Luce JM, Flick MR. An expanded definition of the adult respiratory distress syndrome. Am Rev Respir Dis. 1988;138(3):720–3.
24. Bein T, Grasso S, Moerer O, Quintel M, Guerin C, Deja M, et al. The standard of care of patients with ARDS: ventilatory settings and rescue therapies for refractory hypoxemia. Intensive Care Med. 2016;42(5):699–711.
25. Dellinger RP, Levy MM, Rhodes A, Annane D, Gerlach H, Opal SM, et al. Surviving sepsis campaign: international guidelines for management of severe sepsis and septic shock: 2012. Crit Care Med. 2013;41(2):580–637.
26. Barrientos L, Marin-Esteban V, de Chaisemartin L, Le-Moal VL, Sandre C, Bianchini E, et al. An improved strategy to recover large fragments of functional human neutrophil extracellular traps. Front Immunol. 2013;4:166.
27. Barrientos L, Bignon A, Gueguen C, de Chaisemartin L, Gorges R, Sandre C, et al. Neutrophil extracellular traps downregulate lipopolysaccharide-induced activation of monocyte-derived dendritic cells. J Immunol. 2014;193(11):5689–98.
28. Migdal C, Botton J, El Ali Z, Azoury ME, Guldemann J, Gimenez-Arnau E, et al. Reactivity of chemical sensitizers toward amino acids in cellulo plays a role in the activation of the Nrf2-ARE pathway in human monocyte dendritic cells and the THP-1 cell line. Toxicol Sci. 2013;133(2):259–74.
29. Vandesompele J, De Preter K, Pattyn F, Poppe B, Van Roy N, De Paepe A, et al. Accurate normalization of real-time quantitative RT-PCR data by geometric averaging of multiple internal control genes. Genome Biol. 2002;3(7):RESEARCH0034.
30. Pfaffl MW. A new mathematical model for relative quantification in real-time RT-PCR. Nucleic Acids Res. 2001;29(9):e45.
31. Hellemans J, Mortier G, De Paepe A, Speleman F, Vandesompele J. qBase relative quantification framework and software for management and automated analysis of real-time quantitative PCR data. Genome Biol. 2007;8(2):R19.
32. Allou N, Bronchard R, Guglielminotti J, Dilly MP, Provenchere S, Lucet JC, et al. Risk factors for postoperative pneumonia after cardiac surgery and development of a preoperative risk score. Crit Care Med. 2014;42(5):1150–6.
33. Summers C, Singh NR, White JF, Mackenzie IM, Johnston A, Solanki C, et al. Pulmonary retention of primed neutrophils: a novel protective host response, which is impaired in the acute respiratory distress syndrome. Thorax. 2014;69(7):623–9.
34. Tecchio C, Micheletti A, Cassatella MA. Neutrophil-derived cytokines: facts beyond expression. Front Immunol. 2014;5:508.
35. Scapini P, Cassatella MA. Social networking of human neutrophils within the immune system. Blood. 2014;124(5):710–9.
36. Kangelaris KN, Prakash A, Liu KD, Aouizerat B, Woodruff PG, Erle DJ, et al. Increased expression of neutrophil-related genes in patients with early sepsis-induced ARDS. Am J Physiol Lung Cell Mol Physiol. 2015;308(11):L1102–13.
37. Hoppstadter J, Diesel B, Eifler LK, Schmid T, Brune B, Kiemer AK. Glucocorticoid-induced leucine zipper is downregulated in human alveolar macrophages upon Toll-like receptor activation. Eur J Immunol. 2012;42(5):1282–93.
38. Sharma NS, Wille KM, Zhi D, Thannickal VJ, Brodie DM, Hoopes CW, et al. Use of ECMO in the management of severe acute respiratory distress syndrome: a survey of academic medical centers in the United States. ASAIO J. 2015;61(5):556–63.
39. Maclaren G, Butt W. Extracorporeal membrane oxygenation and sepsis. Crit Care Resusc. 2007;9(1):76–80.
40. Chen Q, Yu W, Shi J, Shen J, Hu Y, Gong J, et al. The effect of extracorporeal membrane oxygenation therapy on systemic oxidative stress injury in a porcine model. Artif Organs. 2014;38(5):426–31.
41. Cheng OZ, Palaniyar N. NET balancing: a problem in inflammatory lung diseases. Front Immunol. 2013;4:1.
42. Yildiz C, Palaniyar N, Otulakowski G, Khan MA, Post M, Kuebler WM, et al. Mechanical ventilation induces neutrophil extracellular trap formation. Anesthesiology. 2015;122(4):864–75.
43. Zhang Y, Wen Z, Guan L, Jiang P, Gu T, Zhao J, et al. Extracellular histones play an inflammatory role in acid aspiration-induced acute respiratory distress syndrome. Anesthesiology. 2015;122(1):127–39.
44. Caudrillier A, Kessenbrock K, Gilliss BM, Nguyen JX, Marques MB, Monestier M, et al. Platelets induce neutrophil extracellular traps in transfusion-related acute lung injury. J Clin Investig. 2012;122(7):2661–71.
45. Wang Y, Ma YY, Song XL, Cai HY, Chen JC, Song LN, et al. Upregulations of glucocorticoid-induced leucine zipper by hypoxia and glucocorticoid inhibit proinflammatory cytokines under hypoxic conditions in macrophages. J Immunol. 2012;188(1):222–9.
46. Lim W, Park C, Shim MK, Lee YH, Lee YM, Lee Y. Glucocorticoids suppress hypoxia-induced COX-2 and hypoxia inducible factor-1alpha expression through the induction of glucocorticoid-induced leucine zipper. Br J Pharmacol. 2014;171(3):735–45.
47. Marwick JA, Dorward DA, Lucas CD, Jones KO, Sheldrake TA, Fox S, et al. Oxygen levels determine the ability of glucocorticoids to influence neutrophil survival in inflammatory environments. J Leukoc Biol. 2013;94(6):1285–92.
48. Ortega-Gomez A, Perretti M, Soehnlein O. Resolution of inflammation: an integrated view. EMBO Mol Med. 2013;5(5):661–74.
49. Sugimoto MA, Vago JP, Teixeira MM, Sousa LP. Annexin A1 and the resolution of inflammation: modulation of neutrophil recruitment, apoptosis, and clearance. J Immunol Res. 2016;2016:8239258.
50. Peters SA, Bots ML, den Ruijter HM, Palmer MK, Grobbee DE, Crouse JR 3rd, et al. Multiple imputation of missing repeated outcome measurements did not add to linear mixed-effects models. J Clin Epidemiol. 2012;65(6):686–95.
51. Kurland BF, Johnson LL, Egleston BL, Diehr PH. Longitudinal data with follow-up truncated by death: match the analysis method to research aims. Stat Sci. 2009;24(2):211.

Venovenous extracorporeal membrane oxygenation devices-related colonisations and infections

Guillemette Thomas[1], Sami Hraiech[1,2], Nadim Cassir[2], Samuel Lehingue[1,2], Romain Rambaud[1,2], Sandrine Wiramus[3], Christophe Guervilly[1], Fanny Klasen[1,2], Mélanie Adda[1], Stéphanie Dizier[1], Antoine Roch[2,4], Laurent Papazian[1,2] and Jean-Marie Forel[1,2*]

Abstract

Background: Nosocomial infections occurring during extracorporeal membrane oxygenation (ECMO) support have already been reported, but few studied infections directly related to ECMO devices. This study aims to evaluate the rate of both colonisations and infections related to ECMO devices at the time of ECMO removal.

Results: We included all consecutive adult patients treated with venovenous ECMO (VV-ECMO) for at least 48 h during a 34-month study. At the time of ECMO removal, blood cultures, swab cultures on insertion cannula site and intravascular cannula extremity cultures were systematically performed. Each ECMO device was classified according to the infectious status into three groups: (1) uninfected/uncolonised ECMO device, (2) ECMO device colonisation and (3) ECMO device infection. Ninety-nine patients underwent 103 VV-ECMO, representing 1472 ECMO days. The ECMO device infection rate was 9.7% (10 events), including 7 ECMO device-related bloodstream infections (6.8%). The ECMO device colonisation rate was 32% (33 events). No difference was observed between the three groups, regarding days of mechanical ventilation, ICU length of stay, ICU mortality and in-hospital mortality. We observed a longer ECMO duration in the ECMO device colonisation group as compared to the uninfected/uncolonised ECMO device group [12 (9–20 days) vs. 5 days (5–16 days), respectively, $p < 0.05$].

Conclusions: At the time of ECMO removal, systematic blood culture and intravascular extremity cannula culture may help to diagnose ECMO device-related infection. We reported a quite low infection rate related to ECMO device. Further studies are needed to evaluate the benefits of systematic strategies of cannula culture at the time of ECMO removal.

Keywords: Venovenous extracorporeal membrane oxygenation, Device-related infections, Device-related colonisation, Infection rate, Colonisation rate

Background

Venovenous extracorporeal membrane oxygenation (VV-ECMO) has become a widely accepted treatment option for life-threatening acute respiratory failure when mechanical ventilation (MV) and adjunctive measures fail to provide adequate gas exchange or when lung rest cannot be achieved due to high ventilator requirements [1, 2]. Over the last two decades, the technique has improved significantly, and several studies have reported encouraging survival rates using VV-ECMO in adults with acute respiratory distress syndrome (ARDS) [3–6]. However, major adverse events have been described, among which infections seem to be the most frequent [1, 6]. In 2011, the Extracorporeal Life Support Organization (ELSO) reported an incidence of 11.7% proven infections in 20,741 ECMO cases for a rate of 15.4 per 1000 ECMO

*Correspondence: jean-marie.forel@ap-hm.fr
[1] Hôpital Nord, Réanimation des Détresses Respiratoires et des Infections Sévères, Assistance Publique–Hôpitaux de Marseille, 13015 Marseille, France
Full list of author information is available at the end of the article

days [7]. To date, most of the studies described nosocomial infections or bloodstream infections (BSI) occurring during ECMO support, but very few studied infections directly related to ECMO devices. Moreover, these studies often mixed venovenous and venoarterial ECMO support, which are very different devices regarding the type of patients, the duration of ECMO and the cannulation procedure [8, 9].

The main objective of this study was to evaluate the rates of both infections and colonisations related to ECMO devices in VV-ECMO adult patients at the time of ECMO removal.

Methods

Study design

An epidemiologic, prospective, observational study was conducted in the 14-bed medical intensive care unit (ICU) of a teaching hospital (Hôpital Nord, Marseille, France), a regional referral centre for the treatment of acute severe respiratory failure. The study was approved by the ethical committee of the «Société de Réanimation de Langue Française». According to French law, no consent for the study was required because it did not modify existing diagnostic or therapeutic strategies.

Patients and ECMO indications

We prospectively included all consecutive adult patients treated with VV-ECMO for at least 48 h during a 34-month study. The ECMO-based programme includes a mobile unit that is able to initiate ECMO in referring hospitals of our region (Provence-Alpes-Côte d'Azur) before transfer to our ECMO referral centre [5].

The decision to initiate ECMO is based on the following: persistent hypoxaemia, defined as $PaO_2/FiO_2 \leq 70$ mmHg for at least 6 h under FiO2 at 1 despite optimisation of mechanical ventilation or $PaO_2/FiO_2 < 100$ mmHg with a Pplat value greater than 35 cmH_2O or respiratory acidosis with $pH \leq 7.15$ despite a respiratory rate greater than 35/min. Exclusion criteria for ECMO included the following: any contraindications to heparin treatment, Sequential Organ Failure Assessment (SOFA) score > 16 [10], moribund patients or those with decisions to limit therapeutic interventions.

ECMO protocol

Venovenous ECMO was instituted using percutaneous cannulation by cardiac surgeons, typically in a femoral–jugular configuration but also in femoral–femoral configuration, especially when ECMO was used as a bridge to lung transplantation. We used centrifugal pumps (Bioconsole 560; Medtronic Perfusion Systems, Minneapolis, MN, USA) with a flow of 3–5 L/min in all patients. Circuits were heparin-coated and composed of Quadrox D with Bioline Coating oxygenators (Maquet, Hirrlingen, Germany), 17–25-Fr cannulae (Edwards Lifesciences, Irvine, CA, USA) and intersept polyvinyl chloride (PVC) class VI tubing (Medtronic, Watford, Hertfordshire, UK).

All cannulas were inserted using strict sterile precautions consistent with Healthcare Infection Control Practices Advisory Committee guidelines (HICPAC guidelines) [11]. For each patient, the cannula insertion site was cleansed with 96% ethanol solution containing 5% povidone-iodine. Sterile drapes were placed over the insertion site. No specific antibioprophylaxis was used at the time of cannulation. Occlusive dressings were used.

A highly trained ICU nursing staff achieved standardised cannula care every 72 h or earlier if clinically indicated (dirty or bloody dressing). If necessary (haemolysis, fibrinolysis), the ECMO circuit was changed using strict sterile precautions as detailed above.

When the ECMO was removed, specimens were systematically collected as follows: (a) blood cultures were sampled from the central venous catheter (CVC), arterial catheter and post-membrane oxygenator. The blood culture vials used for aerobic and anaerobic cultures (Bactec; Becton–Dickinson, Sparks, MD, USA) were incubated for 5 days. After the incubation period and automatic culture detection (Bactec 9240; Becton–Dickinson, Sparks, MD, USA), Gram staining was performed, and the samples were cultured on 5% sheep blood and chocolate agar plates at 37 °C under aerobic and anaerobic atmospheric conditions for all positive blood cultures. (b) Swabs were sampled on the drainage and return cannula site skin just before cleaning with 5% povidone-iodine antiseptic. The culture technique is described as follows. (c) The intravascular extremity of the drainage and return cannula were cut in a sterile manner and analysed by a culture technique described as follows. The extremities of the cannulas, the central venous and the arterial catheter tips when removed, were mixed with tryptic soy broth; 10 μL of each mixture was then cultured on chocolate agar plates at 37 °C under aerobic atmospheric conditions. Swab samples were semi-quantitatively processed immediately by streaking the entire surface of the plates. Identification was performed when a culture yielded at least 10^3 colony-forming units (CFU)/mL. Matrix-assisted laser desorption/ionisation time-of-flight mass spectrometry (MALDI-TOF MS) was used for the bacterial identification as previously described [12].

Definition of ECMO device colonisation and infection

The definitions of ECMO device colonisation or infection were adapted from French and American central line-associated bloodstream infection guidelines [13, 14]. These definitions concern the central line defined as an intravascular catheter that terminates at or close to the heart or in one of the great vessels excluding ECMO devices. Thus, the following definitions were used: (a) cannula colonisation (CC) was defined as a positive quantitative intravascular extremity culture ($\geq 10^3$ CFU). (b) Skin colonisation (SC) was a positive quantitative swab culture ($\geq 10^3$ CFU). (c) Not related ECMO device bacteraemia was defined as one or more positive blood cultures with negative cannula colonisation and another infectious site responsible for bacteraemia. (d) Contamination was defined as one positive blood culture for common skin contaminants [14, 15]. (e) ECMO device infection (ED-I) corresponded to: (e.1) ECMO device-related blood stream infection (EDR-BSI), which was a combination of one or more positive blood cultures (from the CVC, arterial catheter or post-membrane oxygenator) sampled immediately before or within 48 h after ECMO removal, a quantitative intravascular cannula extremity positive culture for the same micro-organism(s) and no other infection explaining the positive blood culture; (e.2) cannula infection (CI), which was considered in cases of a positive quantitative intravascular cannula extremity culture, negative blood culture and systemic infectious signs in the absence of any other infection. CI was also considered in case of a positive quantitative intravascular cannula extremity culture and local infection signs (local purulence or infection signs at insertion site); (e.3) in patients with blood culture and/or quantitative intravascular cannula portion culture positive for coagulase-negative staphylococci, EDR-BSI and CI were considered depending on clinical features (fever, sepsis, septic shock) within 48 h after ECMO removal and on clinical evolution under specific treatment if introduced by the clinician.

An adjudication committee, including one infectious disease specialist and three intensivists, retrospectively classified each case into three categories: (1) uninfected/uncolonised ECMO device (U-I/C ED), including sterile samples, skin colonisation, blood culture contamination and not related ECMO device bacteraemia; (2) ECMO device colonisation (ED-C), including cannula colonisation associated or not with skin colonisation; (3) ECMO device infection (ED-I), including EDR-BSI and CI as previously defined.

Collected data

Prospectively collected data included demographic data; body mass index (BMI); severity of illness as assessed by the Simplified Acute Physiology Score (SAPS) II [16] and SOFA score at ICU admission [10]; major comorbidities; indication for ECMO; site of cannulation; site of ECMO implantation; ECMO system exchange; ECMO transfusion (blood, platelets and plasma), pre- and per-ECMO steroid use; pre- and per-ECMO antibiotics use; duration of both ECMO and mechanical ventilation; outcome (ICU and hospital mortalities, ventilator and ECMO-free days at both day 28 and day 90, ICU length of stay); and nosocomial infections, primary bloodstream infections or fungaemia during ECMO support. Nosocomial infection definitions agreed with those of the Centers for Disease Control and Prevention National Nosocomial Infections Surveillance System [17]. Ventilator-associated pneumonia (VAP) was diagnosed according to previously published criteria [18].

End points

The primary end points were the rates of ECMO device infection or colonisation at the time of ECMO removal. Secondary end points were the rate of skin colonisation and outcomes, such as ICU length of stay, ICU mortality, in-hospital mortality and day-90 mortality, day-28 and day-90 ventilator and ECMO-free days.

Statistical analysis

Descriptive statistics included percentages for categorical variables and medians and interquartile ranges for continuous variables. Comparisons between the three categories (U-I/C ED, ED-C and ED-I) for continuous variables were made using the Kruskal–Wallis test with a post hoc method for multiple comparisons (step-up Simes method to calculate adjusted p value). Comparisons between the three categories (U-I/C ED, ED-C and ED-I) for categorical variables were made using the Pearson Chi-square test for trend. A multinomial logistic regression procedure was performed to identify factors associated with ED-I or ED-C. The U-I/C ED group was used as the reference group. All of the variables with p value < 0.20 (gender, body mass index, statin therapy, per-ECMO plasma transfusion, reason for ECMO, location of ECMO cannulation, type of cannulation, pre-ECMO antibiotic and ECMO duration) were included in the model. The Fleiss' kappa was calculated to evaluate the reliability agreement between the 4 experts regarding the classification of each ECMO case. A p value < 0.05 was considered significant. The statistical analysis was conducted using SPSS, version 20.0 (NY, USA).

Results

Patients

During the study period, 105 patients underwent 109 VV-ECMO (Fig. 1). Four patients underwent 2 VV-ECMO during the same ICU stay with an interval of at least 2 days between each ECMO implantation. Finally, 103 VV-ECMO were analysed (representing 1472 ECMO days). The median age was 49 years (38–62), and the most frequent reason for ECMO was ARDS (77.6%). Fifty-three patients were referred to our ECMO centre

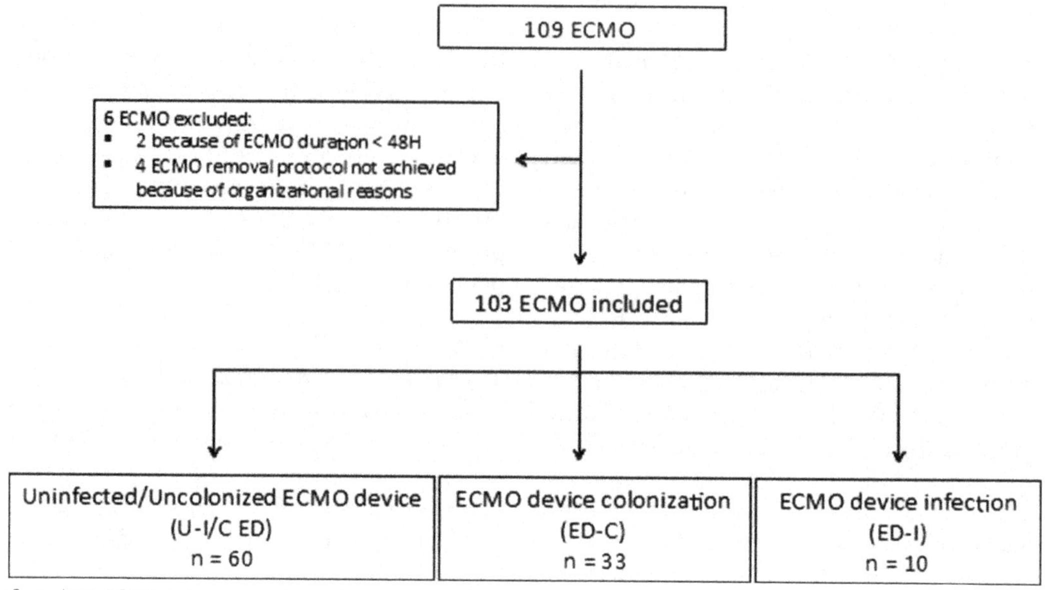

Fig. 1 Study flow chart. ECMO, extracorporeal membrane oxygenation

and transported by our mobile team. The median ECMO duration was 11 days (6–18 days). A total of 63 circuit changes were done in 38 VV-ECMO. General characteristics of each group are provided in Table 1.

ECMO device colonisation and infection (Fig. 2)

At the time of ECMO removal, the rate of ECMO device colonisation (ED-C) was 32% (33 events). The rate of ECMO device infection (ED-I) was 9.7% (10 events), including 7 ECMO device-related bloodstream infections (6.8%). No patient presented with insertion site infectious signs at any moment during ECMO support or within the 48-h period following ECMO removal. The uninfected/uncolonised ECMO device (U-I/C ED) rate was 58.3% (60 of 103). Fleiss' kappa coefficient was 0.94 (standard error, 0.04), corresponding to strong agreement between the experts regarding the classification.

A total of 127 femoral cannulas were inserted. In all, 22% (28 of 127) of the cultures were positive for at least one micro-organism compared with 35.4% of the cultures (28 of 79) regarding the jugular site ($p = 0.052$). Micro-organisms responsible for ED-C and ED-I are detailed in Fig. 3 and Additional file 1: Table S1. Coagulase-negative staphylococcus was the most frequent organism responsible for ED-I (8/10, 80%) and ED-C (20/33, 60.6%). The details of blood culture results are summarised in Additional file 2: Table S2.

We observed a longer ECMO duration in the ED-C group compared with the U-I/C ED group [12 days (9–20 days) versus 5 days (5–16 days), respectively, $p < 0.05$]. Using multivariate analysis, we did not identify any factor associated with ED-C or ED-I (Additional file 3: Table S3).

Skin colonisation

The skin colonisation rate was 23.3% (24 events). When cannula colonisation was observed, concomitant skin colonisation was present in 42.4% of cases (14 of 33), with the same micro-organism in 71.4% of cases (10 of 14). Considering ED-I, no concomitant skin colonisation was observed. No differences were noted regarding skin colonisation between femoral and jugular sites (22/127, 17.3%; 14/79, 17.7%, respectively, $p = 0.91$).

Outcome

Fifty-two patients died in the ICU (50.5%) and 58 during hospitalisation (56.3%). No difference was observed among the three categories (U-I/C ED, ED-C and ED-I) regarding ICU length of stay, ICU mortality, in-hospital mortality and day-90 mortality (Table 2).

A total of 27 patients underwent at least one nosocomial infection other than ED-I, without differences among the three groups ($p = 0.30$). Forty-four nosocomial infections, excluding ED-I, occurred during the 103 VV-ECMO supports, corresponding to 29.9 infectious episodes per 1000 ECMO days. Ventilator-associated pneumonia (VAP) was the most frequent nosocomial infection (45.5%), followed by primary bloodstream infection (36.4%) (Additional file 4: Table S4).

Table 1 General characteristics of ECMO in patients without infected/colonised ECMO device, with ECMO device colonisation and ECMO device infection (at the time of ECMO removal)

Number of ECMO[a]	U-I/C ED 60	ED-C 33	ED-I 10	P value[b]
Age (years)	48 (37–61)	57 (47–63)	43 (41–63)	0.278
Male (*n*, %)	35 (58.3)	23 (69.7)	8 (80)	0.122
BMI (kg/m^2)	24 (22–29)	27 (24–31)	26 (24–27)	0.183
SOFA score[c]	10 (7–12)	9 (7–14)	9 (7–10)	0.607
SAPS II[c]	44 (39–56)	47 (38–57)	46 (36–53)	0.833
Underlying condition				
Diabetes mellitus	9 (15)	4 (12.1)	0	0.233
Renal insufficiency	0	2 (6.1)	0	0.300
Immunocompromised[d]	5 (8.3)	6 (18.2)	1 (10)	0.402
COPD	5 (8.3)	2 (6.1)	0	0.349
Solid tumour	9 (15)	4 (12.1)	2 (20)	0.906
Cirrhosis	2 (3.3)	0	0	0.272
Statin therapy	8 (13.3)	2 (6.1)	0	0.118
ICU stay before ECMO centre admission	2 (0–8)	5 (1–10)	3 (0–4)	0.237
Reason for ECMO[e]				
ARDS	42 (70)	28 (84.8)	10 (100)	0.011*
CAP	18	13	5 (50)	
NP	20	13	4 (40)	
Extrapulmonary	4	2	1 (10)	
Bridge to lung transplantation	2 (6.7)	2 (6.1)	0	0.965
Primary graft dysfunction	14 (23.3)	3 (9.1)	0	0.023*
ECMO characteristics				
Mobile ECMO team	27 (45)	21 (63.6)	5 (50)	0.272
Location of ECMO cannulation				
ICU	44 (73.3)	31 (93.9)	10 (100)	0.005#*
Operating room	16 (26.7)	2 (6.1)	0	
Per-ECMO blood transfusion	9 (4–21)	8 (5–17)	9 (6–16)	0.934
Per-ECMO platelet transfusion	1 (0–4)	1 (0–4)	1 (0–1)	0.651
Per-ECMO plasma transfusion	2 (0–10)	0 (0–4)	0 (0–4)	0.197
Pre-ECMO steroids	14 (23.3)	8 (24.2)	2 (20)	0.903
Per-ECMO steroids	31 (51.7)	15 (45.5)	3 (30)	0.214
Pre-ECMO antibiotics[f]	48 (80)	29 (87.9)	10 (100)	0.085
Per-ECMO antibiotics[g]	58 (96.7)	33 (100)	10 (100)	0.272
Antibiotics at the time of ECMO removal	48 (80)	30 (90.9)	5 (50)	0.314
BSI during ECMO[h]	10 (16.7)	8 (24.2)	2 (20)	0.525
Cannulation				
Femoro–femoral	19 (31.7)	5 (15.2)	0	0.011*
Femoro-jugular	41 (68.3)	28 (84.8)	10 (100)	
ECMO circuit change (≥ 1)	24 (40)	12 (36.4)	2 (20)	0.278
ECMO duration (days)	7.5 (5–16)	12 (9–20)	13 (11–17)	0.021#

Data are provided as no. (%) of ECMO or median value (interquartile range)

ARDS acute respiratory distress syndrome, *BMI* body mass index, *CAP* community-acquired pneumonia, *COPD* chronic obstructive pulmonary disease, *ECMO* extracorporeal membrane oxygenation, *ICU* intensive care unit, *NP* nosocomial pneumonia, *SAPS II* Simplified Acute Physiology Score, *SOFA* sepsis-related organ failure assessment, *U-I/C ED* uninfected/uncolonised ECMO device, *ED-C* ECMO device colonisation, *ED-I* ECMO device infection

* $p < 0.05$, comparison between U-I/C ED and ED-I

# $p < 0.05$, comparison between U-I/C ED and ED-C

[a] Among the 99 patients, 4 underwent 2 ECMO during their ICU stay corresponding to 103 VV-ECMO

[b] *p* value corresponds to the comparison between the three categories (U-I/C ED, ED-C, ED-I)

[c] Calculated at ICU admission

[d] Includes patients with human immunodeficiency virus, solid organ transplantation or haematological malignancy and those receiving chemotherapy, immunosuppressive agents or long-term corticosteroid therapy

[e] For 2 patients, ECMO reason was thoracic surgery

[f] Pre-ECMO antibiotics correspond to antibiotics received for at least 24 h before ECMO implantation

[g] Per-ECMO antibiotics correspond to antibiotics received immediately after ECMO implantation

[h] Bloodstream infection (BSI) under ECMO includes primary and secondary bloodstream infections

Discussion

To our knowledge, this is the first study that systematically analysed ECMO devices at the time of ECMO removal, providing the rate of ECMO device-related infection and colonisation in an adult cohort of venovenous ECMO supports. Our results indicate that the ECMO device infection rate (cannula infections or ECMO device-related bloodstream infections) was 9.7%, and the ECMO device colonisation rate was 32%. Indeed, most of the studies related the incidence of nosocomial infections and bloodstream infections while on venoarterial or venovenous ECMO support, and these studies often used paediatric cohorts [7–9, 19, 20]. The originality of our work was to assess the infection and colonisation rates directly associated with the ECMO device. Schmidt et al. [9] reported a large series of 220 venoarterial ECMO support cases in adult cardiogenic shock and described 21 (9.5%) cannula infections, defined as the association of local signs of infection at the access site with a positive culture of subcutaneous needle aspirate from the cannula site. One major difference with this study is that VA-ECMO cannulation was performed

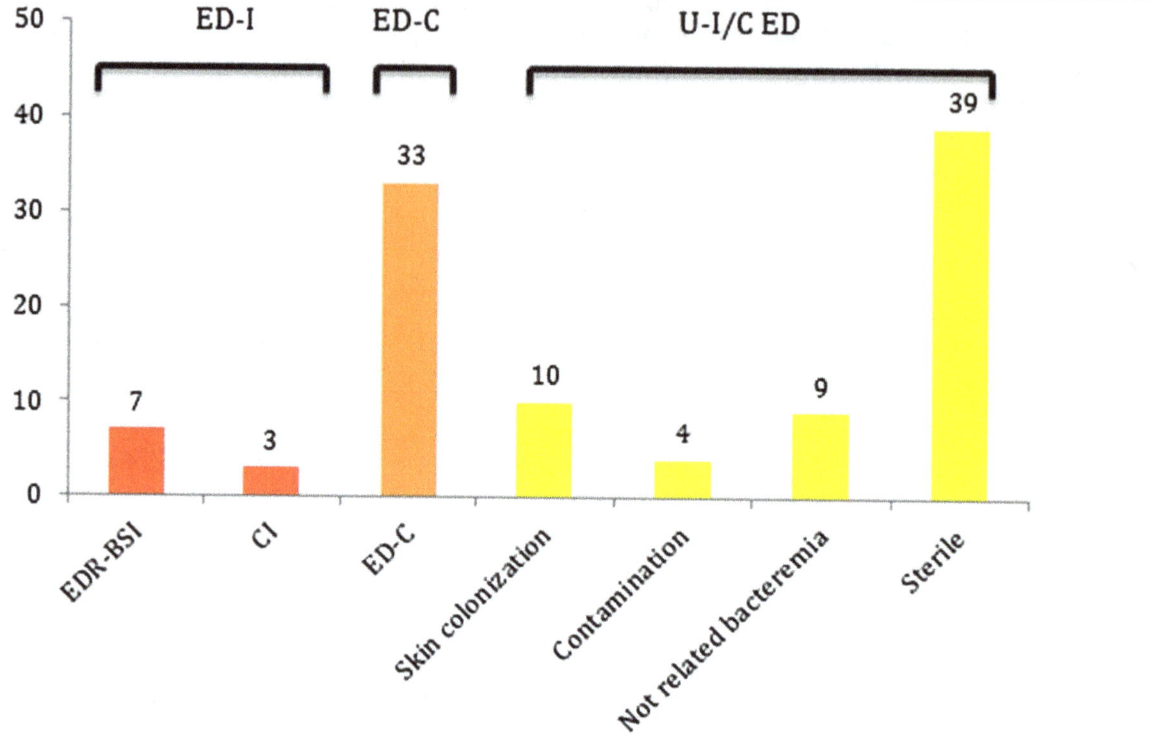

Fig. 2 Details of each ECMO samples leading to different categories: ECMO device infection (ED-I) including ECMO device-related bloodstream infections (EDR-BSI) and cannula infections (CI); ECMO device colonisation (ED-C); uninfected/uncolonised ECMO device (U-I/C ED) including skin colonisation, contamination, not related bacteremia and sterile samples

with an invasive surgical procedure, especially in the case of central VA-ECMO, whereas VV-ECMO cannulation only requires a percutaneous procedure (which was the case for all of our patients). Furthermore, the definition of cannula infection was different and could reflect surgical site infection rather than cannula infection in this study. Of note, none of our patients presented with cannula local infectious signs at any moment during ECMO support and even during the 48 following hours. Lubnow et al. described technical complications leading to system exchange in 265 adult patients treated with VV-ECMO support for acute respiratory failure. Eighty-three patients underwent at least one system change, and 4 of these cases (5%) were due to suspected infection [21]. More recently, Hahne et al. evaluated the culture results of 186 cannulae removed from 94 patients who benefited from extracorporeal circulation for lung or cardiac assistance. Fifteen patients (16%) presented cannula-related infection [22].

ECMO device-related infections may involve the drainage cannula, the return cannula or the membrane oxygenator (MO). Thus, Kuehn et al. [23] hypothesised that the artificial surfaces of the ECMO circuit, particularly the MO, could be the target of microbial adhesion and colonisation, favouring the development of ECMO-related bloodstream infection. The overall patient-based positivity by PCR was 45%. In the present study, membrane oxygenator infection was difficult to assess. We performed post-membranous blood culture on the day of removal (Additional file 4: Table S4), which was positive in 15 cases and allowed the diagnosis of ECMO device-related bloodstream infection (EDR-BSI) in only one case.

Our results revealed a longer ECMO duration in the ED-C group compared with the U-I/C ED group. Catheter duration is a well-known risk factor for catheter colonisation or catheter-related bloodstream infection [24]. Moreover, the prevalence of nosocomial infection increases with ECMO duration [7, 9]. No difference was observed between the U-I/C ED group and ED-I, which is probably due to the small number of patients in this group. At least, skin colonisation was not observed in the 10 ED-I, suggesting that ECMO device-related infections could originate from haematogenous contamination or circuit changes although our data cannot confirm this hypothesis (Table 1).

We reported a higher proportion of primary graft dysfunction, femoro–femoral cannulation and cannulation in the operating room in the U-I/C ED group compared with the ED-C group and/or the ED-I group. This finding

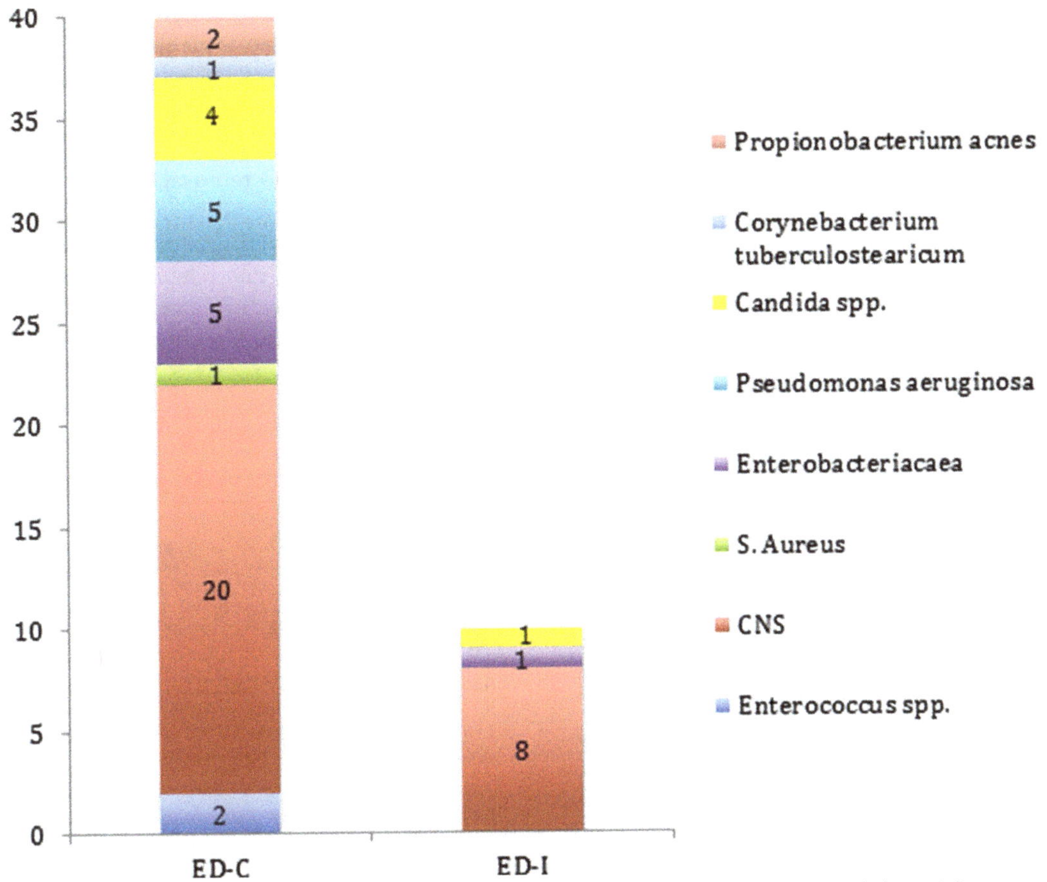

Fig. 3 Micro-organisms associated with ECMO device colonisations and infections. *CNS* Coagulase-negative staphylococci. Seven cannulas were colonised with two different micro-organisms corresponding to 33 cannula colonisations and a total number of 40 micro-organisms

can be easily explained by the fact that all patients with primary graft dysfunction benefited from ECMO cannulation at the end of the lung transplant, in the operating room, and with femoro–femoral cannulation due to surgical technical reasons. Moreover, the duration of ECMO was reduced for primary graft dysfunction indication compared with ARDS indication [5 (4–6) vs. 12 days (7–18), $p < 0.001$ data not shown]. Thus, the differences observed between the different groups are probably the result of significant differences of ECMO duration.

Our study described a very much higher rate of infection with ECMO device than with central venous catheter. During the study period, central venous catheter-related infection rate was 1.2 per 1000 catheter days. ECMO cannula size is bigger (17–25 Fr) and duration of ECMO longer than central venous catheter. Moreover, cannula change is highly problematic because of the few vascular accesses and due to patient's vital dependence on ECMO support.

Antibiotic prophylaxis to prevent nosocomial infections in ECMO patients remains highly controversial due to the emergence of resistance to antibiotics and *Clostridium difficile*-associated colitis [25]. Daily surveillance blood cultures have been proposed as an alternative to antibiotic prophylaxis and remain a routine practice in many ECMO centres, but this strategy is costly and resource consuming [9, 19, 26]. Wide variability in practice is also noted regarding the prevention of nosocomial and bloodstream infections for patients requiring ECMO. In a recent survey of the ELSO members interested in nosocomial bloodstream infection prevention practice, only one-quarter of respondents reported the use of a bundle or checklist during ECMO cannula insertion and less than half utilise a bundle or checklist for cannula maintenance [27]. In our opinion, if daily surveillance blood culture in patients with ECMO support should not be recommended, the systematic culture of vascular cannula portions associated with blood culture performed at the time of removal may help the clinician to make the diagnosis of ECMO device-related infection and guide the antibiotics prescription. Finally, we did not use chlorhexidine antiseptic protocol at the time of

Table 2 Outcome of extracorporeal membrane oxygenation in patients without infected/colonised ECMO device, with ECMO device colonisation and ECMO device infection (at the time of ECMO removal)

Number of ECMO[a]	U-I/C ED 60	ED-C 33	ED-I 10	*p* value
ICU LOS	25 (14–39)	24 (20–33)	30 (23–37)	0.614
ICU mortality	27 (45)	21 (63.6)	4 (40)	0.559
Day-90 mortality	28 (46.7)	22 (66.7)	4 (40)	0.622
In-hospital mortality	32 (53.3)	22 (66.7)	6 (60)	0.896
Days of MV	23 (12–37)	24 (18–32)	28 (23–30)	0.671
VFD day 28	0 (0–1)	0 (0–0)	0 (0–0)	0.385
VFD day 90	1 (0–60)	0 (0–35)	9 (0–52)	0.506
ECMOFD day 28	13 (0–21)	3 (0–18)	7 (0–14)	0.169
ECMOFD day 90	63 (0–83)	9 (0–78)	62 (0–76)	0.156
ECMO weaning	43 (71.7)	17 (51.5)	7 (70)	0.283

Data are provided as no. (%) of ECMO or median value (interquartile range)

ECMO extracorporeal membrane oxygenation, *ECMOFD* ECMO-free day, *ICU* intensive care unit, *LOS* length of stay, *MV* mechanical ventilation, *VFD* ventilator-free day, *U-I/C ED* uninfected/uncolonised ECMO device, *ED-C* ECMO device colonisation, *ED-I* ECMO device infection

[a] Among the 99 patients, 4 underwent 2 ECMO during their ICU stay corresponding to 103 VV-ECMO

cannula insertion and for the standardised cannula care. Chlorhexidine-impregnated dressing for cannula dressing was not used in our study which could be evaluated in the future to evaluate the impact on the rate of ECMO device colonisation and infection.

Our study presents several limitations. There is currently no consensus on the definition of ECMO device-related infection. Indeed, the Centers for Disease Control and Prevention (CDC) guidelines have established a clear definition of central line-related infection or blood stream infections that precisely exclude ECMO devices [14]. Moreover, the definitions that include differential time to blood culture positivity appear to be inappropriate given the impossibility and danger of performing blood culture in ECMO cannulae [13, 28]. We have decided to use the threshold of 10^3 colony-forming unit for the positivity of the device culture, which is derived from catheter infection literature but not validated for the ECMO device so far. At least, our study focused on ECMO device infection and colonisation at the time of removal and not during the ECMO support period. Moreover, the huge majority of our patients were receiving antibiotics at the time of ECMO insertion and during the ECMO run. These two last elements could have led to possible underestimation of the number of infections and colonisations. We did not collected data regarding dressing disruption or changes that might help to explain the differences between the rate of colonisation and the rate of infection. Using a multinomial logistic regression procedure, we failed to establish factors associated with ECMO device colonisation or infection, probably because of the cohort size.

Conclusions

At the time of ECMO removal, systematic blood culture and intravascular extremity cannula culture may help to diagnose ECMO device-related infection. We reported a quite low infection rate related to the devices. Further studies are needed to evaluate the benefits of systematic strategies of cannula culture at the time of ECMO removal.

Additional files

Additional file 1. Table S1. Microorganisms cultured in different samples of 103 Extracorporeal Membrane Oxygenation (at the time of ECMO removal).

Additional file 2. Table S2. Microorganisms cultured in blood culture (at the time of ECMO removal).

Additional file 3. Table S3. Nosocomial infections during ECMO support of Extracorporeal Membrane Oxygenation (ECMO) in patients without infected/colonized ECMO device (U-I/C ED), with EMCO device colonization (ED-C) and ECMO device infection (ED-I) (at the time of ECMO removal).

Additional file 4. Table S4. Multivariate analysis of factors associated with ECMO device infection (ED-I) or colonization (ED-C) at the time of ECMO removal.

Abbreviations

ARDS: acute respiratory distress syndrome; BC: blood culture; BMI: body mass index; BSI: bloodstream infections; CC: cannula colonisation; CI: cannula infection; CFU: colony-forming units; CVC: central venous catheter; ELSO: Extracorporeal Life Support Organization; ECMO: extracorporeal membrane oxygenation; ED-C: ECMO device colonisation; ED-I: ECMO device infection; EDR-BSI: ECMO device-related blood stream infection; HICPAC Guidelines: Healthcare Infection Control Practices Advisory Committee Guidelines; ICU: intensive care unit; MALDI-TOF MS: matrix-assisted laser desorption/ionisation time-of-flight mass spectrometry; MV: mechanical ventilation; PEEP: positive end-expiratory pressure; Pplat: plateau pressure; SAPS: Simplified Acute Physiology Score; SK: akin colonisation; SOFA: Sequential Organ Failure Assessment; U-I/C ED: uninfected/uncolonised ECMO device; VAP: ventilator-associated pneumonia; VT: tidal volume; VV-ECMO: venovenous extracorporeal membrane oxygenation.

Authors' contributions

JMF and GT designed the work. SL, RR, SW, FK and SD collected the data. GT, JMF, LP analysed, interpreted the patient data and wrote the manuscript. SH, NC, MA and CG examined the data to class the type of infection. AR revised the manuscript. All authors read and approved the final manuscript.

Author details

[1] Hôpital Nord, Réanimation des Détresses Respiratoires et des Infections Sévères, Assistance Publique–Hôpitaux de Marseille, 13015 Marseille, France.
[2] URMITE, UMR CNRS 7278, Faculté de Médecine, Aix-Marseille Université,

13005 Marseille, France. [3] Hôpital de la Conception, Réanimation des brulés Assistance Publique–Hôpitaux de Marseille, 13005 Marseille, France. [4] Hôpital Nord, Service des Urgences, Assistance Publique–Hôpitaux de Marseille, 13015 Marseille, France.

Acknowledgements
This manuscript was edited for proper English language, grammar, punctuation, spelling and overall style by one or more of the highly qualified native English-speaking editors at American Journal Experts.

Competing interests
The authors declare that they have no competing interests.

Funding
Not applicable.

References

1. Brodie D, Bacchetta M. Extracorporeal membrane oxygenation for ARDS in adults. N Engl J Med. 2011;365:1905–14. https://doi.org/10.1056/NEJMct1103720.
2. Rehder KJ, Turner DA, Cheifetz IM. Extracorporeal membrane oxygenation for neonatal and pediatric respiratory failure: an evidence-based review of the past decade (2002–2012). Pediatr Crit Care Med J Soc Crit Care Med World Fed Pediatr Intensive Crit Care Soc. 2013;14:851–61. https://doi.org/10.1097/PCC.0b013e3182a5540d.
3. Australia and New Zealand Extracorporeal Membrane Oxygenation (ANZ ECMO) Influenza Investigators. Extracorporeal Membrane Oxygenation for 2009 Influenza A(H1N1) Acute Respiratory Distress Syndrome. JAMA. 2009; 302:1888–1895; https://doi.org/10.1001/jama.2009.1535.
4. Camboni D, Philipp A, Lubnow M, Bein T, Haneya A, Diez C, Schmid C, Müller T. Support time-dependent outcome analysis for veno-venous extracorporeal membrane oxygenation. Eur J Cardio Thorac Surg Off J Eur Assoc Cardio Thorac Surg. 2011;40:1341-1346-1347. https://doi.org/10.1016/j.ejcts.2011.03.062.
5. Roch A, Hraiech S, Masson E, Grisoli D, Forel J-M, Boucekine M, Morera P, Guervilly C, Adda M, Dizier S, Toesca R, Collart F, Papazian L. Outcome of acute respiratory distress syndrome patients treated with extracorporeal membrane oxygenation and brought to a referral center. Intensive Care Med. 2014;40:74–83. https://doi.org/10.1007/s00134-013-3135-1.
6. Fan E, Gattinoni L, Combes A, Schmidt M, Peek G, Brodie D, Muller T, Morelli A, Ranieri VM, Pesanti A, Brochard L, Hodgson C, Van Kiersbilck C, Roch A, Quintel M, Papazian L. Venovenous extracorporeal membrane oxygenation for acute respiratory failure: a clinical review from an international group of experts. Intensive Care Med. 2016;42:712–24. https://doi.org/10.1007/s00134-016-4314-7.
7. Bizzarro MJ, Conrad SA, Kaufman DA, Rycus P. Infections acquired during extracorporeal membrane oxygenation in neonates, children, and adults. Pediatr Crit Care Med J Soc Crit Care Med World Fed Pediatr Intensive Crit Care Soc. 2011;12:277–81. https://doi.org/10.1097/PCC.0b013e3181e28894.
8. Sun H-Y, Ko W-J, Tsai P-R, Sun C-C, Chang Y-Y, Lee C-W, Chen Y-C. Infections occurring during extracorporeal membrane oxygenation use in adult patients. J Thorac Cardiovasc Surg. 2010;140(1125–1132):e2. https://doi.org/10.1016/j.jtcvs.2010.07.017.
9. Schmidt M, Bréchot N, Hariri S, Guiguet M, Luyt C-E, Makri R, Leprince P, Trouillet J-L, Pavie A, Chastre J, Combes A. Nosocomial infections in adult cardiogenic shock patients supported by venoarterial extracorporeal membrane oxygenation. Clin Infect Dis Off Publ Infect Dis Soc Am. 2012;55:1633–41. https://doi.org/10.1093/cid/cis783.
10. Vincent JL, Moreno R, Takala J, Willatts S, De Mendoça A, Bruining H, Reinhart CK, Suter PM, Thijs LG. The SOFA (Sepsis-related Organ Failure Assessment) score to describe organ dysfunction/failure. On behalf of the Working Group on Sepsis-Related Problems of the European Society of Intensive Care Medicine. Intensive Care Med. 1996;22:707–10.
11. O'Grady NP, Alexander M, Burns LA, Dellinger EP, Garland J, Heard SO, Lipsett PA, Masur H, Mermel LA, Pearson ML, Raad II, Randolph AG, Rupp ME, Saint S. Summary of recommendations: guidelines for the prevention of intravascular catheter-related infections. Clin Infect Dis Off Publ Infect Dis Soc Am. 2011;52:1087–99. https://doi.org/10.1093/cid/cir138.
12. Seng P, Drancourt M, Gouriet F, La Scola B, Fournier PE, Rolain JM, Raoult D. Ongoing revolution in bacteriology: routine identification of bacteria by matrix-assisted laser desorption ionization time-of-flight mass spectrometry. Clin Infect Dis Off Publ Infect Dis Soc Am. 2009;49:543–51. https://doi.org/10.1086/600885.
13. Comité technique des infections nosocomiales et des infections liées aux soins, Ministère de la santé, de la jeunesse et des sports DGS/DHOS. http://socialsante.gouv.fr/IMG/pdf/rapport_complet.pdf. Accessed 15 June 2015
14. Centers of Disease Control and Prevention, Healthcare Infection Control Practices Advisory Committee (CDC/HIPAC). http://www.cdc.gov/hicpac/pubs.html. Accessed 15 June 2015.
15. Hall KK, Lyman JA. Updated review of blood culture contamination. Clin Microbiol Rev. 2006;19:788–802. https://doi.org/10.1128/CMR.00062-05.
16. Le Gall JR, Lemeshow S, Saulnier F. A new Simplified Acute Physiology Score (SAPS II) based on a European/North American multicenter study. JAMA. 1993;270:2957–63.
17. Garner JS, Jarvis WR, Emori TG, Horan TC, Hughes JM. CDC definitions for nosocomial infections, 1988. Am J Infect Control. 1988;16:128–40.
18. Papazian L, Roch A, Charles PE, Penot-Ragon C, Perrin G, Roulier P, Goutorbe P, Lefrant JY, Wiramus S, Jung B, Perbet S, Hernu R, Nau A, Baldesi O, Allardet-Servent J, Baumstarck K, Jouve E, Moussa M, Hraiech S, Guervilly C, Forel JM, STATIN-VAP Study Group. Effect of statin therapy on mortality in patients with ventilator-associated pneumonia: a randomized clinical trial. JAMA. 2013;310:1692–700. https://doi.org/10.1001/jama.2013.280031.
19. Kaczala GW, Paulus SC, Al-Dajani N, Jang W, Blondel-Hill E, Dobson S, Cogswell A, Singh AJ. Bloodstream infections in pediatric ECLS: usefulness of daily blood culture monitoring and predictive value of biological markers. The British Columbia experience. Pediatr Surg Int. 2009;25:169–73. https://doi.org/10.1007/s00383-008-2299-1.
20. Burket JS, Bartlett RH, Vander Hyde K, Chenoweth CE. Nosocomial infections in adult patients undergoing extracorporeal membrane oxygenation. Clin Infect Dis Off Publ Infect Dis Soc Am. 1999;28:828–33. https://doi.org/10.1086/515200.
21. Lubnow M, Philipp A, Foltan M, Enger TB, Lunz D, Bein T, Haneya A, Schmid C, Riegger G, Müller T, Lehle K. Technical complications during veno-venous extracorporeal membrane oxygenation and their relevance predicting a system-exchange–retrospective analysis of 265 cases. PLoS ONE. 2014;9:e112316. https://doi.org/10.1371/journal.pone.0112316.
22. Hahne K, Horstmann C, Fischer D, Kock R, Peters G, Lebiedz P. Cannula-related infection in adult medical intensive care unit patients undergoing extracorporeal life support and extracorporeal membrane oxygenation. J Hosp Infect. 2015;91:372–4. https://doi.org/10.1016/j.jhin.2015.08.022.
23. Kuehn C, Orszag P, Burgwitz K, Marsch G, Stumpp N, Stiesch M, Haverich A. Microbial adhesion on membrane oxygenators in patients requiring extracorporeal life support detected by a universal rDNA PCR test. ASAIO J Am Soc Artif Intern Organs. 2013;59:368–73. https://doi.org/10.1097/MAT.0b013e318299fd07.
24. Polderman KH, Girbes ARJ. Central venous catheter use. Part 2: infectious complications. Intensive Care Med. 2002;28:18–28. https://doi.org/10.1007/s00134-001-1156-7.
25. Paterson DL. "Collateral damage" from cephalosporin or quinolone antibiotic therapy. Clin Infect Dis Off Publ Infect Dis Soc Am. 2004;38(Suppl 4):S341–5. https://doi.org/10.1086/382690.
26. Kao LS, Fleming GM, Escamilla RJ, Lew DF, Lally KP. Antimicrobial prophylaxis and infection surveillance in extracorporeal membrane oxygenation

patients: a multi-institutional survey of practice patterns. ASAIO J Am Soc Artif Intern Organs. 2011;57:231–8. https://doi.org/10.1097/MAT.0b013e31820d19ab.

27. Glater-Welt LB, Schneider JB, Zinger MM, Rosen L, Sweberg TM. Nosocomial bloodstream infections in patients receiving extracorporeal life support: variability in prevention practices: a survey of the Extracorporeal Life Support Organization members. J Intensive Care Med. 2015;. https://doi.org/10.1177/0885066615571540.

28. Mermel LA, Allon M, Bouza E, Craven DE, Flynn P, O'Grady NP, Raad II, Rinjders BJA, Sherertz RJ, Warren DK. Clinical practice guidelines for the diagnosis and management of intravascular catheter-related infection: 2009 Update by the Infectious Diseases Society of America. Clin Infect Dis Off Publ Infect Dis Soc Am. 2009;49:1–45. https://doi.org/10.1086/599376.

The association between FABP7 serum levels with survival and neurological complications in acetaminophen-induced acute liver failure

Constantine J. Karvellas[1*], Jaime L. Speiser[2], Mélanie Tremblay[3], William M. Lee[4], Christopher F. Rose[3] and For the US Acute Liver Failure Study Group

Abstract

Background: Acetaminophen (APAP)-induced acute liver failure (ALF) is associated with significant mortality due to intracranial hypertension (ICH), a result of cerebral edema (CE) and astrocyte swelling. Brain-type fatty acid-binding protein (FABP7) is a small (15 kDa) cytoplasmic protein abundantly expressed in astrocytes. The aim of this study was to determine whether serum FABP7 levels early (day 1) or late (days 3–5) level were associated with 21-day mortality and/or the presence of ICH/CE in APAP-ALF patients.

Methods: Serum samples from 198 APAP-ALF patients (nested case–control study with 99 survivors and 99 non-survivors) were analyzed by ELISA methods and assessed with clinical data from the US Acute Liver Failure Study Group (ALFSG) Registry (1998–2014).

Results: APAP-ALF survivors had significantly lower serum FABP7 levels on admission (147.9 vs. 316.5 ng/ml, $p = 0.0002$) and late (87.3 vs. 286.2 ng/ml, $p < 0.0001$) compared with non-survivors. However, a significant association between 21-day mortality and increased serum FABP7 early [log FABP7 odds ratio (OR) 1.16, $p = 0.32$] and late (log FABP7 ~ OR 1.34, $p = 0.21$) was not detected after adjusting for significant covariates (MELD, vasopressor use). Areas under the receiver-operating curve for early and late multivariable models were 0.760 and 0.892, respectively. In a second analysis, patients were grouped based on the presence ($n = 46$) or absence ($n = 104$) of ICH/CE. A significant difference in FABP7 levels between patients with or without ICH/CE at early (259.7 vs. 228.2 ng/ml, $p = 0.61$) and late (223.8 vs. 192.0 ng/ml, $p = 0.19$) time points was not identified.

Conclusion: Serum FABP7 levels were significantly elevated at early and late time points in APAP-ALF non-survivors compared to survivors. However, significant differences in FABP7 levels by 21-day mortality were not ascertained after adjusting for significant covariates (reflecting severity of illness). Our study suggests that FABP7 may not discriminate between patients with or without intracranial complications.

Keywords: Liver-type fatty acid-binding protein, Multiorgan failure, Prognosis, ALFSG index

Background

Acute liver failure (ALF) is defined by the occurrence of hepatic encephalopathy (HE) and hepatic synthetic dysfunction within 26 weeks of the first symptoms of liver disease [1]. Severe coagulopathy, encephalopathy and hemodynamic instability contribute to a picture of multiorgan failure. Currently, the most common cause of ALF in North America is acetaminophen (APAP) [2]. Particularly in APAP-induced ALF, cerebral edema (CE) and intracranial hypertension (ICH) are major causes of morbidity and mortality [3]. The pathogenesis for ICH

*Correspondence: dean.karvellas@ualberta.ca
[1] Division of Gastroenterology (Liver Unit), Department of Critical Care Medicine, University of Alberta, 1-40 Zeidler Ledcor Building, Edmonton, AB T6G-2X8, Canada
Full list of author information is available at the end of the article

and CE in ALF is not fully understood, but astrocyte swelling causing cellular dysfunction as well as increased cerebral blood flow is believed to be implicated [4]. The degree of hyperammonemia has been demonstrated to be associated with ICH [5]. Ammonia, as a gas (NH_3) and ion (NH_4^+), freely crosses the blood–brain barrier and is primarily removed by glutamine synthetase, an enzyme solely found in astrocytes within the brain [6]. Glutamine synthetase catalyzes the amidation of glutamate to glutamine that subsequently leads to hyperosmotic changes and astrocyte swelling. However, studies have shown that hyperammonemia alone does not predict ICH [7].

Given the challenges presented in managing critically ill ALF patients with potential CE/ICH including the consideration for liver transplant (LT), the development of a noninvasive biomarker with the potential to predict ICH would be of great value, especially given the significant bleeding risks of invasive intracranial pressure monitoring in these coagulopathic patients [8].

Fatty acid-binding proteins (FABP) are small (15 kDa) cytoplasmic proteins that are abundantly expressed in tissues with active fatty acid metabolism, such as brain and liver. The primary function of FABPs is the intracellular transport of long-chain fatty acids [9]. The cellular expression of FABPs is responsive to changes in lipid metabolism, which can be induced during pathophysiological conditions, such as ischemia/inflammation or pharmacological stimuli [10]. Brain-type FABP (FABP7) is solely expressed in brain, exclusively in astrocytes [11]. Previous investigations have shown serum levels of FABP7 to be elevated in patients with various neurological diseases including stroke [12] and dementia [13]. While our group recently demonstrated the prognostic value of serum levels of liver-type FABP (FABP1) in ALF, to date FABP7 as a biomarker for the risk of ICH in ALF has not been investigated [14].

This nested case–control study of randomly selected samples from prospectively enrolled patients from the US Acute Liver Failure Study Group (ALFSG) registry aimed to examine levels of FABP7 in APAP-ALF patients. Specifically, our primary objectives were to test the following hypotheses

(a) Higher FABP7 serum levels are significantly associated with 21-day transplant-free mortality (in the absence of transplant) after adjusting for other significant covariates (Analysis 1).
(b) Elevated serum levels of FABP7 in APAP-ALF are significantly associated with ICH/CE after adjusting for other significant covariates (Analysis 2).

Methods

This study is a nested case–control study of prospectively collected data and biosamples of 198 patients enrolled in the US ALFSG registry/biorepository and is outlined in detail in Additional file 1: Figure S1. Between January 1998 and December 2014, 1027 APAP-ALF patients were enrolled in the registry from which 704 patients were alive at day 21 in the absence of LT. We identified 124 survivors with early and late serum samples from which 99 were randomly selected for analysis. Of 224 patients who died in the absence of LT, 87 patients with early and late samples were also included in this analysis. A further 12 patients with exclusively an early sample (of a possible 92) were randomly selected for inclusion in this analysis. Personnel not involved in the analysis of the samples or statistical analysis for the paper performed random selection of patients. All enrolling centers were tertiary academic centers, and all but one were LT centers. The authors' Institutional Review Board (IRB)/Health research ethics boards of all enrolling US ALFSG sites have approved all research, and all clinical investigation has been conducted according to the principles expressed in the 1975 Declaration of Helsinki. Given patients were unable to provide written consent (critical illness, HE), written assent was obtained from the next of kin from each patient. Each center implemented monitoring and therapeutic interventions according to institutional standards of care. Reporting of the analysis of this study followed the STROBE Guidelines for reporting case–control studies [15]. Consistent with ALFSG studies [16], the primary outcome (Analysis 1) was 21-day LT-free survival (no patients included in the analysis received LT). Secondary outcome (Analysis 2) was the development of ICH/CE.

Participants

Inclusion criteria were: (1) evidence of ALF according to the enrollment criteria for the ALFSG (see operational definitions); (2) age $\geq$ 18 years; (3) HE during the first seven days of study admission (West Haven Criteria) [17]; and (4) patients within the ALFSG registry with primary diagnoses of APAP determined by the site investigator. *Exclusion criteria* were: (1) cirrhosis/acute-on chronic liver failure; (2) patients without a primary diagnosis of APAP; and (3) patients who received a LT. Serum samples were analyzed on study admission (early; day 1) and late (either day 3, 4 or 5) where available. Patients who received a LT *were excluded from our study* because listing for transplant is a clinical decision, which is not standardized among ALFSG sites. A further 51 healthy controls were analyzed (University of Alberta) for FABP7 only.

Operational definitions

For the purposes of this study, ALF was defined as INR $\geq$ 1.5 and HE within the first 26 weeks of liver disease in a patient with an acute hepatic insult [18]. HE coma grade was defined by the West Haven Criteria (simplified) as follows: grade 1 ~ any alteration in mentation, grade 2 being somnolent or obtunded but easily rousable or presence of asterixis, grade 3 being rousable with difficulty, and grade 4 being unresponsive to deep pain [17]. In this study, we defined 'low coma grade' as grade 1 or 2 and 'high coma grade' as grade 3 or 4. The KCC [19] predicts poor outcome (death/transplant) if: (a) pH is less than 7.3 or (b) if INR is greater than 6.5, creatinine is greater than 3.4 mg/dl, and coma grade is high (3 or 4). The model for end-stage liver disease (MELD) is defined as 10*(0.957*log(4) + 0.378*log(bilirubin) + 1.12*log(INR)) for dialyzed patients and 10*(0.957*log(creatinine) + 0.378*log(bilirubin) + 1.12*log(INR)) for patients not dialyzed [20].

Laboratory Assays of FABP7

FABP7 was measured in serum samples with a solid-phase enzyme-linked immunosorbent assay (ELISA) following manufacturer's instructions (Biomatik, USA). Briefly, samples were incubated 2 h on a monoclonal anti-FABP7 pre-coated plate. A specific FABP7 biotin-conjugated polyclonal antibody solution was added for 2 h. After washing plates, avidin conjugated to horseradish peroxidase was added for 30 min. Finally, substrate tetramethylbenzidine was added for 15 min. Reactions were stopped by addition of sulfuric acid, and absorbance was read at 450 nm. Standard curve ranges from 0.47 to 30 ng/ml. Samples were performed in duplicate and accepted valid with a variation coefficient less than 25%.

Statistical methods aim one: FABP7 and 21-day survival in APAP-ALF

For differences between outcome groups (APAP-ALF survivors, $n = 99$, APAP-ALF non-survivors, $n = 99$), categorical variables were compared using the Chi-squared test or Fisher's exact test (if $n < 10$ in any cell of the two-by-two table). FABP7 was treated as a continuous variable. Continuous variables were reported as medians with interquartile range (IQR) and compared using the Wilcoxon rank-sum test. Survival was defined as the dichotomous outcome, alive or dead at 21 days after enrollment into the registry (no patients received a LT in this analysis). A two-sided p value of < 0.05 was considered statistically significant for all comparisons (Additional file 2).

In order to control for variables that may confound the effect of FABP7 on 21-day mortality, logistic regression analysis was performed [21]. Aside from FABP7, covariates considered in multivariable modeling included MELD, lactate, vasopressors use, RRT, MV and high coma grade. Separate multivariable (logistic) regression models were derived for FABP7 early (day 1) and late (days 3–5) by including variables, which were significant on univariate analysis and performing backward elimination with a p value threshold of 0.05.

Statistical methods aim two: FABP7 and ICH in APAP-ALF

In this secondary analysis, the outcome of interest examined was intracranial hypertension (ICH) either based on (a) intracranial pressure monitoring with ICP > 25 mm Hg or based on (b) computed tomography (CT) imaging of the brain. CT evidence of cerebral edema was defined as a hypodense signal, effacement of the gray white matter junction, loss of differentiation of the lenticular nucleus and decreased visualization of the sulci, insula and cisterns [22]. Out of the 150 APAP-ALF patients where data were available to determine the presence or absence of ICH, 46 deceased patients had evidence of ICH based on these criteria. Statistical methods for this analysis will be similar to the first analysis except the primary outcome (ICH). Multivariable logistic regression analysis (as described above) was performed [21] to assess independent variables associated with ICH including FABP7. The pre-specified prognostic variables were based on previous publications [5] included at admission into the registry; age, lactate value, MELD [20] score (admission) and other variables with statistical significance on univariable analysis. Model performance for both Aim 1 and Aim 2 was assessed using area under the receiver-operating curve (AUROC) and the Hosmer–Lemeshow test for goodness of fit. SAS software version 9.3 was used for univariate comparisons and multivariable logistic regression modeling.

Results

Analysis one: comparative analysis of 198 APAP-ALF patients

Demographic and clinical outcomes stratified by mortality (alive at day 21, $n = 99$; deceased, $n = 99$) are listed in Table 1. No patients in this analysis received LT. Comparing APAP-ALF survivors and non-survivors at day 21, survivors required significantly less organ support during the 7 days of inpatient study (MV 65 vs. 93%; vasopressors 12 vs. 70%; RRT 27 vs. 45%; $p < 0.008$ for all). Survivors were less likely to achieve high (3 or 4) HE coma grade (62 vs. 93%, $p < 0.0001$) and less likely to receive mannitol for intracranial hypertension (22 vs. 46%, $p = 0.0003$). APAP-ALF survivors were less likely to have complications during the first 7 days of study including seizures (3 vs. 21%, $p < 0.0001$), arrhythmias (25 vs. 38%, $p = 0.047$) or gastrointestinal bleeding (8 vs. 19%, $p = 0.037$). On admission, 7% of APAP-ALF survivors and 16% of non-survivors met KCC ($p = 0.13$). Among the 99 APAP-ALF non-survivors, the most common causes of death reported were multiorgan failure (53%)

Table 1 Demographic, clinical and biochemical parameters in 198 APAP-ALF patients by outcome

	APAP alive day 21 ($n = 99$)		APAP dead day 21 ($n = 99$)		*p* value
	N	Number (%) or median (IQR)	N	Number (%) or median (IQR)	
Age	99	35 (28–43)	99	40 (30–48)	0.084
Sex (female)	99	75 (76%)	99	72 (73%)	0.63
Race					0.23
White	99	83 (84%)	99	79 (80%)	
African-American	99	8 (8%)	99	15 (15%)	
Other	99	8 (8%)	99	5 (5%)	
Organ support (days 1–7)					
Mechanical ventilation	99	64 (65%)	99	93 (93%)	< 0.0001
Vasopressors	99	12 (12%)	99	69 (70%)	< 0.0001
Renal replacement therapy	99	27 (27%)	99	45 (45%)	0.0078
KCC	87	7 (7%)	87	16 (16%)	0.13
Coma grade 3/4 (worst days 1–7)	99	61 (62%)	98	91 (93%)	< 0.0001
ICP-directed therapies (days 1–7)					
ICP monitor	99	12 (12%)	99	21 (21%)	0.086
Mannitol	99	22 (22%)	99	46 (46%)	0.0003
Hypertonic saline	99	11 (11%)	99	14 (14%)	0.52
Barbiturates	99	9 (9%)	99	20 (20%)	0.043
Hypothermia	99	17 (17%)	99	14 (14%)	0.56
Sedatives	99	70 (71%)	99	88 (89%)	0.0014
Blood products (days 1–7)					
Red blood cells	99	34 (34%)	99	50 (51%)	0.021
Fresh-frozen plasma	99	50 (51%)	99	76 (77%)	0.0001
Recombinant VIIA	99	3 (3%)	99	5 (5%)	0.72
Platelets	99	17 (17%)	99	36 (36%)	0.0023
ICU complications (days 1–7)					
Seizures	99	3 (3%)	99	21 (21%)	< 0.0001
Arrhythmias	99	25 (25%)	99	38 (38%)	0.047
GI bleeding	99	8 (8%)	99	19 (19%)	0.037
ARDS	99	0 (0%)	99	3 (3%)	0.25
CT (cerebral edema)	55	7 (13%)	72	32 (44%)	< 0.001
Abnormal CXR	99	88 (89%)	99	83 (84%)	0.30
Bacteremia/blood stream infection	99	7 (7%)	99	10 (10%)	0.61
Cause of death					
Multiorgan failure			99	52 (53%)	
Cerebral edema			99	38 (38%)	
Unknown			99	9 (9%)	

N frequency, *IQR* interquartile range, *ARDS* acute respiratory syndrome, *CT* computed tomography, *CXR* chest x-ray

and neurological complications (38%). Cause of death was unknown in 9% of cases.

Clinical parameters in 198 APAP-ALF patients: admission (early)

Comparisons of clinical parameters on study admission are listed in Table 2. APAP-ALF survivors demonstrated significantly lower MELD scores (23 vs. 29, $p < 0.0001$) than non-survivors on admission. Survivors were significantly less likely to be on organ support (MV 58 vs. 80%, $p = 0.0007$; vasopressors, 9 vs. 42%, $p < 0.0001$) or achieve high HE grade (57 vs. 71%, $p = 0.034$) on admission.

FABP7 levels at admission (early) are listed in Table 2 and graphically shown in Fig. 1. APAP-ALF survivors had significantly lower admission serum FABP7 levels (147.9 vs. 316.5 ng/ml) compared with non-survivors ($p = 0.0002$). In comparison, 52 healthy

Table 2 Demographic, clinical and biochemical parameters in 198 APAP-ALF patients by outcome (admission)

Early (admission)	APAP alive day 21 ($n = 99$)		APAP dead day 21 ($n = 99$)		*p* value
	N	Number (%) or median (IQR)	N	Number (%) or median (IQR)	
Biochemistry					
Hemoglobin (g/dl)	99	10.4 (9.2–12.5)	97	10.9 (9.5–12.2)	0.52
White blood count (10^9/l)	98	8.6 (6.4–11.2)	97	10.9 (7.3–17.5)	0.0008
Platelet count (10^9/l)	98	132.5 (90.0–195.0)	97	110.0 (67.0–160.0)	0.0045
INR	99	2.7 (1.8–4.1)	96	3.4 (2.3–4.8)	0.0023
ALT (IU/l)	98	3380 (1949–6576)	99	3235 (1483–5716)	0.37
Bilirubin (mg/dl)	98	4.1 (2.5–5.6)	99	5.0 (3.6–7.8)	< 0.0001
pH	88	7.4 (7.4–7.5)	88	7.4 (7.3–7.5)	0.22
Ammonia (venous) (µmol/l)	51	92 (73–140)	32	139 (72–205)	0.068
Creatinine (mg/dl)	98	1.4 (0.8–3.0)	98	2.6 (1.2–3.8)	0.0007
Lactate (mmol/l)	71	2.8 (1.7–5.5)	68	7.0 (4.8–11.8)	< 0.0001
Phosphate (mg/dl)	88	2.3 (1.7–3.4)	76	3.2 (2.1–4.5)	0.0061
MELD	98	23.4 (12.7–27.7)	96	29.1 (23.8–34.5)	< 0.0001
High coma grade (3 or 4)	99	56 (57%)	97	69 (71%)	0.034
Organ support					
Mechanical ventilation	99	57(58%)	99	79 (80%)	0.0007
Vasopressors	99	9 (9%)	99	42 (42%)	< 0.0001
Renal replacement therapy	99	19 (19%)	99	24 (24%)	0.39
FABP7 (ng/ml)	99	147.9 (66.6–296.2)	99	316.5 (119.8–562.2)	0.0002
Late ($n = 186$)	**APAP alive day 21 ($n = 99$)**		**APAP dead day 21 ($n = 87$)**		***p* value**
Late (days 3–5)	**N**	**Number (%) or median (IQR)**	**N**	**Number (%) or median (IQR)**	
Biochemistry					
Hemoglobin (g/dl)	94	9.9 (9.0–11.1)	81	10.2 (9.2–10.9)	0.63
White blood count (10^9/L)	94	8.1 (5.9–11.6)	81	11.3 (7.1–15.0)	0.0029
Platelet count (10^9/L)	95	111.0 (68.0–153.0)	81	66.0 (47.0–100.0)	< 0.0001
INR	94	1.5 (1.3–1.8)	75	2.5 (1.8–4.4)	< 0.0001
ALT (IU/L)	94	1172 (612–2007)	78	938 (383–1995)	0.31
Bilirubin (mg/dl)	92	5.5 (2.7–8.2)	78	9.8 (6.7–13.7)	< 0.0001
pH	55	7.4 (7.4–7.5)	76	7.4 (7.3–7.5)	0.042
Ammonia (venous) (µmol/L)	25	62 (44–84)	17	119 (78–133)	0.0038
Creatinine (mg/dl)	94	1.2 (0.7–2.5)	82	2.4 (1.3–4.0)	< 0.0001
Lactate (mmol/L)	31	1.7 (1.0–2.2)	41	3.8 (2.6–6.7)	< 0.0001
Phosphate (mg/dl)	73	2.8 (2.3–3.6)	35	3.3 (2.5–4.5)	0.054
PO_2/FiO_2 ratio	48	3.3 (2.1–4.5)	71	2.5 (1.4–3.9)	0.0087
MELD	87	14.2 (5.4–24.6)	73	29.7 (23.5–35.4)	< 0.0001
High coma grade (3 or 4)[a]	59	35 (59%)	82	72 (88%)	< 0.0001
Organ support					
Mechanical ventilation	99	49 (49%)	88	74 (85%)	< 0.0001
Vasopressors	99	5 (5%)	88	45 (52%)	< 0.0001
Renal replacement therapy	99	10 (19%)	88	27 (31%)	0.062
FABP7 (ng/ml)	99	87.3 (48.0–261.5)	87	286.2 (146.7–536.9)	< 0.0001

N frequency, *IQR* interquartile range, *INR* international normalized ratio, *AST* aspartate aminotransferase, *ALT* alanine aminotransferase, *MELD* model for end-stage liver disease

[a] Hepatic encephalopathy grade according to West Haven criteria

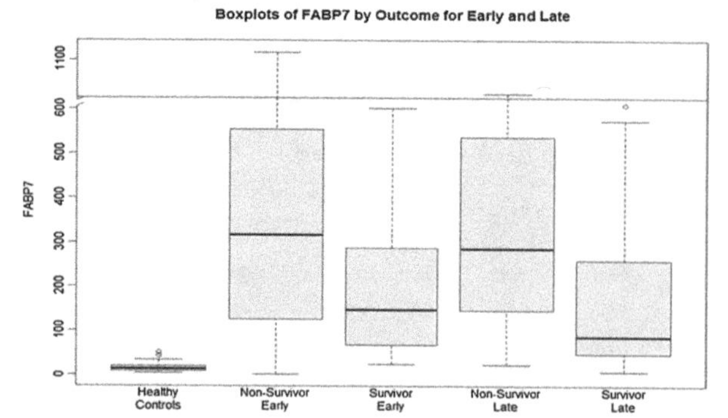

Fig. 1 Serum levels of FABP7 (ng/ml) in healthy controls, non-survivors (early ~ admission), survivors (early), non-survivors (late ~ days 3–5), survivors (late)

controls had median serum levels of 13.5 (8.7–20.2) ng/ml.

Clinical parameters in 186 APAP-ALF patients: days 3–5 (late)

Comparisons of clinical parameters on *days 3–5 (late)* are listed in Table 2. Of the 99 APAP-ALF non-survivors, samples of late time points were available in 87 patients as 12 died before days 3–5. APAP-ALF survivors ($n = 99$) were significantly less likely to be on MV (49 vs. 85%, p < 0.0001) and vasopressors, (5 vs. 52%, p < 0.0001) or achieve high HE grade (59 vs. 88%, p < 0.0001) than non-survivors.

Late (days 3–5) FABP7 are listed in Table 2 and graphically shown in Fig. 1. APAP-ALF survivors had significantly lower late serum FABP7 levels (87.3 vs. 286.2 ng/ml) compared with non-survivors ($p < 0.0001$). FABP7 levels were significantly higher in all ALF patients (survivors and non-survivors) compared to healthy controls for both early and late time points ($p < 0.0001$).

Multivariable analysis: associations with 21-day mortality

In order to adjust for covariates, multivariable logistic regression for 198 APAP-ALF patients to determine associations (adjusted) with 21-day mortality was performed (Table 3). Two models were derived: one on admission (early) and one at days 3–5 (late). Values of serum FABP7 were transformed to their natural logarithm (log FABP1) to comply with the linearity assumption in logistic regression.

Early (admission) model

FABP7 was not associated with 21-day mortality [odds ratio OR 1.001 per increment, 95% CI (1.000, 1.001), $p = 0.18$] after adjusting for significant covariates

Table 3 Early (day 1) and late (days 3–5) predictors of 21-day mortality in 198 APAP-ALF patients

Early	Unadjusted				Multivariable model ($N = 194$), AUROC = 0.766			
	N	OR	95% OR CI	*p* value	Included in Model	OR	95% CI	*p* value
FABP7	198	1.001	(1.000, 1.002)	0.0078	Yes	1.001	(1.000, 1.001)	0.18
MELD	194	1.083	(1.047, 1.119)	< 0.0001	Yes	1.056	(1.020, 1.093)	0.0021
Lactate	132	1.205	(1.095, 1.327)	0.0001	No			
Vasopressors	198	7.368	(3.335, 16.287)	< 0.0001	Yes	4.138	(1.769, 9.677)	0.0011
Renal replacement therapy	198	1.347	(0.683, 2.658)	0.390	No			
Mechanical ventilation	198	2.910	(1.547, 5.475)	0.0009	No			
High coma grade (3 or 4)	196	1.892	(1.047, 3.421)	0.0348	No			
Late (days 3–5)	**Unadjusted**				**Multivariable model ($N = 160$), AUROC = 0.891**			
	N	OR	95% OR CI	*p* value	Included in model	OR	95% CI	*p* value
FABP7	186	1.003	(1.001, 1.004)	0.0001	Yes	1.001	(0.999, 1.003)	0.40
MELD	160	1.115	(1.075, 1.157)	< 0.0001	Yes	1.084	(1.038, 1.132)	0.0003
Lactate	71	6.908	(2.592, 18.406)	0.0001	No			
Vasopressors	186	20.143	(7.462, 54.370)	< 0.0001	Yes	20.419	(6.221, 67.021)	<0.0001
Renal replacement therapy	186	1.895	(0.964, 3.724)	0.0638	No			
Mechanical ventilation	186	5.808	(2.859, 11.802)	< 0.0001	No			
High coma grade (3 or 4)	141	4.936	(2.129, 11.446)	0.0002	No			

Early: lactate ($p = 0.52$), high coma grade ($p = 0.46$), and mechanical ventilator ($p = 0.084$) were not significant on multivariable analysis so not included in the final early model

Late: mechanical ventilation ($p = 0.69$) and high coma grade ($p = 0.53$) were not significant on multivariable analysis so not included in the final late model. Lactate was not included due to missing data including MELD [OR 1.056 (1.020, 1.093) per increment, $p = 0.0021$] and requirement for vasopressors [OR 4.14 (1.77, 9.07), $p = 0.0011$]. This early model demonstrated AUROC of 0.766.

Late (days 3–5) model

FABP7 was not associated with 21-day mortality [OR 1.001 (0.999, 1.003) per increment, $p = 0.40$] after adjusting for significant covariates including MELD [OR 1.084 (1.038, 1.132) per increment, $p = 0.0003$] and requirement for vasopressors [OR 20.42 (6.22, 67.02), $p < 0.0001$]. This late model demonstrated AUROC of 0.891.

Analysis two: comparative analysis of 150 APAP-ALF patients

Demographic and clinical outcomes of 150 patients stratified by the presence ($n = 46$) and absence ($n = 104$) of ICH/CE based on review of subject data (ICP measurements, CT brain, cause of death) are shown in Additional file 3: Table S1. (In 48 patients, the presence or absence of ICH/CE could not be determined.) There were no significant differences in age (36 vs. 39, p = 0.11) or gender (female 74 vs. 69%, $p = 0.56$). During the 7 days of inpatient study, APAP-ALF patients with ICH/CE had higher requirements for ventilation (MV 100 vs. 75%, $p < 0.0001$) and were more likely to achieve high (3 or 4) HE coma grade (100 vs. 72%, $p < 0.0001$). APAP-ALF patients with evidence of ICH/CE were less likely to be alive at day 21 (17 vs. 41%, $p = 0.0049$) but were more likely to be listed for LT (33 vs. 13%, $p = 0.0062$).

Clinical parameters in 150 APAP-ALF patients: admission (early)

Comparisons of clinical parameters on study admission are shown in Additional file 4: Table S2. APAP-ALF patients with ICH/CE had significantly higher serum INR (3.6 vs. 2.9) compared to patients without ICH/CE ($p = 0.024$). On study admission, patients who went on to develop ICH/CE were significantly more likely to be on mechanical ventilation (MV 85 vs. 65%, p = 0.019) and achieve high HE grade (76 vs. 59%, $p = 0.043$). Admission (early) levels of FABP7 are listed in Additional file 4: Table S2 and graphically shown in Fig. 2. There were no significant differences in FABP7 levels on admission between APAP-ALF patients with or without ICH/CE (259.7 vs. 228.2 ng/ml, $p = 0.61$).

Clinical parameters in 186 APAP-ALF patients: days 3–5 (late)

Comparisons of clinical parameters on *days 3–5 (late)* are shown in Additional file 4: Table S2. Patients who developed ICH/CE were significantly more likely to be on mechanical ventilation (MV 95 vs. 63%, $p < 0.0001$) and achieve higher grades of HE (100 vs. 75%, $p = 0.0004$). Days 3–5 (late) levels of FABP7 are shown in Additional file 4: Table S2 and graphically in Fig. 2. There were no significant differences in late FABP7 levels between APAP-ALF patients with or without ICH/CE (223.8 vs. 192.0 ng/ml, $p = 0.19$).

Multivariable analysis: associations with 21-day mortality

Multivariable logistic regression for 198 APAP-ALF to determine associations (adjusted) with the development of ICH/CE was performed (Table 4). Two models were derived; one on admission (early) and one at days 3–5 (late). Values of serum FABP7 were transformed to their natural logarithm (log FABP1) to comply with the linearity assumption in logistic regression.

Early (admission) model

FABP7 was not associated with the development of ICH/CE [OR 1.000 per increment, 95% CI (1.000, 1.001), $p = 0.65$] after adjusting for the only significant covariate, mechanical ventilation [OR 2.880 (1.166, 7.111), $p = 0.022$]. This early model demonstrated AUROC of 0.590.

Late (days 3–5) model

FABP7 was not associated with the development of ICH/CE [OR 1.000 per increment, 95% CI (0.999, 1.001), $p = 0.57$] after adjusting for the only significant covariate, high hepatic coma grade [OR 25.76 (1.40, 472.5), $p = 0.029$]. This late model demonstrated AUROC of 0.641.

Discussion

Key results

In this nested case–control study, we report the first published analysis of FABP7 in a large series of 198

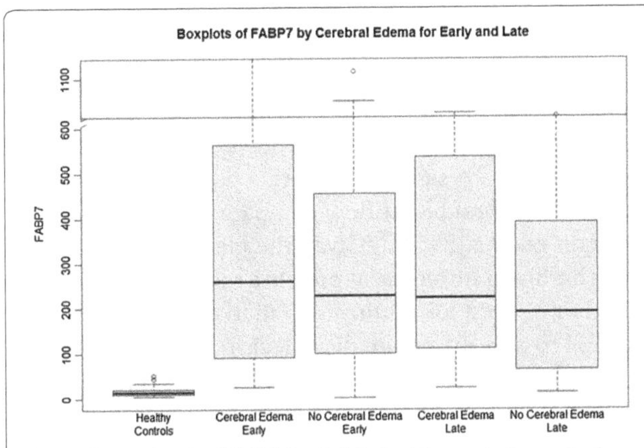

Fig. 2 Serum levels of FABP7 (ng/ml) in healthy controls, cerebral edema (early ~ admission), no cerebral edema (early), cerebral edema (late ~ days 3–5), no cerebral edema (late)

Table 4 Early (admission) and late (days 3–5) predictors of cerebral edema in 150 APAP-ALF patients

Early	Unadjusted				Multivariable model ($N = 148$), AUROC = 0.590			
	N	OR	95% OR CI	*p* value	Included in model	OR	95% CI	*p* value
FABP7	150	1.000	(1.000, 1.001)	0.58	Yes	1.000	(1.000, 1.001)	0.65
MELD	146	1.036	(0.997, 1.078)	0.072	No			
Lactate	100	1.000	(0.997, 1.002)	0.80	No			
Vasopressors	150	0.777	(0.363, 1.660)	0.51	No			
Renal replacement therapy	150	1.313	(0.598, 2.886)	0.50	No			
Mechanical ventilation	150	2.950	(1.199, 7.257)	0.019	Yes	2.880	(1.166, 7.111)	0.022
High coma grade (3 or 4)	148	2.227	(1.017, 4.878)	0.045	No			
Late (days 3–5)	**Unadjusted**				**Multivariable model ($N = 113$), AUROC = 0.641**			
	N	OR	95% OR CI	*p* value	Included in model	OR	95% CI	*p* value
FABP7	138	1.000	(0.999, 1.001)	0.96	Yes	1.000	(0.999, 1.001)	0.57
MELD	118	1.030	(0.994, 1.066)	0.10	No			
Lactate	53	1.031	(0.979, 1.086)	0.25	No			
Vasopressors	138	2.043	(0.947, 4.408)	0.069	No			
Renal replacement therapy	138	1.756	(0.789, 3.909)	0.17	No			
Mechanical ventilation	138	10.115	(2.300, 44.491)	0.0022	No			
High coma grade (3 or 4)*	113	24.324	(1.326, 446.243)	0.0316	Yes	25.759	(1.404, 472.46)	0.029

Early: high coma grade ($p = 0.69$) was not significant on multivariable analysis so not included in the final early model

Late: mechanical ventilation ($p = 0.65$) was not significant on multivariable analysis so not included in the final late model

*Statistically significant on multivariable analysis

well-characterized APAP-ALF patients. Compared with survivors, serum FABP7 levels were significantly higher at serial time points (early and late) in APAP-ALF non-survivors. However, significant differences in FABP7 levels by 21-day mortality were not ascertained after adjusting for significant covariates reflecting severity of illness (MELD, vasopressor dependence). No differences in the FABP7 levels were detected for APAP-ALF patients with and without evidence of ICH/CE.

Comparison with literature

In our study, ICH/CE was the cause of death in 39% of patients, similar to what has been previously reported [16]. ICH/CE arises due to astrocyte swelling, cerebral vasodilatation, dilated cerebral arterioles and altered cerebral blood flow [23, 24]. Furthermore, it has been shown that patients with signs of cerebral edema and ICH have increased cerebral blood flow compared to patients without brain edema [25, 26]. Given the bleeding risks associated with direct intracranial pressure monitoring [8], there is an unmet need for noninvasive markers of brain edema and ICH to help inform medical decisions. In the setting of ALF, astrocyte swelling/injury leads to astrocyte dysfunction and consequently impairs neuronal function leading to HE. However, in parallel, swollen astrocytes release small proteins, molecules and osmolytes in response to astrocyte hypertonicity to reduce swelling. In the past 20 years, several biochemical biomarkers have been investigated for the detection of cerebral injury, including protein S100b [27], neuron-specific enolase (NSE) [27] and glial fibrillary protein (GFAP) [9]. Studies by Strauss et al. [27], as well as Vaquero et al. [28], which included 35 and 54 ALF patients, respectively, concluded that S-100b was not a useful marker of neurological outcome in ALF. Furthermore, despite a consistent increase of S-100b in serum, levels did not correlate with severity of HE, development of brain herniation or outcome. In the same patients, Strauss et al. found that serum levels of NSE were higher in ALF patients with ICH than those who survived without ICH [27]. However, this univariate comparison did not adjust for significant confounding factors/covariates, an important limitation to the study.

Major components of the brain are lipids with brain cells having a high cell membrane/cytoplasm ratio. Cell membranes are formed of lipid bilayers consisting of saturated and unsaturated fatty acids, which can also be oxidized for generating ATP. The primary function of FABPs is to facilitate the transport of intracellular long-chain fatty acids. In the brain, FABP7 and heart FABP (FABP3) are expressed with FABP7 primarily found in astrocytes [29] and FABP3 in neurons [30]. With astrocyte swelling being a neuropathological landmark of ALF along with a hyperdynamic circulation frequently occurring in ALF leading to an increased myocardial demand, FABP3 may be confounded with myocardial injury. Therefore, FABP7 is more specific to brain injury in ALF.

FABP7 has physiological properties that render this protein advantageous as a prognostic biomarker in ALF: (i) it is abundantly present in astrocytes (between approximately 0.8 and 3.1 μg/g of brain tissue), (ii) it has a lower molecular mass (14 kDa); it is smaller than S-100b (21 kDa), enolase (47 kDa) and GFAP (50 kDa) with a much shorter plasma half-life (11 min) [31–33]. Smaller proteins such as FABP7 diffuse more rapidly (via transcytosis) than larger proteins though the interstitial space and cross the blood–brain barrier (BBB).

The release of cerebrovascular proteins into blood plasma is dependent on the status (breakdown) of the BBB, which in ALF is dependent on the underlying mechanisms of cerebral edema, cytotoxic and vasogenic [34]. Astrocyte swelling plays a definitive role in the development of cytotoxic brain edema. In cytotoxic edema, the BBB is intact in the presence of intracellular swelling [35], whereas in vasogenic edema there is breakdown of the BBB and water and plasma constituents accumulate in the extracellular space [36]. Although a complete breakdown of the blood–brain barrier is not evident in ALF, increased permeation to water and other small molecules such as ammonia has been demonstrated resulting from subtle alterations in the protein composition of paracellular tight junctions [37].

Despite elevated levels in ALF patients (survivors and non-survivors) in this analysis, FABP7 did not discriminate between patients who went on to develop significant signs of ICH/CE either on imaging, ICP measurements or at death. One explanation is that variability in BBB permeability during ICH/CE could impact the diffusion rate of FABP7 into the peripheral circulation. In this study, we speculate that heterogeneity in the permeability of the BBB in ALF patients likely impacted the discriminatory ability of serum FABP7 measurements and important neurological outcomes in ALF. While FABP7 in cerebrospinal fluid may be more discriminatory between patients with and without astrocyte swelling/injury, this would not be feasible as a noninvasive biomarker as it would require an interventricular drain.

Limitations

The following limitations of this study warrant consideration. It is a nested case–control study, and as such the event rate of the primary outcome (21-day mortality) was 50%, higher than published in cohort series. Although patients were enrolled and samples were collected prospectively, analysis was performed retrospectively and therefore can comment on association and discrimination (between survivors and non-survivors) and not on the absolute risks of death and intracranial complications according to serum FABP7 levels. To account for potential confounding in the study design, we performed multivariable analysis to adjust for other significant covariates reflecting severity of illness (MELD, vasopressors, mechanical ventilation, hepatic coma grade). To avoid confounding related to LT since transplant listing decisions for APAP-ALF and the organ availability were not consistent between study centers (Simmons et al., ALFSG unpublished data), samples from patients who received a LT were not evaluated in this study. The case–control design of the study may have introduced selection bias, as the primary outcome of survival is automatically unbalanced within the clinical profile of the groups. However, in an attempt to reduce observation bias, data were collected prospectively and within this specific study design, researchers measuring FABP7 were blinded to the clinical and outcome data of patients at the time of patient selection and sample analysis. Finally, we acknowledge that determinations of ICH were done retrospectively using available data from death summaries: cranial imaging and ICP measurements (if a monitor was used), and this may have introduced further bias. The decision to order computed tomography of the brain and the use of ICP monitors were individual decisions made by the practicing clinician, and these were not standardized across the ALFSG registry and may have varied between centers. While renal function may have impacted serum FABP7 levels, we attempted to adjust for this by including renal function (MELD) in multivariable analysis. Nonetheless despite these limitations, we believe these results are robust as they include APAP-ALF cases from across 16 tertiary liver transplant centers comprising the US ALFSG and are the first report of FABP7 in acute liver failure.

Conclusions

Brain FABP levels were elevated in APAP-ALF patients with significantly higher serum levels at early and late time points in APAP-ALF non-survivors. However, significant differences in FABP7 levels by 21-day mortality were not ascertained after adjusting for significant covariates reflecting severity of illness (MELD, vasopressor dependence). No differences in the FABP7 levels were detected for APAP-ALF patients with and without evidence of ICH/CE. FABP7 does not appear to discriminate between patients who did and did not have significant intracranial complications of APAP-ALF.

Abbreviations
ALF: acute liver failure; ALFSG: Acute Liver Failure Study Group; APAP: acetaminophen; FABP7: brain-type fatty acid-binding protein; HE: hepatic encephalopathy; ICU: intensive care unit; INR: international normalized ratio; IQR: interquartile range; KCC: King's College criteria; LT: liver transplantation; MELD: model for end-stage liver disease score; MV: mechanical ventilation; OR: odds ratio; RRT: renal replacement therapy.

Authors' contributions
CJK conceived the study concept and design, performed analysis and interpretation of the data, and drafted the final manuscript. JLS performed statistical analysis and interpretation of data and critically revised the final manuscript. MT performed laboratory analysis and revised the final manuscript. WML supervised the entire US Acute Liver Failure Study Group (U-01 Grant) and critically revised the manuscript for important intellectual content. CFR conceived the idea of the study, assisted in developing study design and interpretation of data and critically revised the final manuscript for important intellectual content. All authors read and approved the final manuscript.

Author details
[1] Division of Gastroenterology (Liver Unit), Department of Critical Care Medicine, University of Alberta, 1-40 Zeidler Ledcor Building, Edmonton, AB T6G-2X8, Canada. [2] Department of Public Health Sciences, Medical University of South Carolina, Charleston, SC, USA. [3] Hepato-Neuro Laboratory, CRCHUM, Université de Montréal, Montreal, Canada. [4] Division of Digestive and Liver Diseases, Department of Internal Medicine, University of Texas Southwestern Medical Center, Dallas, TX, USA.

Acknowledgements
Current members and institutions participating in the Acute Liver Failure Study Group are as follows: W.M. Lee, M.D. (Principal Investigator); Anne M. Larson, M.D., Iris Liou, M.D., University of Washington, Seattle, WA; Michael Schilsky, M.D., Yale University, New Haven, CT; Daniel Ganger, M.D., Northwestern University, Chicago, IL; Robert Fontana, M.D., University of Michigan, Ann Arbor, MI; Brendan McGuire, M.D., University of Alabama, Birmingham, AL; David Koch MD, Medical University of South Carolina, Charleston, SC; R. Todd Stravitz, M.D., Virginia Commonwealth University, Richmond, VA; Constantine J. Karvellas MD, University of Alberta, Edmonton, AB; Jody Olson MD, University of Kansas, Kansas City, KA; Ram Subramanian MD, Emory, Atlanta, GA; James Hanje MD, Ohio State University, Columbus, OH; Bilal Hameed MD, University of California San Francisco, CA.

The University of Texas Southwestern Administrative Group included Grace Samuel, Ezmina Lalani, Carla Pezzia, and Corron Sanders, Ph.D., Nahid Attar, Linda S. Hynan, Ph.D., and the Medical University of South Carolina Data Coordination Unit included Valerie Durkalski, Ph.D., Wenle Zhao, Ph.D., Jaime Speiser, Catherine Dillon, Holly Battenhouse and Michelle Gottfried.

Competing interests
The authors declare that they have no competing interests.

Format
This paper followed the STROBE guideline for reporting cohort studies (BMJ 2007): See Additional file 5.

Funding
The study was sponsored by NIH Grant U-01 58369 (from NIDDK) and a Grant from the University of Alberta Hospital Foundation (UHF).

References

1. O'Grady JG, Williams R. Classification of acute liver failure. Lancet. 1993;342(8873):743.
2. Larson AM, Polson J, Fontana RJ, Davern TJ, Lalani E, Hynan LS, et al. Acetaminophen-induced acute liver failure: results of a United States multicenter, prospective study. Hepatology. 2005;42(6):1364–72.
3. Bernal W, Wendon J. Acute liver failure; clinical features and management. Eur J Gastroenterol Hepatol. 1999;11(9):977–84.
4. Blei AT, Larsen FS. Pathophysiology of cerebral edema in fulminant hepatic failure. J Hepatol. 1999;31(4):771–6.
5. Bernal W, Hall C, Karvellas CJ, Auzinger G, Sizer E, Wendon J. Arterial ammonia and clinical risk factors for encephalopathy and intracranial hypertension in acute liver failure. Hepatology. 2007;46(6):1844–52.
6. Martinez-Hernandez A, Bell KP, Norenberg MD. Glutamine synthetase: glial localization in brain. Science. 1977;195(4284):1356–8.
7. Davern TJ. Predicting prognosis in acute liver failure: ammonia and the risk of cerebral edema. Hepatology. 2007;46(6):1679–81.
8. Karvellas CJ, Fix OK, Battenhouse H, Durkalski V, Sanders C, Lee WM, et al. Outcomes and complications of intracranial pressure monitoring in acute liver failure: a retrospective cohort study. Crit Care Med. 2014;42(5):1157–67.
9. Pelsers MM, Glatz JF. Detection of brain injury by fatty acid-binding proteins. Clin Chem Lab Med. 2005;43(8):802–9.
10. Bass NM, Barker ME, Manning JA, Jones AL, Ockner RK. Acinar heterogeneity of fatty acid binding protein expression in the livers of male, female and clofibrate-treated rats. Hepatology. 1989;9(1):12–21.
11. Glatz JF, van der Vusse GJ. Cellular fatty acid-binding proteins: their function and physiological significance. Prog Lipid Res. 1996;35(3):243–82.
12. Wunderlich MT, Hanhoff T, Goertler M, Spener F, Glatz JF, Wallesch CW, et al. Release of brain-type and heart-type fatty acid-binding proteins in serum after acute ischaemic stroke. J Neurol. 2005;252(6):718–24.
13. Teunissen CE, Veerhuis R, De Vente J, Verhey FR, Vreeling F, van Boxtel MP, et al. Brain-specific fatty acid-binding protein is elevated in serum of patients with dementia-related diseases. Eur J Neurol. 2011;18(6):865–71.
14. Karvellas CJ, Speiser JL, Tremblay M, Lee WM, Rose CF, Group USALFS. Elevated FABP1 serum levels are associated with poorer survival in acetaminophen-induced acute liver failure. Hepatology 2017;65(3):938–49.
15. von Elm E, Altman DG, Egger M, Pocock SJ, Gotzsche PC, Vandenbroucke JP. Strengthening the Reporting of Observational Studies in Epidemiology (STROBE) statement: guidelines for reporting observational studies. BMJ. 2007;335(7624):806–8.
16. Reuben A, Tillman H, Fontana RJ, Davern T, McGuire B, Stravitz RT, et al. Outcomes in adults with acute liver failure between 1998 and 2013: an observational cohort study. Ann Intern Med. 2016;164(11):724–32.
17. Conn HO, Lieberthal MM, editors. The hepatic coma syndromes and lactulose. Baltimore: Williams & Wilkins; 1979.
18. O'Grady JG, Schalm SW, Williams R. Acute liver failure: redefining the syndromes. Lancet. 1993;342(8866):273–5.
19. O'Grady JG, Alexander GJ, Hayllar KM, Williams R. Early indicators of prognosis in fulminant hepatic failure. Gastroenterology. 1989;97(2):439–45.
20. Kamath PS, Wiesner RH, Malinchoc M, Kremers W, Therneau TM, Kosberg CL, et al. A model to predict survival in patients with end-stage liver disease. Hepatology. 2001;33(2):464–70.
21. Li X, Song X, Gray RH. Comparison of the missing-indicator method and conditional logistic regression in 1:m matched case-control studies with missing exposure values. Am J Epidemiol. 2004;159(6):603–10.
22. Shawcross DL, Wendon JA. The neurological manifestations of acute liver failure. Neurochem Int. 2012;60(7):662–71.
23. Larsen FS, Ejlersen E, Hansen BA, Knudsen GM, Tygstrup N, Secher NH. Functional loss of cerebral blood flow autoregulation in patients with fulminant hepatic failure. J Hepatol. 1995;23(2):212–7.
24. Strauss G, Hansen BA, Kirkegaard P, Rasmussen A, Hjortrup A, Larsen FS. Liver function, cerebral blood flow autoregulation, and hepatic encephalopathy in fulminant hepatic failure. Hepatology. 1997;25(4):837–9.
25. Wendon JA, Harrison PM, Keays R, Williams R. Cerebral blood flow and metabolism in fulminant liver failure. Hepatology. 1994;19(6):1407–13.

26. Aggarwal S, Kramer D, Yonas H, Obrist W, Kang Y, Martin M, et al. Cerebral hemodynamic and metabolic changes in fulminant hepatic failure: a retrospective study. Hepatology. 1994;19(1):80–7.
27. Strauss GI, Christiansen M, Moller K, Clemmesen JO, Larsen FS, Knudsen GM. S-100b and neuron-specific enolase in patients with fulminant hepatic failure. Liver Transpl. 2001;7(11):964–70.
28. Vaquero J, Jordano Q, Lee WM, Blei AT. Group USALFS: serum protein S-100b in acute liver failure: results of the US Acute Liver Failure Study group. Liver Transpl. 2003;9(8):887–8.
29. Owada Y, Abdelwahab SA, Kitanaka N, Sakagami H, Takano H, Sugitani Y, et al. Altered emotional behavioral responses in mice lacking brain-type fatty acid-binding protein gene. Eur J Neurosci. 2006;24(1):175–87.
30. Myers-Payne SC, Hubbell T, Pu L, Schnutgen F, Borchers T, Wood WG, et al. Isolation and characterization of two fatty acid binding proteins from mouse brain. J Neurochem. 1996;66(4):1648–56.
31. Ghanem G, Loir B, Morandini R, Sales F, Lienard D, Eggermont A, et al. On the release and half-life of S100B protein in the peripheral blood of melanoma patients. Int J Cancer. 2001;94(4):586–90.
32. Mrozek S, Dumurgier J, Citerio G, Mebazaa A, Geeraerts T. Biomarkers and acute brain injuries: interest and limits. Crit Care. 2014;18(2):220.
33. Wunderlich MT, Ebert AD, Kratz T, Goertler M, Jost S, Herrmann M. Early neurobehavioral outcome after stroke is related to release of neurobiochemical markers of brain damage. Stroke. 1999;30(6):1190–5.
34. Scott TR, Kronsten VT, Hughes RD, Shawcross DL. Pathophysiology of cerebral oedema in acute liver failure. World J Gastroenterol. 2013;19(48):9240–55.
35. Traber PG, Dal Canto M, Ganger DR, Blei AT. Electron microscopic evaluation of brain edema in rabbits with galactosamine-induced fulminant hepatic failure: ultrastructure and integrity of the blood-brain barrier. Hepatology. 1987;7(6):1272–7.
36. Cui W, Sun CM, Liu P. Alterations of blood-brain barrier and associated factors in acute liver failure. Gastroenterol Res Pract. 2013;2013:841707.
37. Nguyen JH, Yamamoto S, Steers J, Sevlever D, Lin W, Shimojima N, et al. Matrix metalloproteinase-9 contributes to brain extravasation and edema in fulminant hepatic failure mice. J Hepatol. 2006;44(6):1105–14.

10

Mortality and detailed characteristics of pre-ICU qSOFA-negative patients with suspected sepsis

Izumi Nakayama[1], Junichi Izawa[2,3*], Hideyuki Mouri[4], Tetsuhisa Kitamura[5] and Junji Shiotsuka[4]

Abstract

Background: Recent studies have suggested that quick Sequential Organ Failure Assessment (qSOFA) scores have limited utility in early prognostication in high-mortality populations. The purpose of this study was to investigate the association between pre-ICU qSOFA scores and in-hospital mortality among patients admitted to the ICU with suspected sepsis. This study also aimed to describe detailed clinical characteristics of qSOFA-negative (< 2) patients.

Methods: This single center, observational study, conducted in a Japanese tertiary care teaching hospital between May 2012 and June 2016, enrolled all consecutive adult patients admitted to the ICU with suspected sepsis. We assessed pre-ICU qSOFA scores with the most abnormal vital signs during the 24-h period before ICU admission. The primary outcome was in-hospital mortality censored at 90 days. We analyzed the association between pre-ICU qSOFA scores and in-hospital mortality.

Results: Among 185 ICU patients with suspected sepsis, 14.1% (26/185) of patients remained qSOFA-negative at the time of ICU admission and 29.2% (54/185) of patients died while in hospital. In-hospital mortality was similar between the groups (qSOFA-positive [≥ 2]: 30.2% [48/159] vs qSOFA-negative: 23.1% [6/26], $p = 0.642$). The Cox proportional hazard regression model revealed that being qSOFA-positive was not significantly associated with in-hospital mortality (adjusted hazard ratio 1.35, 95% confidence interval 0.56–3.22, $p = 0.506$). Bloodstream infection, immunosuppression, and hematologic malignancy were observed more frequently in qSOFA-negative patients.

Conclusions: Among ICU patients with suspected sepsis, we could not find a strong association between pre-ICU qSOFA scores and in-hospital mortality. Our study suggested high mortality and bacterial diversity in pre-ICU qSOFA-negative patients.

Keywords: Intensive care unit, Critical care, Bacteremia, Sepsis, quick Sequential Organ Failure Assessment (qSOFA) score, Infection, Mortality

Background

Early identification and interventions have been shown to improve sepsis outcomes [1, 2]. Recently, the quick Sequential Organ Failure Assessment (qSOFA) score was developed to promptly identify infected patients at risk of mortality. The original study showed that qSOFA-positive (≥ 2) patients had a 3- to 14-fold increase in in-hospital mortality compared to qSOFA-negative (< 2) patients [3]. With its simple and repeatedly measurable property, qSOFA has had a promising role in providing a more effective triage for infected patients [4].

However, recent studies have suggested that qSOFA has limited utility in early prognostication in high-mortality populations. One study showed that almost one-half of patients with infection remained qSOFA-negative even at the time of ICU admission [5]. In studies enrolling patients admitted to the ICU, the mortality of qSOFA-negative patients was greater than 10% [5–9]. Thus, the

*Correspondence: jizawa13@gmail.com
[2] Intensive Care Unit, Department of Anesthesiology, The Jikei University School of Medicine, 3-19-18 Nishi-Shinbashi, Minato-ku, Tokyo 105-8471, Japan
Full list of author information is available at the end of the article

usefulness of qSOFA scores in high-risk populations has remained controversial.

We hypothesized that, for patients with suspected sepsis requiring ICU admission, the prognostic impact of qSOFA-positive was small. The purpose of this study was to investigate the association between pre-ICU qSOFA scores, assessed during the 24-h period before ICU admission, and in-hospital mortality among patients admitted to the ICU with suspected sepsis. Furthermore, we described detailed clinical characteristics of qSOFA-negative patients including clinical diagnosis, primary sites of infection, causative organisms, and comorbidities. Given this description, we aimed to disclose features of patients whose risk of mortality was difficult to estimate using qSOFA.

Methods

Study design, setting, and patients

This was an observational study conducted at the Okinawa Chubu Hospital, a tertiary care teaching hospital with 550 hospital beds and 14 ICU beds in Japan, between May 2012 and June 2016. The hospital institutional review board approved the study protocol (H28-14). Because of the retrospective approach of this study and de-identification of personal data, the board waived the need for informed consent.

We examined data of all adult (≥ 18 years) patients who were admitted to the ICU between May 2012 and June 2016. We identified consecutive patients with suspected sepsis through the following inclusion criteria: the documentation of the reason for ICU admission as 'bacteremia,' 'sepsis,' 'severe sepsis,' or 'septic shock' in the ICU register. Each documentation was based on the clinical judgment as having a severe infection requiring ICU admission. Two attending physicians reviewed the patient data and agreed on the clinical suspicion of infection. We excluded patients with cardiac arrest prior to ICU admission because we did not expect an additional predictive value of qSOFA in these patients.

Data collection

Data for analyses including age, sex, chronic health conditions, location prior to ICU admission, vital signs and qSOFA scores before ICU admission, the presence of rigor ('shaking chills'), primary site of infection, type of organisms, length of ICU stay, the prevalence of bacteremia and in-hospital mortality were collected from patient records. According to a previous report from our institution [10], we routinely classified the qualitative degree of rigor ('chills') as follows: 'mild chills,' feeling cold with the need for an outer jacket; 'moderate chills,' feeling very cold with the need for a thick blanket; and 'shaking chills,' a profound chill with generalized involuntary bodily shaking, even under a thick blanket. Physicians were instructed to record the degree of chills when they suspected bacteremia in daily practice. We described the primary site of infection as bloodstream, respiratory, gastrointestinal, neurological, genitourinary, or musculoskeletal infection based on the clinical context. Bloodstream infection was defined as blood culture-positive infection including infective endocarditis, bacteremia from an unknown origin and catheter-related bacteremia. The primary infection site showed the following organism types, namely gram-negative bacterial infection, gram-positive bacterial infection, polymicrobial infection or fungal infection. Illness severity was assessed using the Acute Physiology and Chronic Health Evaluation (APACHE) II [11] and the Sequential Organ Failure Assessment (SOFA) scores [12] with the most abnormal measurements recorded during the first 24-h period after ICU admission (Additional file 1: Fig. S1). We used the worst SOFA scores and defined sepsis as a SOFA score of ≥ 2 according to the Sepsis-3 definition [4].

Measurement of the main exposure factors (Additional file 1: Fig. S1)

The qSOFA score had three criteria, assigning one point for alteration in mental status (Glasgow Coma Scale < 15), systolic blood pressure ≤ 100 mm, Hg or respiratory rate ≥ 22/min [4]. We evaluated pre-ICU qSOFA scores with the most abnormal vital signs at the time of clinical deterioration during the 24-h period before ICU admission. We set this time window to evaluate the performance value of pre-ICU admission qSOFA scores in prognosticating high-risk patients before ICU transfer. We also aimed to avoid the effect of therapeutic interventions during the ICU stay on qSOFA scores. According to a previous study, we defined qSOFA-positive or qSOFA-negative as a qSOFA score of ≥ 2 or < 2, respectively [3]. We also evaluated pre-ICU systemic inflammatory response syndrome (SIRS) with the most abnormal measurements during the 24-h period before ICU admission. SIRS-positive was defined as two or more of the following: temperature > 38 or < 36 °C, heart rate > 90 beats/min, respiratory rate > 20 breaths/min, or arterial carbon dioxide pressure < 32 mm Hg, white blood cell count > 12,000/μL or < 4000/μL [13]. In addition, we evaluated qSOFA scores and SIRS at the exact moment of ICU arrival using the first measurements of vital signs just after ICU admission.

Outcome measures

The primary outcome measure was in-hospital mortality, which was defined as any cause of death censored at 90 days after ICU admission. Other outcomes included the length of ICU stay, ICU stay ≥ 3 days, bacteremia and in-hospital mortality censored at 28 days after ICU admission. We defined bacteremia as 2 sets of blood culture with the same microorganism or 1 set of blood culture with bacteria, except for possible contaminated resources involving Coagulase-negative *Staphylococci*, *Corynebacterium* species, *Propionibacterium* species, *Bacillus* species, *Aerococcus* species, and *Micrococcus* species [14, 15].

Statistical analysis

Continuous data are presented as medians with interquartile range (IQR) and compared using the Mann–Whitney *U* test. Categorical data are presented as proportions and compared using a *Chi-squared* test or Fisher's exact test when appropriate. We used Kaplan–Meier plots to describe the survival between qSOFA-positive and qSOFA-negative patients and compared the survival curves with the log-rank test. As the primary analysis, the Cox proportional hazard regression model was used to assess the association between being qSOFA-positive before ICU admission and in-hospital mortality censored at 90 days after ICU admission. The hazard ratio (HR) and 95% confidence interval (CI) were calculated. The following variables were incorporated into the primary multivariable models: age, the presence of rigor ('shaking chills'), prior location to the ICU, and chronic health condition with immunosuppression. In the Kaplan–Meier description and the Cox regression analysis, if survival hospital discharge occurs within 90 days after ICU admission, we dealt with it as censoring. We also estimated the performance of pre-ICU qSOFA, pre-ICU SIRS, qSOFA at ICU arrival, and SIRS at ICU arrival in predicting sepsis by the Sepsis-3 and in-hospital mortality censored at 90 days. The crude risk ratios (RRs) with 95% CI and area under receiver operating characteristics (AUROC) were calculated. We used qSOFA scores and SIRS scores as continuous variables for the calculation of AUROCs. All statistical analyses were performed using R (The R Foundation for Statistical Computing, ver.3.2.4) and EZR (Saitama Medical Center, Jichi Medical University, ver.1.32), which is a graphical user interface for R [16]. All tests were two-tailed; *p* values of less than 0.05 were regarded as statistically significant.

Results

The patient flow diagram is presented in Fig. 1. We extracted 188 patients who were admitted to the ICU with suspected sepsis. After excluding 3 patients with prior cardiac arrest, we enrolled 185 patients for our analyses. At least 2 sets of blood cultures were obtained from all participants. The median age was 67 (IQR 57–79), and 61.1% (113/185) of patients were from the emergency room (ER) and 33.5% (62/185) of patients had at least one chronic health condition. Among 185 patients, 85.9% (159/185) were qSOFA-positive and 89.7% (166/185) were SIRS-positive before ICU admission. The median APACHE II and SOFA scores were 21 (IQR 17–28) and 9 (IQR 5–11), respectively. In total, 91.9% (170/185) of patients fulfilled the Sepsis-3 definition, 53.0% (98/185) had positive blood culture, and 29.2% (54/185) died in hospital within 90 days after ICU admission.

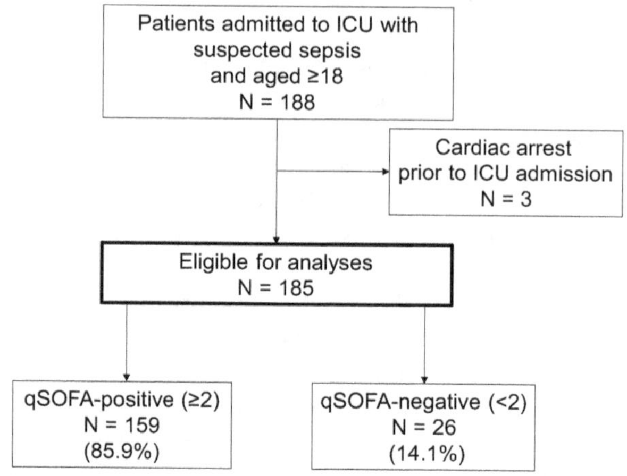

Fig. 1 Flow of patients admitted to the ICU with suspected sepsis from 2012 to 2016. *ICU* denotes intensive care unit, *qSOFA* quick Sequential Organ Failure Assessment

Patient demographics, characteristics at the presentation of infection, and characteristics after ICU admission are presented in Table 1. While qSOFA-positive patients were presented with more deranged vital signs, qSOFA-negative patients were more frequently from the ward (qSOFA-positive: 35.8% [57/159] vs qSOFA-negative: 57.7% [15/26], $p=0.050$) and more frequently had shaking chills (qSOFA-positive: 27.7% [44/159] vs qSOFA-negative: 53.8% [14/26], $p=0.011$). Hematologic malignancy (qSOFA-positive: 5.7% [9/159] vs qSOFA-negative: 15.4% [4/26], $p=0.090$) and immunosuppression (qSOFA-positive: 5.7% [9/159] vs qSOFA-negative: 15.4% [4/26], $p=0.090$) were also observed more frequently in qSOFA-negative patients. The degree of organ dysfunction was similar between the groups in relation to respiration, coagulation, and liver and renal components of the SOFA scores.

The outcomes of qSOFA-negative patients were similar to those of qSOFA-positive patients (Fig. 2 and Table 2). The primary outcome, in-hospital mortality censored at 90 days after ICU admission, was not significantly different between the groups (qSOFA-positive: 30.2% [48/159] vs qSOFA-negative: 23.1% [6/26], $p=0.642$). The other outcomes, ICU length of stay (qSOFA-positive: 3 [2–6] vs qSOFA-negative: 3 [2–5], $p=0.787$),

Table 1 Characteristics before and after ICU admission in patients with suspected sepsis

	qSOFA-positive (≥ 2) (*N* = 159)	qSOFA-negative (< 2) (*N* = 26)	*p* value
Demographics			
Age (median [IQR])	67 [57–79]	68 [63–75]	0.791
Male (%)	95 (59.7%)	16 (61.5%)	1.000
Chronic health condition (%)			
Metastatic cancer	7 (4.4%)	1 (3.8%)	1.000
Chronic dialysis	22 (13.8%)	4 (15.4%)	0.767
Hepatic failure	15 (9.4%)	2 (7.7%)	1.000
Chronic respiratory failure	4 (2.5%)	1 (3.8%)	0.535
Hematologic malignancy	9 (5.7%)	4 (15.4%)	0.090
Immunosuppression	9 (5.7%)	4 (15.4%)	0.090
Characteristics at the presentation of infection			
Location prior to ICU admission (%)			0.050
Emergency room	102 (64.2%)	11 (42.3%)	
General ward	57 (35.8%)	15 (57.7%)	
Vital signs before ICU admission (median [IQR])			
Systolic blood pressure, mm Hg	82 [70–96]	105 [79–120]	0.004
Respiratory rate,/min	28 [24–30]	20 [20–24]	< 0.001
Glasgow coma scale	13 [9–15]	15 [15–15]	< 0.001
Heart rate,/min	116 [101–132]	110 [88–119]	0.047
Body temperature, Celsius	38.2 [37.2–39.1]	38.2 [37.1–39.2]	0.997
Shaking chills (%)	44 (27.7%)	14 (53.8%)	0.011
Characteristics after ICU admission			
APACHE II (median [IQR])	22 [17–29]	20 [15–24]	0.092
SOFA score (median [IQR])	9 [6–12]	6 [3–8]	0.001
SOFA respiration	2 [1–3]	1 [0–3]	0.112
SOFA coagulation	1 [0–2]	1 [0–2]	0.256
SOFA liver	0 [0–1]	0 [0–0]	0.296
SOFA central nervous system	1 [0–3]	0 [0–0]	< 0.001
SOFA renal	1 [0–3]	1 [0–2]	0.887
SOFA cardiovascular	3 [1–4]	1 [0–3]	< 0.001
Lactate, mmol/L (median [IQR])	2.5 [1.5–5.3]	1.5 [0.9–3.5]	0.075

qSOFA scores were assessed with the most abnormal vital signs during the 24-h period before the ICU admission. SOFA and APACHE II scores were calculated with the most abnormal measurements taken during the first 24-h period after the ICU admission

APACHE II Acute Physiology and Chronic Health Evaluation II, *ICU* intensive care unit, *IQR* interquartile range, *qSOFA* quick Sequential Organ Failure Assessment, *SOFA* Sequential Organ Failure Assessment

bacteremia (qSOFA-positive: 53.5% [85/159] vs qSOFA-negative: 50.0% [13/26], $p = 0.833$), and 28-day mortality (qSOFA-positive: 25.2% [40/159] vs qSOFA-negative: 19.2% [5/26], $p = 0.627$) were also similar between the groups. The Kaplan–Meier plots of survival showed no significant difference between the groups ($p = 0.514$). The Cox proportional hazard regression model revealed that pre-ICU qSOFA-positive was not significantly associated with in-hospital mortality (adjusted HR 1.35, 95% CI 0.56–3.22, $p = 0.506$).

Detailed microbiological results are presented in Table 3. Among primary sites of infection, bloodstream infection was more frequent in qSOFA-negative patients (qSOFA-positive: 18.2% [29/159] vs qSOFA-negative: 30.8% [8/26], $p = 0.094$). Among identified organisms, *Staphylococcus aureus* infection was more frequent in qSOFA-negative patients (qSOFA-positive: 8.8% [14/159] vs qSOFA-negative: 15.4% [4/26], $p = 0.290$). Of 26 qSOFA-negative patients, the most common site of infection was bloodstream infection (30.8% [8/26]), followed by genitourinary infection (23.1% [6/26]). Among qSOFA-negative patients who died in the hospital, all the patients had at least one chronic health condition.

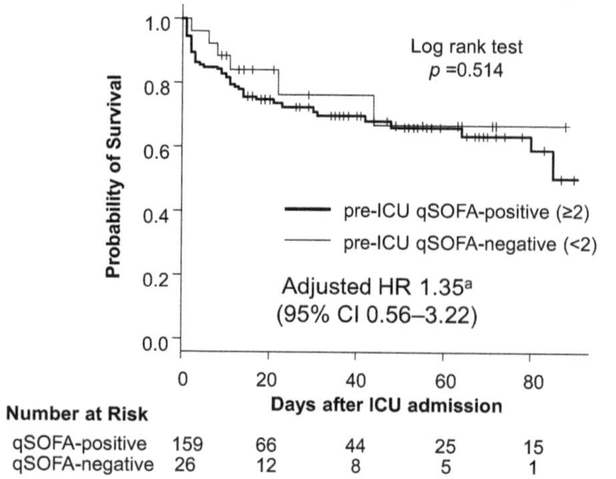

Fig. 2 Kaplan–Meier curves of in-hospital mortality censored at 90 days stratified as pre-ICU qSOFA-positive or qSOFA-negative. [a]Adjusted for age, the presence of rigor ('shaking chills'), prior location to the ICU and chronic health condition with immunosuppression. *CI* confidence interval, *HR* hazard ratio, *ICU* intensive care unit, *qSOFA* quick Sequential Organ Failure Assessment. The vertical tick marks on the curves denote censoring due to survival discharge

The performance of qSOFA and SIRS in predicting sepsis and mortality is shown in Table 4. The association between pre-ICU qSOFA or pre-ICU SIRS and in-hospital mortality censored at 90 days was not significant (qSOFA crude RR 1.38, 95% CI 0.62–2.74, AUROC 0.511; SIRS crude RR 0.92, 95% CI 0.45–1.85, AUROC 0.521). On the other hand, qSOFA at ICU arrival was significantly associated with in-hospital mortality censored at 90 days (crude RR 1.78, 95% CI 1.09–2.89, AUROC 0.586).

Discussion

Our study suggested that the prognostic impact of pre-ICU qSOFA, assessed during the 24-h period before ICU admission, was small among patients with suspected sepsis (HR 1.35, 95% CI 0.56–3.22). In this study, comprised of high-mortality (29.2%) patients, 14% (26/185) of patients remained qSOFA-negative even at the time of ICU admission. Moreover, the difference in in-hospital mortality was small (qSOFA-positive: 30.2% vs qSOFA-negative: 23.1%, $p=0.642$). Importantly, our study suggested that the risk of mortality in patients with bloodstream infection, immunosuppression or hematologic malignancy would be difficult to estimate using qSOFA scores. The results of our study may provide important implications for clinicians in early prognostication of patients with suspected sepsis and for developers of sepsis screening systems.

Among patients with suspected infection outside the ICU, qSOFA scores had greater prognostic accuracy than SIRS [3]. Since 1992, SIRS has gained widespread acceptance as the clinical definition of sepsis [13]. However, the specificity of SIRS ≥ 2 was too low and 70–90% of ICU patients, including non-infected patients, attained SIRS ≥ 2 during their ICU stay [17]. Along with the development of a new definition for sepsis, the qSOFA score has been generated to guide bedside clinicians in identifying infected patients at risk of in-hospital mortality or longer ICU stay [3]. The original study showed that qSOFA-positive patients had a 3- to 14-fold increase in in-hospital mortality compared to qSOFA-negative patients when qSOFA scores were assessed during the 72-h period around the onset of infection. Further external validation studies have shown that qSOFA scores had greater prognostic accuracy than SIRS among patients presenting to the ER [18–20].

However, recent studies have suggested that qSOFA has limited utility in early prognostication in high-mortality populations. In a retrospective analysis of a large adult ICU patient database, qSOFA assessed during the first 24-h following ICU admission had little additional predictive value for mortality over SIRS [6]. In recent studies consisting of patients admitted to the ICU or patients

Table 2 ICU stay and in-hospital mortality in ICU patients with suspected sepsis

	qSOFA-positive (≥ 2) (*N* = 159)	qSOFA-negative (< 2) (*N* = 26)	*p* value
ICU length of stay (median [IQR])	3 [2–6]	3 [2–5]	0.787
ICU stay ≥ 3 days (%)	94 (59.1%)	15 (57.7%)	1.000
Bacteremia (%)	85 (53.5%)	13 (50.0%)	0.833
In-hospital mortality (%)			
28-day mortality	40 (25.2%)	5 (19.2%)	0.627
90-day mortality	48 (30.2%)	6 (23.1%)	0.642

qSOFA scores were assessed with the most abnormal vital signs taken during the 24-h period before the ICU admission

In-hospital mortality was defined as any cause of death censored at 28 days or at 90 days after the ICU admission

ICU intensive care unit, *IQR* interquartile range, *qSOFA* quick Sequential Organ Failure Assessment

Table 3 Microbiological results in ICU patients with suspected sepsis

	qSOFA-positive (≥ 2) (*N*=159)	qSOFA-negative (< 2) (*N*=26)	*p* value
Primary site of infection (%)			
Bloodstream	29 (18.2%)	8 (30.8%)	0.094
Respiratory	31 (19.5%)	3 (11.5%)	0.573
Gastrointestinal	25 (15.7%)	4 (15.4%)	0.770
Neurological	2 (1.3%)	0 (0.0%)	NA
Genitourinary	39 (24.5%)	6 (23.1%)	1.000
Musculoskeletal	19 (11.9%)	1 (3.8%)	0.476
Other	14 (8.8%)	4 (15.4%)	0.290
Type of organisms (%)			
Gram-negative bacterial infection	66 (41.5%)	11 (42.3%)	
Escherichia coli	30 (18.9%)	5 (19.2%)	1.000
Klebsiella pneumoniae	12 (7.5%)	1 (3.8%)	0.697
Pseudomonas aeruginosa	7 (4.4%)	0 (0.0%)	NA
Gram-positive bacterial infection	32 (20.1%)	6 (23.1%)	
Staphylococcus aureus	14 (8.8%)	4 (15.4%)	0.290
Streptococcus pneumoniae	9 (5.7%)	0 (0.0%)	NA
Streptococcus species	4 (2.5%)	1 (3.8%)	0.535
Polymicrobial infection	20 (12.6%)	4 (15.4%)	0.752
Fungal infection	4 (2.5%)	0 (0.0%)	NA
Not specified	37 (23.3%)	5 (19.2%)	0.803

qSOFA scores were assessed with the most abnormal vital signs taken during the 24-h period before the ICU admission

Bloodstream infection was defined as blood culture-positive infection including infective endocarditis, bacteremia from an unknown origin and catheter-related bacteremia

ICU intensive care unit, *NA* not applicable, *qSOFA* quick Sequential Organ Failure Assessment

in the ward, in-hospital mortality of qSOFA-negative patients was higher (13.6–17.4%) compared to mortality in studies consisting of ER patients [5–9]. Therefore, qSOFA was assumed to have limited performance value in prognosticating high-risk patients. Importantly, qSOFA scores assessed after ICU admission were likely to have been affected with therapeutic interventions such as vasopressors and sedative agents [3, 6]. Therefore, pre-ICU qSOFA scores assessed before ICU admission have been evaluated [21].

We focused on patients with suspected sepsis requiring ICU admission and evaluated pre-ICU qSOFA scores assessed during the 24-h period before ICU admission. Our results raise a question as to why the association between pre-ICU qSOFA-positive and mortality was weaker (HR 1.35, 95% CI 0.56–3.22) than that observed in previous studies [3, 18]. To address this question, it is to be noted, first, that our patients were judged as having a severe infection by treating physicians before enrollment. Physicians detected signs of severe infection based not only on vital sign abnormalities such as qSOFA components but also on clinical diagnosis, primary sites of infection, presumed causative organisms and patient comorbidities [22, 23]. Also, some experts have questioned the sensitivity of qSOFA because qSOFA would remain negative until life-threatening organ dysfunction has developed [24]. A previous study showed that qSOFA remained negative even at the time of ICU transfer in one-half of infected patients [5]. In our study, the association between qSOFA and mortality became significant only after ICU admission (Pre-ICU qSOFA: crude RR 1.38, 95% CI 0.62–2.74; qSOFA at ICU arrival: crude RR 1.78, 95% CI 1.09–2.89). Physicians might have detected the risk of further clinical deterioration before qSOFA was determined as positive. As a result, the association between pre-ICU qSOFA and mortality would have attenuated. Our results suggested that qSOFA had little additional predictive value for mortality over clinical judgment (Fig. 2, Table 4). Second, we presented 90-day mortality instead of 28-day mortality. Recent studies have shown that patients with sepsis had increasing mortality beyond the standard 28-day mortality and that the use of long-term outcomes had been postulated to infer the full impact of sepsis [25]. Our study represented long-term outcomes of infected patients requiring ICU admission.

In addition to investigating the association between qSOFA-positive and mortality, we described detailed characteristics in qSOFA-negative patients to disclose

Table 4 Performance of qSOFA and SIRS in predicting sepsis and mortality

	Sepsis by Sepsis-3 definition			In-hospital mortality		
	n/*N* (%)	Crude risk ratio (95% CI)	AUROC	*n*/*N* (%)	Crude risk ratio (95% CI)	AUROC
Pre-ICU qSOFA			0.711			0.511
qSOFA-positive (≥ 2)	149/159 (93.7%)	1.16 (0.96–1.41)		48/159 (30.2%)	1.38 (0.62–2.74)	
qSOFA-negative (< 2)	21/26 (80.8%)	1.00 (ref)		6/26 (23.1%)	1.00 (ref)	
Pre-ICU SIRS			0.710			0.521
SIRS-positive (≥ 2)	155/166 (93.4%)	1.18 (0.93–1.50)		48/166 (28.9%)	0.92 (0.45–1.85)	
SIRS-negative (< 2)	15/19 (78.9%)	1.00 (ref)		6/19 (31.6%)	1.00 (ref)	
qSOFA at ICU arrival			0.624			0.586
qSOFA-positive (≥ 2)	92/98 (93.9%)	1.05 (0.96–1.14)		36/98 (36.7%)	1.78 (1.09–2.89)	
qSOFA-negative (< 2)	78/87 (89.7%)	1.00 (ref)		18/87 (20.7%)	1.00 (ref)	
SIRS at ICU arrival			0.709			0.541
SIRS-positive (≥ 2)	133/139 (95.7%)	1.19 (1.03–1.38)		41/139 (29.5%)	1.04 (0.62–1.77)	
SIRS-negative (< 2)	37/46 (80.4%)	1.00 (ref)		13/46 (28.3%)	1.00 (ref)	

Pre-ICU qSOFA and SIRS scores were assessed with the most abnormal vital signs taken during the 24-h period before the ICU admission. qSOFA and SIRS scores at ICU arrival were assessed with the first measurements just after ICU admission

Sepsis was defined according to the Sepsis-3 definition. In-hospital mortality was defined as any cause of death censored at 90 days after the ICU admission

AUROC area under receiver operating characteristics, *CI* confidence interval, *ICU* intensive care unit, *qSOFA* quick Sequential Organ Failure Assessment, *SIRS* systemic inflammatory response syndrome

features of patients whose risk of mortality was difficult to estimate using qSOFA scores (Table 1, 3). The characteristics, which were more frequently found in qSOFA-negative patients, were hematologic malignancy, immunosuppression, bloodstream infection, and *Staphylococcus aureus* infection. Among 8 bloodstream infections in qSOFA-negative patients, 37.5% (3/8) had chronic dialysis, and 25% (2/8) had hematologic malignancy. We think that the history of comorbidities alerted physicians of further deterioration and prompted physicians to consider ICU transfer before qSOFA scores turned positive. A variety of infections were presented with qSOFA-negative patients in our study. Indeed, we often experienced infective endocarditis, catheter-related bacteremia, pyelonephritis, and bacterial pneumonia in qSOFA-negative patients. Of note, all the patients who died in the qSOFA-negative group had at least one chronic health condition. In these patients, primary sites of infection and comorbidities would be additional useful information for early prognostication.

Our study had several limitations. First, our study was conducted in a single center with a small number of patients. As a result, only 54 in-hospital deaths were observed and the CI for our primary analyses was wide (HR 1.35, 95% CI 0.56–3.22). It is possible that we failed to find an association between pre-ICU qSOFA and in-hospital mortality due to the small sample size. Because no study focused on pre-ICU qSOFA at the time we planned the study, it was difficult to estimate a priori sample size. Second, because we did not observe all the infected patients presented to the ER or the ward, it is possible that we did not accurately estimate the association between qSOFA and mortality in patients not requiring ICU admission. The generalizability of the result of this study might have been attenuated. Currently, however, only a few studies have focused on pre-ICU qSOFA scores and on qSOFA-negative, infected ICU patients [21]. The results of our study provide an important basis for further prospective studies investigating the role of qSOFA in triage decisions for ICU admission. Third, we did not use uniform criteria for ICU admission. The threshold of ICU transfer in each patient largely depends on physicians and hospital-beds availability. Nevertheless, the median APACHE II scores (21, IQR 17–28), SOFA scores (9, IQR 5–11), and mortality (29.2%) of our patients were higher than those of related studies [3, 6, 18] or than in recent multicenter studies enrolling patients with early septic shock (mortality 18%) [26]. Thus, our results reflected the performance value of qSOFA in high-risk populations. Last, due to the retrospective nature of our study, the frequency of qSOFA variable measurements was not standardized. The pre-ICU qSOFA scores in our study were based on the worst vital signs that were obtainable during the 24-h period before ICU admission. There were no missing data regarding qSOFA scores.

Conclusion

In this observational study, among patients admitted to the ICU with suspected sepsis, we could not find a strong association between pre-ICU qSOFA scores and in-hos pital mortality. We described high mortality and bacterial diversity in pre-ICU qSOFA-negative patients. Besides qSOFA scores, primary sites of infection and comorbidities may provide additional useful information for early prognostication in high-risk populations.

Abbreviations

APACHE II: Acute Physiology and Chronic Health Evaluation II; AUROC: area under receiver operating characteristic; CI: confidence interval; ER: emergency room; HR: hazard ratio; ICU: intensive care unit; IQR: interquartile range; qSOFA: quick Sequential Organ Failure Assessment; RR: risk ratio; SIRS: systemic inflammatory response syndrome; SOFA: Sequential Organ Failure Assessment.

Authors' contributions

IN designed the study, analyzed the data, and wrote the first draft of the manuscript. JI reviewed all statistical analyses and critically revised the manuscript. HM extracted the data and critically revised the manuscript. TK supervised the analysis of the data and critically revised the manuscript. JS designed the study and critically revised the manuscript. All the authors read and approved the final manuscript.

Author details

[1] Intensive Care Unit, Department of Internal Medicine, Okinawa Chubu Hospital, 281 Miyazato, Uruma, Okinawa 904-2293, Japan. [2] Intensive Care Unit, Department of Anesthesiology, The Jikei University School of Medicine, 3-19-18 Nishi-Shinbashi, Minato-ku, Tokyo 105-8471, Japan. [3] The Center for Critical Care Nephrology, Clinical Research, Investigation, and Systems Modeling of Acute Illness Center, Department of Critical Care Medicine, University of Pittsburgh School of Medicine, Pittsburgh, PA 15213, USA. [4] Department of Anesthesiology and Critical Care, Jichi Medical University, Saitama Medical Center, 1-847 Amanuma, Oomiya-ku, Saitama, Saitama 330-8503, Japan. [5] Division of Environmental Medicine and Population Sciences, Department of Social and Environmental Medicine, Graduate School of Medicine, Osaka University, 1-1 Yamada-oka, Suita, Osaka 565-0871, Japan.

Acknowledgements

We thank all staff of Okinawa Chubu Hospital. We would like to thank Editage (http://www.editage.jp) for English language editing.

This work was performed at Okinawa Chubu Hospital.

Competing interests

The authors declare that they have no competing interests.

Funding

The authors declare that they have no sources of funding for the research.

References

1. Seymour CW, Gesten F, Prescott HC, Friedrich ME, Iwashyna TJ, Phillips GS, Lemeshow S, Osborn T, Terry KM, Levy MM. Time to treatment and mortality during mandated emergency care for sepsis. N Engl J Med. 2017;376(23):2235–44.
2. Ferrer R, Martin-Loeches I, Phillips G, Osborn TM, Townsend S, Dellinger RP, Artigas A, Schorr C, Levy MM. Empiric antibiotic treatment reduces mortality in severe sepsis and septic shock from the first hour: results from a guideline-based performance improvement program. Crit Care Med. 2014;42(8):1749–55.
3. Seymour CW, Liu VX, Iwashyna TJ, Brunkhorst FM, Rea TD, Scherag A, Rubenfeld G, Kahn JM, Shankar-Hari M, Singer M, et al. Assessment of clinical criteria for sepsis: for the third international consensus definitions for sepsis and septic shock (Sepsis-3). JAMA. 2016;315(8):762–74.
4. Singer M, Deutschman CS, Seymour CW, Shankar-Hari M, Annane D, Bauer M, Bellomo R, Bernard GR, Chiche JD, Coopersmith CM, et al. The third international consensus definitions for sepsis and septic shock (Sepsis-3). JAMA. 2016;315(8):801–10.
5. Churpek MM, Snyder A, Han X, Sokol S, Pettit N, Howell MD, Edelson DP. Quick sepsis-related organ failure assessment, systemic inflammatory response syndrome, and early warning scores for detecting clinical deterioration in infected patients outside the intensive care unit. Am J Respir Crit Care Med. 2017;195(7):906–11.
6. Raith EP, Udy AA, Bailey M, McGloughlin S, MacIsaac C, Bellomo R, Pilcher DV. Prognostic accuracy of the SOFA score, SIRS criteria, and qSOFA score for in-hospital mortality among adults with suspected infection admitted to the intensive care unit. JAMA. 2017;317(3):290–300.
7. Wang JY, Chen YX, Guo SB, Mei X, Yang P. Predictive performance of quick Sepsis-related Organ Failure Assessment for mortality and ICU admission in patients with infection at the ED. Am J Emerg Med. 2016;34(9):1788–93.
8. Giamarellos-Bourboulis EJ, Tsaganos T, Tsangaris I, Lada M, Routsi C, Sinapidis D, Koupetori M, Bristianou M, Adamis G, Mandragos K, et al. Validation of the new Sepsis-3 definitions: proposal for improvement in early risk identification. Clin Microbiol Infect. 2017;23(2):104–9.
9. April MD, Aguirre J, Tannenbaum LI, Moore T, Pingree A, Thaxton RE, Sessions DJ, Lantry JH. Sepsis clinical criteria in emergency department patients admitted to an intensive care unit: an external validation study of quick sequential organ failure assessment. J Emerg Med. 2017;52(5):622–31.
10. Tokuda Y, Miyasato H, Stein GH, Kishaba T. The degree of chills for risk of bacteremia in acute febrile illness. Am J Med. 2005;118(12):1417.
11. Knaus WA, Draper EA, Wagner DP, Zimmerman JE. APACHE II: a severity of disease classification system. Crit Care Med. 1985;13(10):818–29.
12. Ferreira FL, Bota DP, Bross A, Melot C, Vincent JL. Serial evaluation of the SOFA score to predict outcome in critically ill patients. JAMA. 2001;286(14):1754–8.
13. Bone RC, Balk RA, Cerra FB, Dellinger RP, Fein AM, Knaus WA, Schein RM, Sibbald WJ. Definitions for sepsis and organ failure and guidelines for the use of innovative therapies in sepsis. The ACCP/SCCM Consensus Conference Committee. American College of Chest Physicians/Society of Critical Care Medicine. Chest. 1992;101(6):1644–55.
14. Hall KK, Lyman JA. Updated review of blood culture contamination. Clin Microbiol Rev. 2006;19(4):788–802.
15. Chou HL, Han ST, Yeh CF, Tzeng IS, Hsieh TH, Wu CC, Kuan JT, Chen KF. Systemic inflammatory response syndrome is more associated with bacteremia in elderly patients with suspected sepsis in emergency departments. Medicine (Baltimore). 2016;95(49):e5634.
16. Kanda Y. Investigation of the freely available easy-to-use software 'EZR' for medical statistics. Bone Marrow Transpl. 2013;48(3):452–8.
17. Sprung CL, Sakr Y, Vincent JL, Le Gall JR, Reinhart K, Ranieri VM, Gerlach H, Fielden J, Groba CB, Payen D. An evaluation of systemic inflammatory response syndrome signs in the Sepsis Occurrence In Acutely Ill Patients (SOAP) study. Intensive Care Med. 2006;32(3):421–7.
18. Freund Y, Lemachatti N, Krastinova E, Van Laer M, Claessens Y-E, Avondo A, Occelli C, Feral-Pierssens A-L, Truchot J, Ortega M, et al. Prognostic accuracy of Sepsis-3 criteria for in-hospital mortality among patients with suspected infection presenting to the emergency department. JAMA. 2017;317(3):301–8.

19. Singer AJ, Ng J, Thode HC Jr, Spiegel R, Weingart S. Quick SOFA scores predict mortality in adult emergency department patients with and without suspected infection. Ann Emerg Med. 2017;69(4):475–9.
20. Williams JM, Greenslade JH, McKenzie JV, Chu K, Brown AF, Lipman J. Systemic inflammatory response syndrome, quick sequential organ function assessment, and organ dysfunction: insights from a prospective database of ED patients with infection. Chest. 2017;151(3):586–96.
21. Finkelsztein EJ, Jones DS, Ma KC, Pabon MA, Delgado T, Nakahira K, Arbo JE, Berlin DA, Schenck EJ, Choi AM, et al. Comparison of qSOFA and SIRS for predicting adverse outcomes of patients with suspicion of sepsis outside the intensive care unit. Crit Care. 2017;21(1):73.
22. Vincent JL. The clinical challenge of sepsis identification and monitoring. PLoS Med. 2016;13(5):e1002022.
23. Poeze M, Ramsay G, Gerlach H, Rubulotta F, Levy M. An international sepsis survey: a study of doctors' knowledge and perception about sepsis. Crit Care. 2004;8(6):R409–13.
24. Simpson SQ. New sepsis criteria. Chest. 2016;149(5):1117–8.
25. Winters BD, Eberlein M, Leung J, Needham DM, Pronovost PJ, Sevransky JE. Long-term mortality and quality of life in sepsis: a systematic review. Crit Care Med. 2010;38(5):1276–83.
26. The ARISE Investigators, the ANZICS Clinical Trial Group, Peake SL, Delaney A, Bailey M, Bellomo R, Cameron PA, Cooper DJ, Higgins AM, Holdgate A, et al. Goal-directed resuscitation for patients with early septic shock. N Engl J Med. 2014;371(16):1496–506.

11

Assessment of renal hemodynamic toxicity of fluid challenge with 0.9% NaCl compared to balanced crystalloid (PlasmaLyte®) in a rat model with severe sepsis

Pierre-Yves Olivier[1,2,3], François Beloncle[1,2,3], Valérie Seegers[1,4], Maher Tabka[3,5], Mathilde Renou de La Bourdonnaye[3,5], Alain Mercat[1,2], Paul Cales[1,6], Daniel Henrion[3,5], Peter Radermacher[7,8], Lise Piquilloud[1,2], Nicolas Lerolle[1,2,3] and Pierre Asfar[1,2,3*]

Abstract

Background: According to international guidelines, volume expansion with crystalloids is the first-line treatment for hemodynamic management in patients with severe sepsis or septic shock. Compared to balanced crystalloids, 0.9% sodium chloride (0.9% NaCl) induces hyperchloremia and metabolic acidosis and may alter renal hemodynamics and function. We compared the effects of 0.9% NaCl to a less chloride-concentrated fluid, PlasmaLyte® (PL) in targeted fluid resuscitation in a randomized, double-blind controlled study in an experimental model of severe sepsis in rats.

Results: A sepsis with hypotension was induced by cecal ligature and puncture (CLP) in 40 male Wistar rats (20 for each crystalloid). Rats received fluid resuscitation over a period of 200 min for a targeted mean arterial pressure of 90 mm Hg. Animals received similar volumes of 0.9% NaCl or PL. Unlike PL-resuscitated rats, 0.9% NaCl-resuscitated rats experienced hyperchloremia and metabolic acidosis, whereas systemic hemodynamics, renal hemodynamics and renal function were not significantly different between both groups.

Conclusion: In our model of rats with severe sepsis resuscitated with large amounts of crystalloids, 0.9% NaCl-induced hyperchloremic acidosis, but balanced crystalloid did not improve systemic and renal hemodynamics or renal function.

Keywords: Sepsis, Shock, Acute kidney injury, Hemodynamics, Microcirculation, Sodium chloride, PlasmaLyte, Crystalloid, Balanced crystalloid

Background

Arterial hypotension in patients with septic shock and severe sepsis, related to hypovolemia and arterial vasodilation, leads to organ hypoperfusion and ultimately to organ failure. According to the most recent guidelines of the Surviving Sepsis Campaign (SSC), the first-line hemodynamic treatment is to restore blood volume by increasing cardiac preload with crystalloids [1]. The type of crystalloids is not specified, and especially if non-balanced (i.e., 0.9% sodium chloride) or balanced crystalloids should be preferentially used.

The sodium concentration in 0.9% sodium chloride (0.9% NaCl) is close to the sodium plasma concentration (154 vs 135–145 mmol/L, respectively), whereas compared to the chloride concentration in plasma, the 0.9% NaCl chloride concentration is higher (95–105 vs 154 mmol/L, respectively). Hence, when large amounts of 0.9% NaCl are infused in patients with septic shock, a high load of chloride is infused, and both hyperchloremia and subsequently metabolic acidosis may occur as reported in animal models, healthy volunteers and postoperative patients [2–4]. The mechanisms of

*Correspondence: piasfar@chu-angers.fr
[1] CHU d'Angers, 4 rue Larrey, 49000 Angers, France
Full list of author information is available at the end of the article

hyperchloremic-induced acidosis combine the reduction of the anion gap [5] and the dilution of natural proton buffers (albumin and bicarbonates) [6]. Metabolic acidosis is not reported with so-called balanced crystalloid solutions, characterized by a chloride concentration closer to plasma chloride concentration, e.g., Ringer Lactate® (110 mmol/L) or PlasmaLyte® (PL) (98 mmol/L).

The clinical consequences of the metabolic perturbations related to 0.9% NaCl administration are unclear. Several animal studies suggest renal toxicity of hyperchloremic acidosis which leads to renal blood flow and renal filtration rate decrease [7–9], as well as inflammatory and hemodynamic effects [9, 10]. However, the clinical relevance of these models is debatable because of the non-physiological nature of the experimental studied systems (including isolated nephron or deinnervated kidney) and intervention (as infusion of very high concentration of chloride or hydrochloric acid).

A study in healthy volunteers also reported a decrease in renal blood flow after infusion of 0.9 NaCl compared to PL [11]. In patients, potential renal toxicity of hyperchloremic acidosis induced by 0.9% NaCl was reported in two cohort studies [15, 16], but was not confirmed by two small controlled studies [12, 13]. The most recent, large multi-center, controlled study in intensive care units, aimed at comparing 0.9% NaCl to PL used as fluid (SPLIT study [16]), did not report significantly different clinical outcomes between balanced and non-balanced crystalloids. However, the authors and editorialist [17] raised a major limitation of this study, inasmuch as SPLIT study only included a small proportion of patients who were at high risk of acute kidney injury or who required large volumes of intravenous fluids, such as patients with septic shock.

Conclusive data are hence lacking. Therefore, according to the SPLIT investigators' recommendations, we aimed at comparing the renal effects of 0.9% NaCl versus balanced crystalloids in a clinically relevant model of fluid-resuscitated severe sepsis induced by cecal ligature and puncture in rats. In order to understand the putative toxic effect of chloride, we paid special attention to the relationship between systemic hemodynamics, renal blood flow and renal function.

Methods

Experimental model

This protocol received veterinary authority approval (Authorization notification No. 01008.02 from the French Ministry of Higher Education and Research).

We designed a randomized, blind, controlled, experimental prospective study using male Wistar rats (weight: 250–350 g) to compare 0.9% NaCl (Cl [154 mmol/L]) and PL (Cl [98 mmol/L]) used as resuscitation fluids in rats with severe sepsis induced by cecal ligature and puncture.

Surgical preparation

Induction of anesthesia was performed with isoflurane (Piramal Healthcare Inc., Mumbai, India), followed by an intraperitoneal injection of thiopental (Rotex Medica Inc., Trittau, Germany) and ketamine (Renaudin Inc., Paris, France). After additional local anesthesia on the surgical sites (described below), rats were placed on a heating support. Then, they were tracheotomized, ventilated and perfused with a central vein catheter inserted via the left femoral vein. Mean arterial pressure was continuously monitored by a left femoral arterial catheter. The left renal and carotid arteries were isolated, and transit time ultrasound Doppler probes (Transonic System Inc., Ithaca, USA) were placed in contact with them. The bladder was cannulated. Finally, a cecal ligature and puncture (CLP) was performed to induce sepsis. After this surgical preparation was completed (T0, end of preparation), the rats were randomized to 0.9% NaCl or balanced crystalloid (PL) groups.

Blinding and randomization methods

Before the start of the experiment, 0.9% NaCl and PL were sampled in 40 unmarked kits (20 of each fluid) containing 100 mL of 0.9% NaCl or PL and 10 mL of inulin diluted in 0.9% NaCl or PL (1 mg/mL). Kits were numbered randomly and supplied to the investigator who was blinded for the group assignment.

Sepsis induction and monitoring

After sepsis induction by CLP, depending on the randomization arm, the rats were hydrated with 1 mL/H of 0.9% NaCl or PL. Mean arterial pressure was monitored every 10 min until arterial pressure dropped below 90 mm Hg (T1, resuscitation baseline, T0 to T1 = supervision). The rats were then considered hypotensive, and depending on their randomization arm, continuous infusion was increased to 3 mL/H (base infusion). In addition, animals received additional fluid challenges targeted to maintain a mean arterial pressure at 90 mm Hg. The rats were monitored for 200 min from the T1 (T2, end of resuscitation, T1 to T2 = resuscitation) (Fig. 1).

Data collection

Heart rate, mean arterial blood pressure, pressure in the inferior vena cava considered as a surrogate of central venous pressure, left carotid and left renal arteries blood flow, core temperature and urine output were recorded every 10 min.

Doppler probes on left renal and left carotid arteries allowed a continuous monitoring of blood flows

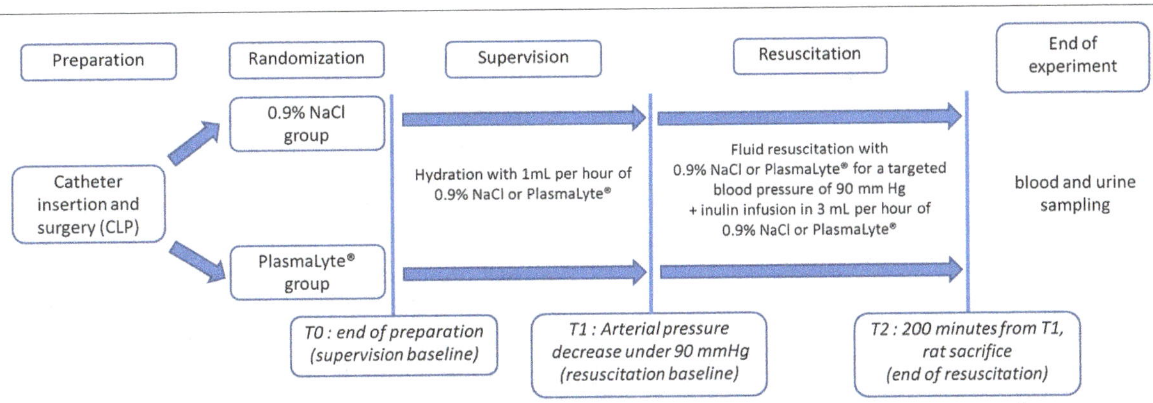

Fig. 1 Experimental design. After catheter insertion and surgical CLP, rats were randomized into the 0.9% NaCl or PlasmaLyte® groups. After randomization (T0, supervision baseline), rats were hydrated with the corresponding crystalloid and were monitored until arterial pressure dropped below 90 mm Hg (T1, end of supervision, resuscitation *baseline*). At that time, they received the allocated crystalloid for 200 min for a targeted blood pressure of 90 mmHg. After 200 min, the animals were killed and their urine and plasma were sampled (T2, end of resuscitation)

(displayed as a numeric mean value in milliliter per minute). The quality of signal was assessed by the adequate pulsatility and the absence of short-term lability (the lack of these criteria led to probe adjustments). The absence of contralateral stenosis, dilatation or renal malformation was controlled after animal killing.

Renal microcirculation was evaluated by measuring velocity in cortical capillaries with Side Dark Field Camera movies (Micro Vision Medical Inc., Amsterdam, the Netherlands). Videos were sampled at T1, T1 + 90 min and T1 + 180 min. Analyses were performed off-line with AVA software (Micro Vision Medical Inc., Amsterdam, the Netherlands). Twenty capillaries (5 capillaries per quadrant) per video were analyzed, and velocities were determined on, at least, three blood cells, as previously described [18].

Renal function was assessed by measuring inulin and creatinine clearance. We used FTIC-labeled inulin (Sigma Inc., Paris, France) diluted in the 3-mL/H base infusion of 0.9% NaCl or PL (depending on the randomization arm), with a 1-mg/mL concentration. Clearance was calculated at the end of the experiment according to the formulae: $U \times V/P$ (U for urine concentration, V for urine volume/time and P for plasma concentration). We used for inulin blood concentration measurement blood sampled at the end of resuscitation and for inulin urine concentration measurement urine sampled from the last hour of resuscitation. The urine volume corresponded to the volume sampled during the last hour of resuscitation. Rats of similar age and weight were supposed to have similar and normal baseline renal function. To reduce blood sampling volume before a severe surgical stress and to assess RIFLE score, we measured baseline blood creatinine in ten training test rats and considered the mean creatinine value for the RIFLE calculation.

Urine was collected at T0 and T2 to measure the concentration of chloride, sodium, potassium, blood urea nitrogen (BUN) and creatinine. Arterial blood was sampled at T2 to measure chloride, sodium, potassium, BUN, creatinine, hematocrit, proteins, pH, phosphate, calcium, bicarbonates, PaO_2 and $PaCO_2$.

Data analysis

Quantitative data are expressed as the mean and standard deviation. A nonparametric Mann–Whitney test was used for intergroup comparisons. For repeated measurements, we used a mixed linear regression model [19]. All statistics were calculated with R software 3.2.2 (free software developed by R Core Team (2008) for the R Foundation for Statistical Computing, Vienna, Austria) and Nlme R package version 3.1-122 (free software developed by Pinheiro J, Bates D, DebRoy S, Sarkar D and R Core Team (2015) for the R Foundation for Statistical Computing, Vienna, Austria). All tests were bilateral, and a p value of <0.05 was considered statistically significant.

Results

Baseline characteristics

Baseline characteristics, at T0 (weight, mean arterial pressure, carotid and renal blood flows, central venous pressure and initial urines analysis), were similar in the groups (Table 1).

Sepsis induction

After cecal ligation and puncture, hypotension occurred within similar time frames in the two groups (205 ± 40 min in the 0.9% NaCl group vs 190 ± 32 min in the PL group, $p = 0.85$). Hemodynamics at hypotension time were similar in both groups (Table 1).

Table 1 Baseline characteristics

	0.9% NaCl $n = 20$	PlasmaLyte® $n = 20$	p
Weight (g)	291 ± 24	293 ± 25	0.80
Mean arterial pressure (mm Hg)			
T0	129 ± 9	126 ± 9	0.30
T1	88 ± 2	86 ± 3	0.17
Mean carotid arterial blood flow (mL/min)			
T0	2.9 ± 0.9	3.0 ± 1.0	0.61
T1	1.8 ± 0.8	1.6 ± 0.5	0.48
Mean renal arterial blood flow (mL/min)			
T0	2.6 ± 1.3	2.1 ± 1.0	0.27
T1	3.0 ± 1.1	2.4 ± 1.2	0.19
Hypotension occurrence delays (min)	176 ± 91	177 ± 74	0.96
T0 urine concentrations (mmol/L)			
Sodium	93 ± 29	88 ± 37	0.52
Chloride	162 ± 56	148 ± 70	0.5
Potassium	172 ± 68	164 ± 66	0.77
BUN	516 ± 144	510 ± 191	0.82
Creatinine	6.0 ± 1.9	6.0 ± 2.9	0.63

Data are presented as mean and standard deviation. There was no significant difference of baseline characteristics between 0.9% NaCl and PlasmaLyte® at the end of preparation or at the time of hypotension occurrence. BUN = blood urea nitrogen. T0: end of preparation and supervision baseline. T1: occurrence of hypotension and resuscitation baseline.

Resuscitation and systemic hemodynamics

During the 200-min resuscitation period, mean arterial blood pressure was successfully maintained above 90 mm Hg during at least 90% of resuscitation time in both groups (Fig. 2). Heart rate, central venous pressure and carotid blood flow increased significantly during the resuscitation period without intergroup differences.

For a similar effect on systemic hemodynamic parameters, both groups required the same fluid volume (20 mL average in addition to 3 mL/H base infusion) to target a mean arterial pressure of 90 mm Hg. The indirect markers of volume expansion such as hematocrit and plasma protein concentration were not significantly different (Table 2).

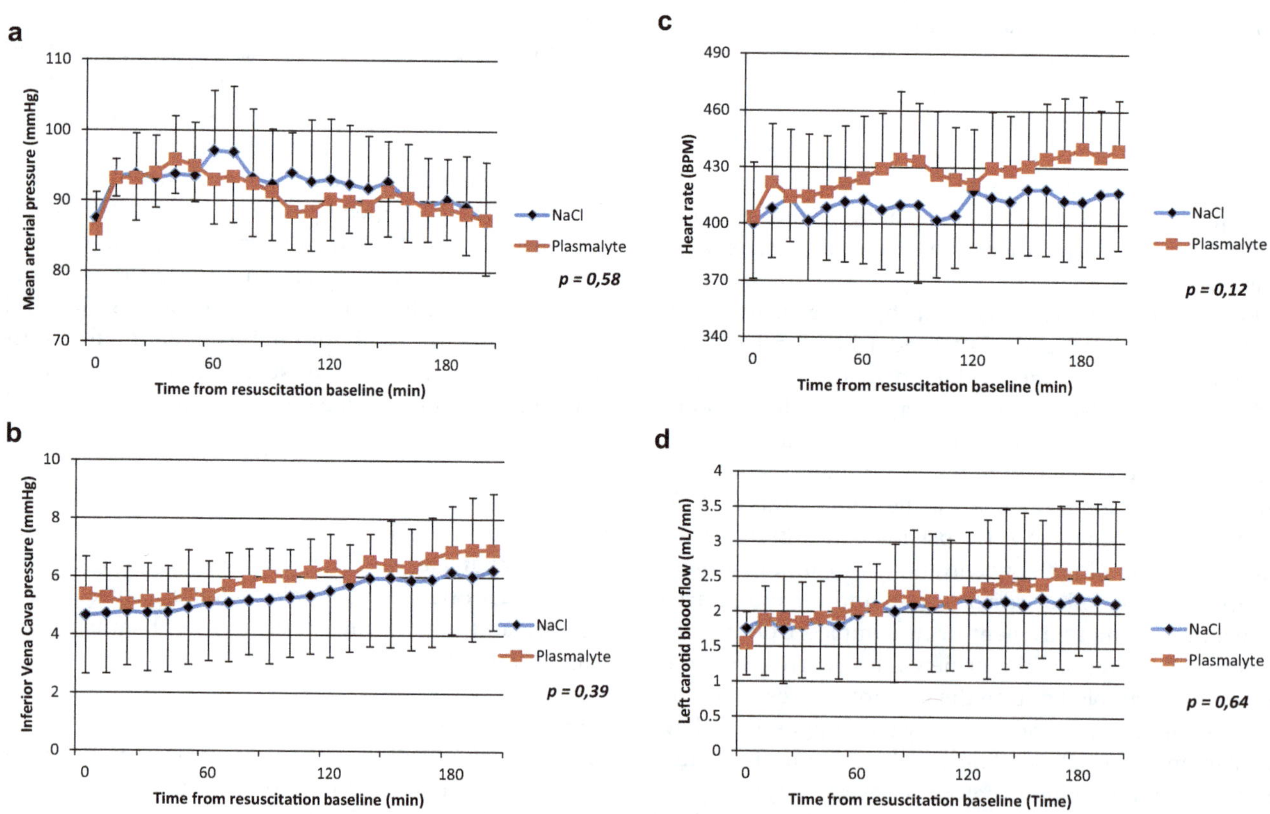

Fig. 2 Systemic hemodynamics during resuscitation. All data are presented as mean and standard deviation. Statistics were performed with a linear regression model. Mean arterial pressure is reported (**a**) and was maintained at approximately 90 mm Hg in both groups. Inferior vena cava (**b**), heart rate (**c**), left carotid blood flow (**d**) were no significantly different between the two groups

Data are presented as mean and standard deviation. Rats in the 0.9% NaCl group had a significant lower arterial pH and HCO^{3-} concentration, higher plasma Na^+, Cl^- and K^+ concentrations and higher plasma osmolarity. There was no significant difference in renal inulin and creatinine clearance between the two groups. BUN = blood urea nitrogen. T2: end of resuscitation. Osmolarity was calculated as follows:

$$(\text{sodium} + \text{potassium}) \times 2 + \text{BUN}.$$

Metabolic data

At the end of the experiment, arterial pH and bicarbonates were significantly lower in the 0.9% NaCl group than in PL-treated rats, whereas $PaCO_2$ was similar in both groups. Sodium, chloride and potassium plasma concentrations were significantly higher in the 0.9% NaCl group compared to the PL group. The other assayed ions did not differ between the groups (Table 2).

Table 2 Plasma, arterial blood gas and urine data at 200 min postresuscitation

	0.9% NaCl $n = 20$	PlasmaLyte® $n = 20$	p
Total fluid requirements (mL) during resuscitation	23 ± 11	23 ± 10	0.99
Plasma at T2			
Sodium (mmol/L)	141 ± 2	138 ± 3	0.017
Chloride (mmol/L)	117 ± 3	104 ± 3	<0.001
Potassium (mmol/L)	6.0 ± 0.6	5.3 ± 0.6	0.004
BUN (mmol/L)	12 ± 3	12 ± 4	0.77
Creatinine (μmol/L)	34 ± 7	36 ± 6	0.27
Phosphate (mmol/L)	3.5 ± 0.5	3.6 ± 0.5	0.36
Calcium (mmol/L)	1.9 ± 0.1	1.9 ± 0.2	0.64
Osmolarity (mmol/L)	306 ± 8	299 ± 8	0.027
Hematocrit (%)	44 ± 6	48 ± 4	0.16
Plasma protein (g/L)	27 ± 3	29 ± 3	0.33
Arterial blood gas			
pH	7.34 ± 0.05	7.44 ± 0.04	<0.001
Bicarbonate (mmol/L)	20 ± 2	26 ± 2	<0.001
$PaCO_2$ (mm Hg)	38 ± 5	39 ± 5	0.62
Urine at T2			
Urine output during resuscitation (mL)	1.7 ± 0.4	2.5 ± 0.6	0.002
Sodium (mmol/L)	52 ± 28	41 ± 15	0.4
Chloride (mmol/L)	182 ± 56	26 ± 6	<0.001
Potassium (mmol/L)	168 ± 48	175 ± 54	0.75
BUN (mmol/L)	533 ± 196	383 ± 161	0.066
Creatinine (mmol/L)	6.0 ± 2.0	4.2 ± 1.3	0.019
Sodium/potassium ratio	0.38 ± 0.24	0.29 ± 0.17	0.44
Measured clearance at T2			
Inulin (mL/min)	5.2 ± 2.9	4.4 ± 1.9	0.49
Creatinine (mL/min)	2.3 ± 1.1	2.3 ± 0.8	0.95

At the end of the experiment, ion urine concentrations were similar in both groups, except for chloride, which was significantly higher in the 0.9% NaCl-treated rats (Table 2).

Renal hemodynamics

Baseline renal arterial blood flow and renal arterial resistances were similar in both groups and remained similar at the end of the experiment. Cortical renal velocities remained stable and similar in the both groups (Fig. 3).

Renal function data

Urine output was significantly higher in the PL group compared to the 0.9% NaCl group (1.65 ± 0.17 vs 2.4 ± 0.28 mL, respectively, $p = 0.002$), but urine was more concentrated in the 0.9% NaCl group (creatinine concentration: 6.2 ± 0.88 vs 4.45 ± 0.57 mmol/L, respectively, $p = 0.019$). Renal function was similarly impaired in both groups, with no significant difference in creatinine and BUN plasma concentrations, inulin and creatinine clearance (Table 2), as well as RIFLE score distribution (Fig. 3).

Discussion

In this experimental study, we aimed at comparing the short-term effects of 0.9% NaCl and PL, a balanced crystalloid, used for fluid resuscitation in hypotensive rats with sepsis, on systemic and renal hemodynamics. To summarize, we found that both crystalloids had similar effects on systemic and renal hemodynamics and on renal function despite the occurrence of hyperchloremic acidosis in 0.9% NaCl group.

As expected, the NaCl 0.9% group showed hyperchloremic acidosis. The occurrence of hyperkalemia, despite the absence of potassium load in 0.9% NaCl group versus a 5-mmol/L load in PL group, was most likely related to acidosis. O'Malley et al. reported a similar effect, in patients with renal graft [13], and hyperkalemia led to premature stop of the trial. Hypernatremia and hyperosmolarity could be explained by the massive load of sodium-rich fluid in 0.9% NaCl.

Conversely, lower urine output in 0.9% NaCl group was not expected. Retrospectively, we hypothesized that the lower osmotic load induced by PL infusion may have favored a lower secretion of antidiuretic hormone, as suggested by Williams et al. [11] and Reid et al. [20], that reported similar higher urine output in healthy volunteers (of note, in these studies, osmotic gap between used balanced solution, Hartmann's solution and 0.9% NaCl was higher than between PL and 0.9% NaCl). The second hypothesis involves a specific action of chloride, leading to a decrease in glomerular filtration rate, as suggested by Wilcox [7] or Ren et al. [8]. However, our hemodynamic

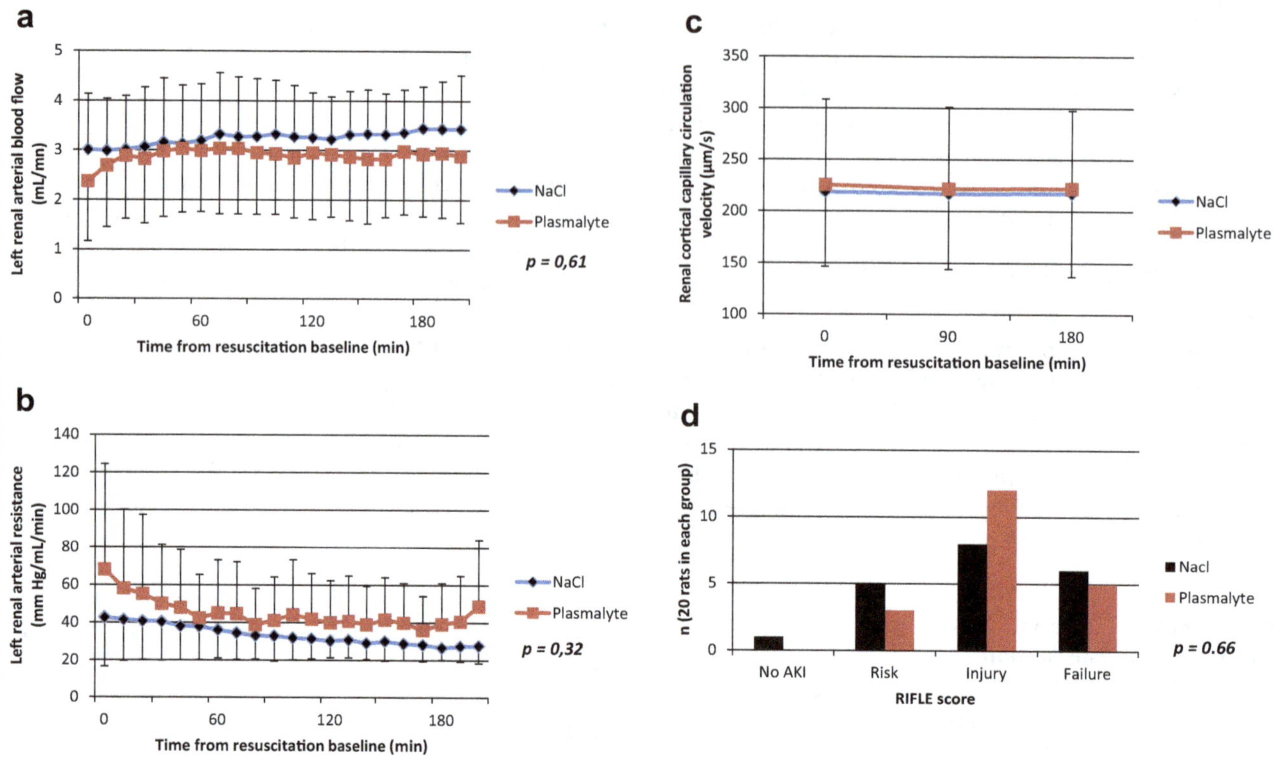

Fig. 3 Renal hemodynamic and renal function during resuscitation. All data are presented as mean and standard deviation; p values were obtained using a mixed linear regression model for **a** and **b** and using the Mann–Whitney test for **c** and **d**. There was no significant difference between the two groups in the left arterial renal rate measured by TTU probes (**a**), *left* renal arterial resistance (**b**) and renal cortical capillary velocity (**c**) measured by Side Dark Field Camera ($p = 0.41$ at resuscitation *baseline* time, $p = 0.54$ at 90 min after resuscitation baseline and $p = 0.51$ at 180 min after resuscitation *baseline*). Distribution in the RIFLE classification (**d**) (based on creatinine plasma concentration, inulin clearance and creatinine clearance) was similar in both groups as shown in **a** ($p = 0.66$ for all classes, $p = 0.34$ for RIFLE score 0, $p = 0.44$ for RIFLE score 1, $p = 0.22$ for RIFLE score 2 and $p = 0.74$ for RIFLE score 3)

and functional renal data did not provide evidence for this mechanism. Finally, due to the short-term design of our study, we cannot exclude that a similar urine output would have been reported in both groups with a longer follow-up.

Tubuloglomerular feedback is thought to play a central role in renal chloride toxicity. In isolated kidneys or nephrons, hyperchloremia and reabsorption of large amounts of chloride by the *macula densa* activate tubular–glomerular feedback as well as the renin angiotensin system, inducing a vasoconstriction of both afferent and efferent glomerular arteries, which, in turn, decreases both renal blood flow and glomerular filtration rate [7–9]. The decrease in renal blood flow consecutive to 0.9% NaCl-induced hyperchloremic acidosis was also reported in healthy volunteers [11].

All these animal studies reported an early renal vasoconstrictor effect of chloride but have used questionable models (isolated nephron, deinnervated kidney, etc.). In order to explore this specific issue of renal hemodynamic effect of chloride, in a more clinically relevant model, we have designed a severe septic fluid-resuscitated model at high risk of renal injury and requiring large crystalloid amounts. By design, due to the severity of the model, it was not possible to assess the long-term effect of chloride renal toxicity. Our study adds new information combining entire animal, large sample for an animal study, large amounts of chloride, severe and pathophysiologically relevant model of sepsis and renal hemodynamics. Our study does not provide evidence for short-term renal vasoconstriction related to high chloride load both at macrocirculatory and at microcirculatory levels.

The study of delayed renal toxicity of chloride related to inflammatory mechanisms was not our purpose, and we do not deny that these mechanisms are involved in renal chloride toxicity. On this topic, Zhou et al. reported a beneficial effect of PL in a less severe model of sepsis in awake rats. In this study, rats were infused with smaller amounts of crystalloids for a longer time [21]. PlasmaLyte® infusion was associated with a better renal function and an attenuated inflammatory response. Our results contrast with Zhou et al. on renal function alteration in the PL group, although our rats seem to present similar metabolic disturbances in the 0.9% NaCl group. In our experimental study, we infused the fourfold amount of crystalloids within a shorter time in anesthetized and ventilated rats. In addition, contrary to Zhou et al., we targeted fluid resuscitation according to mean arterial pressure. The impact of these different experimental designs and severity of hypotension remains speculative. Interestingly, in a more severe hypotensive sepsis model induced by endotoxin injection, Ergin et al. [22] reported no difference either between a balanced experimental crystalloid (Cl^-[119 mmol/L]) and 0.9% NaCl in renal function and renal blood flow.

The clinical relevance of high chloride load and hyperchloremic acidosis remains, respectively, unclear. In surgical patients, the use of 0.9% NaCl, but not balanced crystalloid solutions, was associated with hyperchloremia and metabolic acidosis, however, without significant effects on morbidity, mortality and renal function [14, 15]. These results have led some authors to question the clinical consequences of hyperchloremic acidosis and to challenge the use of balanced crystalloids [23]. Two cohort studies, one retrospective [12] and the other with a before-and-after two-period design [13], fueled the debate in 2012 as they have reported a significant reduction in acute renal failure in postoperative and intensive care patients treated with balanced solutions. These findings were not confirmed by the randomized SPLIT trial [16]. It was argued in the SPLIT trial that the severity of patients mirrored by the mortality rate (7.6 and 8.6% in the PlasmaLyte® and saline groups, respectively) and low fluid requirements was low (2.7 vs 2.6 l, respectively) and may have explained the absence of beneficial effects of PlasmaLyte®. However, two other recent large controlled randomized studies, with higher chloride amounts, in patients presenting high risk of renal acute injury, comparing 3% NaCl to 0.9% NaCl in patients in septic shock for the first one and comparing 0.9% NaCl to PL in patients after cardiac surgery for the second one, reported both hyperchloremic acidosis in patients receiving higher load of chloride but did not reported any detrimental renal effect for these patients [24, 25].

Our study has several limitations. The short duration of our follow-up does not allow us to rule out a delayed detrimental effect. When we designed this study, the available animal data suggested a very early detrimental effect of chloride, supposed to be mediated by short-term mechanisms such as tubuloglomerular feedback and/or renin angiotensin system. Therefore, we designed our study to investigate the early hemodynamic effects and the potential renal functional consequences. We cannot exclude a delayed effect of chloride, but, to the best of our knowledge, there is no clear argument suggesting that this potential delayed effect would not have been preceded by a hemodynamic effect. Zhou et al. investigated the delayed effects of chloride and suggested a delayed toxicity of chloride acidosis, but did not provide data on renal hemodynamic during early phase of resuscitation. However, our study allows the pragmatic conclusion that putative detrimental effect of 0.9% NaCl is neither induced by renal macrocirculatory nor by microcirculatory disturbances. In addition, our study is limited by the absence of cardiac output monitoring, even though this is a major determinant of renal blood flow [26]. As it is a highly invasive surgical procedure in rats, we therefore used carotid blood flow as a surrogate for cardiac output [27]. The risk of bias is also limited as we directly measured renal blood flow in order to check an unexpected alteration in renal blood flow between the two crystalloids. Last limitation is the lack of in vivo assessment of glomerular arteries due to technical reasons, but we measured the cortical microcirculatory velocities which mirror postglomerular microcirculatory blood flow. Therefore, a change in upstream blood flow (i.e., afferent and/or efferent glomerular arteries) should have been detected.

Conclusion

In our model of rats with severe sepsis resuscitated with large amounts of crystalloids, 0.9% NaCl-induced hyperchloremic acidosis, but balanced crystalloid did not improve systemic and renal hemodynamics or renal function.

Abbreviations

BUN: blood urea nitrogen; CLP: cecal ligature and puncture; PL: PlasmaLyte®.

Authors' contributions

PYO contributed to protocol writing, experiment processing, data analysis and manuscript writing. FB helped in protocol writing and manuscript reviewing. VS contributed to statistical analysis, manuscript writing and reviewing. MT participated in experiment processing. MRDLB participated in experiment processing. AM, PC, DH and PR reviewed the manuscript. LP helped in manuscript writing and reviewing. NL and PA helped in protocol writing, manuscript writing and reviewing. All authors read and approved the final manuscript.

Author details

[1] CHU d'Angers, 4 rue Larrey, 49000 Angers, France. [2] Medical Intensive Care Department, University Hospital, Angers, France. [3] BNMI Laboratory, CNRS UMR 6214—INSERM U1083, Angers University, Angers, France. [4] Statistical Department, University Hospital, Angers, France. [5] Faculté de médecine d'Angers, 4 rue haute de reculée, 49000 Angers, France. [6] HIFIH, UPRE-EA 3859, SFR 4208, LUNAM University, Angers, France. [7] Universitätsklinikum, Ulm Helmholtzstr. 8/1, 89081 Ulm, Germany. [8] Institut für Anästhesiologische Pathophysiologie und Verfahrensentwicklung, Universitätsklinikum, Ulm, Germany.

Competing interests

The authors declare that they have no competing interests.

Funding
This study was financed by own funds of the Department of Intensive Care Medicine, University Hospital of Angers.

References

1. Dellinger RP, Levy MM, Rhodes A, Annane D, Gerlach H, Opal SM, et al. Surviving sepsis campaign: international guidelines for management of severe sepsis and septic shock. Crit Care Med. 2013;41(2):580–637.
2. Kellum JA. Saline-induced hyperchloremic metabolic acidosis. Crit Care Med. 2002;30(1):259–61.
3. Kellum J. Fluid resuscitation and hyperchloremic acidosis in experimental sepsis: improved short-term survival and acid-base balance with Hextend compared with saline. Crit Care Med. 2002;30(2):300–5.
4. Doberer D, Funk G-C, Schneeweiss B. Dilutional acidosis: an endless story of confusion. Crit Care Med. 2003;31(1):337–8 **(author reply 338)**.
5. Morgan TJ, Venkatesh B. Designing, "balanced" crystalloids. Crit Care Resusc. 2003;5(4):284–91.
6. Doberer D, Funk G-C, Kirchner K, Schneeweiss B. A critique of Stewart's approach: the chemical mechanism of dilutional acidosis. Intens Care Med. 2009;35(12):2173–80.
7. Wilcox C. Regulation of renal blood flow by plasma chloride. J Clin Invest. 1983;71:726–35.
8. Ren Y, Garvin JL, Liu R, Carretero OA. Role of macula densa adenosine triphosphate (ATP) in tubuloglomerular feedback. Kidney Int. 2004;66(4):1479–85.
9. Marsh J, Margolis TI, Kim D. Mechanism of diminished contractile response to catecholamines during acidosis. Am J Physiol. 1988;254:h20–7.
10. Kellum J. Effects of hyperchloremic acidosis on arterial pressure and circulating inflammatory molecules in experimental sepsis. Chest. 2004;125(1):243–8.
11. Williams EL, Hildebrand KL, McCormick SA, Bedel MJ. The effect of intravenous lactated Ringer's solution versus 0.9% sodium chloride solution on serum osmolality in human volunteers. Anesth Analg. 1999;88(5):999–1003.
12. Shaw AD, Bagshaw SM, Goldstein SL, Scherer LA, Duan M, Schermer CR, et al. Major complications, mortality, and resource utilization after open abdominal surgery: 0.9% saline compared to plasma-lyte. Ann Surg. 2012;255(5):821–9.
13. Yunos NM, Bellomo R, Hegarty C, Story D, Ho L, Bailey M. Association between a chloride-liberal vs chloride-restrictive intravenous fluid administration strategy and kidney injury in critically ill adults. JAMA. 2012;308(15):1566.
14. Wilkes NJ, Woolf R, Mutch M, Mallett SV, Peachey T, Stephens R, et al. The effects of balanced versus saline-based hetastarch and crystalloid solutions on acid-base and electrolyte status and gastric mucosal perfusion in elderly surgical patients. Anesth Analg. 2001;93(4):811–6.
15. O'Malley CMIN, Frumento RJ, Hardy MA, Benvenisty AI, Brentjens TE, Mercer JS, et al. A randomized, double-blind comparison of lactated Ringer's solution and 0.9% NaCl during renal transplantation. Anesth Analg. 2005;100(5):1518–24.
16. Young P, Bailey M, Beasley R, Henderson S, Mackle D, McArthur C, et al. Effect of a buffered crystalloid solution vs saline on acute kidney injury among patients in the intensive care unit: the SPLIT randomized clinical trial. JAMA. 2015;314(16):1701.
17. Kellum JA, Shaw AD. Assessing toxicity of intravenous crystalloids in critically ill patients. JAMA. 2015;314(16):1695.
18. De Backer D, Hollenberg S, Boerma C, Goedhart P, Büchele G, Ospina-Tascon G, et al. How to evaluate the microcirculation: report of a round table conference. Crit Care. 2007;11(5):R101.
19. Laird NM, Ware JH. Random-effects models for longitudinal data. Biometrics. 1982;38:963–74.
20. Reid F, Lobo DN, Williams RN, Rowlands BJ, Allison SP. (Ab)normal saline and physiological Hartmann's solution: a randomized double-blind crossover study. Clin Sci (Lond). 2003;104:17–24.
21. Zhou F, Peng Z-Y, Bishop JV, Cove ME, Singbartl K, Kellum JA. Effects of fluid resuscitation with 0.9% saline versus a balanced electrolyte solution on acute kidney injury in a rat model of sepsis. Crit Care Med. 2014;42(4):e270–8.
22. Ergin B, Zafrani L, Kandil A, Baasner S, Lupp C, Demirci C, et al. Fully balanced fluids do not improve microvascular oxygenation, acidosis and renal function in a rat model of endotoxemia. Shock. 2016;46(1):83–91.
23. Guidet B. A balanced view of balanced solutions. Crit Care. 2010;14:R325.
24. Asfar P, Schortgen F, Boisramé-Helms J, Charpentier J, Guérot E, Megarbane B, et al. Hyperoxia and hypertonic saline in patients with septic shock (HYPERS2S): a two-by-two factorial, multicentre, randomised, clinical trial. Lancet Respir Med. 2017;5(3):180–90.
25. McIlroy D, Murphy D, Kasza J, Bhatia D, Wutzlhofer L, Marasco S. Effects of restricting perioperative use of intravenous chloride on kidney injury in patients undergoing cardiac surgery: the LICRA pragmatic controlled clinical trial. Intensive Care Med. 2017;. doi:10.1007/s00134-017-4772-6.
26. Burban M, Hamel J-F, Tabka M, de La Bourdonnaye M, Duveau A, Mercat A, et al. Renal macro- and microcirculation autoregulatory capacity during early sepsis and norepinephrine infusion in rats. Crit Care 2013;17(4):R139.
27. Langenberg C, Bellomo R, May C, Wan L, Egi M, Morgera S. Renal blood flow in sepsis. Crit Care. 2005;9(4):R363–74.

12

Effect of HA330 resin-directed hemoadsorption on a porcine acute respiratory distress syndrome model

Xuefeng Xu[1,2†], Chune Jia[3†], Sa Luo[3], Yanming Li[1,4], Fei Xiao[1,5], Huaping Dai[3] and Chen Wang[1,3*]

Abstract

Background: Blood purification is an emerging approach to dampening the cytokine storm. This study aims to assess the efficacy of HA330 resin-directed hemoadsorption (HA) on endotoxin-induced porcine acute respiratory distress syndrome (ARDS) model.

Methods: Twenty-four Chinese domestic pigs were allocated into saline group receiving intravenous infusion of saline ($N = 6$) and endotoxin group receiving intravenous infusion of LPS ($N = 18$). When ALI model was initially diagnosed, six pigs in the LPS and saline group were killed for BALF and histopathological analysis. The remaining 12 pigs in LPS group received 3-h HA ($N = 6$) or HA-sham ($N = 6$) treatment, respectively. Following another 5-h observation, animals were killed. Variables on hemodynamics, blood gases and lung mechanics were recorded at a series of time points. Differentially expressed cytokines and proteins were determined by ELISA and proteomics.

Results: HA treatment significantly improved injured oxygenation induced by LPS. HA also partially improved the barrier permeability and reduced lung edema and inflammation/injury induced by LPS infusion. Proteomic analysis showed the differentially expressed proteins between HA- and HA-sham-treated groups mostly belonged to the categories of acute inflammation/immune response, and proteolysis.

Conclusions: Hemoadsorption improved ARDS possibly by blunting the cytokine storm and by restoring homeostasis of the disordered proteome milieu in the exudative phase.

Keywords: ARDS, Cytokine storm, Hemoadsorption, Porcine model, Proteomics

Background

The acute respiratory distress syndrome (ARDS) is a condition with the acute onset of noncardiac respiratory failure that develops in response to a series of insults to the alveolar-capillary barrier [1]. The current mainstay therapy for ARDS is largely supportive [2, 3]. This has been shown to reduce mortality by limiting further iatrogenic injury to the already injured lungs. However, the mortality rate of ARDS is still unacceptably high [4]. ARDS is largely caused by the local alveolar and circulating "cytokine storm" that happens with bacterial/virus infection, burn/trauma and some possible iatrogenic factors, such as high-volume ventilation [5]. This has encouraged the development of several specific targeted pharmacologic therapy directed against single key pathogenic mediators. However, most clinical trials have proven no benefit to disease outcome and were stopped early for futility [6]. Investigators shifted their interests into the extracorporeal blood purification (EBP) modality, which is a nonspecific, broad-spectrum method to blunt the "cytokine storm" by immediately clearing a series of circulating and resident mediators [7].

Until now, there are only some inconsistent preliminary data to investigate the effects of hemofiltration (a modality of EBP) on ARDS animal models [8, 9]. Also, it has been shown that hemoadsorption (HA), another modality of EBP, can improve oxygenation in septic patients

*Correspondence: cyh-birm@263.net
†Xuefeng Xu and Chune Jia contributed equally to this study
[3] Department of Pulmonary and Critical Care Medicine, China-Japan Friendship Hospital, 2 Yinghua Dongjie, Beijing 100029, China
Full list of author information is available at the end of the article

[10, 11]. However, evidences of HA's effects on ARDS patients animal models are scarce. We hypothesize that HA can improve oxygenation, reduce the permeability of alveolar-capillary barrier and alleviate pulmonary edema/damage by blunting the circulating/alveolar cytokines in the process of ARDS. To test this hypothesis, we established an endotoxin-induced ARDS porcine model to explore HA's therapeutic effect by using a HA330 resin cartridge (a new weapon against cytokine storm).

Methods

Research animals and ethical considerations

This study was approved by the Institutional Animal Experiment Committee of Beijing Hospital. All experiments were performed according to the Declaration of Helsinki conventions for the use and care of animals. Twenty-four healthy, 3–4-week-old Chinese domestic white pigs of both sexes were chosen from a local stock routinely used for the experimental research. The average weight of pigs used in this experimental procedure is 43 ± 0.3 kg (mean ± SEM).

Animal preparations

Sedation, anesthesia and muscle relaxation

Detailed information is shown in Additional file 1: Supplement-Methods.

Ventilation and measurements of lung mechanics

Animals were ventilated in a volume-controlled mode. The ventilation protocol at baseline used a tidal volume of 10 ml/kg body weight, a fraction of inspired oxygen (FiO_2) of 0.4 and a positive end-expiratory pressure (PEEP) at 0 cmH_2O. Parameters of lung mechanics were recorded. Detailed information is shown in Additional file 1: Supplement-Methods.

Instrumentation and hemodynamic measurements

Cardiac output (CO), mean arterial pressure (MAP), systematic vascular resistance (SVR), mean pulmonary arterial pressure (MPAP), pulmonary vascular resistance (PVR), pulmonary artery wedge pressure (PAWP), extravascular lung water (EVLW) and pulmonary vascular permeability index (PVPI) were measured with PiCCO and Swan-Ganz systems. Detailed information is shown in Additional file 1: Supplement-Methods.

Experimental protocol

After surgical preparations and instrumentation, all animals were ventilated in prone position and a period of 1 h was left for animal stabilization. Thereafter, baseline (i.e., the time point after 1-h stabilization) parameters including lung mechanics, hemodynamics, blood gases were recorded and venous blood samples were collected. As a next step, lung injury model was produced with i.v. infusion of 50 μg/kg LPS (*Escherichia coli*, serotype O55:B5, Sigma-Aldrich, St. Louis, MO, USA) mixed in 500 ml of saline that was delivered via a volumetric infusion pump (Instrumentation Laboratory, Bedford, MA, USA) for about 2 h [12, 13]. Before the start of the experiment, 24 animals were purchased and randomly divided into four groups according to different conditions: (a) control group ($N = 6$), animals received an i.v. infusion of saline without LPS (LPS-sham); (b) LPS group ($N = 6$), animals received an i.v. infusion of saline with LPS as indicated above. When experimental ARDS was diagnosed in LPS group (PaO_2/FiO_2 is equal or less than 200 mmHg with a PEEP equal to 5 cmH_2O), animals in control and LPS group were all killed for bronchoalveolar lavage fluid (BALF) and histologic assessment in order to aid further diagnosis of lung injury. (c) LPS plus HA-sham group ($N = 6$), animals received an i.v. infusion of saline with LPS. Immediately after ARDS was well established, HA-sham treatment was started by using a hollow fiber membrane hemofilter (Fresenius) with the ultrafiltration line clamped. Two animals in this group were excluded because they died or developed severe sepsis/septic shock and refractory acidosis despite active liquid recovery and vasopressor administration before moderate ARDS diagnosis; (d) LPS plus HA group ($N = 6$), animals received an i.v. infusion of saline with LPS, and real HA treatment was started by using a disposable hemoperfusion cartridge (HA330 resin, styrene divinylbenzene copolymers, with a blood flow of 200–250 ml/min, volume of 185 ml; Jafron Biomedical Co., Ltd., Zhuhai, GuangDong, China; http://www.jafron.com/). Two pigs were also discarded because they died of septic shock and severe disturbance of water, electrolyte and acid base before the establishment of hemoperfusion circulation. HA-sham and HA treatment lasted for 3 h, and thereafter, the animals were monitored for an extended observation period of 5 h and then killed with a bolus injection of 10 ml of 15% KCl. BAL fluid collection and lung tissue harvesting were performed immediately upon exsanguination and sternotomy performance for the measurements of inflammatory markers, proteomes and for histologic evaluation. Parameters of hemodynamics, blood gases and lung mechanics were recorded every hour following the start of LPS or sham LPS infusion until the end of experiment. Plasma samples were also prepared in the corresponding time points. During the experiment, all pigs were continuously infused with Ringer lactate solution or saline at a rate of 12 ml/kg/h at the start of the experiment. The infusion rate was increased to 15–20 ml/kg/h if the MAP was less than 70–50 mmHg. However, if pulmonary artery wedge pressure (PAWP) continuously raised and exceeded 12 mmHg, the rate of infusion should be reduced to prevent fluid overload. Meanwhile, norepinephrine (0.5–1.5 μg/kg/min) was then used to achieve this level of mPAP in LPS-treated pigs. Body temperature was maintained over 36 °C by using a heating blanket. The experimental protocol was summarized in Additional file 2: Fig. S1.

Assessment of the LPS-induced ARDS porcine model

To determine whether ARDS has occurred, at least four main features of ARDS should be assessed: (1) abnormalities of gas exchange. A ratio of the partial pressure of arterial oxygen to the fraction of inspired oxygen (PaO_2/FiO_2) $\leq$ 200 mmHg at PEEP = 5 cmH_2O (clinical diagnostic criteria of moderate ARDS) is the initial evaluating criteria;(2)a remarkable leakage of alveolar barrier as indicated by the significant increase of lung wet-to-dry weight ratio, EWLW and PVPI; (3) a significant infiltration of inflammatory cells and production of inflammatory cytokines in both circulation and lung tissues (plasma and lung IL-6, IL-8, IL-1β, IL-17A and TNF-α levels were measured in our study); (4) diffuse alveolar damage (DAD) as determined by lung histopathological examination [14].

HA330 cartridge-directed hemoadsorption

The HA330 is an electrically neutral microporous resin that is a powerful new weapon in the clearance of "cytokine storm" occurred in sepsis [10]. Detailed information is shown in Additional file 1: Supplement-Methods.

BALF recovery

Sixty milliliter ice-cold saline was used to collect BALF in the left upper, middle and lower lobes. Detailed information is shown in Additional file 1: Supplement-Methods.

Assessment of total protein contents in BALF

BCA (bicinchoninic acid) protein assay reagent kit (Pierce Biotechnology, Rockford, IL, USA) was used. Detailed information is shown in Additional file 1: Supplement-Methods.

Lung tissue collection and histopathological evaluation

The right lower lobe was excised, fixed and sliced for routine hematoxylin and eosin (H&E) staining. ALI scoring was done according to a consensus report published previously [14] (Additional file 3: Table S1). Detailed information is shown in Additional file 1: Supplement-Methods.

Lung water assessed by gravimetric method

Samples from unused right lung lobes were dissected free of non-lung parenchymal tissue, placed in a dish and weighed (wet weight). Then, they were dried in an oven at 80 °C and weighed daily until their weight was maintained unchanged (dry weight). The total water content of the lung was crudely estimated as a wet-to-dry weight ratio (W/D).

Concentrations of proinflammatory mediators in circulation and lung tissues

IL-1β, IL-6, IL-8, TNF-α and IL-17A were measured by ELISA kits (Bluegene Biotech CO., LTD, Shanghai, China). Detailed information is shown in Additional file 1: Supplement-Methods.

Plasma and lung proteome

Protein samples of plasma, BALF and lung tissue in HA or HA-sham treatment group were collected and received iTRAQ-labeled (Applied Biosystems, Foster City, CA, USA) mass spectrometric analysis. Bioinformatics analysis was also performed [15, 16]. Detailed information is shown in Additional file 1: Supplement-Methods.

Statistical analysis

The data are shown as the mean ± SEM. Parametric data between multiple groups were compared by using the Kruskal–Wallis test and followed by Mann–Whitney *U* test if statistically significant. Mann–Whitney *U* test was also used for the comparison between two independent continuous variables. Data were analyzed using the SPSS statistical software package for Windows, version 13.0 (SPSS, Chicago, IL, USA), and $P < 0.05$ was considered as statistically significant.

Results

Intravenous infusion of endotoxin causes sharp changes in physiological parameters

The ratio of PaO_2/FiO_2 and alveolar-arterial oxygen partial pressure difference ($AaDO_2$) in pigs that received LPS infusion declined gradually (from 440 ± 19 to 157 ± 23 mmHg, $P < 0.001$, Fig. 1a; Table 1). After LPS infusion, CO was firstly increased and then decreased when moderate ARDS was diagnosed. However, the changes did not reach statistical difference when compared with saline group. LPS infusion increased MPAP (18.8 ± 1.5 vs. 41.0 ± 1.7 mmHg, $P < 0.001$, Fig. 1b; Table 2) and PVRI (201 ± 13 vs. 781 ± 74 dyn s/cm^5/m^2, $P < 0.001$, Table 2). However, MAP and SVRI continued to decrease (Table 2). In addition, pulmonary mechanics were also damaged as shown by an increase in P_{AW}Peak, P_{AW}Plateau and resistance and a decrease in pulmonary static compliance (Fig. 1c, d; Table 1).

Intravenous infusion of endotoxin causes high-permeability pulmonary edema and lung histologic damages

The EVLWI continuously increased after LPS infusion until ARDS was diagnosed (from 8.0 ± 0.5 ml/kg in

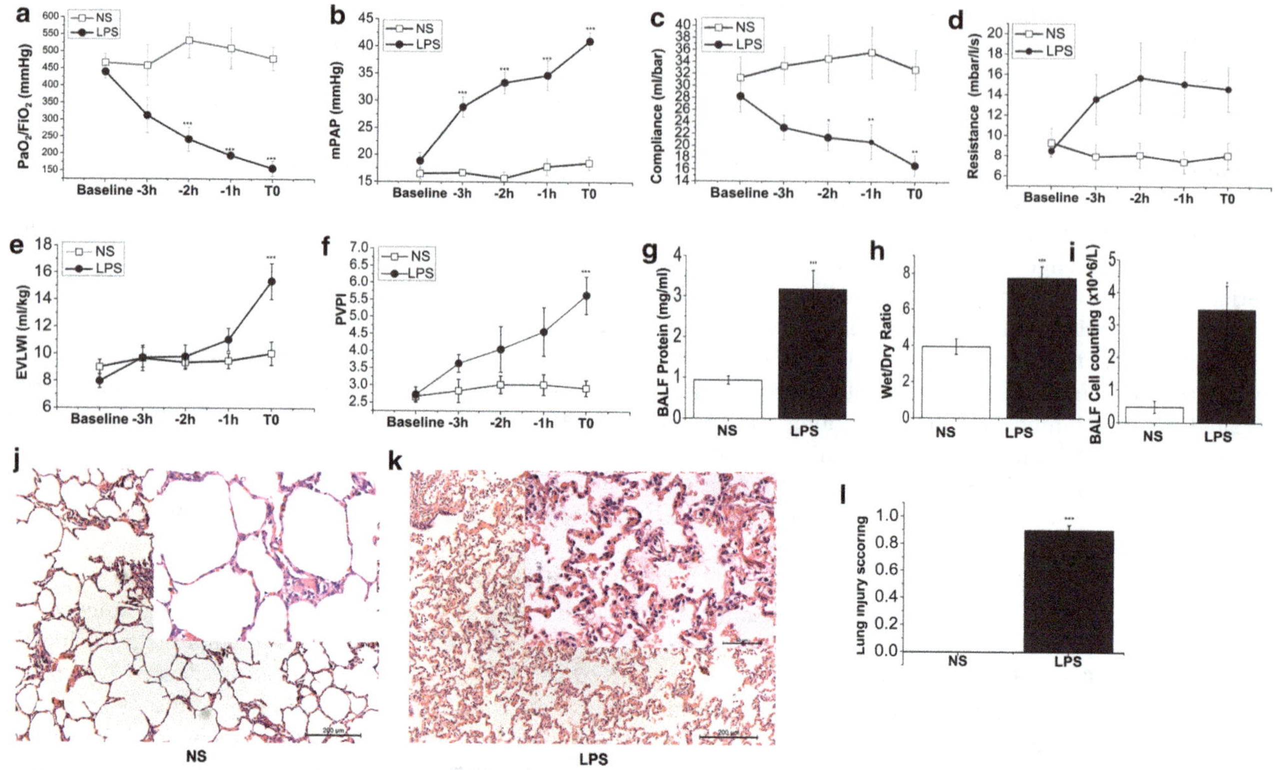

Fig. 1 LPS impairs lung function and alveolar-capillary barriers. Pigs were allocated into intravenous saline and LPS group, respectively. Parameters of oxygenation, hemodynamics and lung mechanics were recorded at different time points from baseline to the end of the experiment (T0). BALF and lung tissues were collected at T0. PaO_2/FiO_2 (**a**) was measured by using blood samples from femoral artery on a blood gas analysis instrument. The value of mPAP (**b**) was gained by Swan-Ganz catheter implantation into jugular vein. Compliance (**c**) and resistance (**d**) were recorded by using Drager Evita 4 ventilator. EVLWI (**e**) and PVPI (**f**) were measured by PiCCO system at baseline and a series of time points until ALI was well established (T0). **g** Whole protein content in the BALF of pigs was detected by using BCA protein assay kit. **h** The ratio of wet/dry lung weight of saline control and LPS challenge pigs. **i** Whole-cell counts in the BALF collected from both groups of pigs. **j** and **k** were the representative histology sections of controls and LPS challenge pigs. HE sections are from one representative animal per group. **l** Lung injury scores were calculated according to ATS report which was in detail described in the "Methods." Data points are expressed as mean ± SEM, $N = 6$ of each group. Statistical significance between saline and LPS group per point of measurement is shown as $^*P < 0.05$; $^{**}P < 0.01$; $^{***}P < 0.001$, respectively

baseline to 15.4 ± 1.3 ml/kg at the end of this experiment when ARDS was established, $P < 0.001$; Fig. 1e). In parallel, there was also a remarkable increase in lung wet/dry ratio in LPS-challenged pigs compared with saline group (Fig. 1h). The alveolar-capillary membrane was also seriously injured by LPS infusion as manifested by a significant increase in both pulmonary vascular permeability index (PVPI) and whole BAL protein concentration (Fig. 1f, g). Infusion of LPS in the endotoxin challenge group was also associated with an increase in the numbers of whole BAL cell counting (Fig. 1i). To determine the histopathological features of ALI model, subset of animals ($N = 6$ in LPS and saline group, respectively) were killed when ARDS model was diagnosed based on oxygenation parameter ($PaO_2/FiO_2 \leq 200$ mmHg at PEEP = 5 cmH_2O). Histologic examinations from animals receiving LPS demonstrated alveolar bleeding, microatelectasis, perivascular edema, marked leukocyte sequestration in alveolar septa and lumen, thickened alveolar walls, and the presence of proteinaceous debris in the alveolar space as compared to control subjects (Fig. 1j–l, Additional file 4: Fig. S2).

Intravenous infusion of endotoxin augments the expressions of systemic and pulmonary inflammatory cytokines

As shown by ELSA assay in Fig. 2, there was no difference in the baseline concentration of plasma IL-1β (Fig. 2a), IL-6 (Fig. 2d), IL-8 (Fig. 2g), TNF-α (Fig. 2j) and IL-17A (Fig. 2m) between LPS and saline groups, but all of these cytokines increased rapidly when challenged with LPS infusion at T0 compared with saline infusion. We also determined the levels of these inflammatory cytokines within BALF and lung homogenates

Table 1 Variables determining oxygenation and lung mechanics in saline controls and LPS-challenged animals

Parameter	Group	Time (h)				
		Baseline	−3 h	−2 h	−1 h	T0
PaO_2/FiO_2 (mmHg)	NS	466 ± 26	458 ± 60	531 ± 51	509 ± 60	479 ± 34
	LPS	440 ± 19	312 ± 51	242 ± 36***	194 ± 10***	157 ± 23***
$PaCO_2$ (mmHg)	NS	35.2 ± 2.8	30.8 ± 2.8	30.5 ± 1.8	32.3 ± 1.1	31.8 ± 1.49
	LPS	36.8 ± 2.4	30.2 ± 1.8	37.5 ± 1.5	36.5 ± 3.0	44.7 ± 5.0**
$AaDO_2$ (mmHg)	NS	47 ± 7	48 ± 14	52 ± 1	51 ± 12	60 ± 4
	LPS	63 ± 5	124 ± 20	143 ± 15**	213 ± 53**	224 ± 48**
P_{AW}Peak (mbar)	NS	16.5 ± 1.8	16.5 ± 1.5	16.5 ± 1.7	17.3 ± 2.0	17.3 ± 1.8
	LPS	21.3 ± 0.9	27.2 ± 1.8**	30.2 ± 2.4***	31.2 ± 2.4***	35.7 ± 2.5***
P_{AW}Plateau (mbar)	NS	12.2 ± 1.8	11.5 ± 1.7	12.2 ± 2.0	13.2 ± 2.3	13.8 ± 2.2
	LPS	15.3 ± 1.2	18.8 ± 1.4	22.3 ± 2.3**	25.7 ± 2.5***	27.3 ± 3.2***
Resistance (mbar/l/s)	NS	9.3 ± 1.4	7.9 ± 1.2	8.1 ± 1.3	7.5 ± 1.1	8.1 ± 1.3
	LPS	8.5 ± 0.4	13.6 ± 2.5	15.7 ± 3.5	15.1 ± 3.2	14.7 ± 2.2
Compliance (ml/mbar)	NS	31.2 ± 3.5	33.3 ± 3.0	34.5 ± 4.0	35.6 ± 4.3	32.8 ± 3.3
	LPS	28.2 ± 2.7	23.0 ± 2.1	21.4 ± 2.3*	20.7 ± 2.9**	16.7 ± 1.8**

Oxygenation and ventilation parameters in saline control and LPS challenge animals at baseline and a series of time points until the end of the experiment when ALI model was diagnosed (data shown are mean ± SEM, $N = 6$ of each group; *$P < 0.05$; **$P < 0.01$; ***$P < 0.001$ versus control group). PaO_2, oxygen partial pressure; FiO_2, inspiratory oxygen fraction; $PaCO_2$, carbon dioxide partial pressure; P_{AW}Peak, peak airway pressure; P_{AW}Plateau, plateau airway pressure

Table 2 Systemic and pulmonary hemodynamic measurements in saline controls and LPS-challenged animals

Parameter	Group	Time (h)				
		Baseline	−3 h	−2 h	−1 h	T0
CO (l/min)	NS	4.1 ± 0.3	4.5 ± 0.4	4.1 ± 0.4	4.2 ± 0.4	4.2 ± 0.4
	LPS	4.1 ± 0.3	4.1 ± 0.5	5.1 ± 0.3	5.0 ± 0.3	3.4 ± 0.3
MAP (mmHg)	NS	105 ± 6	98 ± 6	102 ± 8	101 ± 7	102 ± 8
	LPS	113 ± 3	78 ± 8	56 ± 4***	57 ± 5***	54 ± 5***
SVRI (dyn s/cm^5/m^2)	NS	1783 ± 198	1810 ± 169	1927 ± 148	1822 ± 183	1909 ± 218
	LPS	2399 ± 238	1987 ± 217	1002 ± 111**	952 ± 56**	1160 ± 97*
mPAP (mmHg)	NS	16.5 ± 1.0	16.7 ± 0.5	15.7 ± 1.2	17.8 ± 1.5	18.5 ± 1.2
	LPS	18.8 ± 1.5	28.8 ± 1.9***	3.3 ± 2.0***	34.7 ± 2.7***	41.0 ± 1.7***
PVRI (dyn s/cm^5/m^2)	NS	204 ± 20	193 ± 16	231 ± 48	209 ± 35	201 ± 13
	LPS	364 ± 40	552 ± 115***	542 ± 67**	634 ± 120***	781 ± 74***
PAWP (mmHg)	NS	6.0 ± 1.2	6.5 ± 1.5	6.3 ± 1.4	6.8 ± 1.5	6.8 ± 1.2
	LPS	4.0 ± 1.2	5.5 ± 0.6	8.0 ± 0.6	9.0 ± 0.9	12.2 ± 1.4*
EVLWI (ml/kg)	NS	9.0 ± 0.5	9.7 ± 0.9	9.3 ± 0.5	9.5 ± 0.6	10.0 ± 0.9
	LPS	8.0 ± 0.5	9.7 ± 0.7	9.8 ± 0.9	11.0 ± 0.8	15.4 ± 1.3***
PVPI	NS	2.7 ± 0.1	2.8 ± 0.3	3.0 ± 0.3	3.0 ± 0.3	2.9 ± 0.2
	LPS	2.7 ± 0.2	3.6 ± 0.3	4.0 ± 0.7	4.6 ± 0.7	5.6 ± 0.5***

Hemodynamic parameters are compared between the saline control and LPS-challenged group. (Data are mean ± SEM, $N = 6$ of each group; *$P < 0.05$, **$P < 0.01$, ***$P < 0.001$; versus control group)

CO cardiac output, *MAP* mean arterial pressure, *SVRI* systemic vascular resistance index, *MPAP* mean pulmonary arterial pressure, *PVRI* pulmonary vascular resistance index, *PAWP* pulmonary artery wedge pressure, *EVLWI* extravascular lung water index, *PVPI* pulmonary vascular permeability index

to assess the inflammatory response in the alveolar compartment. ELISA assay showed significant increased levels of these cytokines in BALF and lung homogenates after LPS challenge except IL-17A, which was remarkable increased in BALF but remained unchanged in lung homogenates at T0 (Fig. 2).

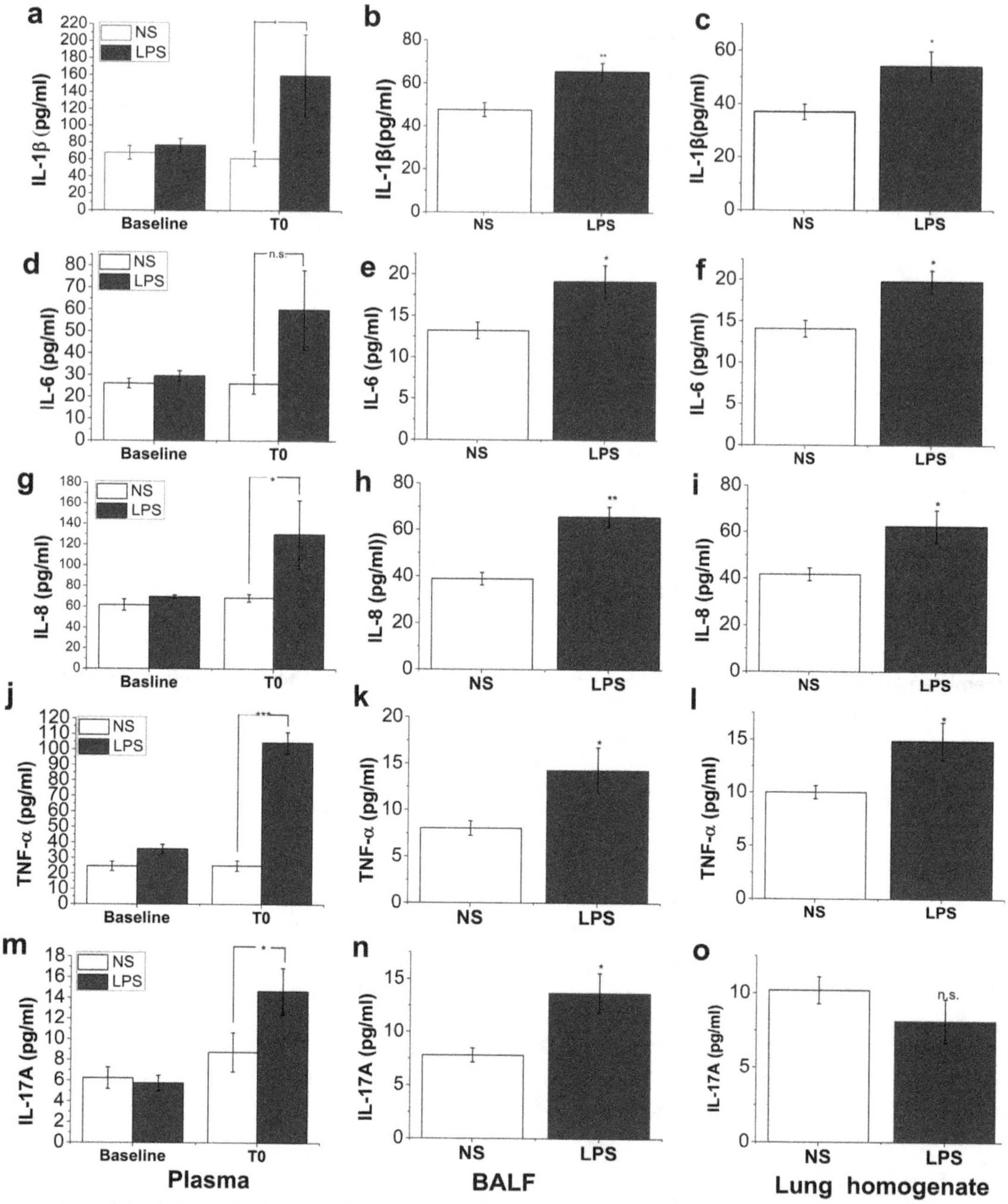

Fig. 2 Concentrations of circulating and pulmonary inflammatory parameters. In LPS group, plasma samples were collected before LPS challenge (baseline) and at the time when ARDS model had been well established (T0). BALF and lung homogenates were also prepared at necropsy. Samples from saline control group were also obtained at the corresponding time points. The level of circulating and pulmonary IL-1β (**a–c**), IL-6 (**d–f**), IL-8 (**g–i**), TNF-α (**j–l**) and IL-17A (**m–o**) was detected by using commercial ELISA kits. Data are presented as mean ± SEM ($N = 6$ of each group). Compared with saline (NS) group, *$P < 0.05$; **$P < 0.01$; ***$P < 0.001$

Hemoadsorption improves oxygenation and lung mechanics in pigs challenged with endotoxin

We found that treatment with HA increased LPS-impaired oxygenation (387 ± 10 mmHg at baseline vs. 183 ± 6 mmHg at T0 vs 315 ± 22 mmHg at 8 h after HA; Fig. 3a; Table 3). In contrast, in endotoxin-challenged pigs that did not receive HA (HA-sham) treatment, the ratio of PaO_2/FiO_2 was only slightly increased at 8 h after HA-sham (Fig. 3a; Table 3). Treatment with HA significantly or showed a trend toward decreasing P_{AW}Peak,

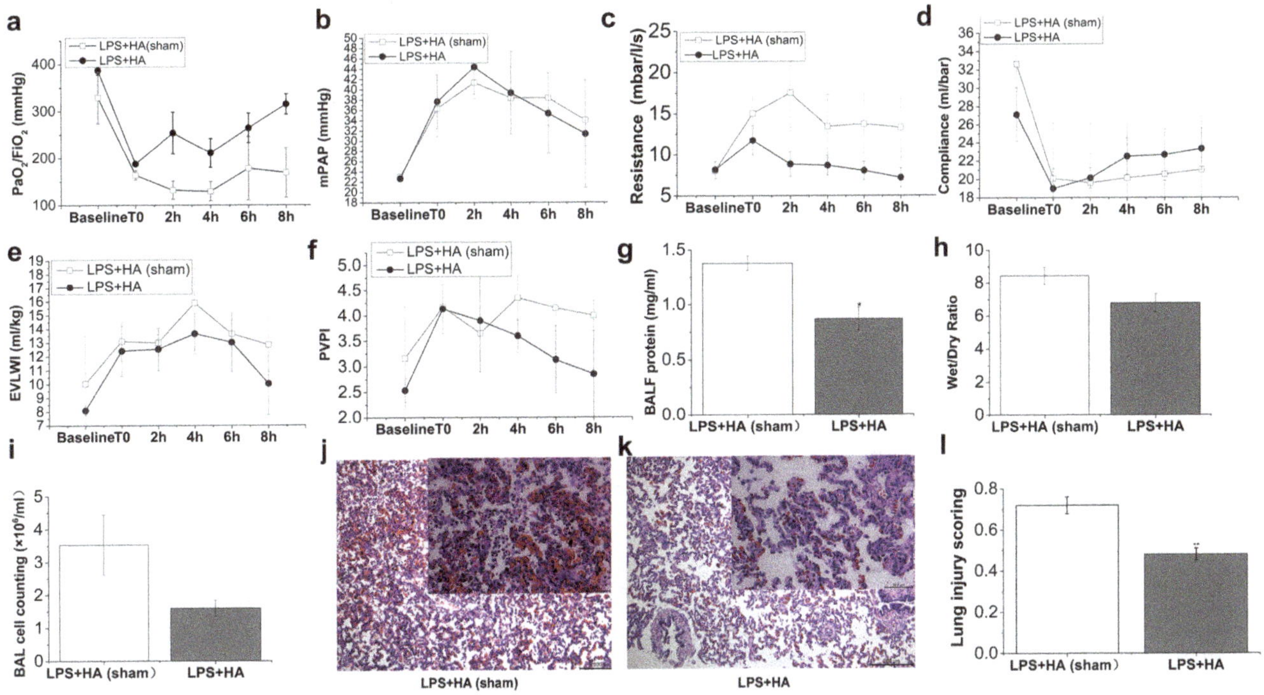

Fig. 3 Effects of HA on oxygenation, lung mechanics and alveolar-capillary barriers. Pigs were challenged with LPS (50 μg/kg) intravenously to recapitulate the features of ARDS. When ARDS was well established (T0), animals received hemoadsorption (HA) or sham-hemoadsorption treatment for 3 h. Following another 5-h observation, animals were killed for BALF and lung tissue processing. At baseline, T0, and a series of time points during (2 h) and after HA (or HA-sham) treatment (4, 6 and 8 h), parameters of oxygenation and lung mechanics were recorded. PaO_2/FiO_2 (**a**) was measured by using blood samples from femoral artery on a blood gas analysis instrument. The value of mPAP (**b**) was gained by Swan-Ganz catheter implantation into jugular vein. Resistance (**c**) and compliance (**d**) were recorded by using Drager Evita 4 ventilator. EVLWI (**e**) and PVPI (**f**) were measured by PiCCO system at indicated time points (baseline, T0, 2, 4, 6 and 8 h following HA or HA-sham treatment). BALF protein (**g**) was assessed at 8 h after HA (or HA-sham) as described in "Methods". **h** The ratio of wet/dry lung weight of animals in both groups was calculated by gravimetric method. **i** Whole-cell counts in the BALF collected from both groups of pigs were numerated by using a counting plate. **j** and **k** were the representative lung histology sections of pigs in LPS + HA (sham) and LPS + HA groups. HE sections are from one representative animal per group. **l** Lung injury scores were calculated according to ATS report which was in detail described in the "Methods." Data points represent as mean ± SEM, $N = 3–4$ of each group and time point. Statistical significance between HA and HA-sham group per point of measurement is shown as $^{*}P < 0.05$

P_{AW}Plateau, lung resistance and the impairment of static compliance induced by endotoxin infusion when all pigs data were pooled together and compared with HA-sham group (Fig. 3c, d; Table 3). However, HA did not alter the impairment of systemic/pulmonary hemodynamic parameters (Fig. 3b; Table 4).

Hemoadsorption blunts lung edema and histopathological signs of ARDS

Compared with LPS + HA-sham group, HA therapy for ARDS pigs caused a decrease in EVLWI, PVPI, lung wet-to-dry weight ratio and BALF cell count (Fig. 3e, f, h, i; Table 4). However, the changes did not reach statistical difference when compared with LPS + HA-sham group. But HA therapy can significantly reduce total BALF protein as compared to HA-sham treatment (Fig. 3g). These beneficial alterations were further reflected by reduced histologic signs of inflammation and injury (Fig. 3j–l).

Hemoadsorption reduces circulating and alveolar cytokine levels

ELISA assay showed that plasma level of IL-1β and IL-6 induced by endotoxin was significantly blunted by HA treatment compared with HA-sham treatment (Fig. 4a, d). HA also elicited a remarkable decrease in the expression of IL-1β and IL-6 in both BALF and lung homogenate (Fig. 4b, c, e, f). Plasma and lung homogenate levels of IL-8 were also decreased (Fig. 4g, i). BALF levels of TNF-α and IL-17A were significantly reduced by HA treatment (Fig. 4k, n).

Hemoadsorption-altered plasma and pulmonary proteome

First, plasma proteome was analyzed. The differentially accumulated proteins (T0 vs baseline) and their dynamic changes after HA/HA-sham treatment (8 h after T0 vs. baseline) are shown in Additional file 5: Fig. S3. These proteins were classified into several categories based on biological process analysis (Tables 5, 6). We identified four

Table 3 Variables determining oxygenation and lung mechanics in LPS + HA (sham)- and LPS + HA-treated animals

Parameter	Group	Time (h)					
		Baseline	T0	2 h	4 h	6 h	8 h
PaO_2/FiO_2 (mmHg)	LPS + HA (sham)	329 ± 55	164 ± 10†	131 ± 20†	129 ± 21†	178 ± 68	169 ± 53
	LPS + HA	387 ± 10	183 ± 6†	254 ± 44*	211 ± 31†	264 ± 31	315 ± 22*§
$PaCO_2$ (mmHg)	LPS + HA (sham)	45 ± 4	40 ± 7	45 ± 17	46 ± 14	46 ± 16	42 ± 14
	LPS + HA	37 ± 5	53 ± 6†	59 ± 9†	54 ± 3†	51 ± 2	45 ± 3
$AaDO_2$ (mmHg)	LPS + HA (sham)	96 ± 24	170 ± 6	363 ± 129	330 ± 103	371 ± 102†	358 ± 96
	LPS + HA	79 ± 10	172 ± 29†	368 ± 68†	368 ± 77†	334 ± 81†	296 ± 66†
P_{AW}Peak (mbar)	LPS + HA (sham)	17.7 ± 1.8	32.0 ± 2.6†	29.7 ± 5.2†	29.7 ± 2.7†	28.3 ± 1.7†	26.7 ± 3.2
	LPS + HA	18.9 ± 1.5	29.0 ± 1.0†	26.3 ± 1.9†	26.3 ± 1.8†	24.7 ± 1.8	24.3 ± 2.3
P_{AW}Plateau (mbar)	LPS + HA (sham)	13.3 ± 0.9	21.0 ± 1.0†	22.7 ± 2.9†	23.3 ± 2.4†	21.0 ± 1.0†	21.7 ± 0.9†
	LPS + HA	15.3 ± 1.8	24.7 ± 1.3†	22.0 ± 1.2†	21.0 ± 1.0†§	20.3 ± 0.9†§	19.0 ± 0.0*†§
Resistance (mbar/l/s)	LPS + HA (sham)	8.0 ± 1.1	15.0 ± 1.8	17.5 ± 4.6	13.4 ± 3.9	13.7 ± 3.6	13.3 ± 4.0
	LPS + HA	8.2 ± 1.0	11.7 ± 1.8	8.8 ± 1.5	8.7 ± 1.2	8.0 ± 1.1	7.2 ± 1.2§
Compliance (ml/mbar)	LPS + HA (sham)	32.6 ± 2.9	20.1 ± 6.1	19.6 ± 7.7	20.2 ± 6.0	20.6 ± 5.0	21.1 ± 5.9
	LPS + HA	27.1 ± 2.9	19 ± 2.2†	20.1 ± 1.1	22.5 ± 2.0	22.7 ± 2.8	23.3 ± 2.3

Oxygenation and ventilation parameters in LPS + HA (sham)- and LPS + HA-treated animals at baseline and a series of time points until the end of the experiment (data are mean ± SEM, $N = 3$–4 of each group; *$P < 0.05$ when compared between groups; †$P < 0.05$ when compared with baseline within per group; §$P < 0.05$ versus T0 within per group). PaO_2, oxygen partial pressure; FiO_2, inspiratory oxygen fraction; $PaCO_2$, carbon dioxide partial pressure; P_{AW}Peak, peak airway pressure; P_{AW}Plateau, plateau airway pressure

Table 4 Systemic and pulmonary hemodynamic measurements compared between LPS + HA (sham) and LPS + HA groups

Parameter	Group	Time (h)					
		Baseline	T0	2 h	4 h	6 h	8 h
CO (l/min)	LPS + HA (sham)	6.36 ± 0.41	5.50 ± 1.98	4.86 ± 1.28	5.35 ± 1.13	5.17 ± 1.10	5.56 ± 1.27
	LPS + HA	4.98 ± 0.48	4.99 ± 0.78	5.34 ± 0.94	6.08 ± 0.97	5.05 ± 0.89	5.15 ± 0.40
MAP (mmHg)	LPS + HA (sham)	125 ± 6	82 ± 3	92 ± 20	106 ± 21	104 ± 25	96 ± 24
	LPS + HA	118 ± 7	85 ± 15	74 ± 9	86 ± 12	82 ± 17	80 ± 16
SVRI (dyn s/cm^5/m^2)	LPS + HA (sham)	1699 ± 59	1120 ± 154	1813 ± 688	1788 ± 468	1681 ± 354	1454 ± 248
	LPS + HA	1992 ± 156	1465 ± 423	1143 ± 231	1210 ± 347	1576 ± 778	1291 ± 461
mPAP (mmHg)	LPS + HA (sham)	23.0 ± 2.6	36.3 ± 5.6	41.3 ± 3.2	38.3 ± 5.8	38.3 ± 5.4	34.0 ± 5.1
	LPS + HA	22.7 ± 0.3	37.7 ± 5.2	44.3 ± 5.2	39.3 ± 8.0	35.3 ± 7.8	31.3 ± 10
PVRI (dyn s/cm^5/m^2)	LPS + HA (sham)	229 ± 31	477 ± 202	518 ± 181	467 ± 85	441 ± 92	343 ± 25
	LPS + HA	248 ± 19	404 ± 60	499 ± 72	421 ± 156	483 ± 196	416 ± 145
PAWP (mmHg)	LPS + HA (sham)	9.7 ± 2.3	12.7 ± 3.2	14.7 ± 3.0	12.0 ± 3.1	14.0 ± 4.2	13.0 ± 2.6
	LPS + HA	8.3 ± 1.2	11.0 ± 1.2	16.3 ± 1.8	13.0 ± 1.7	11.0 ± 2.0	11.7 ± 3.0
EVLWI (ml/kg)	LPS + HA (sham)	10.1 ± 3.5	13.1 ± 1.4	13.0 ± 0.6	15.9 ± 2.5	13.7 ± 1.0	12.9 ± 2.0
	LPS + HA	8.1 ± 0.3	12.4 ± 1.8	12.5 ± 1.5	13.7 ± 1.5	13.0 ± 2.1	10.1 ± 2.3
PVPI	LPS + HA (sham)	3.2 ± 1.0	4.2 ± 0.2	3.7 ± 0.5	4.4 ± 0.5	4.1 ± 0.2	4.0 ± 0.3
	LPS + HA	2.5 ± 0.2	4.1 ± 0.5	3.9 ± 1.0	3.6 ± 0.3	3.1 ± 0.7	2.9 ± 0.9

Hemodynamic parameters are shown in the LPS + HA (sham) and LPS + HA groups. Data are mean ± SEM, $N = 3$–4 of each group; CO, cardiac output; MAP, mean arterial pressure; SVRI, systemic vascular resistance index; MPAP, mean pulmonary arterial pressure; PVRI, pulmonary vascular resistance index; PAWP, pulmonary artery wedge pressure; EVLWI, extravascular lung water index; PVPI, pulmonary vascular permeability index

plasma proteins, i.e., interleukin-1 receptor antagonist protein (IL-1Ra), inter-alpha-trypsin inhibitor heavy chain H4 (ITIH4), matrix metallopeptidase (MMP)-1 and MMP-10, that were up-regulated at T0 in these two groups, but sharply reduced after HA treatment while further increased in HA-sham group (Fig. 5a, b). Differentially expressed proteins (these proteins were comparable at T0 when compared with HA with HA-sham group) after 8-h

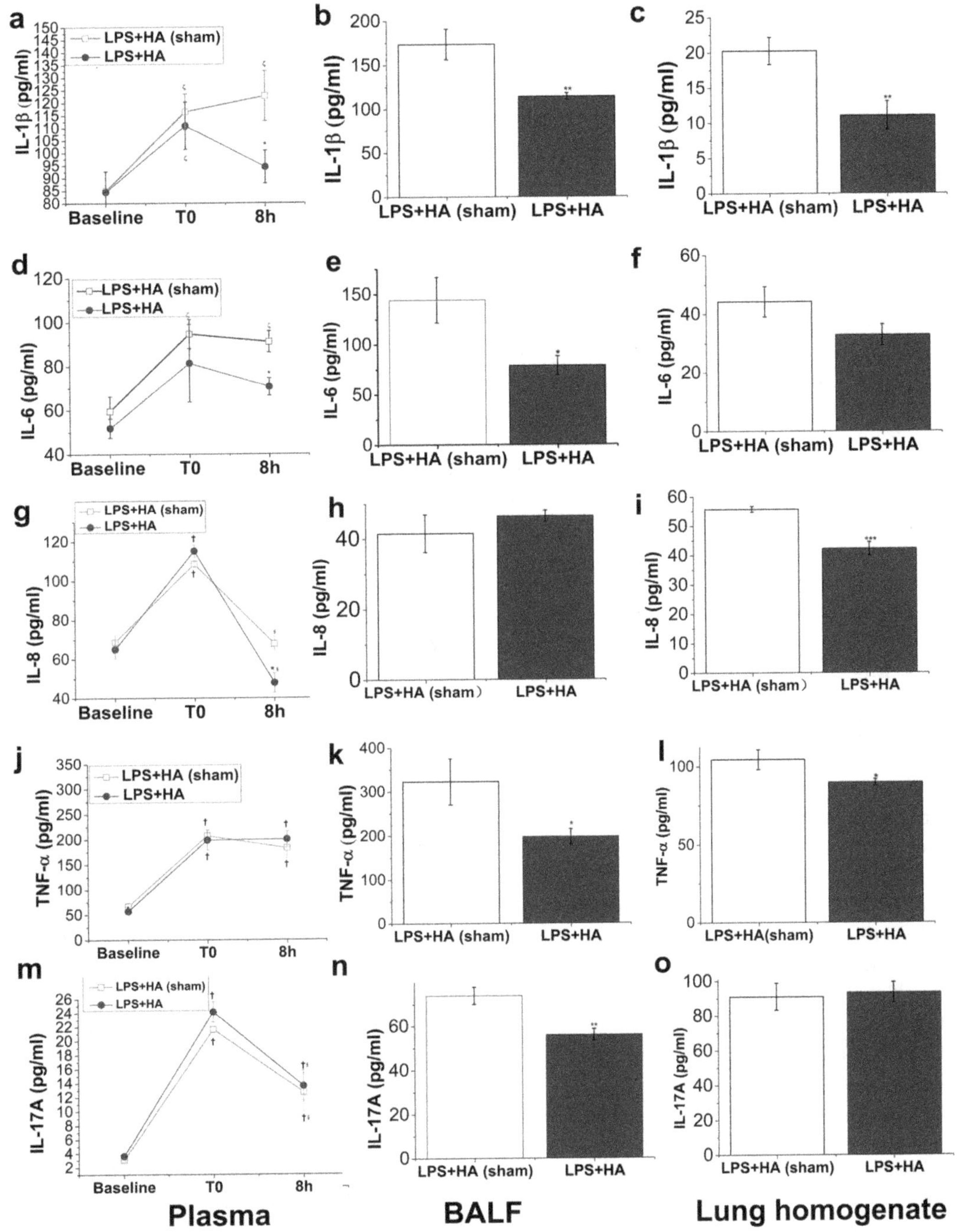

Fig. 4 Effect of HA on the production of LPS-induced circulating and pulmonary inflammatory cytokines. Pigs were allocated into LPS + HA (sham) and LPS + HA groups. Plasma was collected at baseline, and at the time point when ALI model was diagnosed (T0) and the end of the experiment schedule (8 h after T0). BALF and lung homogenates were prepared after pigs were euthanized. The systemic and pulmonary cytokine levels of IL-1β (**a–c**), IL-6 (**d–f**), IL-8 (**g–i**), TNF-α (**j–l**) and IL-17A (**m–o**) were detected by using ELISA kits. Values are mean ± SEM, $N = 4$ of each group. $^{*}P < 0.05$; $^{**}P < 0.01$; $^{***}P < 0.001$ when compared between LPS + HA (sham) and LPS + HA groups; $^{\dagger}P < 0.05$ versus baseline and $^{\S}P < 0.05$ versus T0 when compared within each group

HA or HA-sham treatment, and their GO annotations are also shown in Additional file 6: Table S2 and Additional file 7: Fig. S4. We then analyzed proteome in BALF and lung homogenate samples. Differentially expressed proteins compared between HA and HA-sham groups are shown in Additional file 8: Table S3, Additional file 9: Table

S4, Additional file 10: Table S5, Additional file 11: Table S6. The most five relevant GO categories (*P* value less than 0.05) are shown in Fig. 5c, d. KEGG pathway analysis showed that these differentially expressed proteins were involved in the canonical signaling pathways (Fig. 5e, f).

Discussion

In this current study, we tested the efficacy of "sorbent strategy"-based HA on a porcine ARDS model and found that HA reduced circulating and alveolar levels of proinflammatory cytokines, improved oxygenation and attenuated lung injuries in the exudative phase. This provides some clue that HA330 cartridge may be a novel potential weapon fighting against the "cytokine storm" on the alveolar-capillary membrane barrier.

The most commonly used large-animal models of ARDS include endotoxin infusion, repeated lavage, oleic acid and smoke/burn injury [17]. To reproduce the most known risk factor and etiology for ARDS, which is sepsis [18], we systemically administrated endotoxin (LPS) to mimic the clinically relevant sepsis-induced ARDS. The susceptibility to LPS is highly variable and differs among different animals. Pigs, sheep, calves, and cats are more sensitive to LPS challenge. Low dosage of LPS (μg/kg range) can induce significant ARDS-like features in these animals. In contrast, animals such as rodents or dogs require much higher doses to develop lung injury (mg/kg range). This different vulnerability to LPS may be induced by the pulmonary intravascular macrophages (PIM), a lung resident population of mature macrophage [19]. 8–100 μg/kg of LPS has been used in several previous studies to develop porcine ARDS model [12, 20, 21]. In our study, low amount of LPS (50ug/kg in 500 ml saline for 2 h) can also induce the pigs to develop an abrupt decrease in oxygenation and arterial pressure and a decrease in systemic vascular resistance, needing rapid fluid resuscitation (10–20 ml/kg/h of saline) and the usage of vasopressor infusion (0.5–1.5 μg/kg/min of norepinephrine).

In most recent large-animal studies, the diagnosis of experimental ARDS is ambiguous without definite criteria [12, 18, 21, 22]. To determine whether ARDS really occurred, we adopt the four diagnostic criteria released by ATS official statement on the definition of ARDS in animals [14]. ARDS model was initially diagnosed when PaO_2/FiO_2 is less than 200 mmHg with a PEEP at 5 cmH_2O (criteria (a) moderate ARDS in human beings according to Berlin definition). Then, the ARDS model was further assessed with other criteria listed as follows: (b) permeability. Permeability assessment was performed by using four parameters, i.e., EVLWI, PVPI, BALF protein and the ratio of wet to dry lung weight (W/D ratio). EVLW is the amount of interstitial and alveolar fluid [23]. Previous studies showed that EVLW indexed to body weight (EVLWI) is well correlated with the value obtained by gravimetry and can independently predict mortality in septic and ARDS patients [19]. We found that both EVLWI and W/D ratio were significantly increased after LPS infusion, indicating an exudative edema phase (Fig. 1; Table 2). The permeability of lung epithelium barrier can also be calculated by PVPI [24]. PVPI in this model was increased to 5.6 ± 0.5 at T0 when ARDS was diagnosed (Fig. 1; Table 2), indicating high permeable (rather than hydrostatic) pulmonary edema because it was reported that a PVPI value of 3 can distinguish these two forms of pulmonary edema [24]. Accordingly, BALF protein concentration, another leakage marker [14], was also increased after LPS infusion (Fig. 1g). (c) Histology. To our knowledge, this is the first large-animal study to assess histologic changes at the time point that ARDS was initially diagnosed by oxygenation and ahead of therapy implementation. The major histologic findings are shown in Fig. 1j–l. It is noteworthy that LPS i.v. infusion causes only modest lung edema (perivascular edema, Additional file 4: Fig. S2) as compared to ARDS patients, because the endothelium barrier is more resistant to the damage induced by LPS [19]. (d) Inflammation. We found that both circulating and alveolar inflammatory cytokines were elevated, indicating an acute "cytokine storm" was elicited in systemic and lung milieu by i.v. infusion of LPS.

Thereafter, we conducted subsequent studies to explore the "therapeutic," rather than "prophylactic" effect of hemoadsorption (HA) on the well-established (or far-developed, rather than "immature") ARDS model. HA was performed with the HA330 neutral microporous resin cartridge specially designed for the absorption of medium-sized inflammatory cytokines. First, we found that HA treatment increased PaO_2/FiO_2 gradually (Fig. 3). Several previous studies in septic patients attributed this beneficial effect to the improved hemodynamics [10, 25]. However, a previous experimental study showed that zero-balanced high-volume continuous veno-venous hemofiltration (CVVH) could improve arterial oxygenation without systemic or pulmonary hemodynamics improvement [9]. We also found that animals treated with or without HA330-based hemadsorption did not differ in their levels of MAP, SVRI, MPAP and PVRI (Table 4). Considering that HA therapy elicited a trend in reducing lung water and the permeability of alveolar-capillary membrane barrier (Fig. 3e–i), we assume that oxygenation improvement should be partly due to the reduction of alveolar fluid leakage after clearing the peak concentration of alveolar cytokines, corresponding with the "peak concentration hypothesis" for EBP modality [26]. Lung local cytokines removal may be the result of passive spillover or active transport [26]. Notably, a recent clinical study showed that the

Table 5 Ontology groups and associated differentially expressed plasma proteins in the time points of T0 and 8 h after HA-sham treatment versus baseline

GO biological process	Accession	Protein name	Fold change over baseline[a]	
			T0/baseline	8 h/baseline
Acute-phase response/acute inflammatory response	P79263	Inter-alpha-trypsin inhibitor heavy chain H4	1.22	2.17
	F1SH92	Inter-alpha-trypsin inhibitor heavy chain H4	1.39	2.04
	Q29056	Interleukin-1 receptor antagonist protein	1.49	1.51
	F1SFI7	Alpha-2-HS-glycoprotein (Fragment)	0.76	0.49
	Q29014	Alpha-1 acid glycoprotein (Fragment)	0.68	0.49
	Q8SPS7	Haptoglobin	0.74	0.57
	Q6S4N2	Heat shock 70 kDa protein 1B	0.64	0.65
Regulation of immune system process	P01025	Complement C3	1.45	0.88
	A5PF00	B-factor, properdin	0.75	0.62
	F1RMN7	Hemopexin	0.70	0.63
	Q69DL4	Complement C1qB (Fragment)	0.81	0.60
	A0SEH0	Complement component C6	0.71	0.76
	Q29041	Ficolin-2	0.75	0.69
Defense response/response to stress	P52552	Peroxiredoxin-2 (Fragment)	1.28	1.30
	P32195	Protegrin-2	4.76	2.43
	O02705	Heat shock protein HSP 90-alpha	1.37	2.56
	Q6QR67	Resistin	5.00	3.06
Proteolysis	C9VZX4	Matrix metallopeptidase 1	1.79	3.98
	C9VZX5	Matrix metallopeptidase 10	1.13	1.53
	F2Z528	Proteasome subunit alpha type	1.22	1.22
	F2Z5K2	Proteasome subunit alpha type	1.28	1.21
	I3LQ51	Proteasome subunit beta type	1.49	1.50
	P03974	Transitional endoplasmic reticulum ATPase	1.35	2.27
	Q9GMA6	Alpha-1-antichymotrypsin 2	0.81	0.55
	C4PGL9	Mannan-binding lectin serine peptidase 2	0.79	0.97
	F1SCF0	Alpha-1-antitrypsin	0.81	0.66
Coagulation	F1RPW2	Coagulation factor V	0.66	0.45
	F1RZ36	Coagulation factor VIII	0.64	0.74
	O97507	Coagulation factor XII	0.76	0.66
	K7GQL2	Coagulation factor XIII, A1 polypeptide	0.71	0.79
	F1RX36	Fibrinogen alpha chain	0.83	1.11
	P14460	Fibrinogen alpha chain (Fragment)	1.47	3.12
	P14477	Fibrinogen beta chain (fragment)	1.39	2.30
	P06867	Plasminogen	0.77	0.57
	F1SB81	Plasminogen	0.59	0.59
	B3STX9	Prothrombin	0.68	0.76
Negative regulation of blood coagulation	I3LRJ4	Vitamin K-dependent protein C	0.69	0.57
Metabolic process	Q29214	60S acidic ribosomal protein P0	1.47	2.45
	F1RYZ0	60S acidic ribosomal protein P2	2.17	4.72
	P01965	Hemoglobin subunit alpha	1.39	0.68
	F1RII7	Hemoglobin subunit beta	1.28	0.74
	A0SNU7	Glyceraldehyde-3-phosphate dehydrogenase (fragment)	1.23	1.41
	G9F6X8	Prolyl 4-hydroxylase beta polypeptide	1.45	2.14
	F1SN27	Sorbitol dehydrogenase	1.67	3.13

Table 5 continued

GO biological process	Accession	Protein name	Fold change over baseline[a]	
			T0/baseline	8 h/baseline
Regulation of lipid storage	Q2LE37	Apolipoprotein M	1.25	1.02
	Q29248	Apolipoprotein A-I (Fragment)	0.79	0.79
Cellular metal ion homeostasis	Q8WMN8	Lactoferrin (Fragment)	1.64	0.93
	P09571	Serotransferrin	0.77	0.63
Transport	P04404	Chromogranin-A (Fragment)	1.75	1.89
	Q29545	Inhibitor of carbonic anhydrase	0.67	0.54
	A4US67	Paraoxonase	0.75	0.67
	F1RUN2	Serum albumin	0.76	0.60
	P50390	Transthyretin	0.81	0.76
Positive regulation of cell differentiation	Q0PM28	Pigment epithelium-derived factor	0.70	0.84
Multicellular organismal process	P00761	Trypsin	0.78	0.55
Response to unfolded protein	F1RS36	78 kDa glucose-regulated protein	1.33	1.38
Cytoskeleton organization	I3LVD5	Actin, cytoplasmic 1	1.64	1.09
	A0A0B8RSX6	Filamin A, alpha	1.45	1.71
	B6VNT8	Cardiac muscle alpha actin 1	1.82	1.39
	Q6QA25	Tropomyosin 3	1.59	1.91
	P67937	Tropomyosin alpha-4 chain	1.23	1.29
	Q767L7	Tubulin beta chain	1.37	0.84
	P02543	Vimentin	1.54	5.13
Obsolete GTP catabolic process	Q0PY11	Elongation factor 1-alpha	1.35	1.37
Chromosome organization	P62802	Histone H4	2.50	1.87
Tissue remodeling	Q711S8	Secreted phosphoprotein 24	0.82	0.79
Regulation of biological process	F1S682	Sulfhydryl oxidase	0.80	0.86

[a] Note that changes are expressed as relative abundance of the plasma proteins at T0 or 8 h after HA-sham treatment compared with baseline within the LPS + HA (sham) group. A fold change $\geq$ 1.20, $p < 0.05$ represents more protein abundance in T0 or 8 h versus baseline. By contrast, a fold change $\leq$ 0.83, $p < 0.05$ represents less protein abundance in T0 or 8 h versus baseline

circulating and BALF levels of IL-17A were significantly increased in ARDS patients and predicted an increased influx of alveolar neutrophils, alveolar permeability and organ dysfunction [27]. Thus, reduced BALF level of IL-17A in HA treatment group may be one of the reasons for fewer lung inflammatory cells and decreased acute lung injury. Taken together, by direct/indirect removal of a variety of pathogenic proinflammatory mediators that over-expressed in plasma and lung, HA timely blunted the "cytokine storm" in the process of ARDS and restored immunologic balance at a much lower set-point. These findings were in line with a recent small clinical study on septic-induced ARDS patients [28].

In the last step, we also examined whether HA can effect the whole proteomes in plasma and lung, which has not been previously reported. We found four plasma proteins that were most differentially regulated by HA and HA-sham therapy, i.e., IL-1Ra, MMP-1, MMP-10 and ITIH4 (Fig. 5a, b). Soluble IL-1Ra, an important member in IL-1 family of cytokines [29], was dramatically elevated in ARDS and septic patients [30, 31]. A persistent elevated level of IL-1Ra indicates immunoparalysis, which greatly contributes to the later deaths who survive the initial cytokine storm in ARDS [32]. ITIH4 is a plasma glycoprotein that belongs to a serine protease inhibitor family and acts as an acute-phase protein in several diseases [33]. However, there is a lack of studies aiming to determine the role of ITIH4 as a potential diagnostic or prognostic indicator for ARDS. The matrix metalloproteinases (MMPs) are a family of proteolytic enzymes with the capacity of degrading the extracellular matrix component, thus causing tissue damage in the pathological process [34]. Previous studies were largely focused on the BAL fluid level of MMPs (including MMP2, MMP8 and MMP9) and found an elevated expression pattern [35]. However, the circulating and BALF levels of MMP-1 (interstitial collagenase) and MMP-10 (Stromeolysin 2) in ARDS animals or patients are remained largely unknown. Collectively, we concluded a composite of plasma biomarkers with IL-1Ra, MMPs and ITIH4 may be useful to predict the severity of ARDS. Of course, this hypothesis needs further verification.

Table 6 Ontology groups and associated differentially expressed plasma proteins in the time points of T0 and 8 h after HA treatment versus baseline

GO biological process	Accession	Protein name	Fold change over baseline[a]	
			T0/baseline	8 h/baseline
Acute-phase response/acute inflammatory response	Q29014	Alpha-1 acid glycoprotein (Fragment)	2.70	0.87
	K9J6H8	Alpha-2-macroglobulin	1.82	1.01
	I3L6K3	C-reactive protein	1.43	2.50
	F1RJ76	C-reactive protein	1.27	1.32
	Q8SPS7	Haptoglobin	2.08	1.00
	P79263	Inter-alpha-trypsin inhibitor heavy chain H4	1.89	1.78
	F1SH92	Inter-alpha-trypsin inhibitor heavy chain H4	1.47	1.19
	Q29056	Interleukin-1 receptor antagonist protein	2.44	1.44
	F1S9B8	Serum amyloid A protein	1.64	1.35
Regulation of immune system process	P01025	Complement C3	1.50	1.34
	F1SMJ1	Complement component C7 (Fragment)	1.23	1.07
	A5PF00	B-factor, properdin	2.50	0.95
	F1RMN7	Hemopexin	1.85	1.08
	L8B0S2	IgG heavy chain	1.82	1.00
	L8B0W9	IgG heavy chain	1.30	0.94
	K7ZPU8	IgG heavy chain constant region (Fragment)	1.59	0.72
	Q4Z8N7	Plasma platelet-activating factor acetylhydrolase	1.20	1.38
	P28491	Calreticulin	0.81	1.29
	B0LUW3	Chemerin	0.62	0.79
	F1STZ4	Complement C1q subcomponent subunit A	0.83	0.82
	Q29041	Ficolin-2	0.77	0.72
	A5A758	Keratin 1 (Fragment)	0.53	0.69
	C4PGL9	Mannan-binding lectin serine peptidase 2	0.65	0.75
Defense response/response to stress	A2SW51	Monocyte differentiation antigen CD14	1.64	1.60
	P52552	Peroxiredoxin-2 (Fragment)	1.59	1.64
	P32195	Protegrin-2	1.25	1.05
	B3STX9	Prothrombin	1.28	1.01
	F5XVC2	von Willebrand factor	1.35	1.07
	Q6QR67	Resistin	1.79	1.52
Proteolysis	Q9GMA6	Alpha-1-antichymotrypsin 2	1.47	1.03
	F1SCF0	Alpha-1-antitrypsin	2.04	0.87
	C9VZX4	Matrix metallopeptidase 1	1.47	1.22
	C9VZX5	Matrix metallopeptidase 10	1.43	1.21
Coagulation	P14460	Fibrinogen alpha chain (Fragment)	1.54	3.30
	P14477	Fibrinogen beta chain (Fragment)	1.43	1.78
	F1RQ75	Coagulation factor IX	0.78	0.60
	F1RPW2	Coagulation factor V	0.79	0.67
	Q19AZ7	Coagulation factor VII isoform b protein	0.72	0.81
	K7GQL2	Coagulation factor XIII, A1 polypeptide	0.51	0.54
Negative regulation of blood coagulation	I3LRJ4	Vitamin K-dependent protein C	0.74	0.64
Metabolic process	F1S1G8	Amine oxidase	1.64	1.01
	P01965	Hemoglobin subunit alpha	2.17	1.11
	F1RII7	Hemoglobin subunit beta	1.89	1.22
	Q29052	Inter-alpha-trypsin inhibitor heavy chain H1	1.32	1.08
	F8SIP2	EGF-containing fibulin-like extracellular matrix protein 1	0.80	1.09
	O02668	Inter-alpha-trypsin inhibitor heavy chain H2	0.74	0.64

Table 6 continued

GO biological process	Accession	Protein name	Fold change over baseline[a]	
			T0/baseline	8 h/baseline
	I3LL80	L-lactate dehydrogenase	0.81	0.65
	Q29126	Protein WAP-3	0.31	0.84
Regulation of lipid storage	A0A0F6TNY5	APOB O	1.43	1.09
	Q29433	Apolipoprotein B (Fragment)	2.17	1.21
	Q2LE37	Apolipoprotein M	1.23	1.04
	O97674	Lipoprotein lipase (Fragment)	0.62	0.64
	D3Y264	Apolipoprotein C-II	0.80	0.63
	F1RM45	Apolipoprotein E	0.75	0.89
	Q03472	Apolipoprotein R	0.72	0.60
	Q8WMN7	Plasma phospholipid transfer protein	0.79	0.85
Cellular metal ion homeostasis	I3VKE6	Ceruloplasmin	1.30	1.07
	Q6YT39	Lactotransferrin	1.61	1.33
	P09571	Serotransferrin	2.33	0.91
	D7RK08	Transferrin receptor protein	1.45	1.30
Transport	F1RUN2	Serum albumin	2.08	1.01
	P50390	Transthyretin	1.33	0.89
Positive regulation of cell differentiation	Q0PM28	Pigment epithelium-derived factor	1.32	1.11
Multicellular organismal process	Q711S8	Secreted phosphoprotein 24	0.74	0.72
	O11780	Transforming growth factor-beta-induced protein ig-h3	0.83	0.97
	P67937	Tropomyosin alpha-4 chain	0.81	1.23
	P00761	Trypsin	0.82	0.85

[a] Note that changes are expressed as relative abundance of the plasma proteins at T0 or 8 h after HA treatment compared with baseline within the LPS + HA group. A fold change ≥1.20, $P < 0.05$ represents more protein abundance in T0 or 8 h versus baseline. By contrast, a fold change ≤0.83, $P < 0.05$ represents less protein abundance in T0 or 8 h versus baseline

We also determined the role of HA330 cartridge-based HA on BALF and lung homogenate proteome (Additional file 8: Table S3, Additional file 9: Table S4, Additional file 10: Table S5, Additional file 11: Table S6). Notably, we found that the BALF level of secreted histone H2A, H2B and H4 was significantly blunted after HA therapy compared with HA-sham-treated pigs. Extracellular histones are the constituent of neutrophil extracellular traps (NETs) structures that ensnare and kill bacteria [36]. Elevated extracellular histones in BALF samples from humans with ARDS have been reported [37]. Also, instillation of neutralizing anti-histone H2A/H4 antibody reduced experimental ARDS severity [38]. Because extracellular histones origin from actively secretion by activated inflammatory cells, or from passively release by necrotic cells, we concluded that HA can significantly reduced the BALF level of histones by attenuating inflammatory lung injuries. BALF and lung level of Surfactant protein (SP)-B and SP-C were also significantly up-regulated by HA versus HA-sham treatment. Previous studies showed decreased levels of SP-A, SP-B and SP-C in BALF of ARDS patients [39]. Thus, HA treatment may improve oxygenation by restoring the alveolar levels of surfactant proteins. Collectively, we showed with the first experience that HA330-directed HA performance has a profound impact on plasma and lung proteome in a sepsis-induced ARDS porcine model.

Our studies have some strength. First, we comprehensively assessed the lung histologic features and other

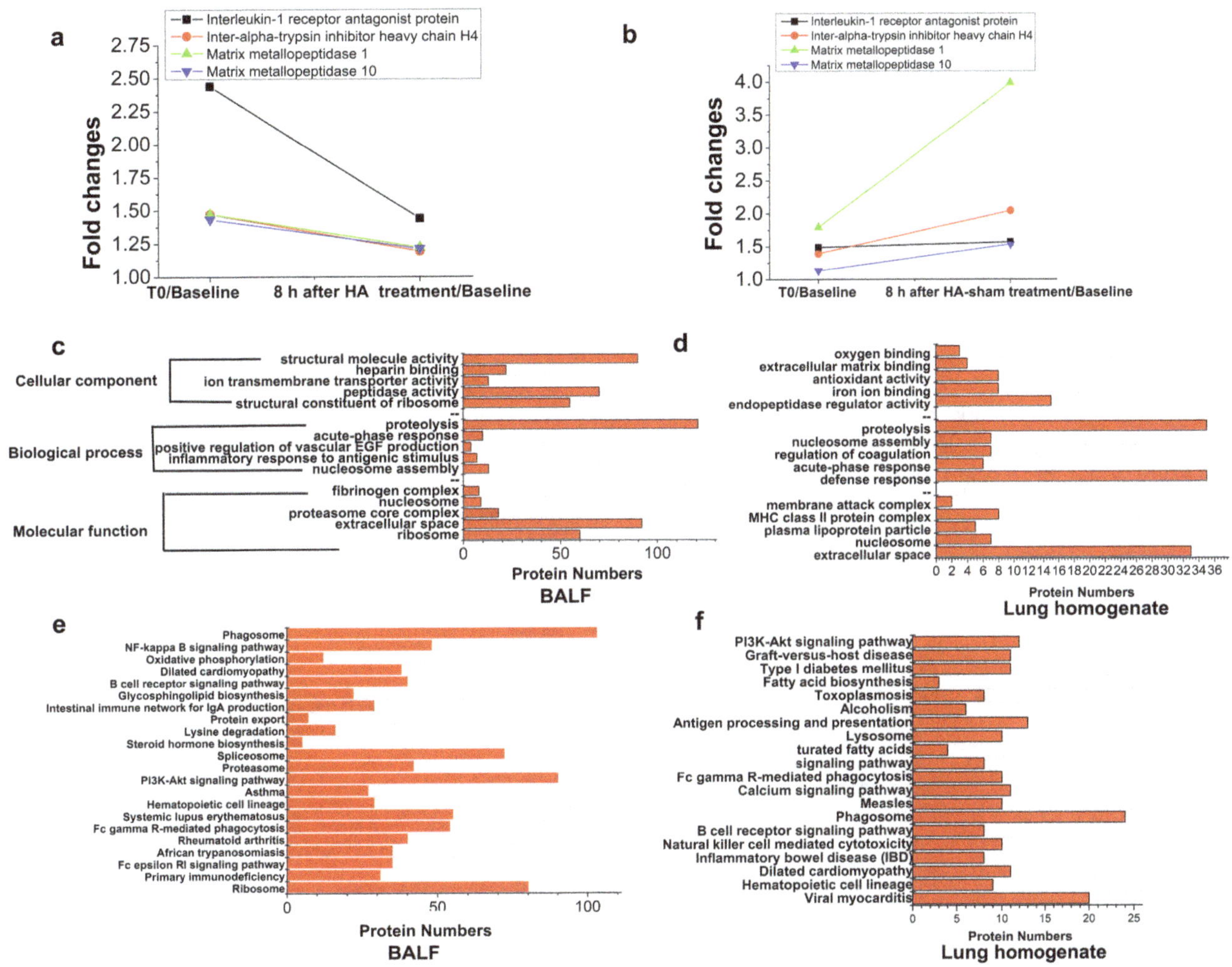

Fig. 5 Differentially expressed plasma, BALF and lung proteins identified with iTRAQ in LPS + HA (sham)- versus LPS + HA-treated pigs. **a** and **b** four plasma proteins that were most differentially expressed after 8-h treatment in LPS + HA (sham)- versus LPS + HA-treated pigs. Note that after LPS infusion, these proteins were up-regulated (T0/baseline); however, after HA treatment, their expression were decreased. By contrast, they were further increased after HA-sham treatment. Functional annotation for differentially expressed BALF (**c**) and lung homogenate (**d**) proteins by HA and HA-sham treatment are shown. *Red bars* represent the numbers of differentially expressed proteins based on three main categories: cellular component, biological process and molecular function. Enriched KEGG pathway analysis for differentially expressed BALF (**e**) and lung homogenate (**f**) proteins by HA and HA-sham treatment are shown. *Red bars* represent the numbers of proteins in a given pathway that differentially expressed between groups

biomarkers when the ARDS model was initially diagnosed by oxygenation. Second, we first assessed the effect of HA on experimental ARDS model by using iTRAQ-labeled proteomic technology. However, our studies also have some limitations. This is a small sample animal study. Also, the effect of HA330 directed HA should be further tested by other ARDS models. Third, the experimental data cannot be directly introduced into the real clinical practice. There is still a long way to go that HA-330 cartridge-based HA can be used in ARDS patients.

Conclusions

In conclusion, HA330 resin-based HA attenuated experimental ARDS by blunting circulating and lung "cytokine storm," improving permeability of alveolar barrier and promoting the recovery of the disordered proteomes.

Additional files

Additional file 1. Supplement-Methods.

Additional file 2: Fig. S1. Experimental protocol. Pigs received surgical preparation for instrumentation and divided into 4 groups. ALI was induced by intravenously infusion of LPS infusion (50 µg/kg over 2 h dissolved in 500 ml saline). Saline control group were challenged by equal amount of saline instead of LPS. When ALI was initially diagnosed ($PaO_2/FiO_2 \leq 200$ mmHg with PEEP = 5 cmH_2O; the time point was set as T0), pigs in LPS and saline groups were sacrificed for BAL and histology examination in order to further assess the ALI model. Other subset of pigs were subsequently treated with either HA-sham (LPS+HA-sham group), or HA (LPS+HA group) performance 3 h. Following this, the observation period was 5 h until the end of the experiment. Pigs in the 2 groups were sacrificed for BAL and histology examination. Physiological variables were recorded as indicated.

Additional file 3: Table S1. Lung injury scoring system.

Additional file 4: Fig. S2. Typical lung pathological changes induced by i.v. infusion of LPS. Representative pig lung sections stained with HE are shown. (A): Note atelectasis and the thickened alveolar walls. The majority of the alveoli are infiltrated with inflammatory cells (40×). (B): Arrow shows patchy neutrophilic infiltrates in alveolar spaces; "†"indicates thickened alveolar walls with septal neutrophils (400×). (C): Note the presence of deposition of pink fibrin strands (asterisk) and septal neutrophils (400×). (D): Note the perivascular edema with interstitial neutrophilic infiltrates (400×).

Additional file 5: Fig. S3. Dynamic expressions of plasma proteins showed with hierarchical cluster analysis. The heatmap represents the log_2 transformed fold change for each protein indicated. Columns represent comparisons between T0/baseline and 8 h after T0/baseline in HA and HA-sham treatment group, respectively; rows represent protein accession numbers. Red colors indicate up-regulated proteins and green colors indicate down-regulated proteins, respectively.

Additional file 6: Table S2. Ontology groups and associated differentially expressed plasma proteins in the time points of 8 h after HA versus HA-sham treatment.

Additional file 7: Fig. S4. Hierarchical clustering of differentially accumulated proteins compared between HA and HA-sham treatment groups. The heatmap represents the log_2 transformed fold change for each protein indicated. Columns represent comparisons between HA and HA-sham treatment groups at T0 and 8 h after T0, respectively; rows represent protein accession numbers. Red colors indicate up-regulated proteins and green colors indicate down-regulated proteins, respectively.

Additional file 8: Table S3. BALF proteins with significantly lower expression in LPS + HA versus LPS+HA (sham)-treated pigs.

Additional file 9: Table S4. BALF proteins with significantly higher expression in LPS + HA- versus LPS+HA (sham)-treated pigs.

Additional file 10: Table S5. Lung homogenate proteins with significantly lower expression in LPS+HA versus LPS + HA (sham)-treated pigs.

Additional file 11: Table S6. Lung homogenate proteins with significantly higher expression in LPS + HA versus LPS + HA (sham)-treated pigs.

Abbreviations

$AaDO_2$: Alveolar–arterial oxygen partial pressure difference; ARDS: Acute respiratory distress syndrome; CO: Cardiac output; CVVH: Continuous venovenous hemofiltration; DAD: Diffuse alveolar damage; EBP: Extracorporeal blood purification; EVLW: Extravascular lung water; HA: Hemadsorption; H4, ITIH4: Inter-alpha-trypsin inhibitor heavy chain; IL-1Ra: Interleukin-1 receptor antagonist protein; PEEP: Positive end-expiratory pressure; MMP: Matrix metallopeptidase; MAP: Mean arterial pressure; MPAP: Mean pulmonary arterial pressure; NETs: Neutrophil extracellular traps; PVPI: Pulmonary vascular permeability index; PIM: Pulmonary intravascular macrophages; PVRI: Pulmonary vascular resistance index; SVRI: Systemic venous resistance index.

Authors' contributions

XX designed, made, analyzed the experiments and drafted the manuscript. CJ designed and made the experiments. L Sa participated in the design and performance of the experiments. F Xiao, Y Li and H Dai participated in the analysis of the data and the critical revision of the article. C Wang contributed to the conception and design of the study, the analysis and interpretation of the data, revision of the article and final approval of the version to be published. All authors read and approved the final manuscript.

Author details

[1] National Clinical Research Centre for Respiratory Diseases, Beijing Hospital, Beijing 100730, China. [2] Department of Surgical Intensive Care Medicine, Beijing An Zhen Hospital, Capital Medical University, No. 2 Anzhen Rd., Chao-Yang District, Beijing 100029, China. [3] Department of Pulmonary and Critical Care Medicine, China-Japan Friendship Hospital, 2 Yinghua Dongjie, Beijing 100029, China. [4] Department of Pulmonary and Critical Care Medicine, Beijing Hospital, Beijing 100730, China. [5] Key Laboratory of Geriatrics, Beijing Hospital and Beijing Institute of Geriatrics, Ministry of Health, Beijing, China.

Acknowledgements

We would like to thank Dr. Mingxu Shang, Dr. Hangyong He, Dr. Xiao Tang and Dr. Bing Sun, Department of Respiratory and Critical Care Medicine, Beijing Chao-Yang Hospital for their for their excellent technical assistance.

Competing interests

The authors declare that they have no competing interests.

Funding

This work was supported by Grants from National Natural Science Foundation of China (Nos. 81490534, 81490530, 81430001).

References

1. Ware LB, Matthay MA. The acute respiratory distress syndrome. N Engl J Med. 2000;342(18):1334–49.
2. Acute Respiratory Distress Syndrome Network, Brower RG, Matthay MA, Morris A, Schoenfeld D, Thompson BT, Wheeler A. Ventilation with lower tidal volumes as compared with traditional tidal volumes for acute lung injury and the acute respiratory distress syndrome. The acute respiratory distress syndrome network. N Engl J Med. 2000;342(18):1301–8.
3. Wiedemann HP, Wheeler AP, Bernard GR, Thompson BT, Hayden D, deBoisblanc B, et al. Comparison of two fluid-management strategies in acute lung injury. N Engl J Med. 2006;354(24):2564–75.
4. Villar J, Blanco J, Kacmarek RM. Current incidence and outcome of the acute respiratory distress syndrome. Curr Opin Crit Care. 2016;22(1):1–6.
5. Walter JM, Wilson J, Ware LB. Biomarkers in acute respiratory distress syndrome: from pathobiology to improving patient care. Expert Rev Respir Med. 2014;8(5):573–86.
6. Pierrakos C, Karanikolas M, Scolletta S, Karamouzos V, Velissaris D. Acute respiratory distress syndrome: pathophysiology and therapeutic options. J Clin Med Res. 2012;4(1):7–16.
7. Panagiotou A, Gaiao S, Cruz DN. Extracorporeal therapies in sepsis. J Intensive Care Med. 2013;28(5):281–95.
8. Su X, Bai C, Hong Q, Zhu D, He L, Wu J, et al. Effect of continuous hemofiltration on hemodynamics, lung inflammation and pulmonary edema in a canine model of acute lung injury. Intensive Care Med. 2003;29(11):2034–42.
9. Ullrich R, Roeder G, Lorber C, Quezado ZM, Kneifel W, Gasser H, et al. Continuous venovenous hemofiltration improves arterial oxygenation in endotoxin-induced lung injury in pigs. Anesthesiology. 2001;95(2):428–36.

10. Huang Z, Wang SR, Su W, Liu JY. Removal of humoral mediators and the effect on the survival of septic patients by hemoperfusion with neutral microporous resin column. Ther Apher Dial. 2010;14(6):596–602.
11. Kushi H, Miki T, Okamaoto K, Nakahara J, Saito T, Tanjoh K. Early hemoperfusion with an immobilized polymyxin B fiber column eliminates humoral mediators and improves pulmonary oxygenation. Crit Care. 2005;9(6):R653–61.
12. Treml B, Neu N, Kleinsasser A, Gritsch C, Finsterwalder T, Geiger R, et al. Recombinant angiotensin-converting enzyme 2 improves pulmonary blood flow and oxygenation in lipopolysaccharide-induced lung injury in piglets. Crit Care Med. 2010;38(2):596–601.
13. Nieman GF, Gatto LA, Paskanik AM, Yang B, Fluck R, Picone A. Surfactant replacement in the treatment of sepsis-induced adult respiratory distress syndrome in pigs. Crit Care Med. 1996;24(6):1025–33.
14. Matute-Bello G, Downey G, Moore BB, Groshong SD, Matthay MA, Slutsky AS, et al. An official American Thoracic Society workshop report: features and measurements of experimental acute lung injury in animals. Am J Respir Cell Mol Biol. 2011;44(5):725–38.
15. Conesa A, Gotz S, Garcia-Gomez JM, Terol J, Talon M, Robles M. Blast2GO: a universal tool for annotation, visualization and analysis in functional genomics research. Bioinformatics. 2005;21(18):3674–6.
16. Kanehisa M, Goto S. KEGG: kyoto encyclopedia of genes and genomes. Nucleic Acids Res. 2000;28(1):27–30.
17. Ballard-Croft C, Wang D, Sumpter LR, Zhou X, Zwischenberger JB. Large-animal models of acute respiratory distress syndrome. Ann Thorac Surg. 2012;93(4):1331–9.
18. Mutz C, Mirakaj V, Vagts DA, Westermann P, Waibler K, Konig K, et al. The neuronal guidance protein netrin-1 reduces alveolar inflammation in a porcine model of acute lung injury. Crit Care. 2010;14(5):R189.
19. Matute-Bello G, Frevert CW, Martin TR. Animal models of acute lung injury. Am J Physiol Lung Cell Mol Physiol. 2008;295(3):L379–99.
20. Albertini M, Clement MG, Lafortuna CL, Caniatti M, Magder S, Abdulmalek K, et al. Role of poly-(ADP-ribose) synthetase in lipopolysaccharide-induced vascular failure and acute lung injury in pigs. J Crit Care. 2000;15(2):73–83.
21. Guo ZL, Lu GP, Ren T, Zheng YH, Gong JY, Yu J, et al. Partial liquid ventilation confers protection against acute lung injury induced by endotoxin in juvenile piglets. Respir Physiol Neurobiol. 2009;167(3):221–6.
22. McVerry BJ, Peng X, Hassoun PM, Sammani S, Simon BA, Garcia JG. Sphingosine 1-phosphate reduces vascular leak in murine and canine models of acute lung injury. Am J Respir Crit Care Med. 2004;170(9):987–93.
23. Jozwiak M, Teboul JL, Monnet X. Extravascular lung water in critical care: recent advances and clinical applications. Ann Intensive Care. 2015;5(1):38.
24. Kushimoto S, Taira Y, Kitazawa Y, Okuchi K, Sakamoto T, Ishikura H, et al. The clinical usefulness of extravascular lung water and pulmonary vascular permeability index to diagnose and characterize pulmonary edema: a prospective multicenter study on the quantitative differential diagnostic definition for acute lung injury/acute respiratory distress syndrome. Crit Care. 2012;16(6):R232.
25. Cruz DN, Antonelli M, Fumagalli R, Foltran F, Brienza N, Donati A, et al. Early use of polymyxin B hemoperfusion in abdominal septic shock: the EUPHAS randomized controlled trial. JAMA. 2009;301(23):2445–52.
26. Rimmele T, Kellum JA. Clinical review: blood purification for sepsis. Crit Care. 2011;15(1):205.
27. Mikacenic C, Hansen EE, Radella F, Gharib SA, Stapleton RD, Wurfel MM. Interleukin-17A is associated with alveolar inflammation and poor outcomes in acute respiratory distress syndrome. Crit Care Med. 2016;44(3):496–502.
28. Huang Z, Wang SR, Yang ZL, Liu JY. Effect on extrapulmonary sepsis-induced acute lung injury by hemoperfusion with neutral microporous resin column. Ther Apher Dial. 2013;17(4):454–61.
29. Palomo J, Dietrich D, Martin P, Palmer G, Gabay C. The interleukin (IL)-1 cytokine family—balance between agonists and antagonists in inflammatory diseases. Cytokine. 2015;76(1):25–37.
30. Parsons PE, Moss M, Vannice JL, Moore EE, Moore FA, Repine JE. Circulating IL-1ra and IL-10 levels are increased but do not predict the development of acute respiratory distress syndrome in at-risk patients. Am J Respir Crit Care Med. 1997;155(4):1469–73.
31. Rogy MA, Coyle SM, Oldenburg HS, Rock CS, Barie PS, Van Zee KJ, et al. Persistently elevated soluble tumor necrosis factor receptor and interleukin-1 receptor antagonist levels in critically ill patients. J Am Coll Surg. 1994;178(2):132–8.
32. Tisoncik JR, Korth MJ, Simmons CP, Farrar J, Martin TR, Katze MG. Into the eye of the cytokine storm. Microbiol Mol Biol Rev. 2012;76(1):16–32.
33. Gonzalez-Ramon N, Hoebe K, Alava MA, Van Leengoed L, Pineiro M, Carmona S, et al. Pig MAP/ITIH4 and haptoglobin are interleukin-6-dependent acute-phase plasma proteins in porcine primary cultured hepatocytes. Eur J Biochem. 2000;267(6):1878–85.
34. Rydlova M, Holubec L Jr, Ludvikova M Jr, Kalfert D, Franekova J, Povysil C, et al. Biological activity and clinical implications of the matrix metalloproteinases. Anticancer Res. 2008;28(2B):1389–97.
35. Davey A, McAuley DF, O'Kane CM. Matrix metalloproteinases in acute lung injury: mediators of injury and drivers of repair. Eur Respir J. 2011;38(4):959–70.
36. Brinkmann V, Reichard U, Goosmann C, Fauler B, Uhlemann Y, Weiss DS, et al. Neutrophil extracellular traps kill bacteria. Science. 2004;303(5663):1532–5.
37. Abrams ST, Zhang N, Manson J, Liu T, Dart C, Baluwa F, et al. Circulating histones are mediators of trauma-associated lung injury. Am J Respir Crit Care Med. 2013;187(2):160–9.
38. Bosmann M, Grailer JJ, Ruemmler R, Russkamp NF, Zetoune FS, Sarma JV, et al. Extracellular histones are essential effectors of C5aR- and C5L2-mediated tissue damage and inflammation in acute lung injury. FASEB J. 2013;27(12):5010–21.
39. Bhargava M, Wendt CH. Biomarkers in acute lung injury. Transl Res. 2012;159(4):205–17.

13

Clinical features and outcome of patients with acute respiratory failure revealing anti-synthetase or anti-MDA-5 dermato-pulmonary syndrome: a French multicenter retrospective study

Constance Vuillard[1], Marc Pineton de Chambrun[2], Nicolas de Prost[3], Claude Guérin[4,5], Matthieu Schmidt[2], Auguste Dargent[6], Jean-Pierre Quenot[6], Sébastien Préau[7], Geoffrey Ledoux[7], Mathilde Neuville[8], Guillaume Voiriot[9], Muriel Fartoukh[9], Rémi Coudroy[10], Guillaume Dumas[11], Eric Maury[11], Nicolas Terzi[12], Yacine Tandjaoui-Lambiotte[13], Francis Schneider[14], Maximilien Grall[15], Emmanuel Guérot[16], Romaric Larcher[17], Sylvie Ricome[18], Raphaël Le Mao[19], Gwenhaël Colin[20], Christophe Guitton[21], Lara Zafrani[22], Elise Morawiec[23], Marie Dubert[24], Olivier Pajot[1], Hervé Mentec[1], Gaëtan Plantefève[1] and Damien Contou[1*]

Abstract

Background: Anti-synthetase (AS) and dermato-pulmonary associated with anti-MDA-5 antibodies (aMDA-5) syndromes are near one of the other autoimmune inflammatory myopathies potentially responsible for severe acute interstitial lung disease. We undertook a 13-year retrospective multicenter study in 35 French ICUs in order to describe the clinical presentation and the outcome of patients admitted to the ICU for acute respiratory failure (ARF) revealing AS or aMDA-5 syndromes.

Results: From 2005 to 2017, 47 patients (23 males; median age 60 [1st–3rd quartiles 52–69] years, no comorbidity 85%) were admitted to the ICU for ARF revealing AS ($n=28$, 60%) or aMDA-5 ($n=19$, 40%) syndromes. Muscular, articular and cutaneous manifestations occurred in 11 patients (23%), 14 (30%) and 20 (43%) patients, respectively. Seventeen of them (36%) had no extra-pulmonary manifestations. C-reactive protein was increased (139 [40–208] mg/L), whereas procalcitonine was not (0.30 [0.12–0.56] ng/mL). Proportion of patients with creatine kinase $\geq 2N$ was 20% ($n=9/47$). Forty-two patients (89%) had ARDS, which was severe in 86%, with a rate of 17% ($n=8/47$) of extra-corporeal membrane oxygenation requirement. Proportion of patients who received corticosteroids, cyclophosphamide, rituximab, intravenous immunoglobulins and plasma exchange were 100%, 72%, 15%, 21% and 17%, respectively. ICU and hospital mortality rates were 45% ($n=21/47$) and 51% ($n=24/47$), respectively. Patients with aMDA-5 dermato-pulmonary syndrome had a higher hospital mortality than those with AS syndrome ($n=16/19$, 84% vs. $n=8/28$, 29%; $p=0.001$).

Conclusions: Intensivists should consider inflammatory myopathies as a cause of ARF of unknown origin. Extra-pulmonary manifestations are commonly lacking. Mortality is high, especially in aMDA-5 dermato-pulmonary syndrome.

Keywords: Inflammatory myositis, Interstitial lung disease, ARDS, Acute respiratory failure, Diagnosis

*Correspondence: damien.contou@ch-argenteuil.fr
[1] Service de Réanimation Polyvalente, Centre Hospitalier Victor Dupouy, 69 rue du Lieutenant Colonel Prudhon, 95100 Argenteuil, France
Full list of author information is available at the end of the article

Background

Identifying the cause of acute respiratory distress syndrome (ARDS) is a crucial step for initiating a targeted treatment and improving prognosis [1, 2]. However, two recent studies [3, 4] showed that 8% of patients with ARDS according to the Berlin criteria [5] lacked exposure to "common" risk factors (e.g., pneumonia, acute pancreatitis, aspiration of gastric content or extra-pulmonary sepsis) with no etiology eventually retrieved in 80% of them [4]. For such atypical ARDS, a comprehensive diagnostic work-up, including specific immunologic tests, is recommended [6] so that to identify immune causes, typically amenable to specific therapeutic interventions (e.g., corticosteroids). Yet, an ancillary analysis [4] of an international, multicenter, prospective cohort study [7] reported that such immunological examinations were performed in only 5% of ARDS without common risk factors.

Anti-synthetase (AS) and anti-melanoma differentiation-associated gene 5 (aMDA-5) syndromes are near one of the other autoimmune inflammatory myopathies [8] potentially responsible for rapidly progressive interstitial lung disease leading to acute respiratory failure and ARDS [9–12]. AS and aMDA-5 dermato-pulmonary syndromes may be clinically indistinguishable one from another, with almost three-quarter of patients with aMDA-5 dermato-pulmonary syndrome exhibiting the clinical attributes of the AS syndrome [8]. When ARF is the initial presentation of AS or aMDA-5 syndromes [9–11, 13–17] or when extra-respiratory manifestations, such as muscular, cutaneous or articular signs are lacking [9, 18–22], the diagnosis is challenging, especially in the intensive care unit (ICU) setting, where many other reasons of acute respiratory failure (ARF) can be discussed. To the best of knowledge, a number of case reports of ARF revealing autoimmune inflammatory myopathies have been previously reported, but an extended case series has not been published as yet.

Therefore, we undertook this retrospective study in order to: (1) describe the clinical features and the outcome of patients admitted to the ICU for ARF revealing either an AS or an aMDA-5 dermato-pulmonary syndrome, and; (2) identify predictive factors of hospital mortality.

Patients and methods

Patients

We conducted a 13-year multicenter retrospective non-interventional study in 35 ICUs in France from January 1, 2005, to December 31, 2017. All patients older than 18 years were included if they met the following criteria: (1) admitted to the ICU for ARF not related to cardiogenic pulmonary edema; (2) no common ARDS risk factor, among pneumonia, acute pancreatitis, aspiration of gastric content, extra-pulmonary sepsis, multiple transfusions, major trauma, pulmonary vasculitis, drowning, severe burns, identified according to the Berlin definition [5]; (3) immunologic test performed during ICU stay, which was positive for anti-synthetase (Jo-1, PL7, PL12, OJ, EJ, KS, Zo, YRS/Tyr/Ha) or anti-MDA-5 autoantibodies; and (4) no alternative diagnosis for ARF. It is worth notifying that in the present study the diagnosis of AS or aMDA-5 dermato-pulmonary syndromes had to be made during the ICU stay. Therefore, those who had a diagnosis of AS or aMDA-5 made before ICU admission were not included.

The investigator of each participating center was responsible for the identification of the patients, either from the hospital medical reports, using the function "research the files in which the key words *MDA-5* or *anti-synthetase* or *myositis* occurs" of Microsoft Windows®, or through a search using the International *Classification of Diseases* (10th Revision) following codes: M608 (autoimmune myositis), M609 (myositis), M332 (polymyositis) and M331 (dermatomyositis). The clinical charts of all identified patients were anonymized before sending to the main investigators (DC and CV). Clinical charts were reviewed in order to check the inclusion criteria.

Data collection

The following data were collected on a standardized anonymized case record form: demographic characteristics (age, gender), severity scores upon ICU admission (Sequential Organ Failure Assessment [23] and Simplified Acute Physiology Score II [24]), main comorbidities, delay between first respiratory sign and ICU admission, clinical examination (respiratory and extra-respiratory manifestations) and laboratory findings at the time of ICU admission (blood leukocytes and platelets counts, serum procalcitonine, C-reactive protein, creatine kinase and creatinine levels, PaO_2/FiO_2 with FiO_2 calculated according to the following formula [25, 26]: $FiO_2 = $ oxygen flow in liter per minute $\times 0.04 + 0.21$ when standard oxygen was used), radiological findings on chest X-ray and CT scan, cytological and bacteriological analyses of broncho-alveolar lavage (BAL) fluid, type of positive autoantibodies (Jo-1, PL7, PL12, OJ, EJ, KS, Zo, YRS/Tyr/Ha or aMDA-5), immunosuppressive treatments received (corticosteroids, cyclophosphamide, rituximab, basiliximab, tacrolimus, cyclosporine, methotrexate, intravenous immunoglobulins or plasma exchange), organ supports in the ICU (invasive mechanical ventilation, extra-corporeal membrane oxygenation (ECMO), renal replacement therapy, vasopressors), ICU and hospital length of stay, ICU and hospital mortality.

Written reports of chest CT scan performed at the time of ICU admission were sent to the main investigators (DC and CV) in order to individualize elementary lesions (ground-glass attenuation, alveolar consolidation, septal thickening, pleural effusion, pneumothorax, pneumomediastinum and mediastinal lymphadenopathy) and their location (lower or upper lobe predominance). Signs of lung fibrosis (honeycombing, traction bronchiectasis and reticulations) were also collected. Cytological analyses of BAL fluid collected at the time of ICU admission were reported, as well as results of open lung, skin or muscle biopsies, if performed.

Statistical analysis

Continuous variables are reported as median [1st–3rd quartiles] and compared by the Mann–Whitney *U* test. Categorical variables are reported as counts and percentage points in groups and compared by using the Fisher's exact test. Survival curves of patients with aMDA-5 and AS syndromes were drawn using the Kaplan–Meier method and compared using the log-rank test. All tests were two-sided, with $p < 0.05$ indicating statistical significance. The statistical analysis was performed by using the RStudio software version 0.99.441 (www.rStudio.com).

Results

Study population and clinical manifestations

From January 1, 2005, to December 31, 2017, 47 patients fulfilled the inclusion criteria, including 28 (60%) with AS syndrome (Jo-1 $n = 13/28$ (47%); PL7 $n = 9/28$ (32%); PL12 $n = 4/28$ (14%); EJ $n = 2/28$ (7%)) and 19 (40%) with aMDA-5 dermato-pulmonary syndrome. All the patients with aMDA-5 dermato-pulmonary syndrome were admitted after January 1, 2010. Demographical characteristics, main comorbidities and clinical manifestations are given in Table 1. Most of the patients had no comorbidity ($n = 40/47$, 85%). Median SAPSII and SOFA scores at the time of ICU admission were 35 [27–53] and 5 [3–8], respectively. The median delay between first respiratory sign and ICU admission was 21 [10–41] days. Most of the patients had central temperature > 38 °C ($n = 27/47$, 57%). Myalgia, arthralgia/arthritis and cutaneous manifestations occurred in 23% ($n = 11/47$), 30% ($n = 14/47$) and 43% ($n = 20/47$) of patients, respectively. About one-third of patients ($n = 17/47$, 36%) had no extra-pulmonary manifestation, in a similar proportion in aMDA-5 and AS groups.

Laboratory and radiological findings

Biological data at the time of ICU admission and radiological findings are reported in Table 2. C-reactive protein levels ($N < 5$ mg/L) were increased (139 [40–208] mg/L), while procalcitonine levels ($N < 0.5$ ng/mL) were not (0.30 [0.12–0.56] ng/mL). The rate of patients having creatine kinase plasma levels greater than 2 times the upper limit of normal laboratory range was 20% ($n = 9/47$) in the whole population, and only 31% ($n = 8/28$) in the AS group. The median PaO_2/FiO_2 ratio at ICU admission was 123 [83–147] mmHg.

Most patients ($n = 45/47$, 96%) had bilateral condensations on chest X-ray, with a predominantly lower location ($n = 46/47$, 98%) (Table 2). All patients underwent a lung CT scan, which showed ground-glass attenuation in 78% ($n = 37/47$) and alveolar condensation in 75% ($n = 35/47$). Signs of lung fibrosis were observed in 36% ($n = 17/47$), while 38% ($n = 18/47$) had mediastinal lymphadenopathies.

Broncho-alveolar fluid analysis and histological data

BAL fluid analyses were available in 89% ($n = 42/47$) of patients and are summarized in Table 2. The cell count was 250 [140–330] × 10^3/mL, and percentages of lymphocytes, neutrophils and macrophages were 11% [4–30], 38% [13–65] and 40% [20–60], respectively. BAL was performed before antibiotic therapy in only 12/42 (29%) patients and was negative for lung infection in every patient. There was no correlation between BAL findings and elementary lesions observed on chest CT scan. In particular, the proportion of patients with > 40% BAL neutrophils did not differ between patients with or without elementary lesions of lung fibrosis on chest CT scan ($n = 8/19$, 42% vs. $n = 11/19$, 58%, $p = 0.72$). An open lung biopsy was performed in 4 (9%) patients and depicted findings consistent with organizing pneumonia ($n = 2$), usual interstitial pneumonitis ($n = 1$) and diffuse alveolar damage ($n = 1$) (Table 2). A total of 13 patients (28%) had a muscle ($n = 7$) or a skin ($n = 6$) biopsy performed during the ICU stay. All muscle biopsies revealed findings consistent with an inflammatory myositis, while skin biopsies were either normal ($n = 1$) or revealed findings consistent with lichenoid dermatitis ($n = 3$) or with dermatomyositis ($n = 2$) (Table 2).

ICU management and outcome

Most patients ($n = 41/47$, 89%) received an antimicrobial therapy upon ICU admission (Table 3). All patients received steroids, after a median delay of 6 [3–12] days following the ICU admission. Other immunosuppressive treatments administered are reported in Table 3.

Table 1 Demographical and clinical manifestations of patients with acute respiratory failure revealing anti-synthetase syndrome or dermato-pulmonary syndrome associated with anti-MDA-5 antibodies

	Missing data	All patients $N=47$	aMDA-5 ARF $N=19$	AS ARF $N=28$	p
Age, years median [IQR]	0	60 [52–69]	60 [51–67]	63 [54–73]	0.51
Male, *n* (%)	0	23 (49)	8 (42)	15 (54)	0.64
SOFA score median [IQR]	0	5 [3–8]	4 [2–8]	5 [3–8]	0.77
SAPSII median [IQR]	0	35 [27–53]	34 [27–53]	38 [27–50]	0.94
Comorbidities, *n* (%)					
Chronic respiratory failure	0	1 (2)	0 (0)	1 (4)	1.00
Congestive heart failure	0	0 (0)	0 (0)	0 (0)	1.00
Cirrhosis	0	1 (2)	0 (0)	1 (4)	1.00
Chronic kidney failure	0	0 (0)	0 (0)	0 (0)	1.00
Active solid cancer or malignant hemopathy	0	0 (0)	0 (0)	0 (0)	1.00
HIV	0	0 (0)	0 (0)	0 (0)	1.00
Diabetes mellitus	0	5 (11)	1 (5)	4 (14)	0.64
Obesity (body mass index ≥ 30 kg/m^2)	0	1 (2)	0 (0)	1 (4)	1.00
No comorbidities	0	40 (85)	18 (95)	22 (79)	0.60
Active or former tobacco use, *n* (%)	0	20 (43)	7 (37)	13 (46)	0.73
Respiratory manifestations, *n* (%)					
Delay first respiratory sign—ICU admission, days	2	21 [10–41]	21 [11–43]	21 [10–41]	0.73
Dry cough	0	23 (49)	8 (42)	15 (54)	0.64
Chest pain	0	0 (0)	0 (0)	0 (0)	1.00
Hemoptysis	0	1 (2)	0 (0)	1 (4)	1.00
Bilateral crackles	5	34 (81)	13 (77)	21 (84)	0.69
Fever (> 38 °C)	0	27 (57)	9 (47)	18 (64)	0.40
Extra-respiratory manifestations, *n* (%)					
Myalgia	0	11 (23)	2 (11)	9 (32)	0.16
Muscles weakness	0	6 (13)	1 (5)	5 (18)	0.38
Arthralgia/arthritis	0	14 (30)	6 (32)	8 (29)	1.00
Cutaneous manifestations	0	20 (43)	13 (68)	7 (25)	0.008
Mechanic's hand	0	8 (17)	3 (15)	5 (19)	1.00
Raynaud's phenomenon	0	3 (6)	1 (5)	2 (7)	1.00
Facial erythema	0	12 (26)	9 (47)	3 (11)	0.007
Gottron's papules	0	5 (11)	5 (26)	0 (0)	0.008
Ulcerations	0	3 (6)	3 (16)	0 (0)	0.06
Trunk rash	0	7 (15)	5 (26)	2 (7)	0.10
No extra-respiratory manifestations	0	17 (36)	6 (31)	11 (39)	0.81

aMDA-5 anti-MDA-5 antibodies, *AS* anti-synthetase, *ARF* acute respiratory failure, *HIV* human immunodeficiency virus, *ICU* intensive care unit, *IQR* inter-quartile range, *SAPS2* simplified acute physiology score, *SOFA* sepsis-related organ failure assessment

Almost all patients ($n=42/47$, 89%) had ARDS, categorized as severe ($PaO_2/FiO_2 \leq 100$ mmHg with PEEP ≥ 5 mmH_2O) in 86% ($n=36/47$), with 17% ($n=8/47$) of them requiring ECMO. ICU and hospital mortality rates were 45% ($n=21/47$) and 51% ($n=24/47$), respectively. Patients with aMDA-5 dermato-pulmonary syndrome had a higher ICU mortality than those with AS syndrome ($n=16/19$, 84% vs. $n=5/28$, 18%; $p<0.001$). Among the 26 ICU survivors, 5 (19%) were diagnosed with a cancer (colorectal $n=3$, pharyngeal $n=1$, melanoma $n=1$) during the 279 [158–500] days post-ICU stay follow-up.

Comparison between hospital survivors and non-survivors

Compared to patients who survived at the hospital discharge, those who died were more likely to have an aMDA-5 autoantibody ($n=16/24$, 67% vs. $n=3/23$, 13%; $p=0.001$), had a higher rate of ground-glass attenuation

Table 2 Biological, radiological and cytological findings in patients with acute respiratory failure revealing anti-synthetase syndrome or dermato-pulmonary syndrome associated with anti-MDA-5 antibodies

	Missing data	All patients $N=47$	aMDA-5 ARF $N=19$	AS ARF $N=28$	p
Biological data at ICU admission, median [IQR]					
Leukocytes count ($10^3/mm^3$)	1	11.5 [8.5–17]	8.4 [6.7–9.8]	16.0 [12.1–21.1]	< 0.001
C-reactive protein (mg/L)	9	139 [40–208]	38 [22–99]	187 [128–262]	0.30
Procalcitonine (ng/mL)	9	0.30 [0.12–0.56]	0.32 [0.11–0.48]	0.30 [0.13–1.42]	< 0.001
Creatininemia (µmol/L)	14	63 [51–78]	59 [51–73]	64 [51–80]	0.04
Creatine kinase (UI/L)	3	157 [69–256]	127 [75–186]	192 [69–932]	0.76
Creatine kinase $\geq 2N$	3	9 (20)	1 (6)	8 (31)	0.02
$PaCO_2$ (mmHg)	1	34 [31–41]	34 [32–42]	33 [31–41]	0.06
PaO_2/FiO_2 (mmHg)	3	123 [83–147]	139 [91–174]	117 [78–144]	0.82
Chest X-ray, *n* (%)					
Bilateral opacities	0	45 (96)	19 (100)	26 (93)	0.51
Lower lobe location	0	46 (98)	19 (100)	27 (96)	1.00
Number of quadrants on chest X-ray, *n*					
1	0	1 (3)	0 (0)	1 (4)	0.30
2		27 (68)	10 (59)	17 (74)	
4		12 (30)	7 (41)	5 (22)	
Chest CT scan, *n* (%)					
Performed	0	47 (100)	19 (100)	28 (100)	1.00
Ground-glass attenuation	0	37 (78)	18 (96)	19 (68)	0.03
Alveolar consolidations	0	35 (75)	13 (68)	22 (79)	0.51
Septal thickening	0	12 (26)	8 (42)	4 (14)	0.05
Pleural effusion	0	13 (28)	3 (16)	10 (36)	0.24
Pneumothorax	0	4 (9)	3 (16)	1 (3.6)	0.29
Pneumomediastinum	0	1 (2)	1 (5)	0 (0)	0.40
Mediastinal lymphadenopathy	0	18 (38)	7 (37)	11 (39)	1.00
Signs of lung fibrosis	0	17 (36)	6 (32)	11 (39)	0.82
Traction bronchiectasis	0	17 (36)	6 (32)	11 (39)	0.82
Reticulations	0	12 (26)	4 (21)	8 (29)	0.78
Honeycombing	0	5 (10)	1 (5)	4 (14)	0.64
Broncho-alveolar lavage (BAL), *n* (%) or median [IQR]					
Performed	0	42 (89)	16 (84)	26 (93)	0.38
Delay ICU admission—BAL	0	1 [0–3]	0 [− 1.5–1.0]	2 [1–4]	0.08
Total cell count (10^3/mL)	8	250 [140–330]	250 [128–390]	250 [160–290]	0.42
Lymphocytes (%)	1	11 [4–30]	22 [8–34]	5 [3–17]	0.06
Neutrophils (%)	2	38 [13–65]	15 [6–36]	51 [20–80]	0.001
Macrophages (%)	2	40 [20–60]	53 [39–73]	29 [15–83]	0.009
Eosinophils (%)	6	0 [0–2]	0 [0–1]	0 [0–2]	0.154
Presence of siderophages	5	2 (4)	1 (6)	1 (4)	1.00
Lung biopsy, *n* (%)	0	4 (9)	1 (5)	3 (11)	–
Diffuse alveolar damage		1	0	1	
Usual interstitial pneumonitis		1	0	1	
Organizing pneumonia		2	1	1	
Skin biopsy, *n* (%)	0	6 (13)	5 (26)	1 (4)	–
Normal		1	0	1	
Lichenoïd dermatitis		3	3	0	
Dermatomyositis		2	2	0	
Muscle biopsy, *n* (%)	0	7 (15)	4 (21)	3 (11)	–
Inflammatory myositis		7	4	3	

aMDA-5 anti-MDA-5 antibodies, *AS* anti-synthetase, *ARF* acute respiratory failure, *BAL* broncho-alveolar lavage, *ICU* intensive care unit, *IQR* inter-quartile range

Table 3 ICU management and outcome of patient with acute respiratory failure revealing anti-synthetase syndrome or dermato-pulmonary syndrome associated with anti-MDA-5 antibodies

	Missing data	All patients $N=47$	aMDA-5 ARF $N=19$	AS ARF $N=28$	p
Treatment, n (%) or median [IQR]					
Antibiotics therapy at ICU admission	0	41 (89)	15 (79)	26 (96)	0.14
Immunosuppressive treatment	0	47 (100)	19 (100)	28 (100)	1.00
Delay ICU-IS treatment (days)	0	6 [3–12]	4 [1.5–11]	6 [4–16]	0.25
Corticosteroids pulses	0	47 (100)	19 (100)	28 (100)	1.00
Cyclophosphamide	0	34 (72)	16 (84)	18 (64)	0.24
Rituximab	0	7 (15)	6 (32)	1 (4)	0.01
Cyclosporine	0	2 (4)	2 (10)	0 (0)	0.16
Tacrolimus	0	2 (4)	2 (11)	0 (0)	0.16
Basiliximab	0	2 (4)	2 (11)	0 (0)	0.16
Intravenous immunoglobulins	0	10 (21)	5 (26)	5 (18)	0.50
Plasma exchange	0	8 (17)	7 (37)	1 (4)	0.005
Number of immunosuppressive treatments	0	2 [2, 3]	3 [2–4]	2 [1, 2]	< 0.001
Ventilatory support, n (%)					
Noninvasive ventilation before intubation	0	14 (30)	4 (21)	10 (36)	0.45
High-flow nasal cannula oxygen before intubation	0	21 (45)	11 (58)	10 (36)	0.23
Tracheal intubation	0	43 (92)	18 (95)	25 (89)	0.64
ARDS	0	42 (89)	18 (95)	24 (86)	0.64
Mild ($200 < PaO_2/FiO_2 \leq 300$ mmHg)	0	1 (2)	1 (6)	0 (0)	0.43
Moderate ($100 < PaO_2/FiO_2 \leq 200$ mmHg)	0	5 (12)	0 (0)	5 (21)	0.06
Severe ($PaO_2/FiO_2 \leq 100$ mmHg)	0	36 (86)	17 (94)	19 (79)	0.21
Nitric oxide inhalation	0	23 (50)	14 (74)	9 (33)	0.02
Neuromuscular blocking agents	0	36 (78)	17 (90)	19 (70)	0.16
Prone position	0	26 (57)	12 (63)	14 (52)	0.64
Veno-venous ECMO	0	8 (17)	6 (32)	2 (7)	0.05
Extra-ventilatory support, n (%)					
Renal replacement therapy	0	8 (17)	4 (21)	4 (14)	0.70
Vasopressors	0	37 (79)	17 (90)	20 (71)	0.17
Outcome, n (%) or median [IQR]					
Duration of invasive mechanical ventilation (days)	0	21 [14–35]	19 [9–26]	23 [17–37]	0.34
Length of ICU stay (days)	0	26 [19–38]	22 [17–36]	28 [21–38]	0.20
Length of hospital stay (days)	0	38 [22–67]	22 [19–44]	44 [33–70]	0.015
ICU mortality	0	21 (45)	16 (84)	5 (18)	< 0.001
Hospital mortality	0	24 (51)	16 (84)	8 (29)	0.001

aMDA-5 anti-MDA-5 antibodies, *AS* anti-synthetase, *ARDS* acute respiratory distress syndrome, *ARF* acute respiratory failure, *ECMO* extra-corporal membrane oxygenation, *ICU* intensive care unit, *IQR* inter-quartile range, *IS* immunosuppressive treatment

($n=22/24$, 92% vs. 15/23, 65%; $p=0.04$) and a lower rate of alveolar condensation ($n=14/24$, 58% vs. 21/23, 91%; $p=0.02$) on chest CT scan, and were given 3 [2, 3] versus 2 [1, 2] different immunosuppressive regimens during the ICU stay ($p=0.002$) (Table 4). After adjustment on syndrome (anti-synthetase or aMDA-5 dermato-pulmonary syndrome), the presence of ground-glass attenuations on chest CT scan was no longer associated with in-hospital mortality ($p=0.24$). The Kaplan–Meier graph showed a lower probability of survival 90 days after ICU admission in patients with aMDA-5 antibody than in patients with AS antibody (Fig. 1; $p<0.0001$ log-rank test).

Discussion

We are herein reporting the first large cohort of patients admitted to ICU for ARF revealing either AS or aMDA-5 dermato-pulmonary syndrome. The main findings are: (1) clinical manifestations may be nonspecific with the

Table 4 Comparison between hospital survivors and non-survivors

	Non-survivors $N=24$	Survivors $N=23$	p
Clinical, biological and immunological characteristics, n (%) or median [IQR]			
Age	65 [59–70]	55 [50–64]	0.062
Male	9 (38)	14 (61)	0.19
SOFA	5 [2–8]	5 [3–8]	0.73
SAPSII	32 [28–53]	41 [27–54]	0.82
Type of autoantibodies			
Anti-MDA-5	16 (67)	3 (13)	0.001
Anti-synthetase antibody	8 (33)	20 (87)	0.001
JO-1	3 (13)	10 (44)	0.04
PL7	3 (13)	6 (26)	0.28
PL12	1 (4)	3 (13)	0.35
EJ	1 (4)	1 (4)	1
Delay first respiratory sign—ICU admission, days	21 [10–43]	20 [10–39]	0.31
Creatine kinase $\geq 2N$	3 (13)	6 (29)	0.27
PaO_2/FiO_2 upon ICU admission	126 [90–149]	117 [82–147]	0.65
Chest X-ray and CT scan, n (%)			
Number of quadrants on chest X-ray			
1	1 (5)	0 (0)	0.74
2	13 (62)	14 (74)	
4	7 (33)	5 (26)	
Ground-glass attenuation on chest CT scan	22 (92)	15 (65)	0.04
Alveolar consolidations on chest CT scan	14 (58)	21 (91)	0.02
Signs of lung fibrosis on chest CT scan	9 (38)	8 (35)	1.00
Broncho-alveolar lavage (BAL), n (%) or median [IQR]			
Total cell count (10^3/mL)	250 [80–370]	260 [189–293]	0.36
Lymphocytes percentage	17 [5–31]	7 [3–18]	0.33
Lymphocytes > 10%	12 (55)	9 (45)	0.76
Lymphocytes > 25%	8 (36)	4 (20)	0.41
Neutrophils percentage	20 [10–52]	49 [18–73]	0.12
Neutrophils > 40%	8 (38)	11 (55)	0.44
Neutrophils > 65%	3 (14)	7 (35)	0.16
Management in ICU, n (%) or median [IQR]			
Immunosuppressive (IS) treatment			
Delay ICU admission—IS treatment	4 [3–12]	6 [3–16]	0.63
Number of IS treatments	3 [2, 3]	2 [1, 2]	0.002
Corticosteroids	24 (100)	23 (100)	1.00
Cyclophosphamide	20 (83)	14 (61)	0.16
Rituximab	6 (25)	1 (4)	0.10
Basiliximab	2 (8)	0 (0)	0.49
Cyclosporine	1 (4)	1 (4)	1.00
Tacrolimus	2 (8)	0 (0)	0.19
Intravenous immunoglobulins	7 (29)	3 (13)	0.29
Plasma exchange	6 (25)	2 (9)	0.25
Tracheal intubation	24 (100)	19 (83)	0.05
ARDS	23 (96)	19 (83)	0.19
Severe ($PaO_2/FiO_2 \leq 100$ mmHg)	22 (96)	14 (74)	0.07
Moderate ($100 < PaO_2/FiO_2 \leq 200$ mmHg)	1 (4)	4 (21)	0.16
Mild ($200 < PaO_2/FiO_2 \leq 300$ mmHg)	0 (0)	1 (5)	0.45
Nitric oxide inhalation	18 (78)	5 (22)	< 0.001
Veno-venous ECMO	6 (25)	2 (9)	0.25

Table 4 (continued)

	Non-survivors N=24	Survivors N=23	p
Vasopressors	21 (88)	16 (70)	0.17
Renal replacement therapy	5 (21)	3 (13)	0.70

ARDS acute respiratory distress syndrome, *CI* confidence interval, *ECMO* extra-corporeal membrane oxygenation, *ICU* intensive care unit, *IQR* inter-quartile range, *IS* immunosuppressive, *OR* odds ratio

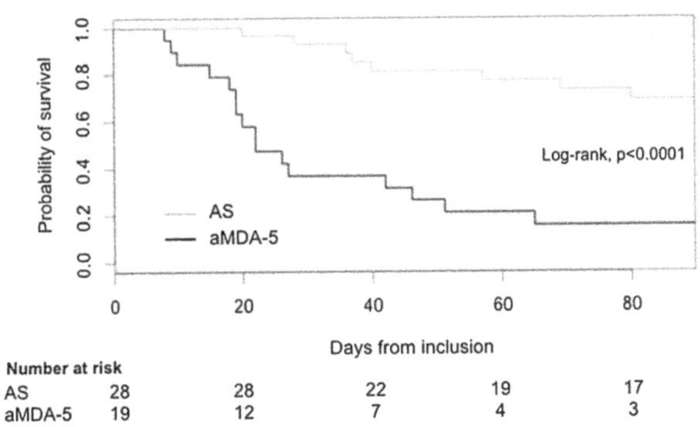

Fig. 1 Kaplan–Meier graph of the probability of survival from ICU admission to day 90 in patients with dermato-pulmonary syndrome associated with anti-MDA-5 antibodies (black curve) and patients with anti-synthetase syndrome (gray curve)

absence of extra-pulmonary manifestations of inflammatory myositis in one-third of patients; (2) hypoxemia is severe with a high rate of severe ARDS and rescue maneuvers; and (3) hospital mortality is high, especially in dermato-pulmonary syndrome associated with aMDA-5 autoantibodies.

AS and aMDA-5-associated dermato-pulmonary syndromes are two near each of the other inflammatory myopathies that may be responsible for severe acute interstitial lung diseases [9–11]. The diagnosis is easy to consider when extra-pulmonary manifestations are present. In AS syndrome, the main extra-pulmonary manifestations include myositis with elevated creatine kinase levels, non-erosive arthritis, Raynaud's phenomenon and thick cracked skin over the tips and sides of the fingers called "mechanic's hands" [27–32]. However, there is a wide heterogeneity in clinical manifestations depending on the causative AS autoantibody [33, 34]. In aMDA-5-associated dermato-pulmonary syndrome, the cutaneous manifestations (skin ulcerations or necrosis, facial erythema, mechanic's hands, periungual telangiectasia, Gottron's papules, Raynaud's phenomenon) are in the forefront [10, 11, 35] and usually contrast with the absence of clinical signs of myositis (clinically "amyopathic myositis"). Demographical and clinical findings in our patients were in line with those recently reported in non-ICU patients with AS [22, 32, 34] or with aMDA-5 dermato-pulmonary syndromes [10].

Both in AS and aMDA-5 dermato-pulmonary syndromes, extra-pulmonary manifestations may be lacking [9, 10] rendering the diagnosis difficult to make. In our series, more than one-third of patients had no extra-pulmonary manifestations with a similar proportion in AS and aMDA-5 patients. This rate contrasts with the 10% rate recently reported [10] in patients with aMDA-5 dermato-pulmonary syndrome, reflecting the lack of training of intensivists for the clinical assessment of these patients and highlighting the need for a multidisciplinary approach. Considering the high proportion of patients lacking extra-pulmonary manifestations, the clinical presentation may mimic that of a "bilateral pneumonia without microbiological documentation." Hence, 89% of our patients received antibiotic therapy at ICU admission. The presence of an intense inflammatory syndrome with increased C-reactive protein levels contrasting with the lack of elevation of serum procalcitonine could help intensivists appreciating the probability of an infectious process, this dissociation being highly suggestive of a non-infectious inflammatory process.

In our series, BAL was performed in 89% of patients. Unlike a recent work [3] showing that a lymphocytic BAL fluid was associated with better ICU survival in ARDS patients with no common risk factor, our study failed to identify any predictive role of BAL cytology on hospital survival. BAL fluid analysis does not seem a useful diagnostic tool for AS or aMDA-5 dermato-pulmonary syndromes, but should nevertheless be performed to rule out an alternative diagnosis, such as diffuse alveolar hemorrhage or active infection.

All included patients underwent chest CT scan. Interestingly, CT chest findings predominate in the lower lobes, which is consistent with a previous report [36]. CT scan signs of lung fibrosis have been recently shown to be associated with a poor outcome in patients with ARF related to interstitial lung diseases [37]. In our study, CT scan signs of lung fibrosis were not associated with hospital mortality, probably because of a lack of adequate power. While ground-glass opacities are usually considered as potentially reversible lung lesions during idiopathic pulmonary fibrosis [38, 39], these lesions were associated with in-hospital mortality in our study, probably because they were more frequently observed during aMDA-5 dermato-pulmonary syndromes. Indeed, this association was no longer observed after adjustment on the type of positive antibody (anti-synthetase or aMDA-5).

Our series underlines the severity of AS and aMDA-5 dermato-pulmonary syndrome, since 89% of patients fulfilled the Berlin criteria for ARDS [5], categorized as severe ($PaO_2/FiO_2 \leq 100$ mmHg with PEEP ≥ 5 mmH_2O) in 86% of cases. Anti-MDA-5 dermato-pulmonary syndromes exhibited a significantly higher mortality than AS syndromes, with almost all these patients dying in the ICU of refractory ARDS despite a high rate of ECMO (32%). Moreover, aMDA-5 patients had a much higher mortality than those with severe ARDS included in the lung safe study [7], highlighting the irreversibility of lung lesions despite immunosuppressive treatments. These results are in line with previous series, showing that refractory ARDS is the leading cause of mortality in aMDA-5 patients [10].

Whether our patients had a true ARDS (i.e., presence of diffuse alveolar damage (DAD), the histological hallmark of ARDS) or simply fulfilled the Berlin criteria while having a non-DAD histology is unknown. In fact, the Berlin definition of ARDS is not fully reliable for diagnosing DAD, and several non-DAD histological entities (such as lung fibrosis, organizing pneumonia, diffuse alveolar hemorrhage or lung tumoral infiltration) have been reported in patients fulfilling the clinical and radiological criteria for ARDS [1, 40–42]. Regarding the onset of lung injury, the Berlin definition of ARDS stipulates that "respiratory signs should occur (or worsen) within 7 days after an exposure to a common ARDS risk factor" (e.g., pneumonia, acute pancreatitis, aspiration of gastric content or extra-pulmonary sepsis). In our patients, the absence of a common risk factor for ARDS according to the Berlin definition together with delay between first respiratory sign and ICU admission exceeding 7 days (21 days) advocate more for an ARDS mimicker rather than for a real ARDS. However, a recent histological study revealed that 50% of patients with an acute decompensation of AS syndrome due to JO-1 autoantibody exhibited histological lesions of DAD [43].

In non-ICU patients, the prognosis of inflammatory myopathies depends on the severity of lung involvement [10, 22, 32, 44]. Treatment of interstitial lung disease associated with AS and aMDA-5 dermato-pulmonary syndromes is not standardized and based on case reports. Numerous immunosuppressive therapies are available (e.g., cyclophosphamide, methotrexate, azathioprine, mycophenolate mofetil, cyclosporine, tacrolimus, rituximab, basiliximab, intravenous immunoglobulins or plasma exchange) [9, 11, 14, 21, 45, 46], but high-dose corticosteroids remain the first-line therapy. Our study underlines the wide variations in the choice of immunosuppressive treatment even if the association corticosteroids–cyclophosphamide was administered in almost 3 over 4 patients. Patients with aMDA-5 received significantly more immunosuppressive drugs highlighting a higher severity.

Of note, 19% of ICU survivors developed cancer, in line with previous series of AS patients [47].

Limitations

Our study suffers from several limitations. First, we included a limited number of patients, inherent to the rarity of the disease. However, this is the first series on ARF revealing AS or aMDA-5 syndromes in an ICU context and our findings are consistent with previous reports. This limited number of patients precluded performing multivariable analyses and thus did not allow for adjusting the observed association between some variables and mortality with potential confounders. Second, the relationship between positive AS or aMDA-5 autoantibody and ARF is not proven. We therefore cannot exclude that some patients had a fortuitously positive autoantibody and that inflammatory myopathy was not the cause of ARF. However, this hypothesis appears unlikely since an alternative diagnosis for ARF had to be excluded, and all patients were treated with immunosuppressive therapies underlining the high degree of clinician's suspicion. Third, because the patients were recruited over a 13-year period in 35 centers, ICU procedures were inevitably heterogeneous. Fourth, the prevalence of aMDA-5 dermato-pulmonary syndromes may have been underestimated during the study period since detection of aMDA-5 autoantibody was first described in 2005 [48] and was therefore routinely available only from 2010 in most of participating centers. Last, several classical predictors of mortality related to ventilation (tidal volume or driving pressure [49]) were not available as a result of a long-term retrospective design.

Clinical implications

Considering the high proportion of patients lacking extra-pulmonary manifestations and the nonspecific presentation mimicking that of a bilateral community-acquired pneumonia, we believe that ARF related to autoimmune inflammatory myopathies may be underdiagnosed. Hence, de Prost et al. recently showed that the diagnostic work-up performed in ARDS patients with no common risk factor was not comprehensive, with only 5% of patients having immunological tests [4]. The lack of screening for AS or aMDA-5 autoantibodies is probably one of the reasons why these diseases are underestimated. Therefore, when the etiology of ARF appears unclear, we recommend a more aggressive diagnostic work-up [6], including immunological tests in order to identify patients amenable to specific therapies.

A careful assessment of extra-pulmonary manifestations, such as cutaneous or articular signs, is crucial. While the presence of extra-pulmonary manifestations is highly suggestive, the 3-week delay between first respiratory signs and ICU admission, the absence of an obvious etiology for ARF, the presence of bi-basal consolidations on chest X-ray with an intense inflammatory process, contrasting with a low procalcitonin level together with the lack of microbiological documentation are the main clues to consider the diagnosis of AS or aMDA-5 syndromes in a patient without extra-pulmonary manifestation. To better assess the relevance of these signs, further prospective studies aiming at systematically screen for autoantibodies in ARDS without risk factors are needed. Once the diagnosis is made, the management is difficult and requires a multidisciplinary approach involving intensivists, pulmonologists, internists and rheumatologists in order to decide the best-individualized therapeutic strategy.

Conclusions

Intensivists should consider inflammatory myopathies, such as anti-synthetase syndrome and dermato-pulmonary syndrome associated with anti-MDA-5 antibodies, as a cause of acute respiratory failure when the etiology appears unclear. Extra-pulmonary manifestations are commonly lacking and an isolated lung involvement may reveal the disease. Hospital mortality is high, especially in aMDA-5 dermato-pulmonary syndrome.

Abbreviations

ARDS: acute respiratory distress syndrome; ARF: acute respiratory failure; AS: anti-synthetase; aMDA-5: anti-MDA-5 autoantibody; BAL: broncho-alveolar lavage; DAD: diffuse alveolar damage; ECMO: extra-corporeal membrane oxygenation; ICU: intensive care unit.

Authors' contributions

DC had full access to all the data in the study and takes responsibility for the integrity of the data and the accuracy of the data analysis. DC made substantial contribution to the study design, data collection and analysis and manuscript writing. CV contributed to data collection and interpretation, and drafting of the manuscript. MPC, NdP, AD, J-PQ, SP, GL, MN, GV, MF, RC, GD, EM, NT, YT-L, FS, MG, EG, RL, SR, RLM, GC, CG, LZ and EM contributed to patients identification in each center, data collection and manuscript writing. MD contributed to the data analysis, statistical analysis and manuscript revision. NdP, CG, OP, HM and GP contributed to the manuscript writing and revision, and provided important intellectual content. All authors read and approved the final manuscript.

Author details

[1] Service de Réanimation Polyvalente, Centre Hospitalier Victor Dupouy, 69 rue du Lieutenant Colonel Prudhon, 95100 Argenteuil, France. [2] Service de Réanimation Médicale, Centre Hospitalier Universitaire Pitié-Salpétrière – Assistance Publique Hôpitaux de Paris, 47-83 boulevard de l'Hôpital, 75013 Paris, France. [3] Service de Réanimation Médicale, Centre Hospitalier Universitaire Henri Mondor – Assistance Publique Hôpitaux de Paris, 51 avenue du Maréchal de Lattre de Tassigny, 94010 Créteil, France. [4] Service de Réanimation Médicale, Hôpital de la Croix-Rousse, 103 Grande rue de la Croix-Rousse, 69004 Lyon, France. [5] INSERM 955, Créteil, France. [6] Service de Médecine Intensive Réanimation, Centre Hospitalier Universitaire François Mitterrand de Dijon, 14 rue Paul Gaffarel, 21000 Dijon, France. [7] Service de Réanimation, Centre Hospitalier Régional Universitaire de Lille, 2 avenue Oscar Lambret, 59000 Lille, France. [8] Service de Réanimation Médicale, Centre Hospitalier Universitaire Bichat Claude-Bernard – Assistance Publique Hôpitaux de Paris, 46 rue Henri Huchard, 75877 Paris, France. [9] Service de Réanimation médico-chirurgicale, Centre Hospitalier Universitaire Tenon – Assistance Publique Hôpitaux de Paris, 5 rue de la Chine, 75020 Paris, France. [10] Service de Réanimation médicale, Centre hospitalier universitaire de Poitiers, 2 rue de la Milétrie, 86021 Poitiers, France. [11] Service de Réanimation médicale, Centre Hospitalier Universitaire Saint-Antoine – Assistance Publique Hôpitaux de Paris, 184 rue du Faubourg Saint-Antoine, 75012 Paris, France. [12] Service de Réanimation, Centre Hospitalier Universitaire de Grenoble Alpes, avenue Maquis du Grésivaudan, 38700 La Tronche, France. [13] Service de Réanimation médico-chirurgicale, Centre Hospitalier Universitaire Avicennes – Assistance Publique Hôpitaux de Paris, 125 rue de Stalingrad, 93000 Bobigny, France. [14] Service de Réanimation, Centre Hospitalier Universitaire de Strasbourg, 1 avenue Molière, 67200 Strasbourg, France. [15] Service de Réanimation Médicale, Centre Hospitalier Universitaire de Rouen, 1 rue de Germont, 76000 Rouen, France. [16] Service de Réanimation Médicale, Centre Hospitalier Universitaire Hôpital Européen Georges-Pompidou – Assistance Publique Hôpitaux de Paris, 20 rue Leblanc, 75015 Paris, France. [17] Service de Réanimation Médicale, Centre Hospitalier Universitaire de Montpellier, 191 avenue du Doyen Gaston Giraud, 34000 Montpellier, France. [18] Service de Réanimation Polyvalente, Centre Hospitalier Robert-Ballanger, Boulevard Robert Ballanger, 93600 Aulnay-sous-Bois, France. [19] Service de Réanimation médicale, Centre Hospitalier Régional Universistaire de Brest, Site La Cavale Blanche, Boulevard Tanguy Prigent, 29200 Brest, France. [20] Service de réanimation médico-chirurgicale, Centre Hospitalier Départemental de Vendée, Les Oudairies, 85925 La Roche sur Yon Cedex 9, France. [21] Service de Réanimation médico-chirurgicale, Centre Hospitalier du Mans, 194 avenue Rubillard, 72037 Le Mans, France. [22] Service de Réanimation médicale, Hôpital Saint-Louis, Assistance Publique Hôpitaux de Paris, 1 avenue Claude Vellefaux, 75010 Paris, France. [23] Unité de Réanimation et de Surveillance continue, Service de Pneumologie et Réanimation médicale, Groupe hospitalier Pitié-Salpêtrière, 47-83 bd de l'hôpital, 75651 Paris, France. [24] Service d'Immunologie Clinique, Hôpital Saint-Louis, Assistance Publique Hôpitaux de Paris, 1 avenue Claude Vellefaux, 75010 Paris, France.

Acknowledgements

We thank Jonathan Messika (Réanimation, Hôpital Louis Mourier, Colombes), Frédéric Pène (Réanimation médicale, Hôpital Cochin, Paris), Morgan Benaïs (Réanimation médico-chirurgicale, Saint Denis), Jérémy Rosman (Réanimation polyvalente, Charleville), David Schnell (Réanimation médico-chirurgicale, Angoulême), Sébastien Jochmans (Réanimation Polyvalente, Melun), Sami Hraiech and Jérémy Bourenne (Réanimations, Marseille), Guillaume Schnell (Réanimation médico-chirurgicale, Le Havre), Damien Du Cheyron (Réanimation médicale, Caen), Aude Gibelin (Réanimation médico-chirurgicale, Hôpital Tenon, Paris), Cédric Bruel (Réanimation Polyvalente, Hôpital Saint-Joseph, Paris), Kamel Toufik (Réanimation médico-chirurgicale, Orléans) and Jérémie Lemarié (Réanimation, Nancy) for having searched for eligible patients.

Competing interests

The authors declare that they have no competing interests.

Funding

This study did not receive funding from external or internal sources.

References

1. Papazian L, Doddoli C, Chetaille B, Gernez Y, Thirion X, Roch A, et al. A contributive result of open-lung biopsy improves survival in acute respiratory distress syndrome patients. Crit Care Med. 2007;35:755–62.

2. Vincent JL, Santacruz C. Do we need ARDS? Intensive Care Med. 2012;42:282–3.
3. Gibelin A, Parrot A, Maitre B, Brun-Buisson C, Mekontso Dessap A, Fartoukh M, et al. Acute respiratory distress syndrome mimickers lacking common risk factors of the Berlin definition. Intensive Care Med. 2015;42:164–72.
4. de Prost N, Pham T, Carteaux G, Mekontso Dessap A, Brun-Buisson C, Fan E, et al. Etiologies, diagnostic work-up and outcomes of acute respiratory distress syndrome with no common risk factor: a prospective multicenter study. Ann Intensive Care. 2017;7:69.
5. Ranieri VM, Rubenfeld GD, Thompson BT, Ferguson ND, Caldwell E, Fan E, et al. Acute respiratory distress syndrome: the Berlin definition. JAMA. 2012;307:2526–33.
6. Papazian L, Calfee CS, Chiumello D, Luyt CE, Meyer NJ, Sekiguchi H, et al. Diagnostic workup for ARDS patients. Intensive Care Med. 2016;42:674–85.
7. Bellani G, Laffey JG, Pham T, Fan E, Brochard L, Esteban A, et al. Epidemiology, patterns of care, and mortality for patients with acute respiratory distress syndrome in intensive care units in 50 countries. JAMA. 2016;315:788–800.
8. Hall JC, Casciola-Rosen L, Samedy LA, Werner J, Owoyemi K, Danoff SK, et al. Anti-melanoma differentiation-associated protein 5-associated dermatomyositis: expanding the clinical spectrum. Arthritis Care Res (Hoboken). 2013;65:1307–15.
9. Tillie-Leblond I, Wislez M, Valeyre D, Crestani B, Rabbat A, Israel-Biet D, et al. Interstitial lung disease and anti-Jo-1 antibodies: difference between acute and gradual onset. Thorax. 2008;63:53–9.
10. Uzunhan Y, Nunes H, Leroux G, Miyara M, Benveniste O, Allenbach Y. Dermato-pulmonary syndrome associated with MDA-5 antibodies. Eur Respir J. 2016;48(suppl 60):2138.
11. Chaisson NF, Paik J, Orbai AM, Casciola-Rosen L, Fiorentino D, Danoff S, et al. A novel dermato-pulmonary syndrome associated with MDA-5 antibodies: report of 2 cases and review of the literature. Medicine (Baltimore). 2012;91:220–8.
12. Grasselli G, Vergnano B, Pozzi MR, Sala V, D'Andrea G, Scaravilli V, et al. Interstitial pneumonia with autoimmune features: an additional risk factor for ARDS? Ann Intensive Care. 2017;7:98.
13. Bizien N, Renault A, Boles JM, Delluc A. Acute interstitial lung disease revealing antisynthetase syndrome. Rev Pneumol Clin. 2011;67:367–70.
14. Guglielmi S, Merz TM, Gugger M, Suter C, Nicod LP. Acute respiratory distress syndrome secondary to antisynthetase syndrome is reversible with tacrolimus. Eur Respir J. 2008;31:213–7.
15. Kim SH, Park IN. Acute respiratory distress syndrome as the initial clinical manifestation of an antisynthetase syndrome. Tuberc Respir Dis (Seoul). 2016;79:188–92.
16. Clawson K, Oddis CV. Adult respiratory distress syndrome in polymyositis patients with the anti-Jo-1 antibody. Arthritis Rheum. 1995;38:1519–23.
17. Piroddi IM, Ferraioli G, Barlascini C, Castagneto C, Nicolini A. Severe respiratory failure as a presenting feature of an interstitial lung disease associated with anti-synthetase syndrome (ASS). Respir Investig. 2016;54:284–8.
18. Friedman AW, Targoff IN, Arnett FC. Interstitial lung disease with autoantibodies against aminoacyl-tRNA synthetases in the absence of clinically apparent myositis. Semin Arthritis Rheum. 1996;26:459–67.
19. Shi J, Li S, Yang H, Zhang Y, Peng Q, Lu X, et al. Clinical profiles and prognosis of patients with distinct antisynthetase autoantibodies. J Rheumatol. 2017;44:1051–7.
20. Kinebuchi S, Mizuno K, Moriyama H, Ooi H, Hasegawa T, Yoshizawa H, et al. Two cases of interstitial pneumonia with anti-Jo-1 antibodies in the absence of myositis. Nihon Kokyuki Gakkai Zasshi. 2003;41:739–45.
21. Sauty A, Rochat T, Schoch OD, Hamacher J, Kurt AM, Dayer JM, et al. Pulmonary fibrosis with predominant CD8 lymphocytic alveolitis and anti-Jo-1 antibodies. Eur Respir J. 1997;10:2907–12.
22. Hervier B, Wallaert B, Hachulla E, Adoue D, Lauque D, Audrain M, et al. Clinical manifestations of anti-synthetase syndrome positive for anti-alanyl-tRNA synthetase (anti-PL12) antibodies: a retrospective study of 17 cases. Rheumatology (Oxford). 2010;49:972–6.
23. Vincent JL, Moreno R, Takala J, Willatts S, De Mendonca A, Bruining H, et al. The SOFA (Sepsis-related Organ Failure Assessment) score to describe organ dysfunction/failure. On behalf of the Working Group on Sepsis-Related Problems of the European Society of Intensive Care Medicine. Intensive Care Med. 1996;22:707–10.
24. Le Gall JR, Lemeshow S, Saulnier F. A new simplified acute physiology score (SAPS II) based on a European/North American multicenter study. JAMA. 1993;270:2957–63.
25. Wettstein RB, Shelledy DC, Peters JI. Delivered oxygen concentrations using low-flow and high-flow nasal cannulas. Respir Care. 2005;50:604–9.
26. Coudroy R, Frat JP, Boissier F, Contou D, Robert R, Thille AW. Early identification of acute respiratory distress disorder in the absence of positive pressure ventilation: implications for revision of the berlin criteria for acute respiratory distress syndrome. Crit Care Med. 2017;46:540–6.
27. Connors GR, Christopher-Stine L, Oddis CV, Danoff SK. Interstitial lung disease associated with the idiopathic inflammatory myopathies: what progress has been made in the past 35 years? Chest. 2010;138:1464–74.
28. Imbert-Masseau A, Hamidou M, Agard C, Grolleau JY, Cherin P. Antisynthetase syndrome. Joint Bone Spine. 2003;70:161–8.
29. Schmidt WA, Wetzel W, Friedlander R, Lange R, Sorensen HF, Lichey HJ, et al. Clinical and serological aspects of patients with anti-Jo-1 antibodies—an evolving spectrum of disease manifestations. Clin Rheumatol. 2000;19:371–7.
30. Hengstman GJ, van Engelen BG, van Venrooij WJ. Myositis specific autoantibodies: changing insights in pathophysiology and clinical associations. Curr Opin Rheumatol. 2004;16:692–9.
31. Marguerie C, Bunn CC, Beynon HL, Bernstein RM, Hughes JM, So AK, et al. Polymyositis, pulmonary fibrosis and autoantibodies to aminoacyl-tRNA synthetase enzymes. Q J Med. 1990;77:1019–38.
32. Marie I, Josse S, Decaux O, Diot E, Landron C, Roblot P, et al. Clinical manifestations and outcome of anti-PL7 positive patients with antisynthetase syndrome. Eur J Intern Med. 2013;24:474–9.
33. Vazquez-Abad D, Rothfield NF. Sensitivity and specificity of anti-Jo-1 antibodies in autoimmune diseases with myositis. Arthritis Rheum. 1996;39:292–6.
34. Marie I, Josse S, Decaux O, Dominique S, Diot E, Landron C, et al. Comparison of long-term outcome between anti-Jo1- and anti-PL7/PL12 positive patients with antisynthetase syndrome. Autoimmun Rev. 2012;11:739–45.
35. Fiorentino D, Chung L, Zwerner J, Rosen A, Casciola-Rosen L. The mucocutaneous and systemic phenotype of dermatomyositis patients with antibodies to MDA5 (CADM-140): a retrospective study. J Am Acad Dermatol. 2010;65:25–34.
36. Zamora AC, Hoskote SS, Abascal-Bolado B, White D, Cox CW, Ryu JH, et al. Clinical features and outcomes of interstitial lung disease in anti-Jo-1 positive antisynthetase syndrome. Respir Med. 2016;118:39–45.
37. Zafrani L, Lemiale V, Lapidus N, Lorillon G, Schlemmer B, Azoulay E. Acute respiratory failure in critically ill patients with interstitial lung disease. PLoS ONE. 2014;9:e104897.
38. Gay SE, Kazerooni EA, Toews GB, Lynch JP 3rd, Gross BH, Cascade PN, et al. Idiopathic pulmonary fibrosis: predicting response to therapy and survival. Am J Respir Crit Care Med. 1998;157:1063–72.
39. Wells AU, Desai SR, Rubens MB, Goh NS, Cramer D, Nicholson AG, et al. Idiopathic pulmonary fibrosis: a composite physiologic index derived from disease extent observed by computed tomography. Am J Respir Crit Care Med. 2003;167:962–9.
40. Thille AW, Esteban A, Fernandez-Segoviano P, Rodriguez JM, Aramburu JA, Penuelas O, et al. Comparison of the Berlin definition for acute respiratory distress syndrome with autopsy. Am J Respir Crit Care Med. 2013;187:761–7.
41. Patel SR, Karmpaliotis D, Ayas NT, Mark EJ, Wain J, Thompson BT, et al. The role of open-lung biopsy in ARDS. Chest. 2004;125:197–202.
42. Gerard L, Bidoul T, Castanares-Zapatero D, Wittebole X, Lacroix V, Froidure A, et al. Open lung biopsy in nonresolving acute respiratory distress syndrome commonly identifies corticosteroid-sensitive pathologies, associated with better outcome. Crit Care Med. 2018;46:907–14.

43. Yousem SA, Gibson K, Kaminski N, Oddis CV, Ascherman DP. The pulmonary histopathologic manifestations of the anti-Jo-1 tRNA synthetase syndrome. Mod Pathol. 2010;23:874–80.
44. Marie I, Hachulla E, Cherin P, Dominique S, Hatron PY, Hellot MF, et al. Interstitial lung disease in polymyositis and dermatomyositis. Arthritis Rheum. 2002;47:614–22.
45. Witt LJ, Curran JJ, Strek ME. The diagnosis and treatment of antisynthetase syndrome. Clin Pulm Med. 2016;23:218–26.
46. Zou J, Li T, Huang X, Chen S, Guo Q, Bao C. Basiliximab may improve the survival rate of rapidly progressive interstitial pneumonia in patients with clinically amyopathic dermatomyositis with anti-MDA5 antibody. Ann Rheum Dis. 2014;73:1591–3.
47. Castaneda-Pomeda M, Prieto-Gonzalez S, Grau JM. Antisynthetase syndrome and malignancy: our experience. J Clin Rheumatol. 2011;17:458.
48. Sato S, Hirakata M, Kuwana M, Suwa A, Inada S, Mimori T, et al. Autoantibodies to a 140-kd polypeptide, CADM-140, in Japanese patients with clinically amyopathic dermatomyositis. Arthritis Rheum. 2005;52:1571–6.
49. Amato MB, Meade MO, Slutsky AS, Brochard L, Costa EL, Schoenfeld DA, et al. Driving pressure and survival in the acute respiratory distress syndrome. N Engl J Med. 2015;372:747–55.

Practical approach to diastolic dysfunction in light of the new guidelines and clinical applications in the operating room and in the intensive care

F. Sanfilippo[1*], S. Scolletta[2], A. Morelli[3] and A. Vieillard-Baron[4]

Abstract

There is growing evidence both in the perioperative period and in the field of intensive care (ICU) on the association between left ventricular diastolic dysfunction (LVDD) and worse outcomes in patients. The recent American Society of Echocardiography and European Association of Cardiovascular Imaging joint recommendations have tried to simplify the diagnosis and the grading of LVDD. However, both an often unknown pre-morbid LV diastolic function and the presence of several confounders—i.e., use of vasopressors, positive pressure ventilation, volume loading—make the proposed parameters difficult to interpret, especially in the ICU. Among the proposed parameters for diagnosis and grading of LVDD, the two tissue Doppler imaging-derived variables *e'* and *E/e'* seem most reliable. However, these are not devoid of limitations. In the present review, we aim at rationalizing the applicability of the recent recommendations to the perioperative and ICU areas, discussing the clinical meaning and echocardiographic findings of different grades of LVDD, describing the impact of LVDD on patients' outcomes and providing some hints on the management of patients with LVDD.

Keywords: Diastolic function, Systolic function, Weaning failure, Sepsis, Critical care

Background

The study of left ventricular (LV) diastolic function and the impact of decreased LV compliance and impaired relaxation has received growing interest. This is certainly due to not only the high incidence of LV diastolic dysfunction (LVDD) in the general population and its sensible impact on patients outcomes [1], but also the growing use of echocardiography, which remains the sole clinical tool allowing the estimation of LV diastolic function. A cross-sectional survey of over 2000 randomly selected Minnesota residents aged 45 years or older found an incidence of LVDD almost five times higher than LV systolic dysfunction (28 vs. 6%, respectively), which was a strong predictor of mortality (hazard ratio ranging from 8.3 for mild LVDD to 10.2 for at-least-moderate LVDD) [1]. Up to 50% of patients presenting to the hospital with pulmonary edema and hypertension have unchanged LV systolic function and normal mitral valve apparatus, when compared during and after the acute episode [2]. Similarly, the incidence of isolated LVDD may be higher than 50% in patients hospitalized for heart failure (HF) [3].

The importance of LVDD is strongly emerging in the perioperative setting [4] and in critically ill patients [5–8], and the present review highlights the knowledge in the field. Moreover, since pharmacological strategies for improving LV diastolic function are limited and are more likely to produce results only in the long term [9], we provide a focused summary of the literature followed by key approaches that may help clinicians in the optimization and management of the patient with LVDD.

*Correspondence: filipposanfi@yahoo.it
[1] Department of Anesthesia and Intensive Care, IRCCS-ISMETT (Istituto Mediterraneo per i Trapianti e Terapie ad alta specializzazione), Palermo, Italy
Full list of author information is available at the end of the article

Main text

Recent guidelines and their applicability in the perioperative and intensive care settings

The most recent American Society of Echocardiography and European Association of Cardiovascular Imaging (ASE/EACVI) joint recommendations for the diagnosis and assessment of LVDD [10] made substantial changes compared with the previous recommendations [11]. One of the main aims of the new guidelines was to simplify the approach of clinicians to grading of LVDD, which in the previous version was deemed too complex because many parameters were included. Such recently revised guidelines have changed the methodology for determining LVDD, recommending an assessment mainly based on the following four variables: tricuspid regurgitation (TR) jet velocity, left atrial (LA) volume, e' wave and E/e' ratio. The e' and E/e' ratio are two parameters derived by tissue Doppler imaging (TDI) analysis, measuring longitudinal fiber lengthening during early diastole at level of mitral valve annulus using a modified pulsed wave Doppler setting (high amplitude, low velocity). The e' maximal velocity reflects LV relaxation rate, while E/e' correlates with the LV filling pressures and a ratio above 13–15 is associated with pulmonary arterial occlusion pressures > 18 mmHg [10]. The cutoffs for the four variables recommended by the guidelines are summarized in Table 1.

In patients with normal LV systolic function, abnormalities of more than half of measurable parameters (i.e., a patient may have no TR) define the presence of LVDD. On the other hand, the new guidelines support that patients with structural abnormalities, known ischemic heart disease or abnormal LV systolic function will have impaired myocardial relaxation, and thus, echocardiography examination may focus on the assessment of LV filling pressures and diastolic dysfunction grade.

Once diagnosis of LVDD is made, the following step is to proceed with grading of the dysfunction itself. The four parameters indicated in Table 1 and the E/A ratio are used to grade LVDD and can be found in the recently published recommendations [10], but LVDD grading is not the aim of the present review, which is not intended for cardiologists or experts in echocardiography. Of note, an interesting retrospective cohort study by Almeida and Colleagues conducted on 1000 individuals aged ≥ 45 years and with normal systolic function found poor concordance between the new and the previous versions of the guidelines (published in 2009) for the evaluation of LV diastolic function [10, 11]. In this study, the new guidelines resulted in a significantly lower incidence of LVDD (1.4 vs. 38.1% of 2009 recommendations) [12].

Unfortunately, assessing LVDD is not always easy and the guidelines' authors themselves state "*...the guidelines are not necessarily applicable to children or in the perioperative setting.*" The fact that applicability of these guidelines to the perioperative setting represents a challenge is not surprising. Indeed, patients undergoing major surgery are mechanically ventilated and exposed to drugs with vasoactive effects, and they easily fluctuate from hyper- to hypovolemia due to perioperative fasting, fluid shift, hemorrhage, etc. Moreover, the use of transthoracic echocardiography (TTE) is limited in the operating room, and the applicability of e' and E/e' ratio with transesophageal echocardiography (TEE) should consider the importance of obtaining a good alignment of TDI signal.

On the other hand, it is somewhat surprising that the authors did not mention the limitations of such new guidelines in the critically ill patients. Same limitations as the ones described in the perioperative setting may be also present. Moreover, in this population of patients, the TR jet velocity may worsen under the negative influence of mechanical ventilation on right ventricular (RV) function and there are a large number of factors that may increase pulmonary pressure at pre-capillary level, making the reliability of TR jet velocity at least questionable. Among these factors, pulmonary vascular resistances may increase with elevated airway pressures, although it should be kept in mind that the transmission of pleural pressure itself is reduced when lung compliance is low (i.e., acute respiratory distress syndrome). Additionally, the effects of mechanical ventilation on LV diastolic function are not negligible, and one study in cardiac surgery patients showed that increasing levels of positive end-expiratory pressure (PEEP) reduced significantly both septal and lateral e' values, possibly representing an impaired LV relaxation due to worse RV function (and possibly RV dilatation) [13]. In other words, the observed LVDD may not be related to the disease itself, but driven by the conditions of mechanical ventilation. One could say that LVDD is associated with a worst prognosis when reflecting a specific injury of the myocardium, while probably this is not the case when LVDD is mainly induced by ventilation settings and clinical management.

With respect to the second parameter listed in Table 1, the LA volume is influenced by loading conditions and critically ill patients are certainly exposed to sudden changes of circulating volume for either absolute or relative hypovolemia (i.e., trauma and/or sepsis). More importantly, patients with sepsis or septic shock are characterized not only by vasoplegia with reduction in LV afterload, but they also show myocardial depression (septic cardiomyopathy) [14]. Furthermore, as clarified in the recent guidelines, LA enlargement is observed when LVDD is chronic and cannot probably be used in more acute situations, as frequently observed in the intensive care unit (ICU). How acutely the LA can dilate during

Table 1 Four main parameters used to define left ventricular diastolic dysfunction and their cutoffs

Parameter	Abnormal value	Mode of measurement	Limitation/confounders
TR jet velocity	> 2.8 m/s	Parasternal and apical 4-ch view with CFD to get highest velocity aligned with CWD. Adjust gain and contrast to display complete spectral envelope (no signal spikes or feathering) Analysis: peak modal velocity during systole at leading edge of spectral waveform	Indirect estimate of LA pressure; adequate recording of full envelope not always possible; in some cases accuracy of calculation is dependent on reliable estimation of right atrial systolic pressure
LA volume	> 34 mL/m^2	Apical 4-ch and 2-ch: acquire freeze frames (1-2 frames before MV opening). LA volume measured in dedicated views (length and transverse diameters maximized) Analysis: method of disks or area-length method; correct for body surface area. Do not include LA appendage or pulmonary veins in tracings	LA dilatation is seen in bradycardia, high-output states, heart transplants, atrial flutter/fibrillation, significant MV disease, despite normal LV diastolic function; LA dilatation occurs in well-trained athletes; suboptimal image quality (i.e., foreshortening) precludes accurate tracings; it can be difficult to quantify in patients with aortic aneurysms or in patients with large inter-atrial septal aneurysms
e′	Septal < 7 cm/s Lateral < 10 cm/s	Apical 4-ch view: PWD sample volume (usually 5–10 mm axial size) at lateral or septal basal regions. Use ultrasound system presets for wall filter and lowest signal gain. Optimal spectral waveforms should be sharp (no signal spikes, feathering or ghosting) Analysis: peak modal velocity in early diastole at the leading edge of spectral waveform	Limited accuracy in patients with CAD and RWMAs, significant MAC, surgical rings or prosthetic MV, pericardial disease; need to sample at least two sites; different cutoffs depending on sampling site; age dependent (decreases with aging)
E/e′ ratio	Average > 14 Septal > 15 Lateral > 13	E wave: apical 4-ch with CFD imaging for optimal alignment of PWD with blood flow. PWD sample volume (1–3 mm axial size) between mitral leaflet tips. Use low wall filter setting (100–200 MHz) and low signal gain. Optimal spectral waveforms should not display spikes or feathering Analysis: peak modal velocity in early diastole at the leading edge of spectral waveform *e′*: see above Analysis: E velocity divided by *e′* velocity	Not accurate in normal subjects, patients with MAC, pericardial disease; "gray zone" of values in which LV filling pressures are indeterminate; accuracy reduced in CAD and RWMAs; different cutoff values depending on the site used for measurement

4-ch, four-chamber; 2-ch, two-chamber; CAD, coronary artery disease; CFD, color flow Doppler; CWD, continuous wave Doppler; LA, left atrium; LV, left ventricle; MAC, mitral annulus calcifications; MV, mitral valve; PWD, pulsed wave Doppler; RWMAs regional wall motion abnormalities; TR, tricuspid regurgitation

the early stages of critical illness is a matter of future research. A recent study evaluated early changes in LA volume after acute myocardial infarction. At 4-month follow-up the authors found that 35% of patients had LA remodeling, defined as LA volume index ≥ 10 ml/m^2. However, at 1-month follow-up there was a mean change of 6 ml/m^2, with no significant differences between patients with or without LA remodeling [15]. Therefore, it seems that changes in LA volume can happen in a relatively short-term but not so acutely as it matters in the case of critically ill patients. Interestingly, another study demonstrated that magnitude and pattern of LA appendage emptying/filling velocities are dependent on loading conditions and that velocities are influenced mainly by changes in LV rather than in LA appendage function [16]. In light of the above, estimation of LA volume as for the prediction of acute changes of LV diastolic function in critically ill patients seems a physiologically imprecise parameter. Moreover, it is important to note that the LA volume is not precisely quantifiable with TEE, which adds further limitations for patients necessitating an echocardiographic assessment but having poor acoustic windows for a transthoracic examination, for whatever reason (i.e., due to mechanical ventilation). Another significant issue in the ICU regards the inability of echocardiographic evaluation to diagnose whether the LVDD is a new acute finding, mainly related to the critical illnes (e.g. sepsis for instance) and then possibly reversible, or if LVDD pre-existed to the ICU admission, considering the amount of admission of older and older patients carrying a significant burden of comorbidities. The only way to differentiate between both is to repeat echocardiographic evaluation longitudinally until the discharge and maybe after full recovery, but this approach would be very time- and resource-consuming. However, observing a LA dilatation could help physicians determine whether diastolic dysfunction existed prior to admission in the ICU.

For the above reasons it becomes challenging the assessment of sepsis-related changes in LV diastolic function according to fluctuations in LA volume and/or TR jet velocities, while the two TDI parameters (e' and E/e', see Table 1) probably remain the only reliable approach, due to their relative independency from the loading state [17]. Importantly, a recent meta-analysis by Sanfilippo et al. [5] showed that such parameters are associated with survival in septic patients.

Clinical and echocardiographic findings of different grades of LVDD

Hereby, we provide a simplified interpretation to the progression from normal LV diastolic function to different degrees of LVDD. In this context, it should be kept in mind that LV diastolic properties and LV filling pressure are closely related. In particular, Fig. 1 shows the relationship between left-sided pressures (LA and LV, Fig. 1a) and the corresponding echocardiographic findings for each stage in terms of transmitral blood flow (Fig. 1b) and of TDI mitral annular displacement (Fig. 1c). In the outpatient setting, once diagnosis of LVDD is made (i.e., patients with reduced LV systolic function and/or structural cardiomyopathy and/or fulfilling 3–4 parameters shown in Table 1), the grading of dysfunction is assessed according to the E/A ratio (and eventually E wave velocity). Figure 2 shows an algorithm for grading of LVDD in the outpatients according to the ASE/EACVI 2016 guidelines.

From physiological perspectives, in patients with normal LV diastolic function, the LV fills smoothly in the presence of low LA pressures and thus with a relatively small LA-to-LV gradient (in the order of few mmHg). The corresponding echocardiographic appearance in the transmitral blood flow is a dominant early (E) wave over the atrial (A or late) wave, and the corresponding TDI e' and a' waves demonstrate a similar ratio (first column from the left in Fig. 1).

With regard to the interpretation of transmitral blood flow, at initial stages of LVDD the LV becomes stiffer with impaired LV relaxation and the LA-to-LV gradient becomes smaller. Therefore, the early filling wave gradually decreases and the atrial wave becomes dominant ($E < A$ wave): This is the classical features of LVDD grade I (second column from the left in Fig. 1).

The subsequent progression of LVDD with further relaxation impairment causes physiological mechanisms of adaptation (i.e., fluid retention and changed loading conditions) with a consequent increase in LA pressure in order to restore a "pseudo-normal" LA-to-LV gradient (LVDD grade II). Thus, during this stage of LVDD there is a "pseudo-normalization" of transmitral flow pattern ($E > A$ wave) due to the reactive increase in LA pressures in response to worsening LVDD (third column from the left in Fig. 1).

Finally, when the LV chamber becomes poorly compliant and increasingly stiff (LVDD grade III), only a certain amount of blood can flow from the LA to the LV at each diastole. Importantly, such reduced amount of blood flowing into the LV during the early phase of diastole (E wave) quickly boosts the LV end-diastolic pressure at very high level so that the subsequent atrial contraction is unable to generate a decent filling (usually in the order of very few ml of blood). Consequently, the E wave is very dominant and the E/A ratio is usually > 2 (last column from the left in Fig. 1). The LVDD grade III has been further divided into reversible and irreversible, but performing such distinction is challenging, it requires patient's collaboration (i.e.,

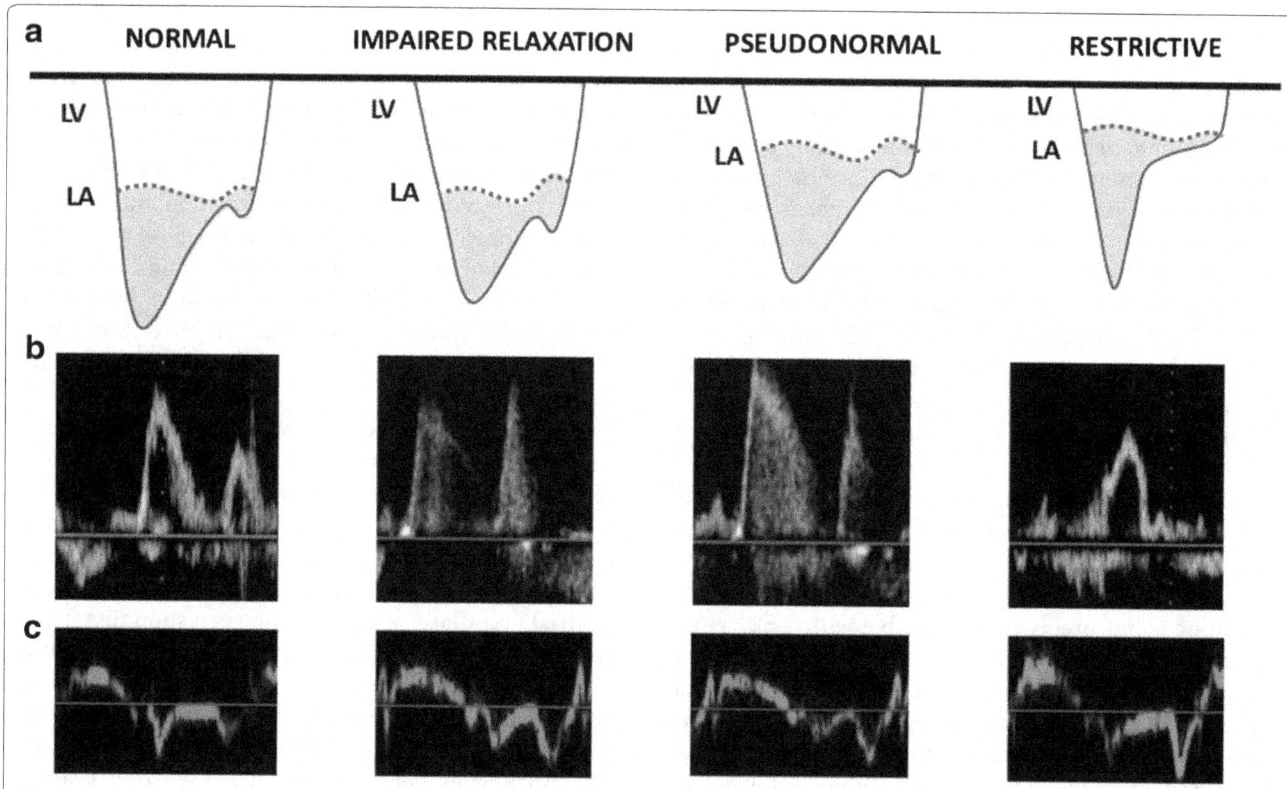

Fig. 1 Progression from normal diastolic function to worsening degrees of left ventricular diastolic dysfunction (LVDD). The top row **a** illustrates the respective changes in left atrial (LA) and left ventricular (LV) pressures with the progression of LVDD. The middle and bottom rows show examples of the patterns of transmitral blood flow (**b**) and of tissue Doppler imaging of the mitral annulus (**c**). These patterns are shown for each stage of LVDD, with corresponding changes of the *E* and *e*′ (early), and *A* and *a*′ (atrial) waves. From left to right, 2a: normal diastolic function ($E > A$; $e' > a'$); 2b: LVDD grade I ($E < A$; $e' < a'$); 2c: LVDD grade II ($E > A$; $e' < a'$); 2d: LVDD grade III ($E \gg A$; $e' \ll a'$)

performing Valsalva manoeuver), and more importantly it is probably more useful in the cardiology outpatient setting rather than in the operating room or in the ICU patients.

On the other hand, as shown in Fig. 1c, changes in TDI waves e' and a' are more unidirectional with the development of LVDD. The a' is an excellent marker of global atrial contraction and has similar values at septal and lateral levels [18]. It correlates very well with LA ejection fraction, LA ejection force and LA kinetic energy [19], being independent from the flow of blood filling the LV. For this reason the a' does not become smaller, but rather increases with progression of LV diastolic dysfunction and with more vigorous LA contraction in adaptation to the increased pressures. Only with advanced LA dilatation reaching a threshold of fiber length, LA shortening and contractility begin to decline, similar to what happens for the LV (Frank–Starling curve) [20–23]. On the other hand, the decline in *A* wave is likely to happen earlier in the progression of LVDD, because it is related to the reduction in transmitral blood flow in the presence of very high LV filling pressure.

Therefore, there is a progressive decrease in e' and a consequent increase in a' so that the e'/a' ratio moves gradually from >1 to <1 values; however, while $e'/a' > 1$ usually denotes a normal LV diastolic function and $e'/a' \ll 1$ is of restrictive pattern, it is more difficult to use the e'/a' ratio for the distinction between LVDD grades I and II.

In general, this paragraph provides a summary that may help readers in understanding the relationships between the LA-to-LV gradient and the changes in transmitral blood flow and mitral annular TDI displacement. It is mandatory to keep in mind that the interpretation of such parameters should take into account factors like patient's history (i.e., chronic atrial fibrillation—AF—may cause LA enlargement) and physiological factors (i.e., age influences cutoff for *E* wave). Moreover, the assessment becomes even more challenging in the ICU where the echocardiographic parameters can be affected by several confounders. For instance, the heart rate (especially tachycardia) and the use of vasopressors and/or inotropes influence the LV

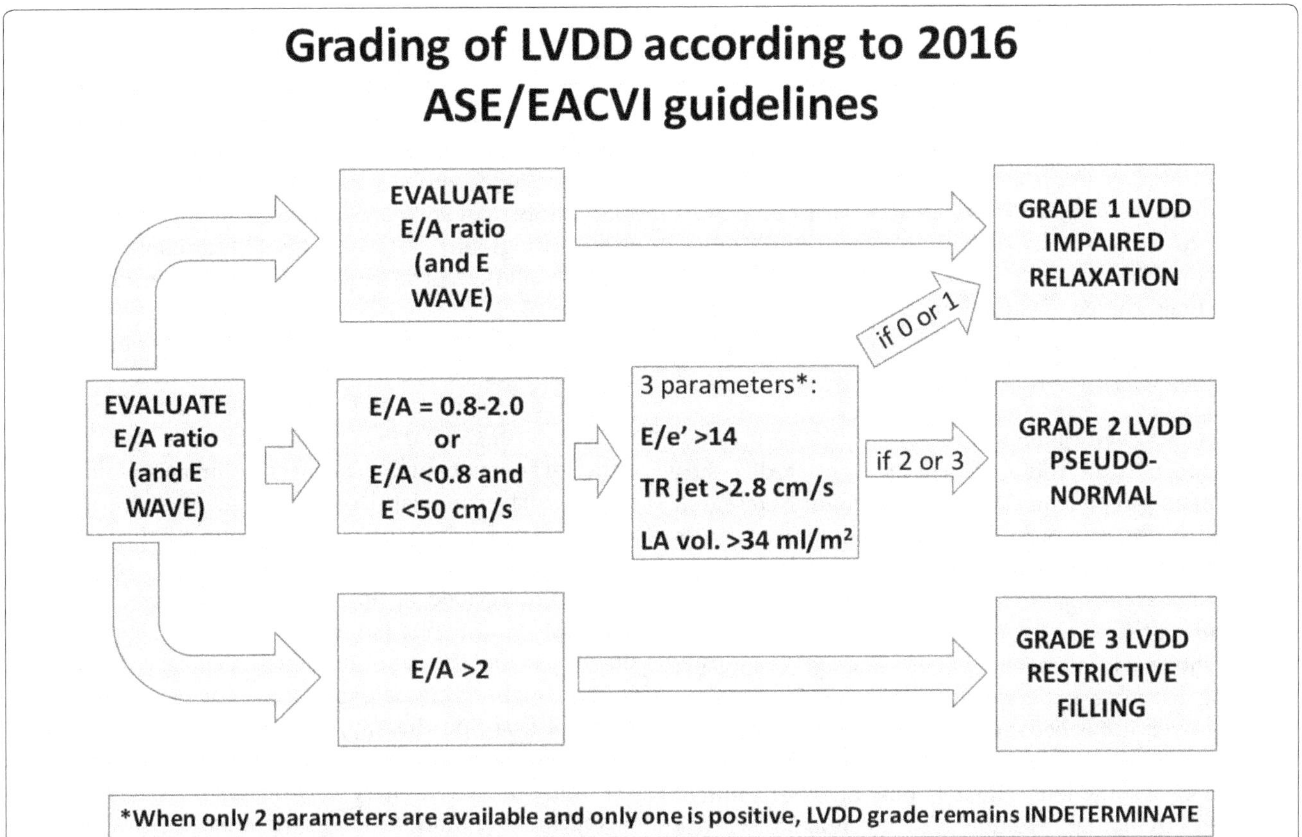

Fig. 2 Algorithm for grading of left ventricular diastolic dysfunction (LVDD) in outpatients according to the 2016 American Society of Echocardiography and European Association of Cardiovascular Imaging (ASE/EACVI) guidelines

diastolic properties; the *E/A* ratio may vary according to non-hemodynamic factors such as mechanical ventilation; and it is also of limited value in patients with significant mitral and/or aortic valve disease, or before fluid resuscitation has been carried out in critically ill patients.

Impact of LVDD in the perioperative setting

Nowadays, surgery is performed without a true "age cut-off" with older and older patients undergoing surgical procedures. Such patients have a large burden of comorbidities, including LVDD. However, the vast majority of literature of LVDD in the perioperative setting includes patients undergoing cardiac surgery or vascular surgery, since these patients generally present a larger spectrum of comorbidities, especially from cardiovascular perspectives. Moreover, such patients are frequently monitored perioperatively with TEE and thus real-time estimation and monitoring of LVDD could be feasible, although it should be kept in mind that TDI measures have not yet been fully validated with TEE.

In patients undergoing cardiac surgery, LVDD correlates with difficult weaning from cardiopulmonary bypass and higher inotropic needs [24, 25]. Moreover, there is some evidence of correlation between advanced LVDD and postoperative AF after cardiac surgery [26, 27].

In patients undergoing major vascular surgery, preoperative isolated LVDD is more frequent than isolated LV systolic dysfunction (43 vs. 8%, respectively) and, importantly, LVDD is an independent predictor of postoperative HF and prolonged hospital stay, and it is associated with postoperative adverse cardiovascular events and long-term cardiovascular mortality [28, 29].

While the impact of preoperative LVDD in these high-risk surgical specialties is not unexpected, more uncertainty reigns on the importance of LVDD in patient's outcome in other surgical specialties. In this regard, one of the issues is the ethical concerns and potential value in performing intraoperative TEE in patients with isolated LVDD undergoing non-high-risk surgery. Cabrera-Schulmeyer and Arriaza conducted an interesting study in patients with cardiac comorbidities and undergoing non-cardiac/non-vascular (abdominal, urological and orthopedic) surgery. The authors stratified patients according to preoperative normal (< 8), borderline (8–15) and high (> 15) *E*/*e*′ ratio. Patients with borderline and high *E*/*e*′

had a higher incidence of perioperative complications (higher incidence of pulmonary edema at 24 h and 48 h, arrhythmias) and longer ICU stay and hospital stay than patients with normal E/e'. Moreover, patients with high E/e' had significantly higher mortality as compared to normal ratio (8 vs. 0%, respectively) [4].

While preoperative LVDD correlates with outcome, a postoperative evaluation of patient's diastolic function should consider ruling out first the influence of stressors that may worsen diastolic function (i.e., pain-related tachycardia reduces diastolic time, hypo- and hypervolemia may influence LV filling pressures, etc.).

Impact of LVDD in the intensive care

With respect to the role of LVDD in (non-cardiac surgery) critically ill patients, the greater amount of research is related to the role of LVDD in the outcome of sepsis and in the weaning from mechanical ventilation.

LVDD and sepsis

Septic shock is characterized by intense vasoplegia requiring vasoactive therapy to restore blood pressure [30]; however, it has become more evident over the past years that septic patients are affected by pronounced myocardial dysfunction, which is possibly the result of increased circulating cytokine and catecholamine levels [14, 31]. We emphasize that, in case of overt septic shock and in the absence of signs of other causes of shock, fluid resuscitation should not be delayed in order to get information on LV diastolic function from an advanced critical care echocardiography examination or by requesting cardiology consultation. It is also likely that in patients with pronounced hypovolemia (and vasoplegia), the parameters used for the evaluation of LV diastolic function will undergo dramatic changes according to fluid resuscitation and/or the start of vasopressor infusion. It is pivotal understanding that assessment of LV diastolic function cannot be dissociated from evaluation of LV filling pressure, which in certain group of patients undergoes sudden clinical variations.

The so-defined septic cardiomyopathy may involve either the LV, the RV, or both, affecting systolic and/or diastolic function. With all the limitations coming from the use of LV ejection fraction (LVEF) for the evaluation of systolic function, a meta-analysis found no association between LV or RV systolic dysfunction and mortality in patients with severe sepsis or septic shock [32]. On the other hand, a subsequent meta-analysis demonstrated a strong association between LVDD and mortality in the same population of critically ill patients and confirmed also the absence of association between LV systolic dysfunction and mortality [6, 7]. Moreover, the same group of authors recently showed that worse TDI parameters (lower e' and higher E/e' ratio) are associated with mortality in septic patients [5]. Interestingly, another meta-analysis investigated the value of speckle tracking echocardiography in the prognostic evaluation of septic cardiomyopathy, showing that worse values of LV strain are associated with negative outcome in septic patients [33]. More research is warranted for speckle tracking echocardiography to understand if it could represent a better marker of intrinsic LV function in critically ill patients.

The association between LVDD and outcome in patients with severe sepsis and septic shock may be explained looking at the pathophysiology of sepsis. In patients with LVDD, the LV filling benefits from maintenance of adequate preload, sinus rhythm and avoidance of tachycardia, while sepsis causes sequential disturbances at such levels since patients become relatively hypovolemic, tachycardic and frequently develop arrhythmias, with AF described in up to 23% of patients with septic shock [34, 35]. Septic patients are relatively hypovolemic due to vasoplegia and increased capillary permeability and higher venous capacitance. In fact, the recommended first-line therapy for the treatment of sepsis is to restore preload. In patients with LVDD and increased LV filling pressures there is probably a narrow window for optimizing fluid status. In these patients, even under condition of theoretical "fluid-responsiveness," a little amount of fluid may precipitate pulmonary edema or cause a hemodynamic collapse. Therefore, without any delay in the initial fluid resuscitation of septic patients, the subsequent preload optimization may benefit by the knowledge of his/her LVDD conditions, too, which should be integrated with other variables. For instance, patients with acute respiratory distress syndrome and/or acute or pulmonale may not benefit from fluid due to both hydrostatic worsening of non-cardiogenic pulmonary edema and further RV dilatation. Patients with severe RV dysfunction may suffer from extra amount of fluids because the RV dilatation together with paradoxical septal motion hampers LV filling creating a "LVDD-like" condition by pushing the septal region and reducing LV compliance. However, using an experimental model of lung injury and high airway pressures, Katira et al. [36] reported very low augmentation of LV filling pressure as a consequence of RV failure, possibly as a consequence of decreased venous return and/or increased pulmonary vascular permeability.

Similarly, patients with at-least-moderate mitral regurgitation may worsen their pulmonary function if an extra amount of fluid is administered [37]. Not only preload but afterload too affects negatively the evaluation of LV diastolic function. In this regard, LV diastolic function worsens as a consequence of increased afterload due to hypertension [38] or related pharmacological [39] and non-pharmacological (increased intra-abdominal pressure [40]) factors. However, the main issues in this matter are represented by the difficulty of directly and reliably quantifying the LV afterload with echocardiography.

Another factor that further worsens LV filling is tachycardia, mainly disproportionally reducing the LV diastolic time. Although healthy individuals compensate for by accelerating the LV relaxation process (frequency-dependent acceleration of relaxation [41]), this process is impaired during sepsis [42]. The LV filling is further worsened by the development of AF and the consequent loss of efficacious atrial contraction. In this respect, although speculative, it is possible that the use of beta-blockade may produce more benefits in septic patients with LVDD for their ability to reduce heart rate and for their anti-arrhythmic properties [43, 44]. Another hypothesis which has to be evaluated in the future is the fact that septic patients with LVDD may have a worst tolerance to fluid expansion.

Concerning the incidence of LVDD in sepsis, it is worth noting that a recent study by Clancy et al. [45] found that the application of new guidelines for the evaluation of LV diastolic function identified a significantly higher incidence of LVDD as compared to the previous 2009 guidelines. This finding is interesting since a study in the general population found opposite results (much lower incidence of LVDD with new guidelines as compared to the 2009 version), as previously discussed [12].

LVDD and weaning from mechanical ventilation

During mechanical ventilation, LV preload and afterload are decreased, and the transition from positive to negative pressure (spontaneous breathing) creates unfavorable LV loading conditions and may also trigger myocardial ischemia [46]. There is growing evidence that the largest amount of weaning failures are of cardiac origin.

A recent study investigated the value of a combined integrated thoracic sonographic evaluation (respiratory, cardiac and diaphragmatic) in predicting early post-extubation respiratory distress. The detection of lung interstitial water was the most relevant parameter detected during thoracic ultrasound, while among factors studied by echocardiography, the estimation of LV filling pressure was predictive of post-extubation distress. On the contrary, indexes of systolic function and diaphragmatic excursion had poor impact over the prediction of respiratory failure [47].

One study showed an association between weaning failure and both lower LVEF and higher E/e' [48], but another one failed to show an association between LVEF and weaning failure [49]. The presence of LVDD seems more strongly associated with weaning failure as shown by several studies. Konomi et al. [50] found an independent association between LVDD and weaning failure (odds ratio 11.2), while Papanikolaou et al. [51] found lateral E/e' as the only factor independently associated with weaning failure possibly reflecting the association between a higher degree of LVDD and weaning failure. Moschietto et al. [49] found higher E/e' and lower e' in the failing group and interestingly that e' velocity increased in patients successfully weaned, while it remained unchanged in those failing.

The largest study on this topic recently showed that the vast majority of patients failing a spontaneous breathing trial (SBT) and weaning from mechanical ventilation develop weaning-induced pulmonary edema (WiPO) and that structural cardiopathy, chronic obstructive pulmonary disease and obesity are the main risk factors for WiPO [52]. In a subgroup of patients with cardiac output monitoring, the authors were able to show that WiPO is associated with *preload-independence* and that a subsequent SBT is more likely to succeed after diuretic therapy and a more negative fluid balance (achieving *preload-dependence*). This study found similar LVEF and fluid balance between patients with WiPO and non-WiPO, but the first group had significantly higher E/e' ratio, possibly reflecting a worse diastolic function [8]. In support of this hypothesis, WiPO failure patients monitored with cardiac output showed an increase in both global end-diastolic volume and extra-vascular lung water as compared to non-WiPO failures where these remained unchanged. Such findings highlight the risk of the transition from positive to negative pressure ventilation, where an increase in LV preload cannot be accommodated in patients with high LV filling pressures.

How to manage the patient with LVDD

The management of patients with LVDD can be challenging, and unfortunately, there is no magic bullet that rapidly improves LV diastolic function, pharmacologically or non-pharmacologically. A graphical summary of suggestions to manage the critically ill patients with LVDD is provided in Fig. 3. Moreover, no study exists to demonstrate that improving LVDD in the critically ill patients could beneficially impact the prognosis. Only few drugs have shown some improvements of LVDD. Among them beta-blockers are an example. Indeed, it is known their ability to ameliorate LVDD in HF with preserved LVEF [9], and beta-blockade also improves LV filling pressures and coronary flow reserve in patients with uncomplicated arterial hypertension [53]. It is worth noting the results of the first large randomized study on beta-blockers in patients with septic shock, with beneficial effects of esmolol infusion as shown by a significant improvement in cardiac performance, lower inotropic requirements and higher survival as compared to placebo. Both negative chronotropic and anti-arrhythmic effects of esmolol may have had positive influence on LV diastolic function, although the authors did not present echocardiographic data and this hypothesis remains speculative.The same group of authors recently showed an improved LV filling pattern and ventriculo-arterial coupling after esmolol infusion in septic patients [54]; moreover, immune, metabolic and coagulative effects of beta-blockers treatment may result advantageous in patients with sepsis [44]. Another therapeutically plausible option for patients with heart failure could be represented by the use of angiotensin-converting enzyme inhibitors, which may reduce LV remodeling and improve diastolic function [55–58]. However, the effects of this class of drugs are evident in the long run only and their efficacy is not demonstrated for LVDD in the acute setting. A potentially interesting drug that may ameliorate the hemodynamic profile of septic patients may be represented by dexmedetomidine (α-2 agonist), a sedative drug that has shown a possible reduction in catecholamines release associated with increased blood pressure response to exogenous vasopressors in experimental models of septic shock [59–62]. A clinical study has completed its enrollment (ClinicalTrials.gov Identifier: NCT02638545), but more research is warranted before drawing any conclusion. Another drug that has shown improvements of LV diastolic function is levosimendan [63], and its properties are unique if compared to catecholamines (which usually worsen LV diastolic function [64]) and phosphodiesterase inhibitors (LV diastolic function remaining grossly unchanged) [65]. However, levosimendan has specific pharmacokinetic and pharmacodynamic properties that make it not ideal when the effect is needed rapidly.

In general, although LVDD can be potentially reversed or reduced in its magnitude with appropriate treatment in the long run, this seems rather difficult in the acute critically ill patients; since the pharmacological approach to the optimization of diastolic function does not offer rapid solutions at present, clinicians should probably focus on the maintenance of the best loading conditions for the patient with established LVDD. From a clinical perspective, patients with LVDD grade I are usually more easy to manage, but the dominance of the atrial filling ($E<A$, see Fig. 1) makes them very sensible to the loss of atrial filling (i.e., AF) in case of baseline reduced LVEF. Therefore, particular attention should be devoted to the avoidance of AF [66].

In case of patients with LVDD grade II, clinicians should carefully evaluate the volume status. Indeed, such patients are prone to develop pulmonary edema under condition of hypervolemia; on the other hand, in case of hypovolemia the LA pressure decreases and patients lose their compensatory mechanism to maintain a "normal" LA-to-LV gradient, and this situation can be further aggravated by AF (loss of atrial contribution).

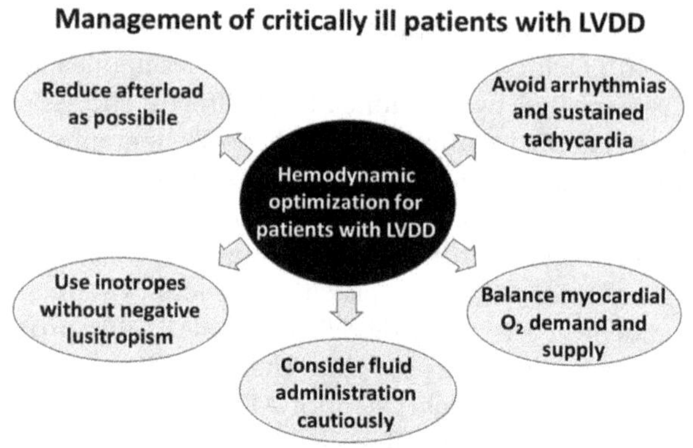

Fig. 3 Suggestions for the management of critically ill patients with left ventricular diastolic dysfunction (LVDD)

Patients with LVDD grade III are generally very frail patients and, for instance, severe abnormalities in LV filling pattern can explain the case of patients with HF with preserved LVEF, where patients are symptomatic despite no gross alteration in LVEF. In the outpatients, these individuals benefit from cardiology consultation and optimization, and they may also be considered for cardiac resynchronization therapy in case of prolonged QRS [67]. However, this option may not be easy in the acute phase of critical illness [68]. It is the authors' opinion that, if an urgent intervention is needed, such patients should be possibly managed by anesthesiologists with experience in the cardiac setting and optimized using echocardiography across the perioperative period.

Finally, because diastolic function is affected early during myocardial ischemia (earlier than systolic function) [69], attention should be paid to the factors associated with myocardial hypoperfusion. Ensuring an appropriate oxygen delivery to the LV by maintaining adequate diastolic blood pressure (with careful approach especially in patients with reduced arterial elastance and with risk factors for—or known for—coronary artery disease), possibly reducing the heart rate and thus the myocardial oxygen demand, and balancing the right level of LV afterload should all be part of the clinician's considerations when approaching the patient with LVDD.

Conclusion

There is growing evidence on the contribution of diastolic function to patients' outcome both in the perioperative setting and in the ICU. The assessment and grading of diastolic dysfunction remains challenging in these patients, and the guidelines used in the outpatient setting are not fully applicable. While pharmacological optimization remains difficult, especially with time constraints (urgency/emergency cases), a proactive management aiming at maintaining adequate loading conditions and an appropriate balance between myocardial oxygen demand and delivery could be the best strategies in managing patients with left ventricular diastolic dysfunction.

Abbreviations

LV: left ventricle; LVDD: left ventricular diastolic dysfunction; HF: heart failure; ASE: American Society of Echocardiography; EACVI: European Association of Cardiovascular Imaging; TR: tricuspid regurgitation; LA: left atrium; TDI: tissue Doppler imaging; TTE: transthoracic echocardiography; TEE: transesophageal echocardiography; RV: right ventricle; PEEP: positive end-expiratory pressure; AF: atrial fibrillation; LVEF: left ventricular ejection fraction; SBT: spontaneous breathing trial; WiPO: weaning-induced pulmonary edema.

Authors' contributions

All the authors discussed the idea of writing a review on this topic. FS wrote the first draft of the review. SS designed the figures. FS amended the draft according to the feedback from SS, AM and AVB. All authors read and approved the final manuscript.

Author details

[1] Department of Anesthesia and Intensive Care, IRCCS-ISMETT (Istituto Mediterraneo per i Trapianti e Terapie ad alta specializzazione), Palermo, Italy. [2] Unit of Intensive Care Medicine, Department of Medical Biotechnologies, University of Siena, Siena, Italy. [3] Department of Anaesthesiology and Intensive Care, University of Rome, "La Sapienza", Rome, Italy. [4] Hospital Ambroise Paré, Assistance Publique-Hôpitaux de Paris, Boulogne, France.

Acknowledgements

None.

Competing interests

The authors declare that they have no competing interests.

References

1. Redfield MM, Jacobsen SJ, Burnett JC Jr, Mahoney DW, Bailey KR, Rodeheffer RJ. Burden of systolic and diastolic ventricular dysfunction in the community: appreciating the scope of the heart failure epidemic. JAMA. 2003;289:194–202.
2. Gandhi SK, Powers JC, Nomeir AM, Fowle K, Kitzman DW, Rankin KM, Little WC. The pathogenesis of acute pulmonary edema associated with hypertension. N Engl J Med. 2001;344:17–22.
3. Yancy CW, Lopatin M, Stevenson LW, De Marco T, Fonarow GC, Committee ASA. Investigators: clinical presentation, management, and in-hospital outcomes of patients admitted with acute decompensated heart failure with preserved systolic function: a report from the Acute Decompensated Heart Failure National Registry (ADHERE) Database. J Am Coll Cardiol. 2006;47:76–84.
4. Cabrera Schulmeyer MC, Arriaza N. Good prognostic value of the intraoperative tissue Doppler-derived index E/e' after non-cardiac surgery. Minerva Anestesiol. 2012;78:1013–8.
5. Sanfilippo F, Corredor C, Arcadipane A, Landesberg G, Vieillard-Baron A, Cecconi M, Fletcher N. Tissue Doppler assessment of diastolic function and relationship with mortality in critically ill septic patients: a systematic review and meta-analysis. BJA: Br J Anaesth. 2017;119:583–94.
6. Sanfilippo F, Corredor C, Fletcher N, Landesberg G, Benedetto U, Foex P, Cecconi M. Erratum to: Diastolic dysfunction and mortality in septic patients: a systematic review and meta-analysis. Intensive Care Med. 2015;41:1178–9.
7. Sanfilippo F, Corredor C, Fletcher N, Landesberg G, Benedetto U, Foex P, Cecconi M. Diastolic dysfunction and mortality in septic patients: a systematic review and meta-analysis. Intensive Care Med. 2015;41:1004–13.
8. Sanfilippo F, Santonocito C, Burgio G, Arcadipane A. The importance of diastolic dysfunction in the development of weaning-induced pulmonary oedema. Crit Care. 2017;21:29.
9. Bergstrom A, Andersson B, Edner M, Nylander E, Persson H, Dahlstrom U. Effect of carvedilol on diastolic function in patients with diastolic heart failure and preserved systolic function. Results of the Swedish Doppler-echocardiographic study (SWEDIC). Eur J Heart Fail. 2004;6:453–61.
10. Nagueh SF, Smiseth OA, Appleton CP, Byrd BF III, Dokainish H, Edvardsen T, Flachskampf FA, Gillebert TC, Klein AL, Lancellotti P, Marino P, Oh JK, Alexandru Popescu B, Waggoner AD. Recommendations for the evaluation of left ventricular diastolic function by echocardiography: an update from the American Society of Echocardiography and the European Association of Cardiovascular imaging. Eur Heart J Cardiovasc Imaging. 2016;29:277–314.
11. Nagueh SF, Appleton CP, Gillebert TC, Marino PN, Oh JK, Smiseth OA, Waggoner AD, Flachskampf FA, Pellikka PA, Evangelisa A. Recommendations for the evaluation of left ventricular diastolic function by echocardiography. Eur J Echocardiogr. 2009;10:165–93.
12. Almeida JG, Fontes-Carvalho R, Sampaio F, Ribeiro J, Bettencourt P, Flachskampf FA, Leite-Moreira A, Azevedo A. Impact of the 2016 ASE/EACVI recommendations on the prevalence of diastolic dysfunction in the general population. Eur Heart J Cardiovasc Imaging. 2017;19:380–6.
13. Juhl-Olsen P, Hermansen JF, Frederiksen CA, Rasmussen LA, Jakobsen CJ, Sloth E. Positive end-expiratory pressure influences echocardiographic measures of diastolic function: a randomized, crossover study in cardiac surgery patients. Anesthesiology. 2013;119:1078–86.
14. Vieillard-Baron A, Cecconi M. Understanding cardiac failure in sepsis. Intensive Care Med. 2014;40:1560–3.
15. Bakkestrom R, Andersen MJ, Ersboll M, Bro-Jeppesen J, Gustafsson F, Kober L, Hassager C, Moller JE. Early changes in left atrial volume after acute myocardial infarction. Relation to invasive hemodynamics at rest and during exercise. Int J Cardiol. 2016;223:717–22.
16. Hoit BD, Shao Y, Gabel M. Influence of acutely altered loading conditions on left atrial appendage flow velocities. J Am Coll Cardiol. 1994;24:1117–23.
17. Ho CY, Solomon SD. A clinician's guide to tissue Doppler imaging. Circulation. 2006;113:e396–8.
18. Lindstrom L, Wranne B. Pulsed tissue Doppler evaluation of mitral annulus motion: a new window to assessment of diastolic function. Clin Physiol. 1999;19:1–10.
19. Khankirawatana B, Khankirawatana S, Peterson B, Mahrous H, Porter TR. Peak atrial systolic mitral annular velocity by Doppler tissue reliably predicts left atrial systolic function. J Am Soc Echocardiogr. 2004;17:353–60.
20. Blondheim DS, Osipov A, Meisel SR, Frimerman A, Shochat M, Shotan A. Relation of left atrial size to function as determined by transesophageal echocardiography. Am J Cardiol. 2005;96:457–63.
21. Okamoto M, Tsubokura T, Morishita K, Nakagawa H, Yamagata T, Kawagoe T, Hondo T, Tsuchioka Y, Matsuura H, Kajiyama G. Effects of volume loading on left atrial systolic time intervals. J Clin Ultrasound. 1991;19:405–11.
22. Prioli A, Marino P, Lanzoni L, Zardini P. Increasing degrees of left ventricular filling impairment modulate left atrial function in humans. Am J Cardiol. 1998;82:756–61.
23. Triposkiadis F, Tentolouris K, Androulakis A, Trikas A, Toutouzas K, Kyriakidis M, Gialafos J, Toutouzas P. Left atrial mechanical function in the healthy elderly: new insights from a combined assessment of changes in atrial volume and transmittal flow velocity. J Am Soc Echocardiogr. 1995;8:801–9.
24. Bernard F, Denault A, Babin D, Goyer C, Couture P, Couturier A, Buithieu J. Diastolic dysfunction is predictive of difficult weaning from cardiopulmonary bypass. Anesth Analg. 2001;92:291–8.
25. Licker M, Cikirikcioglu M, Inan C, Cartier V, Kalangos A, Theologou T, Cassina T, Diaper J. Preoperative diastolic function predicts the onset of left ventricular dysfunction following aortic valve replacement in high-risk patients with aortic stenosis. Crit Care. 2010;14:R101.

26. Chua SK, Shyu KG, Lu MJ, Hung HF, Cheng JJ, Lee SH, Lin CH, Chao HH, Lo HM. Association between renal function, diastolic dysfunction, and postoperative atrial fibrillation following cardiac surgery. Circ J. 2013;77:2303–10.
27. Lacalzada J, Jimenez JJ, Iribarren JL, de la Rosa A, Martin-Cabeza M, Izquierdo MM, Mari-Lopez B, Garcia-Gonzalez MJ, Jorge-Perez P, Barragan A, Laynez I. Early transthoracic echocardiography after cardiac surgery predicts postoperative atrial fibrillation. Echocardiography. 2016;33:1300–8.
28. Flu WJ, van Kuijk JP, Hoeks SE, Kuiper R, Schouten O, Goei D, Elhendy A, Verhagen HJ, Thomson IR, Bax JJ, Fleisher LA, Poldermans D. Prognostic implications of asymptomatic left ventricular dysfunction in patients undergoing vascular surgery. Anesthesiology. 2010;112:1316–24.
29. Matyal R, Hess PE, Subramaniam B, Mitchell J, Panzica PJ, Pomposelli F, Mahmood F. Perioperative diastolic dysfunction during vascular surgery and its association with postoperative outcome. J Vasc Surg. 2009;50:70–6.
30. Antonelli M, Bonten M, Chastre J, Citerio G, Conti G, Curtis JR, De Backer D, Hedenstierna G, Joannidis M, Macrae D, Mancebo J, Maggiore SM, Mebazaa A, Preiser JC, Rocco P, Timsit JF, Wernerman J, Zhang H. Year in review in Intensive Care Medicine 2011. II. Cardiovascular, infections, pneumonia and sepsis, critical care organization and outcome, education, ultrasonography, metabolism and coagulation. Intensive Care Med. 2012;38:345–58.
31. Beesley SJ, Weber G, Sarge T, Nikravan S, Grissom CK, Lanspa MJ, Shahul S, Brown SM. Septic cardiomyopathy. Crit Care Med. 2018;46:625–34.
32. Huang SJ, Nalos M, McLean AS. Is early ventricular dysfunction or dilatation associated with lower mortality rate in adult severe sepsis and septic shock? A meta-analysis. Crit Care. 2013;17:R96.
33. Sanfilippo F, Corredor C, Fletcher N, Tritapepe L, Lorini FL, Arcadipane A, Vieillard-Baron A, Cecconi M. Left ventricular systolic function evaluated by strain echocardiography and relationship with mortality in patients with severe sepsis or septic shock: a systematic review and meta-analysis. Crit Care. 2018;22:183.
34. Kuipers S, Klein Klouwenberg PM, Cremer OL. Incidence, risk factors and outcomes of new-onset atrial fibrillation in patients with sepsis: a systematic review. Crit Care. 2014;18:688.
35. Makrygiannis SS, Margariti A, Rizikou D, Lampakis M, Vangelis S, Ampartzidou OS, Katsifa K, Tselioti P, Foussas SG, Prekates AA. Incidence and predictors of new-onset atrial fibrillation in noncardiac intensive care unit patients. J Crit Care. 2014;29(697):e1–5. https://doi.org/10.1016/j.jcrc.2014.03.029 **Epub 2014 Apr 4**.
36. Katira BH, Giesinger RE, Engelberts D, Zabini D, Kornecki A, Otulakowski G, Yoshida T, Kuebler WM, McNamara PJ, Connelly KA, Kavanagh BP. Adverse heart–lung interactions in ventilator-induced lung injury. Am J Respir Crit Care Med. 2017;196:1411–21.
37. Sanfilippo F, Scolletta S. Fluids in cardiac surgery: sailing calm on a stormy sea? Common sense is the guidance. Minerva Anestesiol. 2017;83:537–9.
38. Krzesinski P, Uzieblo-Zyczkowska B, Gielerak G, Stanczyk A, Kurpaska M, Piotrowicz K. Global longitudinal two-dimensional systolic strain is associated with hemodynamic alterations in arterial hypertension. J Am Soc Hypertens. 2015;9:680–9.
39. Ros M, Azevedo ER, Newton GE, Parker JD. Effects of nitroprusside on cardiac norepinephrine spillover and isovolumic left ventricular relaxation in the normal and failing human left ventricle. Can J Cardiol. 2002;18:1211–6.
40. Alfonsi P, Vieillard-Baron A, Coggia M, Guignard B, Goeau-Brissonniere O, Jardin F, Chauvin M. Cardiac function during intraperitoneal CO2 insufflation for aortic surgery: a transesophageal echocardiographic study. Anesth Analg. 2006;102:1304–10.
41. Janssen PM, Periasamy M. Determinants of frequency-dependent contraction and relaxation of mammalian myocardium. J Mol Cell Cardiol. 2007;43:523–31.
42. Joulin O, Marechaux S, Hassoun S, Montaigne D, Lancel S, Neviere R. Cardiac force-frequency relationship and frequency-dependent acceleration of relaxation are impaired in LPS-treated rats. Crit Care. 2009;13:R14.
43. Morelli A, Ertmer C, Westphal M, Rehberg S, Kampmeier T, Ligges S, Orecchioni A, D'Egidio A, D'Ippoliti F, Raffone C, Venditti M, Guarracino F, Girardis M, Tritapepe L, Pietropaoli P, Mebazaa A, Singer M. Effect of heart rate control with esmolol on hemodynamic and clinical outcomes in patients with septic shock: a randomized clinical trial. JAMA. 2013;310:1683–91. https://doi.org/10.1001/jama.2013.278477.
44. Sanfilippo F, Santonocito C, Morelli A, Foex P. Beta-blocker use in severe sepsis and septic shock: a systematic review. Curr Med Res Opin. 2015;31:1817–25.
45. Clancy DJ, Scully T, Slama M, Huang S, McLean AS, Orde SR. Application of updated guidelines on diastolic dysfunction in patients with severe sepsis and septic shock. Ann Intensive Care. 2017;7:121.
46. Dres M, Teboul JL, Anguel N, Guerin L, Richard C, Monnet X. Passive leg raising performed before a spontaneous breathing trial predicts weaning-induced cardiac dysfunction. Intensive Care Med. 2015;41:487–94.
47. Silva S, Ait Aissa D, Cocquet P, Hoarau L, Ruiz J, Ferre F, Rousset D, Mora M, Mari A, Fourcade O, Riu B, Jaber S, Bataille B. Combined thoracic ultrasound assessment during a successful weaning trial predicts postextubation distress. Anesthesiology. 2017;127:666–74.
48. Caille V, Amiel JB, Charron C, Belliard G, Vieillard-Baron A, Vignon P. Echocardiography: a help in the weaning process. Crit Care. 2010;14:R120.
49. Moschietto S, Doyen D, Grech L, Dellamonica J, Hyvernat H, Bernardin G. Transthoracic echocardiography with Doppler tissue imaging predicts weaning failure from mechanical ventilation: evolution of the left ventricle relaxation rate during a spontaneous breathing trial is the key factor in weaning outcome. Crit Care. 2012;16:R81.
50. Konomi I, Tasoulis A, Kaltsi I, Karatzanos E, Vasileiadis I, Temperikidis P, Nanas S, Routsi CI. Left ventricular diastolic dysfunction—an independent risk factor for weaning failure from mechanical ventilation. Anaesth Intensive Care. 2016;44:466–73.
51. Papanikolaou J, Makris D, Saranteas T, Karakitsos D, Zintzaras E, Karabinis A, Kostopanagiotou G, Zakynthinos E. New insights into weaning from mechanical ventilation: left ventricular diastolic dysfunction is a key player. Intensive Care Med. 2011;37:1976–85.
52. Liu J, Shen F, Teboul JL, Anguel N, Beurton A, Bezaz N, Richard C, Monnet X. Cardiac dysfunction induced by weaning from mechanical ventilation: incidence, risk factors, and effects of fluid removal. Crit Care. 2016;20:369.
53. Galderisi M, D'Errico A, Sidiropulos M, Innelli P, de Divitiis O, de Simone G. Nebivolol induces parallel improvement of left ventricular filling pressure and coronary flow reserve in uncomplicated arterial hypertension. J Hypertens. 2009;27:2108–15.
54. Morelli A, Singer M, Ranieri VM, D'Egidio A, Mascia L, Orecchioni A, Piscioneri F, Guarracino F, Greco E, Peruzzi M, Biondi-Zoccai G, Frati G, Romano SM. Heart rate reduction with esmolol is associated with improved arterial elastance in patients with septic shock: a prospective observational study. Intensive Care Med. 2016;42:1528–34.
55. Chang NC, Shih CM, Bi WF, Lai ZY, Lin MS, Wang TC. Fosinopril improves left ventricular diastolic function in young mildly hypertensive patients without hypertrophy. Cardiovasc Drugs Ther. 2002;16:141–7.
56. Siegmund T, Schumm-Draeger PM, Antoni D, Bibra HV. Beneficial effects of ramipril on myocardial diastolic function in patients with type 2 diabetes mellitus, normal LV systolic function and without coronary artery disease: a prospective study using tissue Doppler. Diab Vasc Dis Res. 2007;4:358–64.
57. Yalcin F, Aksoy FG, Muderrisoglu H, Sabah I, Garcia MJ, Thomas JD. Treatment of hypertension with perindopril reduces plasma atrial natriuretic peptide levels, left ventricular mass, and improves echocardiographic parameters of diastolic function. Clin Cardiol. 2000;23:437–41.
58. Zhang Q, Chen Y, Liu Q, Shan Q. Effects of renin-angiotensin-aldosterone system inhibitors on mortality, hospitalization, and diastolic function in patients with HFpEF. A meta-analysis of 13 randomized controlled trials. Herz. 2016;41:76–86.
59. Geloen A, Chapelier K, Cividjian A, Dantony E, Rabilloud M, May CN, Quintin L. Clonidine and dexmedetomidine increase the pressor response to norepinephrine in experimental sepsis: a pilot study. Crit Care Med. 2013;41:e431–8.
60. Hernandez G, Tapia P, Alegria L, Soto D, Luengo C, Gomez J, Jarufe N, Achurra P, Rebolledo R, Bruhn A, Castro R, Kattan E, Ospina-Tascon G,

Bakker J. Effects of dexmedetomidine and esmolol on systemic hemodynamics and exogenous lactate clearance in early experimental septic shock. Crit Care. 2016;20:234.
61. Lankadeva YR, Booth LC, Kosaka J, Evans RG, Quintin L, Bellomo R, May CN. Clonidine restores pressor responsiveness to phenylephrine and angiotensin II in ovine sepsis. Crit Care Med. 2015;43:e221–9.
62. Miranda ML, Balarini MM, Bouskela E. Dexmedetomidine attenuates the microcirculatory derangements evoked by experimental sepsis. Anesthesiology. 2015;122:619–30.
63. Malik V, Subramanian A, Hote M, Kiran U. Effect of levosimendan on diastolic function in patients undergoing coronary artery bypass grafting: a comparative study. J Cardiovasc Pharmacol. 2015;66:141–7.
64. Tarvasmaki T, Lassus J, Varpula M, Sionis A, Sund R, Kober L, Spinar J, Parissis J, Banaszewski M, Silva Cardoso J, Carubelli V, Di Somma S, Mebazaa A, Harjola VP. Current real-life use of vasopressors and inotropes in cardiogenic shock—adrenaline use is associated with excess organ injury and mortality. Crit Care. 2016;20:208.
65. Couture P, Denault AY, Pellerin M, Tardif JC. Milrinone enhances systolic, but not diastolic function during coronary artery bypass grafting surgery. Can J Anaesth. 2007;54:509–22.
66. Vieillard-Baron A, Boyd J. Non-antiarrhythmic interventions in new onset and paroxysmal sepsis-related atrial fibrillation. Intensive Care Med. 2018;44:94–7.
67. Cleland JG, Daubert JC, Erdmann E, Freemantle N, Gras D, Kappenberger L, Tavazzi L. The effect of cardiac resynchronization on morbidity and mortality in heart failure. N Engl J Med. 2005;352:1539–49.
68. Rinaldi C, Auricchio A, Prinzen F. Left ventricular endocardial pacing for the critically ill. Intensive Care Med. 2018;44:915–7.
69. Schwarzl M, Huber S, Maechler H, Steendijk P, Seiler S, Truschnig-Wilders M, Nestelberger T, Pieske BM, Post H. Left ventricular diastolic dysfunction during acute myocardial infarction: effect of mild hypothermia. Resuscitation. 2012;83:1503–10.

15

Evaluation of emotional excitation during standardized endotracheal intubation in simulated conditions

Nicolas S. Marjanovic[1,2,3], Christelle Teiten[4], Nicola Pallamin[5] and Erwan L'Her[6,7*]

Abstract

Objective: To assess how stressful conditions in endotracheal intubation could induct emotional excitation in a population of acute care physicians.

Materials and methods: Two situations were randomly tested: one in standard and easy intubation conditions the other under difficult conditions presumed to induce stress (monitoring alarms, manikin lying on the floor, difficult intubation). Emotional excitation was assessed using several physiological (cardiac patterns, electrodermal activity and eye-tracking) and psycho-cognitive patterns. Auto-evaluations of video recordings and mental workload were performed immediately after simulation.

Results: Significant physiological parameter modifications were observed under the stressful intubation conditions (SDNN 35 ± 15 vs. 42 ± 21; $p = 0.035$—AVNN 514 ± 94 vs. 548 ± 110; $p < 0.0001$). Emotional excitation was demonstrated to lead a higher mental workload (NASA-TLX = 39 ± 18 vs. 63 ± 15; $p = 0.001$), frustration and effort dimensions being its determinant components ($p < 0.01$). Video recording auto-evaluations depicted significant emotional excitation occurrence under the difficult conditions, with few differences according to the operator's experience.

Conclusion: This study highlights the fact that a stress condition during ETI on a simulation model leads to an important emotional excitation as compared to the neutral condition.

Keywords: Patient simulation, Laryngoscopy, Emergency medicine, Emotional excitation, Stress

Background

Endotracheal intubation (ETI) is a standard procedure for the airway management. In emergency medicine (EM), anesthesiology and critical care, it is a challenging procedure associated with severe life-threatening complications, including cardiac arrest. These complications vary according to the operator expertise and depend on several factors, notably in prehospital EM, i.e., unstable medical conditions, environmental requirements, unknown patient medical history [1] and emotional excitation.

Technical skills training has traditionally been modeled on an apprenticeship system, where trainees operated under direct supervision from their seniors. Over recent years, this system has evolved, taking into account security concepts developed in the aerospace sector with simulation and healthcare guidelines from national authorities [2, 3]. Simulation is increasingly used in this setting, and different learning programs exist between juniors and seniors [4].

Emotional excitation that is frequently and improperly called "stress" can be considered as a psychological status that may affect physicians' performance [5]. While a certain degree of emotional excitation may improve task performance (positive impact), it can also become a threat when the perceived demand outweighs individual resources (negative impact, i.e., "stress").

*Correspondence: erwan.lher@chu-brest.fr
[6] Department of Intensive Care Medicine, University Hospital of Brest - La Cavale Blanche, Boulevard Tanguy Prigent, 29609 Brest Cedex, France
Full list of author information is available at the end of the article

We made the hypothesis that stress conditions to IOT would induce a high level of emotional excitation as compared toneutral conditions and that the experience could lead to a lower level of stress.

The main objective of this study was to assess how stressful conditions in ETI could induct emotional excitation in a population of acute care physicians. A second objective was to assess how emotional excitation varied among seniors and juniors.

Materials and methods

Study design

This prospective, crossover, randomized study was conducted in situ by the CESIM Santé—LATIM INSERM UMR 1101 research unit at Brest University Hospital (France) between April and May 2016.

A block randomization was used to determine the scenario's order.

The study was approved by our local ethics committee, and participants were asked to complete a demographic questionnaire and to sign informed consent.

Participants

The study was conducted with acute care medicine juniors and seniors. Seniors had to be at least one-year experienced, but juniors could have no prior or a few experience in endotracheal intubation on real patients.

Intubation management

Intubation was performed using an endotracheal tube with 7.0 mm of internal diameters (Mallinckrodt, Dublin, Ireland). The direct laryngoscopy was performed using a Macintosh blade (Size 4). Participants could use a flexible mandrel if needed.

The success of the intubation was secondarily confirmed by an experienced practitioner by a visual control and a lungs' auscultation.

Scenarios

Two scenarios of drug overdose were designed and tested before prior to the study, to ensure reproducibility and realistic environmental conditions.

ETI was performed using standard devices of our hospital. All subjects, juniors included, were familiar with these devices. We used an ALS Kelly manikin (Laerdal, Stavanger, Norway) and two standardized recordings of the patient's monitoring system simulator evolution (LLEAP, Laerdal, Stavanger, Norway):

(1) *Neutral condition* The manikin was lying supine on a stretcher that could be adjusted by participants. Vital signs were considered stable [heart rate (HR) = 90 bpm, blood pressure = 120/80 mmHg, oxygen saturation (SpO2) = 98%, normal sinus rhythm]. Endotracheal intubation was to be free of any difficult intubation-associated factors. No evolution of the scenario was to occur during the intubation procedure.

(2) *Stress condition* The manikin was lying supine on the floor, in a corner of the room, with reduced available space. Patient's clinical condition was to deteriorate gradually within 2 min: from tachycardia, to atrial fibrillation and ventricular tachycardia; hypoxemia was present at the beginning of the scenario, despite adequate preoxygenation, and was to deteriorate (SpO2 decrease from 92 to 70%). The tongue of the manikin was blown up to Cormack class IV. Deterioration of physiological parameters was to trigger the monitor's range alarms after a 15-s period, and the alarm volume was set to be very loud.

Physicians handled the scenarios consecutively, in a randomized and crossover design. Participants were informed that ETI was the main purpose of the study and that global care was not required. Preoxygenation and rapid sequence induction were considered already carried out. ECG and pulse oximetry monitor, and all necessary devices were placed beside the manikin, and if required, operators could ask for a gum elastic bougie.

A limit of two unsuccessful attempts and/or a maximum duration of 5 min were considered to define ETI failure.

Emotional excitation assessment

Emotional excitation was assessed using various physiological and psycho-cognitive parameters:

(1) Heart rate variability (HRV). HRV offers a noninvasive indicator of autonomic nervous system activity [6] and was recorded using a two-lead electrocardiogram attached to the upper chest. The signal was sampled at 1000 Hz using a Biopac® MP36R system and analyzed using AcqKnowledge software (*Biopac Systems Inc, Santa Barbara, CA, USA*). All data were visually checked for quality control. Time-domain and frequency-domain analyses of beat-to-beat RR intervals were performed according to the following parameters [7]:

- Heart rate (HR), the average of RR intervals.
- Maximum heart rate (maxHR).
- Standard deviation of RR intervals (SDNN). SDNN reflects all the cyclic components responsible for variability in the period of recording and therefore represents total variability.

- Average of all RR intervals (AVNN).
- LF/HF ratio, ratio of low (LF) to high (HF) frequency power. HF is the power spectral density of series of the RR intervals between 0.15 and 0.40 Hz due to parasympathetic activity, and LF is the power spectral density for intervals between 0.04 and 0.15 Hz due to sympathetic activity. LF/HF ratio. LF/HF ratio was proposed as an index of sympathetic to parasympathetic balance of heart rate fluctuation [8].

(2) Electrodermal activity (EDA). EDA can also be used to examine implicit emotional responses that may occur with or without conscious awareness (i.e., threat, anticipation) [9]. An Embrace wristband (Empatica, Cambridge, MA, USA) was used to monitor EDA via skin conductance level (SCL). SCL is a tonic level of electrical skin conductivity in EDA activity [10] and is presumed to reflect sympathic nervous system activity.

(3) Eye-tracking. Eye-tracking is a technique that provides an objective, quantifiable and measurable link between an individual and his immediate environment [11]. SMI eye-tracking glasses (SensoMotoric Instruments GmbH, Teltow, Germany) recorded saccades, blinking and eye fixations using iView ETG 2.2 and BeGaze 3.5.101 software (SensoMotoric Instruments GmbH, Teltow, Germany) to record and export data into video and text formats. SMI glasses were adjusted and calibrated individually, before each simulation. Calibration was carried out by aligning the focus circle as displayed on the output screen of the eye tracking notebook with the actual fixation focus of the participant. Data were subsequently analyzed using a proprietary software. Blinks and fixations were recorded in the central vision. Periods with excessive noise, usually due to movement, were eliminated from analysis. Blinks and fixations were expected higher in a stress condition.

Psycho-cognitive evaluations

Psycho-cognitive evaluations were performed using three different methods after each scenario:

(1) Likert-type scale. Each practitioner evaluated stress level using a Likert-type scale, from 1—none—to 10—very important stress

(2) Mental workload. Mental workload estimation was assessed using the National Aeronautics and Space Administration Task Load Index (NASA-TLX) [12, 13]. This questionnaire is regularly used to evaluate different medical and surgical procedures and to assess human–machine interface (HMI).

(3) Self-assessment stress evaluation. It was carried out immediately after each scenario, while viewing back-recorded video sequences. The participant was asked to quantify his stress level from 0 to 100 using a haptic 3D wheel navigator (3Dconnexion Space Navigator) and a proprietary software (Autoconfrontation V1.0.4, BCom, Brest, France).

Statistical analysis

Statistical analysis and data entry were performed using SPSS 23.0 software (IBM Corporation, Armonk, NY, USA). Continuous quantitative data are presented as means ± STD. Non-normally distributed data are presented using median and extreme values, categorical variables by a percentage. Statistical analysis was performed using the Wilcoxon test in between groups and the two scenarios for the same population. P-values equal or below 0.05 were considered significant.

Results

Twenty-six acute care physicians were recruited (16 seniors, 10 juniors). Their general characteristics are depicted inTable 1. Physiological patterns are shown in Table 2 and Fig. 1, and psycho-cognitive and subjective assessments are shown in Table 3 and Fig. 2.

Emotional excitation between scenarios

Physiological patterns as HR, maxHR, SDNN and AVNN differed statistically between neutral and stress

Table 1 Population characteristics

Age (years)	32.5 ± 6.8
Male *n* (%)	11 (42)
Position	
Seniors *n* (%)	16 (62)
Juniors *n* (%)	10 (38)
Initial formation	
Emergency physician	19 (73)
Anesthesiologist	3 (12)
Intensivist	4 (15)
Intubation experience	
Seniors (years)	11.2 ± 3.7
Juniors (years)	2.4 ± 2.3
Drugs consumption *n* (%)	
Caffeine in the previous 2 h	16 (62)
Anxiolytics	0 (0)
Beta-blockers	0 (0)

Values are provided as mean + STD, or number and percentage

Table 2 Physiological measurement of emotional excitation during scenarios

	Overall			Senior			Junior		
	Neutral	Stress	*p*	Neutral	Stress	*p*	Neutral	Stress	*p*
Heart rate variation (HRV)									
HR mean value	114.1 ± 21	120.7 ± 19.9	*0.002*	111.1 ± 21.6	117.2 ± 21.5	*0.007*	119.8 ± 19.8	127 ± 15.8	0.235
HR maximal value	127.1 ± 20.5	140.1 ± 20.6	*0.003*	123.1 ± 21.1	137.8 ± 23.8	*0.005*	134.6 ± 18.3	144.3 ± 13.6	0.362
SDNN (ms)	41.7 ± 21.3	35.1 ± 14.8	*0.035*	41.9 ± 22.2	38.1 ± 15.5	0.307	41.3 ± 21	29.7 ± 12.4	*0.017*
AVNN (ms)	547.9 ± 110.1	514 ± 94.2	*< 0.0001*	563.8 ± 116.8	532.4 ± 103.9	*0.003*	517.9 ± 96.2	481.1 ± 67	0.069
LF/HF ratio	3.5 ± 0.3	3.5 ± 0.2	0.1	3.5 ± 0.3	3.5 ± 0.2	0.256	3.5 ± 0.3	3.6 ± 0.1	0.208
SCL electrodermal activity (ms)	1.8 ± 3.1	1.9 ± 3.1	0.259	2.3 ± 3.8	2.6 ± 3.7	0.721	0.9 ± 0.7	0.7 ± 0.7	0.108
Eye-tracking									
Blink (*n*)	1537 ± 2173	4109 ± 3750	*0.03*	1722 ± 2544	5081 ± 4086	*0.013*	1085 ± 1149	2407 ± 1191	*0.025*
Fixation (*n*)	2451 ± 1752	3806 ± 2249	*0.03*	2023 ± 1423	4002 ± 2381	*0.011*	3339 ± 1980	3537 ± 1951	0.779

Values are provided as mean ± STD or number and percentage

A *p* value ≤ 0.05 was considered statistically significant (in italics)

According to our results, the intubation stress sequence was associated with different HRV parameters, an increase in eye-blinking and fixation episodes in stress condition, as compared to the neutral condition

HR heart rate, *HRV* heart rate variability, *SDNN* standard deviation of all NN intervals, *AVNN* average of all NN intervals, *LF/HF ratio* ratio of low (LF) to high (HF) frequency power, *SCL* skin conductance level, *Blink* the overall number of eye links during the measurement periods, *Fixation* the overall number of eye fixations during the measurement periods

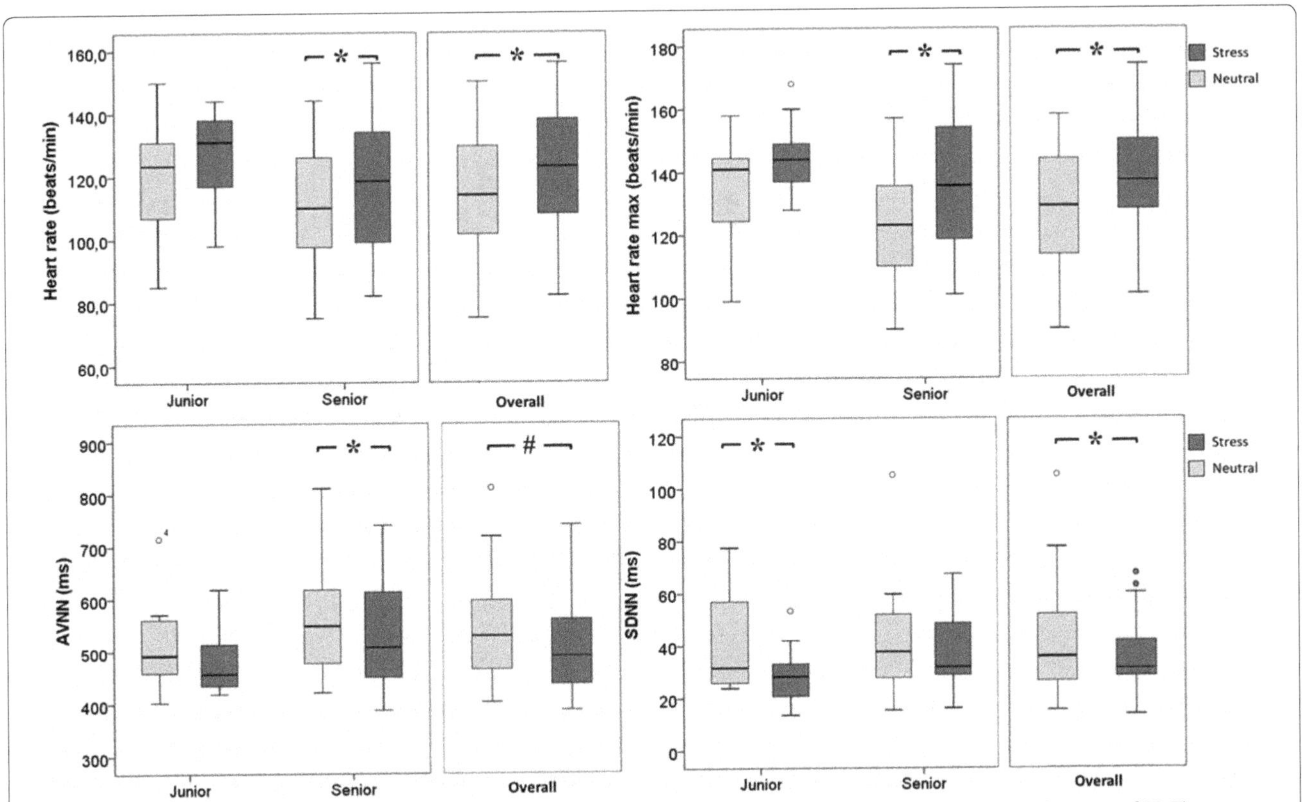

Fig. 1 Heart rate and heart rate variability measurement. AVNN is the average of RR interval, and SDNN is the standard deviation of RR. There was a difference in heart rate, max heart rate and AVNN for overall participants and for seniors, between stress and neutral scenarios. For juniors, there was a difference only for SDNN. *$p < 0.01$ # $p < 0.0001$. HRV is primarily dependent on the parasympathetic autonomic nervous system. Overall, there was a lower HRV between the 2 scenarios with the acceleration of HR, a SDNN and AVNN lower values. Statistical analysis shows significant results in different HRV parameter but not always at the same time

Table 3 Psycho-cognitive and subjective emotional excitation assessment

	Overall			Senior			Junior		
	Neutral	Stress	*p*	Neutral	Stress	*p*	Neutral	Stress	*p*
Global mental workload	38.8±18	63.5±15.1	*<0.0001*	38.5±19.7	65±16.6	*0.002*	39.2±15.7	61.3±12.9	*0.015*
Mental workload	9.2±8.3	8.5±9.4	0.922	8.8±9.4	7.6±9.4	0.78	9.9±6.6	9.8±9.8	0.678
Physical workload	3.1±4.2	6.1±5.5	0.023	3.3±4.2	5.8±5.6	0.133	2.7±4.2	6.7±5.7	0.069
Temporal workload	11.2±8.2	15.7±7.5	*0.005*	10.2±8.2	15.5±7.8	*0.036*	12.8±8.3	16±7.4	*0.038*
Performance	7.5±6.7	11.8±8.2	0.089	7.5±7.6	14±8	*0.041*	7.4±5.1	8.3±7.6	0.674
Effort	5.5±3.4	11.5±7	*0.0003*	5.9±3.9	10.8±6.5	*0.003*	4.8±2.4	12.6±8	*0.036*
Frustration	2.4±4.6	10±9.6	*0.003*	2.9±5.5	11.4±9.8	*0.013*	1.5±2.3	7.9±9.4	0.068
Stress measurement									
Likert scale	2.4±1.7	5.3±2.5	*0.00002*	2.3±1.9	5±2.8	*0.009*	2.6±1.6	5.8±2.2	*0.007*
Stress mean	22.3±18.2	45±22.1	*0.000036*	20.2±17.3	44.4±22.3	*0.001*	25.8±20	45.8±22.9	*0.009*
Stress max	38.7±24.6	67.7±26	*0.000033*	35.8±25.8	66.8±26.1	*0.001*	43.2±23	69.3±27.4	*0.009*

In NASA-TLX assessment, each dimension could be analyzed as follows: mental workload: mental and perceptual activity required during task. Physical workload: physical (muscle) activity required. Temporal workload: time pressure felt during task. Performance: feeling of success. It is important to indicate that the performance scale is inversed. The higher the performance dimension, the lower the feeling of performance. Effort: global difficulty (physically and mentally) to accomplish the task. Frustration: level of irritation stress and frustration. The first three dimensions (mental workload, physical and temporal demands) are related to constraints imposed on the subject by the task; the subsequent three other dimensions are related to interactions of the subject with the task. Stress level was assessed according a Likert scale from 1 to 10, and by a video recording auto-evaluation scale from 1—minimum—to 100—maximum

Significant *p* values are highlighted in italics

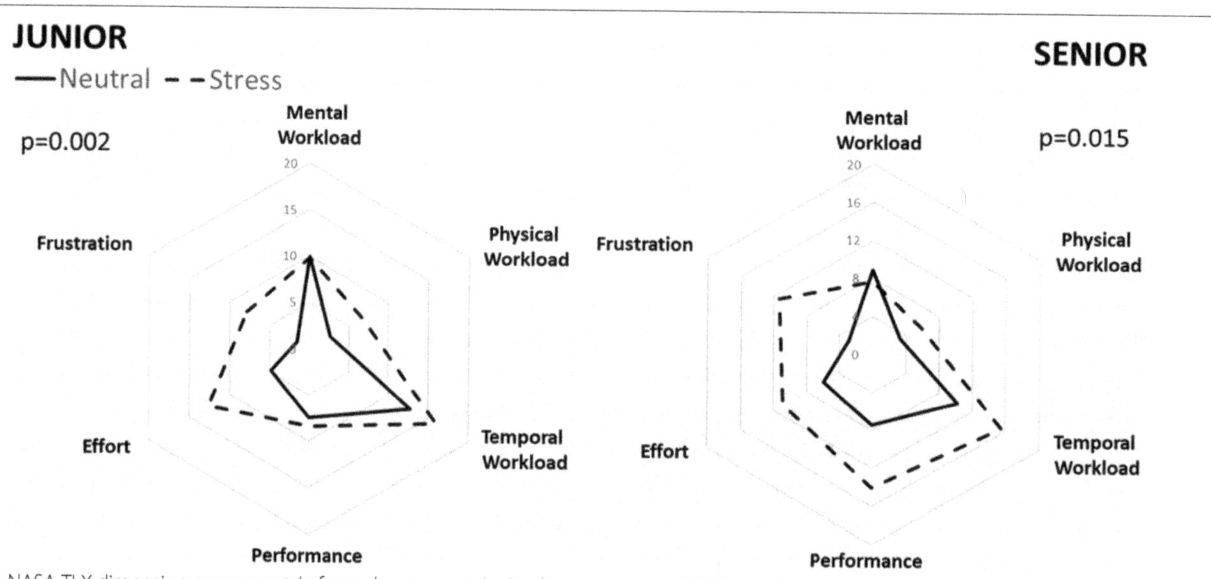

Fig. 2 NASA-TLX dimension assessment. Left graph represents juniors' assessment, and right graph senior's assessment. Plain line represents measurements during neutral scenario, and dotted line measurements during stress scenario. *p* value compared NASA-TLX between each scenarios and for each group. There was a difference of NASA-TLX between neutral and stress scenario for juniors (38.5±19.7 vs. 65±16.6; $p=0.002$) and for seniors (39.2±15.7 vs. 61.3±12.9; $p=0.015$)

condition (Table 2, Fig. 1). SCL did not differ between scenarios. The number of blinks and eye fixations was statistically higher in stress condition.

Task load index significantly differed, and subjective assessment of stress felt during scenarios was statistically higher during stress condition.

Emotional excitation in each group

HR, maxHR and AVNN differed statistically between neutral and stress conditions for seniors (Table 2). We did not observe a difference in HRV patterns between neutral and stress condition for juniors, except with SDNN.

SCL did not differ between scenarios for seniors and juniors, and the number of eye fixations was statistically higher in stress condition for seniors.

In the TLX assessment, temporal workload and effort dimensions were higher during stress condition for juniors, while performance and frustration dimensions likewise differed for seniors as compared to neutral condition.

Intubation success

In neutral condition, 96% of the participants succeed to perform intubation after the first attempt and 100% after the second attempt. In stress condition, 15.5% succeed after the first attempt, 61.5% after the second attempt, and 23% failed to perform intubation.

Discussion

This study highlights the fact that a stress condition during ETI on a simulation model leads to an important emotional excitation as compared to the neutral condition. While emotional excitation yet occurred for all participants, unlike studies performed in surgery [14], the data collected in this study suggest that in such conditions, experience has a limited impact on emotional excitation.

Acute care medicine can be considered as a complex system where emotional excitation is one element, interacting with other components such as task performance, such interactions being responsible for human errors [15]. Medical simulation is a powerful tool to assess the different features of emotional excitation and to measure-interactions between practitioners and tasks. Our study design depicts a comprehensive approach of emotional excitation, where each physiological and psycho-cognitive data enable to explore specific responses to stress.

HR reflects emotional excitation among practitioners [15]. HR is higher during the first few minutes of the simulation [15–17] and subsequently decreases, possibly due to the practitioner's getting used to the simulation exercise. It is worthwhile to note that most of the practitioners had high HR, even exceeding 80% of their theoretical maximal value. In our study, HR was significantly higher during stress condition than neutral condition which is consistent with the literature [18]. Heart rate variability (HRV) is a physiological phenomenon, which is a suitable assessment of the autonomous nervous system controlling the heart functions, thus exploring another aspect of HR in emotional excitation.

Considering that cardiovascular activity is directly influenced by the autonomic nervous system, LF/HF ratio has been proposed as an index of sympathetic to parasympathetic balance of heart rate fluctuation. HF is driven by respiration and appears to be an indicator of the parasympathetic activity, while LF is derived from both parasympathetic and sympathetic activity. HRV was also explored through AVNN and SDNN measurements, which are presumed to be less dependent from emotional excitation. Our data therefore suggest a disturbed autonomic nervous system function during simulation [19]. Such a phenomenon has been associated with mental stress [20] and suggested to indicate inability to respond to physiological variability [21]. Senior HRV tends to be higher than junior ones, which may raise the hypothesis that experience is responsible for a more tranquil behavior, as also observed in other studies [18, 19, 21]. During HRV frequency analysis, low HR values were responsible for a higher LF/HF ratio, the persistence of this indicator within scenarios indicating sympathetic system activation, even in a neutral situation [22]. Short-lasting exposure to psychosocial stressors has been described to indicate parasympathetic withdrawal and increased sympathetic activity [23].

Emotional excitation induces an increase in the sweat gland activity and therefore a modification of the electrical properties of the skin (EDA), which can be assessed by SCL [24]. However, SCL values did not differ in between scenarios within our study. Wachtel et al. reported that in the event of stress, some participants were slower to respond to peripheral stimuli [25]; it could therefore be considered that the delay in between the scenarios was too short in our study. While 10–25% of our participants were estimated as non-responders in terms of EDA [26], some participants may have cardiovascular abnormalities, which may lead to EDA rhythmic artefacts [9]. Finally, it is not possible to obtain high-quality EDA measurements from some individuals, especially in simulation conditions with movement artefacts [9].

Another way to assess stress is eye-tracking techniques, which provides an objective, quantifiable and measurable link between an individual and his immediate environment [11]. Because links between the focus of vision and the focus of cognition have been established [27], eye-tracking may provide useful information for studying situational awareness [28]. As expected, eye fixation and number of blinks were higher in stress conditions, suggesting an enhanced encoding of the environment [29] in order to improve performance. However, juniors had more eye fixation in neutral conditions than experienced practitioners, and they did not experience more fixation during stress condition. As compared to juniors, seniors had more eye fixations in stress conditions. Herten et al. showed that emotional excitation leads to a memory enhancement and to promote attentional narrowing toward relevant stimuli at the expense of irrelevant data, associated with more eye fixation [29]. Schulz et al. have demonstrated that juniors were spending more time looking at the patients' monitoring devices than experts [30]. They suggested than experienced practitioners might be able to maintain sufficient situation awareness without spending more time in monitoring tasks and could actively direct their attention toward manual and relevant tasks [30]. Our results suggested stress condition was not associated with a memory enhancement for juniors, probably due to their inexperience. In normal condition, we suspect than eye fixation was linked with an inappropriate attentional narrowing on irrelevant data. By contrast, because of emotional excitation, seniors were able to better optimize their memory to improve their performance than juniors, resulting with more eye fixation in stress condition. Attentional narrowing in a stressful situation may be related to a greater fixation [31, 32], thus being a predictor of memory performance [33]. While stress seems to prepare the organism for accurate attentional processing of relevant stimuli, eye-tracking technology has the potential to transform the way clinical simulation is evaluated, thereby helping to improve patient safety [34]. Its standardized use may lead to the development of training protocols to improve students' education.

According to our participants, the stress condition generated more emotional excitation and more mental workload than neutral condition. Task load index, assessed by NASA-TLX, is a psycho-cognitive scale measuring difficulty to perform a task [13]. In the NASA-TLX measurement, TLX is influenced by two types of dimension: (1) dimensions depending on human–machine interface (mental, physical and temporal workload) and (2) dimensions depending on the task and on the environment of the task (effort, performance and frustration). Within our study, the importance of each dimension differed in between groups. For seniors, the difference mainly concerned the performance and frustration, while for juniors there was a trend toward physical workload increase. These results could be explained by the fact that experience diverts the focus of participants when they are subjected to emotional excitation. Juniors are concerned by procedure itself, while seniors are concerned by success, which can generate frustration.

Our study suffers from limitations. First, while this was an exploratory study, no power calculation was performed to assess sample size and a post hoc analysis may consider that the observed power was insufficient to allow conclusion on the secondary objectives of the study. Moreover, while practitioners were recruited at their workplace, individual stress factors independent from our study could have been exerted on participants. Second, heart rate variations might be influenced by physiological demand that could differ between scenarios. However, this does not seem to be a major problem for results analysis while: (1) HRV variations are not strictly correlated with heart rate values; (2) physiological demand during the difficult intubation scenario was calibrated to be as lower as possible for the physicians. Furthermore, other recorded parameters (that cannot be correlated with physiological demand) were consistent with an increased emotional excitation in between the two different scenarios: (1) eye-tracking assessment of blinking and eye fixation; (2) psycho-cognitive scoring using Likert scales and NASA-TLX. Third, the motion sensor clusters distributed among the practitioners were a key factor limiting their freedom of movement; the participant was alone to perform the task, while in clinical routine he will be provided some help and use several other difficult intubation equipment. Finally, the choice and interpretation of our sensors results could also be discussed. Concerning eye-tracking, Lotfus et al. concluded that attention and eye fixation could be dissociated [34]. Beside these limitations, our study has some strengths. To the best of our knowledge, this study provides various aspects of emotional excitation, including physiological measurement (HR, eye-tracking and SCL), psycho-cognitive evaluation and subjective stress assessment. Thus, our model is the first to allow a global and comprehensive model assessing emotional excitation due to stressful conditions in acute care medicine procedure.

In conclusion, an isolated analysis of intubation during a simulation is an important source of stressfor seniors and juniors when it is presented as a difficult intubation according to prehospital criteria. According to the Yerkes–Dodson law, subjects may need some part of stress to improve performance, while a too high level of stress may decrease performance [35]. Our study depicts significant physiological and psycho-behavioral changes between ETI conditions. Medical simulation taking into account emotional excitation sensors may enable an enhancement of practitioners' performance while improving teaching.

Abbreviations

AVNN: average of RR intervals; EDA: electrodermal activity; EM: emergency medicine; ETI: endotracheal intubation; HMI: human machine interface; HRV: heart rate variability; maxHR: maximum heart rate; MWL: mental workload; SCL: skin conductance level; SDNN: standard deviation of HRV; TLX: task load index.

Author's contributions

CT and ELH conceived the study. CT, NM, ELH and NP acquired data. ELH and NM provided statistical expertise. CT, NM and ELH wrote the manuscript. All authors read and approved the final manuscript.

Author details

[1] Emergency Department and Prehospital Care, University Hospital of Poitiers, 86000 Poitiers, France. [2] CIC1402 U5 ALIVE – University Hospital of Poitiers, 86000 Poitiers, France. [3] ABS-Lab – Laboratory of Anatomy, Biomechanics and Simulation, Poitiers University, School of Medicine, 86000 Poitiers, France. [4] Emergency Department, University Hospital of Brest - La Cavale Blanche,

29609 Brest Cedex, France. [5] B-com, Institute of Research and Technology, Brest University, 29609 Brest Cedex, France. [6] Department of Intensive Care Medicine, University Hospital of Brest - La Cavale Blanche, Boulevard Tanguy Prigent, 29609 Brest Cedex, France. [7] CeSIM/LaTIM UMR 1101, Western Brittany University – School of Medicine, Rue Camille Desmoulins, 29200 Brest, France.

Acknowledgements
The authors would like to acknowledge all the physicians who agreed to participate in this study. The authors wish to thank Jeffrey Arsham, an American medical translator, for reviewing and editing our original English language manuscript.

Competing interests
ELH is a consultant for Smiths Medical, General Electrics; he is the co-founder of Oxynov Inc., a Canadian R&D company dedicated to automation of respiratory care processes. NM received honoraria from Weinmann medical and Airliquide healthcare for lectures. CT and NP do not declare any conflict of interest.

Funding
No funding was received for this study.

Prior presentations
The following work was presented to the American Thoracic Society 2017 congress: Stress Evaluation During Endotracheal Intubation on a Simulation Model, May 22, 2017, Washington, DC, USA.

References

1. Combes X, Wang HE, Kupas DF, Paris PM, Bates RR, Costantino JP, Yealy DM. Multivariate predictors of failed prehospital endotracheal intubation. Acad Emerg Med. 2003;10:717–24.
2. Health French Authority. Assessment and improvement of practices. Health simulation's good practice; 2012.
3. Neale G, Woloshynowych M, Vincent C. Exploring the causes of adverse events in NHS hospital practice. J R Soc Med. 2001;94:322–30.
4. Bond WF, Deitrick LM, Arnold DC. Using simulation to instruct emergency medicine residents in cognitive forcing strategies. Acad Med. 2004;79:438–46.
5. Daglius Dias R, Scalabrini Neto A. Stress levels during emergency care: a comparison between reality and simulated scenarios. J Crit Care. 2016;33:8–13.
6. Berntson GG, Bigger JT Jr, van der Molen MW. Heart rate variability: origins, methods, and interpretive caveats. Psychophysiology. 1997;34:623–48.
7. Guidelines heart rate variability standards of measurement, physiological interpretation, and clinical use task force of the European Society of Cardiology and the North American Society of Pacing and Electrophysiology. Eur Heart J. 1996;17:354–81.
8. Pagani M, Lombardi F, Guzzetti S, Rimoldi O, Furlan RA, Pizzinelli P, et al. Power spectral analysis of heart rate and arterial pressure variabilities as a marker of sympatho-vagal interaction in man and conscious dog. Circ Res. 1986;59:178–93.
9. Braithwaite JJ, Watson DG, Jones R, Rowe M. A guide for analysing electrodermal activity (EDA) and skin conductance responses (SCRs) for psychological experiments. Psychophysiology. 2015;49:1017–34.
10. Boucsein W, Fowles DC, Grimnes S, Ben Shakhar G, Roth WT, Dawson ME, Filion DL. Publication recommendations for electrodermal measurements. Psychophysiology. 2012;49:1017–34.
11. Mele ML, Federici S. Gaze and eye-tracking solutions for psychological research. Cogn Process. 2012;13:261–5.
12. NASA Task Load Index (TLX) V 1.0 users manual, Human Systems Information Analysis Center; 1988.
13. Hart SG, Staveland LE. Development of NASA-TLX (task load index): results of experimental and theoretical research. Hum Ment Workload. 1988;52:139–83.
14. Wetzel CM, Black SA, Hanna GB, Athanasiou T, Kneebone RL, Nestel D, Wolfe JH, Woloshynowych M. The effects of stress and coping on surgical performance during simulations. Ann Surg. 2010;25(1):171–6.
15. Kohn LT, Corrigan JM, Donaldson MS, editors. Institute of Medicine (US) Committee on Quality of Health Care in America. To err is human: building a safer health system. Washington, DC: National Academies Press (US); 2000.
16. Arora S, Sevdalis N, Nestel D, Woloshynowych M, Darzi A, Kneebone R. The impact of stress on surgical performance: a systematic review of the literature. Surgery. 2010;147:318–30.
17. Mills B, Carter O, Rudd C, Claxton L, O'Brien R. An experimental investigation into the extent social evaluation anxiety impairs performance in simulation-based learning environments amongst final-year undergraduate nursing students. Nurse Educ Today. 2016;45:9–15.
18. Rieger A, Stoll R, Kreuzfeld S, Behrens K, Weippert M. Heart rate and heart rate variability as indirect markers of surgeons' intraoperative stress. Int Arch Occup Environ Health. 2014;87:165–74.
19. Horsten M, Ericson M, Perski A, Wamala SP, Schenck-Gustafsson K, Orth-Gomér K. Psychosocial factors and heart rate variability in healthy women. Psychosom Med. 1999;61:49–57.
20. Myrtek M, Weber D, Brugner G, Muller W. Occupational stress and strain of female students:results of physiological, behavioural, and psychological monitoring. Biol Psychol. 1996;42:379–91.
21. Brosschot JF, Van Dijk E, Thayer JF. Daily worry is related to low heart rate variability during waking and the subsequent nocturnal sleep period. Int J Phychophysiol. 2007;63:39–47.
22. Clays E, De Bacquer D, Crasset V, et al. The perception of work stressors is related to reduced parasympathetic activity. Int Arch Occup Environ Health. 2011;84:185–91.
23. Delaney JPA, Brodie DA. Effects of short-term psychological stress on the time and frequency domains of heart-rate variability. Percept Mot Skills. 2000;91:515–24.
24. Naveteur J, Buisine S, Gruzelier JH. The influence of anxiety on electrodermal responses to distractors. Int J Psychophysiol. 2005;56:261–9.
25. Wachtel PL. Anxiety, attention and coping with threat. J Abnorm Psychol. 1968;73:137–43.
26. Figner B, Murphy RO. Using skin conductance in judgment and decision making research. In: Schulte-Mecklenbeck M, Kuehberger A, Ranyard R, editors. A handbook of process tracing methods for decision research. New York: Psychology Press; 2011.
27. Just MA, Carpenter PA. Eye fixations and cognitive processes. Cogn Psychol. 1976;8:441–80.
28. Williams B, Quested A, Cooper S. Can eye-tracking technology improve situational awareness in paramedic clinical education? OAEM. 2013;5:23–8.
29. Herten N, Otto T, Wolf OT. The role of eye fixation in memory enhanced under stress—an eye tracking study. Neurobiol Learn Mem. 2017;140:134–44.
30. Schulz CM, Schneider E, Schneider G. Visual attention of anaesthetists during simulated critical incidents. Br J Anaesth. 2011;106:807–13.
31. Chajut ED, Algom D. Selective attention improves under stress: implications for theories of social cognition. J Per Soc Psychol. 2003;85:231–48.
32. Christianson SA, Loftus EF, Hoffman H, Loftus GR. Eye fixations and memory for emotional events. J Exp Psychol Learn Mem Cogn. 1991;17:693–701.
33. Loftus GR. Eye fixations and recognition memory for pictures. Cogn Psychol. 1972;3:525–51.
34. Posner MI. Orienting of attention. Q J Exp Psychol A. 1980;32:3–25.
35. Yerkes R, Dodson J. The relation of strength of stimulus to rapidity of habit-formation. J Comp Neurol Psychol. 1908;18:459–82.

Usefulness of video-laryngoscopy with the Airway Scope for intubation performance and learning: an experimental manikin controlled study

Pierre-Louis Declercq[1], Michael Bubenheim[2], Stéphanie Gelinotte[1], Kévin Guernon[1], Jean-Baptiste Michot[1], Vincent Royon[1], Dorothée Carpentier[1], Gaëtan Béduneau[1,3], Fabienne Tamion[1] and Christophe Girault[1,3,4*]

Abstract

Background: Different video-laryngoscopes (VDLs) for endotracheal intubation (ETI) have recently been developed. We compared the performance of the VDL Airway Scope (AWS) with the direct laryngoscopy by Macintosh (DLM) for ETI success, time and learning.

Methods: We performed an experimental manikin controlled study. Twenty experienced (experts) and 40 inexperienced operators (novices) for DLM-ETI were enrolled. None of them had experience with the use of AWS-VDL. Novices were assigned to start learning with DLM or AWS, and two sub-groups of 20 novices were formed. Experts group constituted the control group. Each participant performed 10 ETI attempts with each device on the same standard manikin. The primary endpoint was the ETI success probability. Secondary endpoints were ETI time, technical validity and qualitative evaluation for each technique. We also assessed the learning order and the successive attempts effects for these parameters.

Results: Overall, 1200 ETI attempts were performed. ETI success probability was higher with the AWS than with the DLM for all operators (98 vs. 81 %; $p < 0.0001$) and for experts compared to novices using devices in the same order (97 vs. 83 %; $p = 0.0002$). Overall ETI time was shorter with the AWS than with the DLM (13 vs. 20 s; $p < 0.0001$) and for experts compared to novices using devices in the same order (11 vs. 21 s; $p < 0.0001$). Among novices, those starting learning with AWS had higher ETI success probability (89 vs. 83 %; $p = 0.03$) and shorter ETI time (18 vs. 21 s; $p = 0.02$). Technical validity was found better with the AWS than DLM for all operators. Novices expressed global satisfaction and device preference for the AWS, whereas experts were indifferent.

Conclusions: AWS-VDL permits faster, easier and more reliable ETI compared to the DLM whatever the previous airway ETI experience and could be a useful device for DLM-ETI learning.

Keywords: Intubation, Video-laryngoscopy, Airway Scope, Macintosh, Simulation, Learning

Background

Endotracheal intubation (ETI) is a routine life-saving procedure for airway management, and direct laryngoscopy with the Macintosh laryngoscope (DLM) is probably the most common way to perform ETI. Nevertheless, ETI using DLM (DLM-ETI) is a high-risk procedure, which can lead to vital complications, particularly in intensive care unit (ICU) patients [1, 2]. These risks are related to the critical setting as well as the underlying disease (hypoxemia, hemodynamic instability) and technical conditions of ETI [3]. Furthermore, learning and regular

*Correspondence: Christophe.Girault@chu-rouen.fr
[4] Service de Réanimation Médicale, Hôpital Charles Nicolle, Centre Hospitalier Universitaire-Hôpitaux de Rouen, 1, Rue de Germont, 76031 Rouen Cedex, France
Full list of author information is available at the end of the article

training are needed to sufficiently acquire skills and experience with the DLM technique [4–7].

In the past few years, new devices called video-laryngoscopes (VDLs) have been developed for improving airway management. With optical or video technique, most of these instruments allow to indirectly visualize the larynx and control the endotracheal tube (ETT) passing throughout the glottis [8]. To date, these different VDLs have been mainly used in the operating and emergency room or prehospital setting [7, 8]. Although VDL has been more recently applied in ICU setting [9–16], some authors have shown that ETI with VDL (VDL-ETI) could be associated with longer ETI time, lower oxygen saturation and even higher mortality as compared to conventional DLM-ETI [9, 13]. In fact, due to their technical conception, VDL may have their respective advantages and pitfalls, and their place may be still controversial in the ICU where airway management appears more hazardous and insufficiently studied [17].

Therefore, there is a need to rigorously assess each VDL device on an experimental and clinical basis in order to optimize ETI success. The Airway Scope (AWS®, Pentax Corp., Tokyo, Japan) is a new VDL device first reported in 2006 (Fig. 1) [18]. We hypothesized that ETI success rate, time and learning to perform a reliable ETI could be optimized by the use of the AWS as compared to the DLM, in experienced and inexperienced operators.

Methods

We conducted an experimental manikin controlled study to compare the AWS and DLM performance for ETI success and time, as well as ETI learning between experienced and inexperienced operators. All operators agreed to participate in this manikin study, and as it was a teaching study, which enrolled no patients and did not evaluate physiopathological process, our local ethics committee (Comité de Protection des Personnes du Nord Ouest I) stated that no ethical approval and no consent were required (conclusion date February 20, 2015, chairperson address: Pr F. Bauer, Hôpital Charles Nicole, Centre Hospitalier-Universitaire de Rouen, 1 rue de Germont 76031, France). No company sponsored the study nor supplied any device used. Experienced operators, named "experts," were 20 senior ICU physicians ($n = 9$) or anesthesia residents ($n = 11$) who had previously performed more than 100 DLM-ETI but with no prior experience

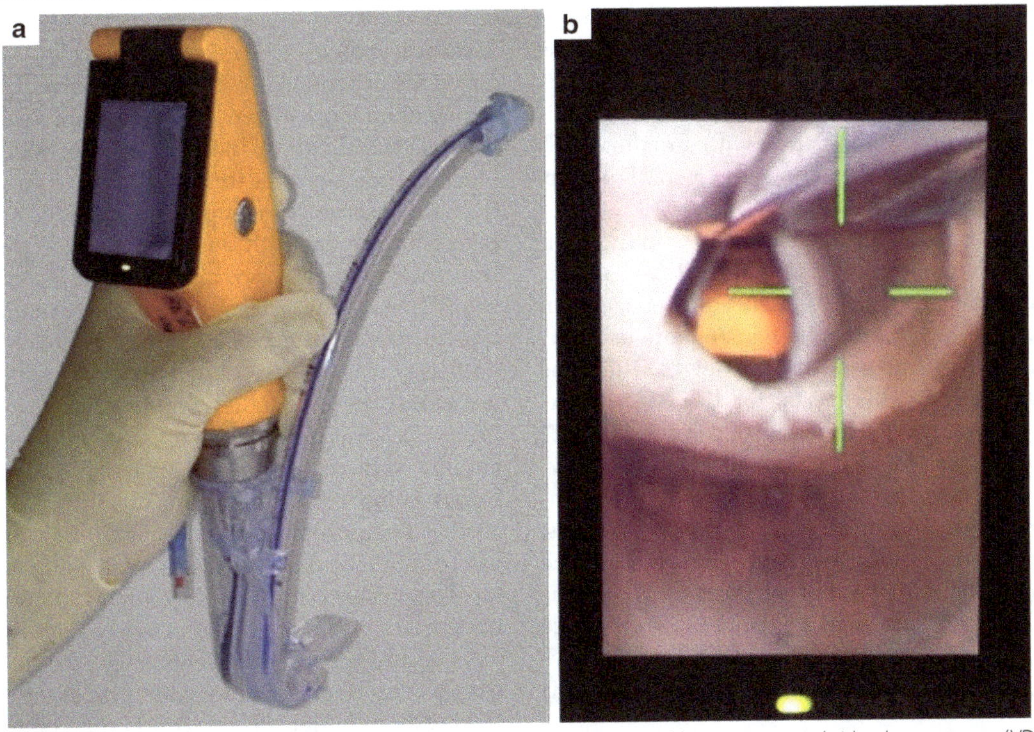

Fig. 1 Airway Scope® (AWS; Pentax Corp., Tokyo, Japan) device. **a** The AWS is a portable and battery-operated video-laryngoscope (VDL) with an integrated and wide-viewing-angle (180°) liquid crystal display (LCD) monitor (6.1 cm) providing an indirect laryngoscopy of the airway via a charged coupled device attached to the blade tip of the AWS. The single-use intlock blade has a specific tube guide to accept the ETT (internal diameter between 6.5 and 8 mm). AWS-ETI requires to load and lift the epiglottis with the AWS blade tip. **b** Once the target signal on the LCD monitor is aligned with the glottis opening, the ETT is passed through the vocal cords (**a**). Then, the AWS is removed laterally, leaving the ETT in place

with AWS-ETI. Inexperienced operators, named "novices," were 40 medical students with no prior experience with either of the two ETI techniques. Male and female participants were equally distributed for each novice sub-group (10 vs. 10), except for the expert sub-group (13 vs. 7, respectively).

ETI was performed on a simple manikin head (Cparlene®, Adult Airway Larry manikin, CPR Savers & First Aid Supply, Scottsdale, USA) without any difficult ETI criteria, either with the DLM (blade size no. 3) or with the AWS. The AWS is a portable and battery-operated VDL with an integrated and wide-viewing-angle (180°) liquid crystal display (LCD) monitor (6.1 cm) providing an indirect laryngoscopy of the airway via a charged coupled device attached to the blade tip of the AWS. The single-use intlock blade has a specific tube guide to accept the ETT (Fig. 1a). Concerning AWS-ETI, in contrast to DLM-ETI, the ETT must be preloaded on the tube guide and ETI requires to load and lift the epiglottis with the blade tip. Once the target signal on the LCD monitor is aligned with the glottis opening, the ETT is passed through the vocal cords (Fig. 1b). Then, the AWS is removed laterally, leaving the ETT in place. For AWS-ETI, the ETT was already preload in the blade-side channel before starting the ETI attempt. All ETI were performed with no introducer and a lubricated low-pressure cuffed ETT (Portex®, Smiths Medical, St Paul, USA) with an internal diameter of 7.5 mm. The manikin head was maintained in a neutral position, i.e., not in improved Jackson's position. The good ETT position was confirmed by lung inflation with a manual self-inflating bag (AMBU® Mark IV, Ambu Corp., Ballerup, Denmark).

All inexperienced students underwent 30-min theoretical and practical training, including an ETI demonstration with each device by one experienced investigator in both techniques. During this training, students had only one attempt on the manikin with each device. The same program was given to all experts, for the AWS alone. Then, each participant performed 10 consecutive ETI attempts on the manikin with both devices. The novice operators were assigned to two different study sub-groups according to the device order of the 10 attempts, whereas the experts group performed all attempts in the same order. Therefore, three sub-groups of 20 operators were organized according to their ETI experience and device order, i.e., expert (DLM then AWS), novice 1 (DLM then AWS) and novice 2 (AWS then DLM) sub-groups.

The primary endpoint of the study was the ETI success probability with each technique. ETI success was defined as an ETI performed within 60 s, with ETT in place in the trachea. Consequently, ETI failure could have been either due to a delayed ETI (>60 s) or due to esophageal intubation. Several secondary endpoints were assessed. The ETI time was defined as the time taken from the blade (DLM or AWS) first passing the incisors until ETT passage through the vocal cords. We also reported the time between the ETT passage through the vocal cords and lung inflation. The ETI technical validity for each attempt with both devices was scored and visually assessed by collecting the following adverse events: for the DLM: dental trauma based on the excessive pressure exerted by the blade on the upper incisors, epiglottis loading and default of epiglottis traction due to a lack of handle traction up and forward; for the AWS: ETT dislodgment (mobilization outside the blade channel or ablation when removing the AWS laterally), epiglottis not loaded and epiglottis luxation as well as blade malposition in the glottis. The number of esophageal intubations for both devices and the Cormack and Lehane grade for the DLM were also recorded [19].

After performing 10 ETI attempts with each device, all participants were asked to rate the following qualitative evaluation criteria using a 5-point Likert scale: ease of assembly of the device, difficulty with ETT manipulation, force of traction required for ETI, as well as the global satisfaction with the technique. It was also asked for their preference regarding the techniques for everyday use.

Statistical analysis

Given the dependence between successive attempts of the same volunteer, a mixed-effect logistic regression model was used [20]. As operator's selection was based on a block design, sex was treated as a random block effect. Because observed times appeared skewed, a mixed-effect regression model with auto-correlated errors was used with time being lognormal. Point and interval estimates were then retransformed using the exponential function to present the results in conventional units. Since no failure was observed in all operator groups at several occasions, the p value for differences between attempts using AWS was derived by comparing the results of each attempt with respect to the first one, the one with the lowest number of successes for this device, and then correcting for multiple testing using Holm's procedure. In case of undefined logits, the sign test was carried out for local testing and simple logistic regression was used in all other cases.

As regards technical events, the number per operator was described using median, first and third quartiles [$Q1$–$Q3$]. In order to assess whether operator groups differed with respect to the occurrence of these events, Freeman–Halton's test was used when results were heavily tied, i.e., events happened to less than 8 operators, otherwise the Kruskal–Wallis test was taken. In order to come to know whether operators assessed both devices differently, the sign test was used.

A p value less than 0.05 was considered statistically significant.

Results

Sixty participants performed 20 ETI attempts each, yielding 400 ETI attempts for each sub-group, i.e., a total of 1200 ETI attempts were assessed.

Considering all ETI attempts, we observed 111 failures with the DLM and 14 with the AWS (Table 1). In univariable analysis, the overall ETI success probability was significantly higher for the AWS compared to the DLM (98 vs. 81 %; $p < 0.0001$), for experts compared to novices 1 (97 vs. 83 %; $p = 0.0002$) and for novices 2 compared to novices 1 (89 vs. 83 %; $p = 0.03$). No significant learning effect of successive attempts was observed for ETI success. These findings were confirmed by multivariable analysis with independent factors (Table 1). As regards univariable analysis, ETI time was significantly shorter with AWS compared to DLM for all operators (13 vs. 20 s; $p < 0.0001$), for experts compared to novices 1 (11 vs. 21 s; $p < 0.0001$) and for novices 2 compared to novices 1 (18 vs. 21 s; $p = 0.02$) (Table 2). When compared to the first attempt, ETI time was significantly reduced at the third attempt (21 vs. 17 s; $p = 0.003$) and for all further attempts (Table 2). Multivariable analysis with independent factors led to the same conclusions (Table 2).

All experts succeeded their 10 AWS-ETI attempts, whereas 9 novices failed at least once (3 and 6 novices in sub-groups 1 and 2, respectively). Fourteen experts (70 %) succeeded all DLM-ETI attempts in contrast to 3 (15 %) and 7 (35 %) novices in sub-groups 1 and 2, respectively (data not shown).

Empirical ETI learning curves are shown separately for AWS (Figs. 2, 3) and DLM (Figs. 4, 5). The AWS-ETI success proportion curves for novices are close to that of experts (Fig. 2). Looking at AWS alone and noting that no failure was observed for several attempts, no evidence was found for an effect of experience, learning order and successive attempts (Fig. 2). ETI time for AWS alone was significantly shorter for experts when compared to novices 1 (9 vs. 16 s; $p < 0.0001$), when learning order began with AWS instead of DLM (13 vs. 16 s; $p = 0.0001$) and with increasing number of attempts (10 and 19 s, at first and tenth attempts, respectively; $p < 0.0001$) (Fig. 3). Learning curves were different for each sub-group with DLM (Figs. 4, 5). When considering DLM alone, DLM-ETI success proportion was significantly higher for experienced operators as compared to novices 1 (95 vs. 82 %; $p = 0.0002$), when learning started with AWS as compared to DLM (82 vs. 68 %; $p = 0.002$), but no significant effect of successive attempt was found (Fig. 4). ETI time for DLM alone changed significantly between the first and the tenth attempts (24 and 18 s, respectively; $p = 0.048$) and was shorter for experts (13 vs. 28 s; $p < 0.0001$) and for novices 2 (23 vs. 28 s; $p = 0.0002$) as compared to novices 1 (Fig. 5).

In univariable analysis, the time between the ETT passage through the vocal cords and lung inflation was found significantly shorter for all operators when the DLM was used as compared to AWS (9 vs. 11 s; $p < 0.0001$), when ETI was performed by experts (7 vs. 13 s; $p < 0.0001$) or by novices 2 (12 vs. 13 s; $p = 0.005$) as compared to novices 1, and with increasing number of attempts (12 and 9 s, at first and tenth attempts, respectively; $p < 0.001$). All these findings were confirmed by multivariable analysis (data not shown).

ETI technical validity and adverse events are reported in Tables 3 and 4. The DLM-ETI technical validity appeared higher for experts than for both novice sub-groups ($p = 0.0005$; Table 3). All adverse events occurred more frequently in these two sub-groups, and dental pressure was the main event reported. There were few adverse events with the AWS-ETI and virtually no difference in technical validity between the three sub-groups (Table 4). The main events reported were epiglottis luxation for experts ($p = 0.04$) and delayed ETI time for both novice sub-groups ($p = 0.04$).

Concerning qualitative assessment of ETI technique (data not shown), DLM was considered easier to assemble than the AWS by expert and novice 2 sub-groups. ETT manipulation with DLM was considered easier by experts although novices reported no difference. All sub-groups agreed that DLM-ETI required more force than did AWS-ETI. ETI global satisfaction and preference were in favor of the AWS in both novice sub-groups, whereas experts were indifferent.

Discussion

To our knowledge, this is the largest controlled manikin study comparing a new device, AWS-VDL, with the DLM technique for ETI. The AWS allowed faster, easier and more reliable ETI performance than the DLM whatever the previous airway ETI experience. Interestingly, novice operators who started with the AWS performed DLM-ETI more efficiently than those starting with the DLM, which suggests AWS to be a useful device for DLM-ETI learning. Furthermore, there was no effect of successive attempts on ETI success probability with both devices. This could mean that for novice operators, AWS-ETI learning on manikin is achieved after the first attempts. By contrast, and as demonstrated in previous studies [4–6], 10 ETI attempts were found insufficient for novice operators to perform DLM-ETI with reliably. Finally, our results demonstrate that AWS-ETI acquisition may require less operator skill than the DLM.

Table 1 Factors potentially influencing endotracheal intubation success probability

	All attempts ($n = 1200$)		Univariable analysis*					Multivariable analysis***				
			Success** probability	95 % CI limits				Success probability for novices 1	95 % CI limits			
	Number of attempts, *n*	Failure attempts, *n* (%)		Lower	Upper	Odds ratio	*p* value		Odds ratio	Lower	Upper	*p* value
ETI device	1200	125 (10.4)										
DLM	600	111 (18.5)	0.81	0.67	0.90	1.00	<0.0001	0.69	–	0.005	1.00	<0.0001
AWS	600	14 (2.3)	0.98	0.94	0.99	9.57		0.96	–	0.09	1.00	
Operator sub-group (device order)												
Experts (DLM then AWS)	400	10 (2.5)	0.97	0.94	0.99	8.04	0.0002	–	9.06	4.17	19.71	<0.0001
Novices 1 (DLM then AWS)	400	70 (17.5)	0.83	0.72	0.90	1.00	–	–	1.00	–	–	–
Novices 2 (AWS then DLM)	400	45 (11.3)	0.89	0.81	0.94	1.68	0.03	–	1.80	1.12	2.89	0.02
Attempt number in the series of 10 attempts												
1	120	17 (14.2)	0.87	0.73	0.94	1.00	Reference	–	–	–	–	–
2	120	18 (15)	0.85	0.71	0.93	0.89	0.70	–	–	–	–	–
3	120	12 (10)	0.90	0.79	0.96	1.41	0.39	–	–	–	–	–
4	120	17 (14.2)	0.86	0.72	0.93	0.95	0.88	–	–	–	–	–
5	120	8 (6.7)	0.93	0.84	0.97	2.21	0.08	–	–	–	–	–
6	120	13 (10.8)	0.89	0.77	0.95	1.29	0.52	–	–	–	–	–
7	120	11 (9.2)	0.91	0.80	0.96	1.56	0.28	–	–	–	–	–
8	120	8 (6.7)	0.93	0.84	0.97	2.21	0.08	–	–	–	–	–
9	120	10 (8.3)	0.92	0.82	0.97	1.73	0.19	–	–	–	–	–
10	120	11 (9.2)	0.90	0.79	0.96	1.42	0.35	–	–	–	–	–

ETI endotracheal intubation, *DLM* direct laryngoscopy with Macintosh, *AWS* video-laryngoscopy with Airway Scope®

* Univariable analysis, all of the 1200 attempts have been analyzed separately according to 3 variables: ETI device (DLM vs. AWS), operator sub-group (experts vs. novices 1 and novices 1 vs. novices 2) and the attempt number in the series of 10 attempts

** Probability of a single successful attempt for one operator

*** Novices 1 is the reference sub-group of the multivariable analysis, i.e., the simultaneous analysis of 2 variables: ETI device (DLM vs. AWS) and operator sub-group (experts vs. novices 1 and novices 1 vs. novices 2). For example, the probability of a successful attempt is 9.06 higher for an expert than a novice 1

Table 2 Factors potentially influencing endotracheal intubation time

	All attempts ($n = 1200$)		Univariable analysis*				Multivariable analysis**				
			ETI Time (s)	95 % CI limits		*p* value	ETI time at first attempt for novices 1 (s)	Time multiplier***	95 % CI limits		*p* value
	Number of attempts, *n*	Sample arithmetic mean time (s)		Lower	Upper				Lower	Upper	
ETI device	1200	19.63									
DLM	600	24.52	20.44	16.18	25.83	<0.0001	35.65	–	29.61	42.93	<0.0001
AWS	600	14.73	12.72	10.08	16.06		22.51	–	18.75	27.02	
Operator sub-group (device order)											
Experts (DLM then AWS)	400	12.53	11.01	9.28	13.07	<0.0001	–	0.54	0.49	0.58	<0.0001
Novices 1 (DLM then AWS)	400	25.35	20.51	17.29	24.32		–	1.00	–	–	–
Novices 2 (AWS then DLM)	400	21.00	18.37	15.49	21.79	0.02	–	0.83	0.77	0.90	<0.0001
Attempt number in the series of 10 attempts											
1	120	24.92	20.99	16.42	26.84	Reference	–	1.00	–	–	–
2	120	23.63	19.44	15.16	24.92	0.16	–	0.91	0.83	1.01	0.08
3	120	20.62	17.09	13.33	21.93	0.003	–	0.80	0.71	0.89	0.0001
4	120	19.56	15.92	12.41	20.42	<0.0001	–	0.74	0.66	0.84	<0.0001
5	120	18.76	15.22	11.87	19.51	<0.0001	–	0.71	0.63	0.80	<0.0001
6	120	18.22	14.87	11.59	19.09	<0.0001	–	0.69	0.62	0.77	<0.0001
7	120	18.65	15.34	11.94	19.72	<0.0001	–	0.71	0.63	0.80	<0.0001
8	120	17.81	14.59	11.35	18.75	<0.0001	–	0.68	0.60	0.76	<0.0001
9	120	17.03	14.06	10.96	18.03	<0.0001	–	0.65	0.58	0.73	<0.0001
10	120	17.06	13.69	10.61	17.66	<0.0001	–	0.63	0.57	0.70	<0.0001

ETI endotracheal intubation, *DLM* direct laryngoscopy with Macintosh, *AWS* video-laryngoscopy with Airway Scope®

* Univariable analysis, all the 1200 attempts have been analyzed separately according to 3 variables: ETI device (DLM vs. AWS), operator sub-group (experts vs. novices 1 and novices 1 vs. novices 2) and the attempt number in the series of 10 attempts

** Novices 1 at the first attempt serve as reference situation of the multivariable analysis, i.e., the simultaneous analysis of 3 variables: ETI device (DLM vs. AWS), operator sub-group (experts vs. novices 1 and novices 1 vs. novices 2) and the attempt number in the series of 10 attempts

*** Multiplicative factor allowing to estimate ETI time from the novices 1 ETI time for the others situations. For example, ETI time for an expert using AWS at first attempt is estimated to be 12.16 s, i.e., $22.51 \times 0.54 \times 1$

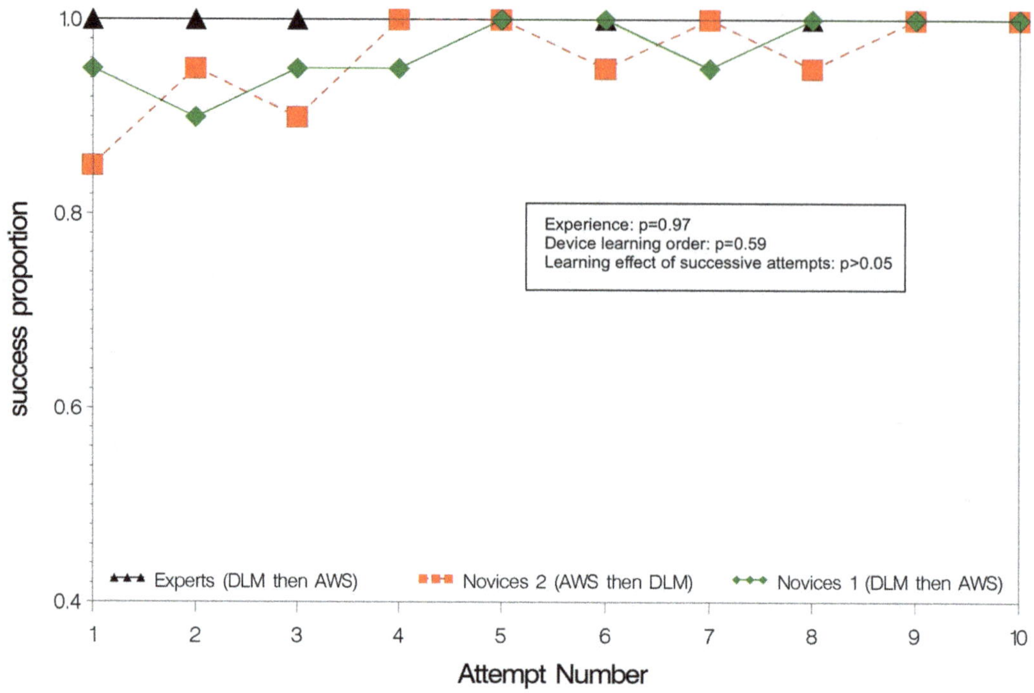

Fig. 2 AWS-ETI learning curves according to ETI success rate by attempt and operator sub-group. *ETI* endotracheal intubation, *DLM* direct laryngoscopy with Macintosh, *AWS* video-laryngoscopy with Airway Scope®. Success proportion is the observed number of successes among 100 attempts for the 3 study sub-groups (experts, novices 1 and novices 2) according to the attempt number in a series of ten attempts and the device used (DLM or AWS). *p* values refer to homogeneity tests for experience (experts compared to novices 1), device learning order (novices 1 compared to novices 2), and to the global test for any difference between attempts, which evaluate the learning effect of successive attempts

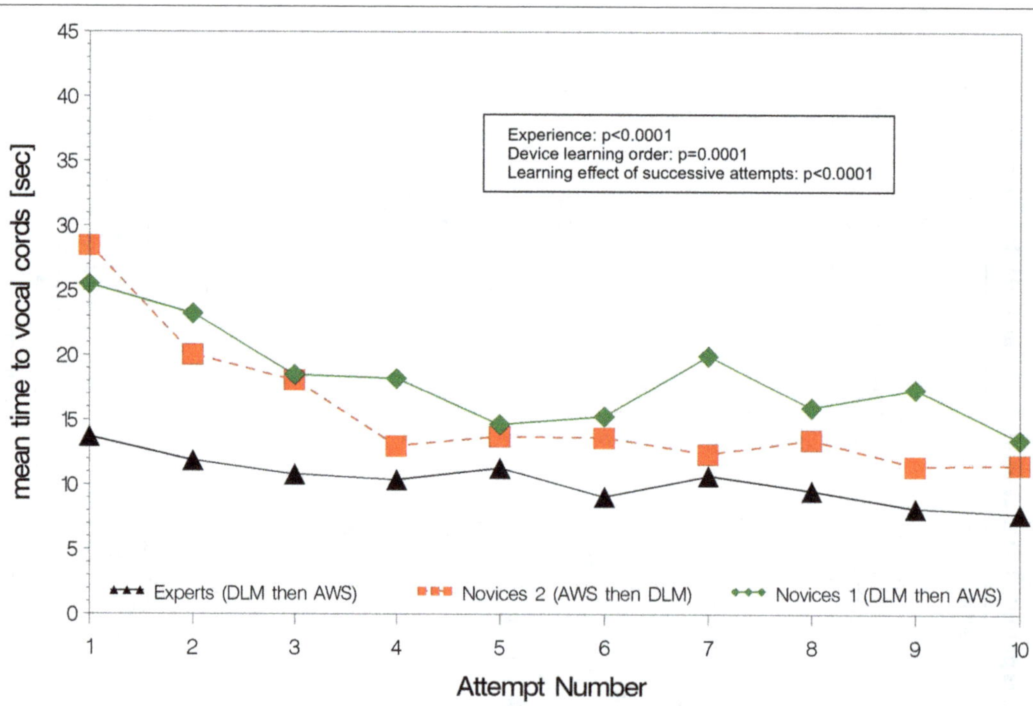

Fig. 3 AWS-ETI learning curves according to ETI time by attempt and operator sub-group. *ETI* endotracheal intubation, *DLM* direct laryngoscopy with Macintosh, *AWS* video-laryngoscopy with Airway Scope®. Mean time to vocal cords corresponds to ETI time (time taken from the blade (DLM or AWS) first passing the incisors until ETT passage through the vocal cords) in seconds according to the attempt number in a series of ten attempts and the device used (DLM or AWS). *p* values refer to homogeneity tests for experience (experts compared to novices 1), device learning order (novices 1 compared to novices 2), and to the global test for any difference between attempts, which evaluate the learning effect of successive attempts

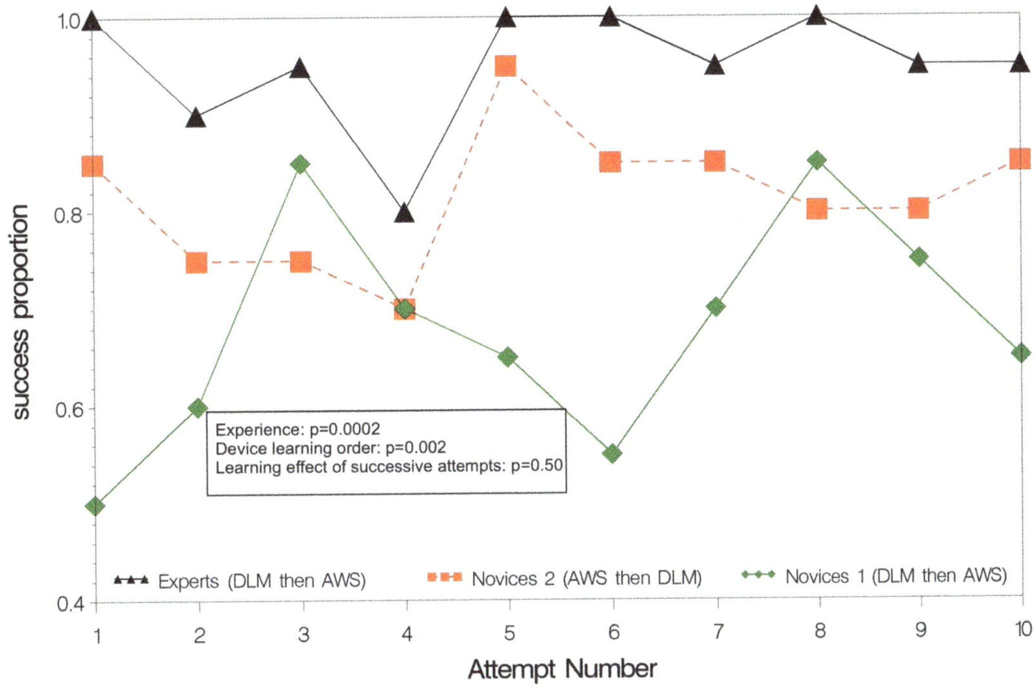

Fig. 4 DLM-ETI learning curves according to ETI success rate by attempt and operator sub-group. *ETI* endotracheal intubation, *DLM* direct laryngoscopy with Macintosh, *AWS* video-laryngoscopy with Airway Scope®. Success proportion is the observed number of successes among 100 attempts for the 3 study sub-groups (experts, novices 1 and novices 2) according to the attempt number in a series of ten attempts and the device used (DLM or AWS). *p* values refer to homogeneity tests for experience (experts compared to novices 1), device learning order (novices 1 compared to novices 2), and to the global test for any difference between attempts, which evaluate the learning effect of successive attempts

Our results for AWS-ETI performance are in agreement with those of one previous manikin study comparing the AWS with DLM in 31 inexperienced nurses [21]. Two prospective randomized clinical studies reported that the AWS allowed to decrease ETI time and failure by inexperienced residents as compared to DLM [22, 23]. In routine anesthesia, the AWS was also able to significantly improve the laryngeal view being more reliable in case of unanticipated difficult ETI as compared to DLM [24].

The time between the ETT passage through the vocal cords and lung inflation was found shorter with the DLM for all operators. The device itself could explain this finding in part. Indeed, the DLM can be more easily removed than the AWS, since the operator has to take care not to accidentally remove the tube inserted in the AWS side channel (Fig. 1a) while he removes the AWS blade laterally [18]. This adverse event occurred three times in six hundred ETI attempts with AWS in our study. In addition, the time required to remove the AWS from the mouth should not delay the lung inflation. In practice, it is possible to ventilate the more hypoxemic patients manually before removing the AWS device. The time between ETI and lung inflation was also found shorter for experts compared to novices. This could be explained by the experts' greater experience to manage cuff inflation as well as manual self-inflating ventilation.

Technical validity and adverse events with both devices, closely related to ETI acquisition and performance, have been poorly reported [21, 25]. We found a better ETI technical validity and less adverse events with the AWS, although epiglottis luxation and AWS blade malposition were frequently reported for experts and novices, respectively. In a clinical study, ETT impingement onto the laryngeal structures has also been observed in 4 % of 320 ETI, but this could be easily managed by adjusting the AWS blade direction [24]. Unlike previous manikin and clinical studies [21–24], we observed two cases of esophageal intubation by novice operators with the AWS. Numerous adverse technical events, a higher Cormack and Lehane grade and delayed DLM-ETI were expected with the DLM in inexperienced sub-groups and reflected the difficulty to acquire the DLM-ETI technique [4–6]. Interestingly, the DLM-ETI failure rate was not negligible (2.5 %) for experienced operators with a significant amount of dental pressure. This could be related to manikin head rigidity, which can be more difficult to intubate than patients [21, 25]. Furthermore, dental pressure by the DLM could have been overestimated as it was

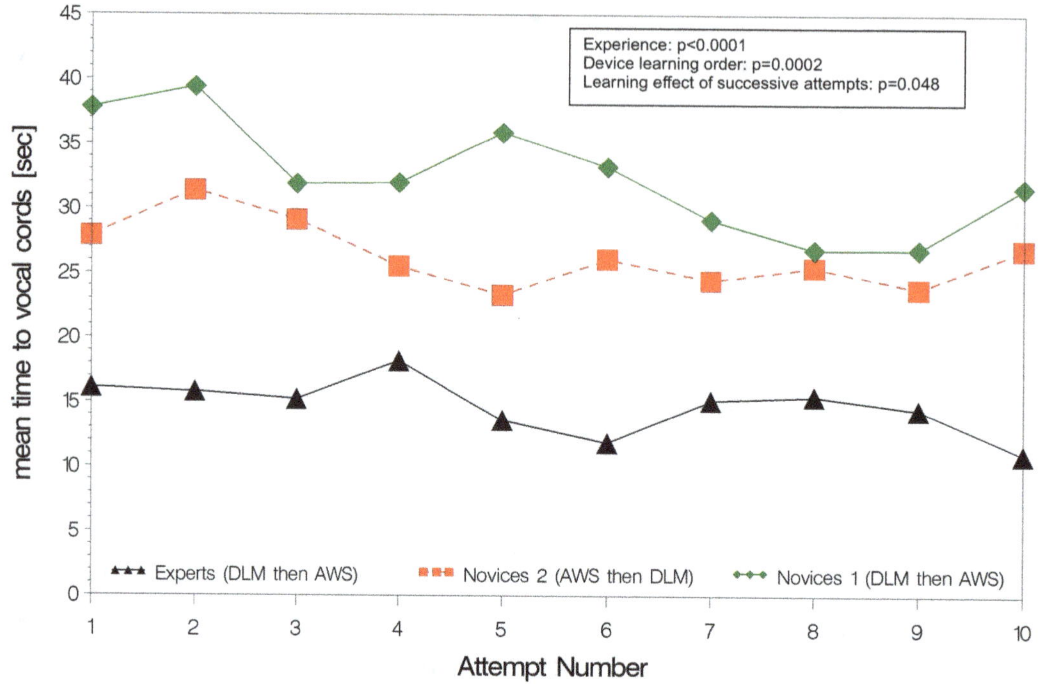

Fig. 5 DLM-ETI learning curves according to ETI time by attempt and operator sub-group. *ETI* endotracheal intubation; *DLM* direct laryngoscopy with Macintosh, *AWS* video-laryngoscopy with Airway Scope®. Mean time to vocal cords corresponds to ETI time (time taken from the blade (DLM or AWS) first passing the incisors until ETT passage through the vocal cords) in seconds according to the attempt number in a series of ten attempts and the device used (DLM or AWS). *p* values refer to homogeneity tests for experience (experts compared to novices 1), device learning order (novices 1 compared to novices 2), and to the global test for any difference between attempts, which evaluate the learning effect of successive attempts

subjectively evaluated and not based on the number of audible teeth clicks [21, 25] or video-recording. Indeed, a video-recording for each attempt would have been useful to improve attempts analysis and their technical validity as well as limit the potential subjective interpretation of investigators, especially for DLM-ETI. Furthermore, watching video-recordings would have allowed to operators to see and understand their potential mistakes and therefore to improve themselves. However, such video-recordings would have been very time-consuming for all the 1200 ETI attempts.

The simplicity and facility of AWS use were confirmed by an ETI qualitative evaluation by all operators including global satisfaction and preference. Nevertheless, AWS assembly and ETT manipulation were considered to be slightly more difficult by expert and novice 1 subgroups. One explanation could be that AWS assembling can be less intuitive as the blade requires to be attached and locked to the monitor by a metallic collar and clip, and the ETT must be maintained in place while the AWS blade is removed laterally [18]. It is noteworthy that all operators considered that the DLM-ETI required more force of traction than did the AWS-ETI. This finding could explain, in part, the significant frequency of excessive dental pressure reported with the DLM including expert operators, as well as the higher ETI failure rate and longer ETI time for novices. Our findings on global satisfaction for the AWS confirm those of previous studies in inexperienced operators [7, 26, 27]. They also showed that DLM-ETI experts may rapidly appropriate the AWS-ETI technique.

AWS-ETI performance and easiness could probably be explained by its technical features. First, the disposable AWS blade is anatomically designed to conform to the shape of the mouth and pharynx and to pass over the tongue dorsum, with the minimal displacement of soft tissues. Second, unlike the DLM, the AWS does not require alignment of the oral, pharyngeal and tracheal axes to visualize the vocal cords [18]. Third, once inserted into the mouth, the AWS requires minimal adjustment of its position, whereas the DLM requires coordinated movements to expose the glottis [21, 24]. Fourth, imposed by the anatomic shape of the blade, epiglottis loading with the AWS blade tip allows to get the best glottis view to perform reliable ETI. By contrast, the DLM-ETI does not require epiglottis loading, but the blade tip must be placed into the glossoepiglottic fold in order to tract epiglottis and getting direct view of the glottis space

Table 3 Technical validity and adverse events for endotracheal intubation with the DLM by operator sub-group

	Operator sub-group (device order)						*p* value*
	Experts (DLM then AWS) *n* = 20		Novices 1 (DLM then AWS) *n* = 20		Novices 2 (AWS then DLM) *n* = 20		
	Events ** (out of 200 attempts)	Median [Q1–Q3]***	Events** (out of 200 attempts)	Median [Q1–Q3]***	Events ** (out of 200 attempts)	Median [Q1–Q3]***	
Technically valid attempts, *n*	146	9 [7–9]	61	2 [1–4]	84	4 [2–6]	0.0005
Adverse technical events							
Esophageal intubation, *n*	6	0 [0–0]	34	1 [0–2]	21	0 [0–2]	0.02
Delayed ETI time (>60 s), *n*	4	0 [0–0]	30	1 [0–2]	16	0 [0–1]	0.003
Dental pressure, *n*	49	1 [0–3]	78	4 [2–5]	76	3 [2–5]	0.02
Epiglottis loading, *n*	1	0 [0–0]	26	1 [0–2]	25	1 [0–2]	0.0001
Lack of traction, *n*	3	0 [0–0]	35	1 [0–4]	15	0 [0–1]	0.002
Cormack–Lehane grade (median)	–	1 [1, 2]	–	2 [1, 2]	–	2 [1, 2]	0.008

ETI endotracheal intubation, *DLM* direct laryngoscopy with Macintosh, *AWS* video-laryngoscopy with Airway Scope®

* Kruskal–Wallis test

** Total number of each event on 200 attempts in each sub-group with DLM

*** Median [1st–3rd quartile] per operator of the number of events on 10 attempts with DLM in each sub-group

Table 4 Technical validity and adverse events for endotracheal intubation with the AWS by operator sub-group

	Operator sub-group (device order)						*p* value
	Experts (DLM then AWS) *n* = 20		Novices 1 (DLM then AWS) *n* = 20		Novices 2 (AWS then DLM) *n* = 20		
	Events* (out of 200 attempts)	Median [Q1–Q3]**	Events* (out of 200 attempts)	Median [Q1–Q3]**	Events* (out of 200 attempts)	Median [Q1–Q3]**	
Technically valid attempts, *n*	179	9 [8–10]	177	9 [9, 10]	184	9 [9, 10]	0.59****
Adverse technical event							
Esophageal intubation, *n*	0	0 [0–0]	1	0 [0–0]	1	0 [0–0]	1.0***
Delayed ETI time (>60 s.), *n*	0	0 [0–0]	5	0 [0–0]	7	0 [0–0]	0.04***
Epiglottis luxation, *n*	21	1 [0–2]	13	0 [0–1]	8	0 [0–1]	0.04****
Epiglottis unloaded, *n*	0	0 [0–0]	2	0 [0–0]	0	0 [0–0]	0.32***
ETT dislodgment, *n*	0	0 [0–0]	0	0 [0–0]	3	0 [0–0]	0.1***
Blade malposition in glottis, *n*	0	0 [0–0]	9	0 [0–0]	5	0 [0–0]	0.43***

ETI endotracheal intubation, *DLM* direct laryngoscopy with Macintosh, *AWS* video-laryngoscopy with Airway Scope®

* Total number of each event on 200 attempts in each sub-group with AWS

** Median [1st–3rd quartile] per operator of the number of events on 10 attempts with AWS in each sub-group

*** Freeman–Halton's test

**** Kruskal–Wallis test

[28]. This technical features, notably the need for loading the epiglottis or not, could explain in part the difference between both devices regarding ETI performance such as handling and the risk of adverse events or injuries. Therefore, the entire ETI procedure being performed under visual control with the AWS monitor, ETI could be more secured and supervised.

Simulation program and manikin studies are now essential for operator's skill acquisition of life-saving procedures like ETI in the ICU environment [29–31]. Anyway, clinical studies are obviously needed. A recent meta-analysis, involving nine clinical ICU studies, demonstrated that VDL-ETI in ICU could be useful to decrease difficult ETI, esophageal intubation, Cormack 3/4 grades, and increase first-attempt success, but did not reduce severe complications [16]. However, these results should be interpreted with caution due to the between study heterogeneity depending on the outcome analyzed, operator experience and different VDL devices used. In fact, these ICU studies primarily assessed the GlideScope (GVL®; Verathon Medical, Bothell, WA, USA) [16], a VDL with a different conception and operating mode, mainly due to a deported screen and the use of a separate preformed metal stylet inserted into the ETT. In contrast, two prospective randomized clinical cohort studies performed by inexperienced providers outside the ICU found better performances for the AWS [22, 23]. Furthermore, due to their technical conception, the best glottis view provided by different VDL may not always match ETI outcomes [9, 13]. AWS advantages result from its integrated monitor and ETT side channel into the handle and blade, respectively, allowing to facilitate the ETT insertion and to visualize its entire progression [24]. These features are useful to avoid the difficulties due to the necessary coordination between a separate monitor and/or the use of an additional stylet. In addition, other VDL may partially blind the ETT progression and result in serious complications [32]. It must be underlined that our experimental manikin study has been conducted with a non-difficult airway head, and results cannot be expanded in cases of difficult ETI. Experimental and clinical studies have previously shown, however, that AWS-ETI could be a reliable technique in different difficult airways such as pharyngeal obstruction, cervical spine rigidity, tongue edema [26, 33] and limited mouth opening ($\approx$20 mm) [34]. AWS can also be used according to a multimodal approach combining a flexible stylet or a fiberoptic bronchoscope, particularly if nasal ETI is required [35].

Nevertheless, there are some situations at risk of AWS-ETI difficulty or failure. The blade introduction in the mouth can be difficult due to the device length. However, the AWS blade introduction first, and secondarily connect to the AWS handle, may permit to introduce the entire device in the mouth. Despite a specific blade-side channel for introducing an aspiration catheter, abundant pharyngeal secretions can also obstruct the LCD glottis view, as well as condensation on the blade extremity [24]. In rare cases, the larynx can be difficult to reach due to a shorter length of the blade [36]. Finally, the minimum mouth opening required for the AWS-VDL insertion appears to be 20–25 mm [34], and AWS usefulness in cases of sub-glottic tumors needs to be assessed, likely in association with fiberoptic bronchoscope [37].

Therefore, all these features are strong arguments to initially perform manikin studies and to conduct then prospective clinical studies with each type of VDL, in no difficult as well as difficult ETI settings, before to determine the VDL-ETI's place in the ICU [38].

Some limitations must be underlined in our study. First, it was a manikin study that may not strictly reproduce the human clinical conditions for ETI, particularly in the ICU regarding the underlying disease and technical circumstances. However, the manikin's airway has been recognized as an acceptable and realistic condition for ETI evaluation [29–31]. Second, as it was obviously not possible to perform a blind study, a potential bias may exist, particularly for experts and investigators. Nevertheless, this bias was probably reduced, as our main endpoints were clearly defined. Lastly, we used subjective qualitative criteria as secondary endpoints for which the evaluation may widely change. However, this was probably unlikely as we found a good agreement between these criteria and our objective endpoints, particularly for ETI success and time.

Conclusions

This large experimental manikin controlled study demonstrates that the AWS allowed faster, easier and more reliable ETI than did the DLM whatever the previous airway ETI experience. It also confirms that DLM-ETI needs a prolonged learning, whereas AWS-ETI requires less operator skill than does the DLM to effectively and rapidly secure the airway. Our results further suggest that the AWS may be a useful device for ETI learning with the DLM. Nevertheless, further randomized clinical studies are still warranted to determine the respective place of different VDL devices for ETI practice, particularly in the ICU setting.

Abbreviations

AWS: Airway Scope; AWS-ETI: Endotracheal intubation with Airway Scope; AWS-VDL: Airway Scope video-laryngoscope; DLM: Direct laryngoscopy with Macintosh; DLM-ETI: Endotracheal intubation with Macintosh laryngoscope; ETI: Endotracheal intubation; ETT: Endotracheal tube; ICU: Intensive care unit; VDL: Video-laryngoscope; VDL-ETI: Endotracheal intubation with video-laryngoscope.

Authors' contributions

PLD contributed to conception and design of the study, acquisition of data, analysis and interpretation of data, drafted the submitted article and provided final approval of the version to be published. MB contributed to analysis and interpretation of the data, performed the statistical analysis, drafted the submitted article and provided final approval of the version to be published. SG, KG, JBM, VR, DC and FT contributed to data analysis and interpretation, critical revision of the manuscript for important intellectual content and provided final approval of the version to be published. CG was at the study's origin, contributed to study design and conception, study supervision, data analysis and interpretation and provided final approval of the version to be published. All authors read and approved the final manuscript.

Author details

[1] Department of Medical Intensive Care, Rouen University Hospital, Rouen Cedex, France. [2] Department of Clinical Research Support, Biostatistics Unit, Rouen University Hospital, Rouen Cedex, France. [3] UPRES EA 3830-IRIB, Institute for Biomedical Research, Rouen University, Rouen Cedex, France. [4] Service de Réanimation Médicale, Hôpital Charles Nicolle, Centre Hospitalier Universitaire-Hôpitaux de Rouen, 1, Rue de Germont, 76031 Rouen Cedex, France.

Competing interests

All the authors declare that they have no competing interests.

References

1. Jaber S, Amraoui J, Lefrant JY, Arich C, Cohendy R, Landreau L, et al. Clinical practice and risk factors for immediate complications of endotracheal intubation in the intensive care unit: a prospective, multiple-center study. Crit Care Med. 2006;34:2355–61.
2. Cook TM, Woodall N, Harper J, Benger J. Major complications of airway management in the UK: results of the Fourth National Audit Project of the Royal College of Anaesthetists and the Difficult Airway Society. Part 2: intensive care and emergency departments. Br J Anaesth. 2011;106:632–42.
3. De Jong A, Molinari N, Terzi N, Mongardon N, Arnal J-M, Guitton C, et al. Early identification of patients at risk for difficult intubation in the intensive care unit: development and validation of the MACOCHA score in a multicenter cohort study. Am J Respir Crit Care Med. 2013;187:832–9.
4. Konrad C, Schupfer G, Wietlisbach M, Gerber H. Learning manual skills in anesthesiology: Is there a recommended number of cases for anesthetic procedures? Anesth Analg. 1998;86:635–9.
5. Mulcaster JT, Mills J, Hung OR, MacQuarrie K, Law JA, Pytka S, et al. Laryngoscopic intubation: learning and performance. Anesthesiology. 2003;98:23–7.
6. Garza AG, Gratton MC, Coontz D, Noble E, Ma OJ. Effect of paramedic experience on orotracheal intubation success rates. J Emerg Med. 2003;25:251–6.
7. Griesdale DE, Liu D, McKinney J, Choi PT. Glidescope_video-laryngoscopy versus direct laryngoscopy for endotracheal intubation: a systematic review and meta-analysis. Can J Anesth. 2012;59:41–52.
8. Niforopoulou P, Pantazopoulos I, Demestiha T, Koudouna E, Xantos T. Video-laryngoscopes in the adult airway management: a topical review of the literature. Acta Anaesthesiol Scand. 2010;54:1050–61.
9. Griesdale DE, Chau A, Isac G, Ayas N, Foster D, Irwin C, et al. Video-laryngoscopy versus direct laryngoscopy in critically ill patients: a pilot randomized trial. Can J Anaesth. 2012;59:1032–9.
10. Noppens RR, Geimer S, Eisel N, David M, Piepho T. Endotracheal intubation using the C-MAC_video laryngoscope or the Macintosh laryngoscope: a prospective, comparative study in the ICU. Crit Care. 2012;16:R103.
11. Kory P, Guevarra K, Mathew JP, Hegde A, Mayo PH. The impact of video laryngoscopy use during urgent endotracheal intubation in the critically ill. Anesth Analg. 2013;117:144–9.
12. Lakticova V, Koenig SJ, Narasimhan M, Mayo PH. Video laryngoscopy is associated with increased first pass success and decreased rate of esophageal intubations during urgent endotracheal intubation in a medical intensive care unit when compared to direct laryngoscopy. J Intensive Care Med. 2015;30:44–8.
13. Yeatts DJ, Dutton RP, Hu PF, Chang YW, Brown CH, Chen H, et al. Effect of video laryngoscopy on trauma patient survival: a randomized controlled trial. J Trauma Acute Care Surg. 2013;75:212–9.
14. De Jong A, Clavieras N, Conseil M, Coisel Y, Moury PH, Pouzeratte Y, et al. Implementation of a combo videolaryngoscope for intubation in critically ill patients: a before-after comparative study. Intensive Care Med. 2013;39:2144–52.
15. Mosier JM, Whitmore SP, Bloom JW, Snyder LS, Graham LA, Carr GE, et al. Video laryngoscopy improves intubation success and reduces esophageal intubations compared to direct laryngoscopy in the medical intensive care. Crit Care. 2013;17:R237.
16. De Jong A, Molinari N, Conseil M, Coisel Y, Pouzeratte Y, Belafia F, et al. Video laryngoscopy versus direct laryngoscopy for orotracheal intubation in the intensive care unit: a systematic review and meta-analysis. Intensive Care Med. 2014;40:629–39.
17. Cook T, Behringer EC, Benger J. Airway management outside the operating room: hazardous and incompletely studied. Curr Opin Anaesthesiol. 2012;25:461–9.
18. Koyama J, Aoyama T, Kusano Y, Seguchi T, Kawagishi K, Iwashita T, et al. Description and first clinical application of Airway Scope for tracheal intubation. J Neurosurg Anesthesiol. 2006;18:247–50.
19. Cormack RS, Lehane J. Difficult tracheal intubation in obstetrics. Anaesthesia. 1984;39:1105–11.
20. Hedeker D, Gibbons RD. Longitudinal data analysis. Hoboken: Wiley; 2006.
21. Miki T, Inagawa G, Kikuchi T, Koyama Y, Goto T. Evaluation of the Airway Scope, a new video laryngoscope, in tracheal intubation by naive operators: a manikin study. Acta Anaesthesiol Scand. 2007;51:1378–81.
22. Hirabayashi Y, Seo N. Tracheal intubation by non-anaesthetist physicians using the Airway Scope. Emerg Med J. 2007;24:572–3.
23. Hirabayashi Y, Seo N. Tracheal intubation by non-anesthesia residents using the Pentax-AWS Airway Scope and Macintosh laryngoscope. J Clin Anesth. 2009;21:268–71.
24. Suzuki A, Toyama Y, Katsumi N, Kunisawa T, Sasaki R, Hirota K, et al. The Pentax-AWS rigid indirect video laryngoscope: clinical assessment of performance in 320 cases. Anaesthesia. 2008;63:641–7.
25. Malik MA, Hassett P, Carney J, Higgins BD, Harte BH, Laffey JG. A comparison of the Glidescope, Pentax AWS, and Macintosh laryngoscopes when used by novice personnel: a manikin study. Can J Anaesth. 2009;56:802–11.
26. Koyama Y, Inagawa G, Miyashita T, Kikuchi T, Miura N, Miki T, et al. Comparison of the Airway Scope, gum elastic bougie and fiberoptic bronchoscope in simulated difficult tracheal intubation: a manikin study. Anaesthesia. 2007;62:936–9.
27. Lewis AR, Hodzovic I, Whelan J, Wilkes AR, Bowler I, Whitfield R. A paramedic study comparing the use of the Airtraq, Airway Scope and Macintosh laryngoscopes in simulated prehospital airway scenarios. Anaesthesia. 2010;65:1187–93.
28. Henderson JJ. Questions about the Macintosh laryngoscope and technique of laryngoscopy. Eur J Anaesthesiol. 2000;17:2–5.
29. Hesselfeldt R, Kristensen MS, Rasmussen LS. Evaluation of the airway of the SimMan full-scale patient simulator. Acta Anaesthesiol Scand. 2005;49:1339–45.
30. Piquette D, Tarshis J, Regehr G, Fowler RA, Pinto R, LeBlanc VR. Effects of clinical supervision on resident learning and patient care during simulated ICU scenarios. Crit Care Med. 2013;41:2705–11.
31. Kennedy CC, Cannon EK, Warner DO, Cook DA. Advanced airway management simulation training in medical education: a systematic review and meta-analysis. Crit Care Med. 2014;42:169–78.
32. Cooper RM. Complications associated with the use of the GlideScope videolaryngoscope. Can J Anaesth. 2007;54:54–7.
33. Kariya T, Inagawa G, Nakamura K, Fujimoto J, Aoi Y, Morita S, et al. Evaluation of the Pentax-AWS(®) and the Macintosh laryngoscope in difficult intubation: a manikin study. Acta Anaesthesiol Scand. 2011;55:223–7.

34. Komatsu R, Kamata K, Hoshi I, Sessler DI, Ozaki M. Airway Scope and gum elastic bougie with Macintosh laryngoscope for tracheal intubation in patients with simulated restricted neck mobility. Br J Anaesth. 2008;101:863–9.
35. Xue FS, Xiong J, Yuan YJ, Wang Q, Asai T. Pentax-AWS video laryngoscope for awake nasotracheal intubation in patients with a difficult airway. Br J Anaesth. 2010;104:505–6.
36. Sasano N, Yamauchi H, Fujita Y. Failure of the Airway Scope to reach the larynx. Can J Anaesth. 2007;54:774–5.
37. Gaszyński T. A combination of KingVision video-laryngoscope and flexible fibroscope for awake intubation in patient with laryngeal tumor-case report and literature review. Anaesthesiol Intensive Ther. 2015;47:433–5.
38. Apfelbaum JL, Hagberg CA, Caplan RA, Blitt CD, Connis RT, Nickinovich DG, et al. Practice guidelines for management of the difficult airway: an updated report by the American Society of Anesthesiologists Task Force on management of the difficult airway. Anesthesiology. 2013;118:251–70.

17

Plasma microRNAs levels are different between pulmonary and extrapulmonary ARDS patients

Yi Zheng[1,2], Song-qiao Liu[1], Qin Sun[1], Jian-feng Xie[1], Jing-yuan Xu[1], Qing Li[1], Chun Pan[1], Ling Liu[1] and Ying-zi Huang[1*]

Abstract

Background: Mesenchymal stem cells (MSC) obviously alleviate the damage of the structure and function of pulmonary vascular endothelial cells (VEC). The therapeutic effects of MSC are significantly different between pulmonary ARDS (ARDSp) and extrapulmonary ARDS (ARDSexp). MicroRNAs (miRNAs), as important media of MSC regulating VEC, are not studied between ARDSp and ARDSexp. We aimed to explore the plasma levels difference of miRNAs that regulate VEC function and are associated with MSC (*MSC-VEC*-miRNAs) between ARDSp and ARDSexp patients.

Methods: *MSC-VEC*-miRNAs were obtained through reviewing relevant literatures screened in PubMed database. We enrolled 57 ARDS patients within 24 h of admission to the ICU and then collected blood samples, extracted plasma supernatant. Patients' clinical data were collected. Then, plasma expression of *MSC-VEC*-miRNAs was measured by real-time fluorescence quantitative PCR. Simultaneously, plasma endothelial injury markers VCAM-1, vWF and inflammatory factors TNF-α, IL-10 were detected by ELISA method.

Results: Fourteen miRNAs were picked out after screening. A total of 57 ARDS patients were included in this study, among which 43 cases pertained to ARDSp group and 14 cases pertained to ARDSexp group. Plasma miR-221 and miR-27b levels in ARDSexp group exhibited significantly lower than that in ARDSp group (miR-221, 0.22 [0.12–0.49] vs. 0.57 [0.22–1.57], $P = 0.008$, miR-27b, 0.34 [0.10–0.46] vs. 0.60 [0.20–1.46], $P = 0.025$). Plasma vWF concentration in ARDSexp group exhibited significantly lower than that in ARDSp group (0.77 [0.29–1.54] vs. 1.80 [0.95–3.51], $P = 0.048$). Significant positive correlation was found between miR-221 and vWF in plasma levels ($r = 0.688$, $P = 0.022$). Plasma miR-26a and miR-27a levels in non-survival group exhibited significantly lower than that in survival group (miR-26a, 0.17 [0.08–0.20] vs. 0.69 [0.24–2.33] $P = 0.018$, miR-27a, 0.23 [0.16–0.58] vs. 1.45 [0.38–3.63], $P = 0.021$) in ARDSp patients.

Conclusion: Plasma miR-221, miR-27b and vWF levels in ARDSexp group are significantly lower than that in ARDSp group. Plasma miR-26a and miR-27a levels in non-survival group are significantly lower than that in survival group in ARDSp patients.

Keywords: Pulmonary ARDS, Extrapulmonary ARDS, MicroRNA, Vascular endothelial cell

Background

Acute respiratory distress syndrome (ARDS) is a common critical disease in intensive care unit (ICU). In recent years, although mechanical ventilation, liquid management, extracorporeal membrane oxygenation and other therapeutic technologies have improved significantly, ARDS is associated with high morbidity and mortality in critically ill patients [1]. Endothelial dysfunction is a key characteristic of ARDS, giving rise to increasing vascular permeability and then pulmonary edema and respiratory failure [2, 3]. The biological underpinnings

*Correspondence: yz_huang@126.com
[1] Department of Critical Care Medicine, Zhongda Hospital, School of Medicine, Southeast University, No. 87, Dingjiaqiao Road, Gulou District, Nanjing 210009, China
Full list of author information is available at the end of the article

manipulating the development of endothelial dysfunction in ARDS are incompletely cognized and represent the inevitable course to precision diagnosis and treatment.

Patients with ARDS which is a heterogeneous syndrome have variant etiologies and pathologies and respond differently to therapeutic interventions [4]. One approach to reducing ARDS heterogeneity is to subclassify patients as ARDSp (originating from pulmonary disease) or ARDSexp (originating from extrapulmonary disease) [5]. In the early stages of ARDS, there were significant differences in damage degree of endothelial cells between ARDSp and ARDSexp [6, 7]. When lung morphology was analyzed by computed tomography (CT), ARDSp was characterized by prominent consolidation, while ARDSexp was characterized by prominent ground-glass opacification [8]. The two subtypes of ARDS respond differently to therapeutic interventions such as alterations in positive end-expiratory pressure, prone ventilation, and recruitment maneuvers [9–13]. Nevertheless, the underlying mechanism governing this difference needs further research.

Mesenchymal stem cells (MSC), protecting adherens junction (VE-cadherin and β-catenin), reducing the lung endothelial cell apoptosis, improve pulmonary vascular endothelial cells (VEC) permeability of ARDS [14–18]. However, the therapeutic effects of MSC are significantly different between ARDSp and ARDSexp [19]. This is similar to bone marrow-derived mononuclear cell more effectively improving survival, lung mechanics and histology in ARDSexp than these in ARDSp [20]. The mechanism of difference is not entirely clear.

MicroRNAs (miRNAs), a group of small (19–25 nucleotides) non-coding segments of RNA, regulate gene expression by binding to target mRNA to inhibit their translation. MiRNAs also play an important role in the regulation of gene expression in the pathogenesis of ARDS. Previous studies [21, 22] showed that MSC control activity of pulmonary VEC through regulating microRNAs (miRNAs) levels. Herein, we tentatively defined *MSC-VEC*-miRNAs as a group of miRNAs which are associated with MSC, have regulatory effects on VEC and have previously been studied in ARDS. Then, levels of *MSC-VEC*-miRNAs can be different in patients with ARDSp and ARDSexp.

Yet, so far, no study has tested whether *MSC-VEC*-miRNAs may serve as biomarkers distinguish between ARDSp and ARDSexp. In this study, 14 *MSC-VEC*-miRNAs were filtrated through relevant literatures. Further, we have examined the expression levels of these *MSC-VEC*-miRNAs in plasma collected from patients diagnosed as ARDSp and ARDSexp. Our purpose is to explore the plasma levels difference of *MSC-VEC*-miRNAs between ARDSp and ARDSexp which is probably helpful for the study in pathogenesis and clinical diagnosis of ARDSp and ARDSexp.

Methods

Screening of *MSC-VEC*-miRNA

Using the combination of keywords and MeSH terms for "endothelial cell" and "microRNA", we searched PubMed for articles that describe associations between the miRNAs and endothelial cell. Each article was reviewed and associated miRNAs ("miRNAs cluster 1") were recorded. Then, we searched each miRNA in "miRNAs cluster 1" individually in conjunction with mesenchymal stromal cell (e.g., "miR-21" and "mesenchymal stromal cell") and reviewed each article to get miRNAs ("miRNAs cluster 2") associated with mesenchymal stromal cell from "miRNAs cluster 1". Using the same method, we obtained *MSC-VEC*-miRNAs, eligible microRNAs that were associated with MSC, has regulatory effects on VEC and has previously been studied in ARDS (Additional file 1: Table S1).

Subject recruitment and sample acquisition

All new ICU admissions at Zhongda Hospital Affiliated to Southeast University from January 2016 to September 2016 were screened for the presence of ARDS based on acute respiratory distress syndrome: the Berlin Definition [23]. Additional inclusion criteria included 18 years $\leq$ age $\leq$ 89 years and admission into the ICU within the previous 24 h. We excluded immunocompromised patients including history of stem cell transplant, immunosuppressive medication using and excluded patients with malignant tumor and pregnant women.

After signing informed consent, subjects had blood drawn via venipuncture or from pre-existing intravascular catheters. Blood samples from enrolled patients were obtained within 24 h of admission to the ICU. Samples were centrifuged at 1900*g* for 10 min, and the plasma supernatant was extracted and stored in refrigeratory at − 80 degrees Celsius.

Patients data collection

Demographic and clinical data from eligible patients was abstracted from the electronic medical record. Demographic data: gender, age, actual height, actual weight, etc. Patient's condition: main diagnosis, acute physiology and chronic health evaluation (APACHE) II scores, sequential organ failure assessment (SOFA) scores, ARDS etiology. ARDS severity: arterial blood PO_2/FiO_2 ratio, Murray lung injury score. The style of oxygen therapy and parameters: noninvasive ventilation, invasive ventilation and ventilator parameters. Clinical outcomes: ICU and hospital length of stay, 28-day mortality, occurrence of shock (defined by clinician), occurrence of acute kidney injury [KDIGO Clinical Practice Guideline for Acute Kidney Injury].

RNA isolation

The frozen plasma was taken out from refrigeratory and incubated at 37 °C in a water bath until samples are completely thawed. Prolonged incubation should be avoided, which may compromise RNA integrity. RNAs were isolated from plasma samples using miRNeasy serum/plasma kits (Qiagen). The miRNeasy Serum/Plasma Spike-In Control, a *Caenorhabditis elegans* miR-39 miRNA mimic, was chosen as the normalized internal control. 3.5 μl miRNeasy Serum/Plasma Spike-In Control (1.6×10^8 copies/μl working solution) was added to the tube containing the lysate before adding chloroform in the RNA extraction process.

Real-time PCR

After total RNA isolation, quantitative real-time PCR (qRT-PCR) was performed with a miScript System (Qiagen, USA). All procedures were performed according to the instructions provided by the manufacturer. Reverse transcription (RT) was done in a reaction component of 20 μl, which contained 2 μl miScript Reverse Transcriptase Mix, 2 μl miScript Nucleics Mix, 4 μl miScript HiSpec Buffer, a certain volume of template RNA containing 100 ng total RNA and a little RNase-free water increasing reaction volume to 20 μl. The mixture was incubated 37 °C for 60 min and 95 °C for 5 min. The 20 μl RT product was diluted into 100 μl. Reaction system of quantitative real-time PCR contained 10 μl SYBR Green PCR Master Mix, 2 μl miScript specific primer, 2 μl miScript universal primer, 2 μl cDNA and 4 μl RNase-free water. qRT-PCR used an Applied Biosystems StepOne detection system at 95 °C for 15 min, followed by 40 cycles of 95 °C for 15 s, 55 °C for 30 s, 70 °C for 30 s. All qRT-PCRs were performed in triplicate, and the raw Ct (threshold cycle) of each sample was the mean value of three Ct values. The data were analyzed by the $2^{-\Delta\Delta CT}$ method.

Statistical analysis

Baseline characteristics and clinical condition indicator of human subjects were compared between ARDSp and ARDSexp. Expression levels of selected miRNAs detected by qRT-PCR were normalized to miR-39 and analyzed using the $2^{-\Delta\Delta CT}$ method. Results for normally distributed continuous variables are presented as mean ± SD and compared between groups by Student's *t* tests. Results for non-normally distributed continuous variables are summarized as medians [interquartile ranges] and were compared by Mann–Whitney *U* tests. Results for categorical variables are presented as sample rate (constituent ratio) and were compared Chi-squared test or Fisher exact test. Logistic regression analysis was carried out to determine the variables that were associated independently with the death of ARDSp patients. We examined whether miR-26a and miR-27a were independent risk factors for the death after adjustment for age and APACHE II score. All tests were two-sided, and *P* values < 0.05 were considered statistically significant.

Results

Screening result of *MSC-VEC*-miRNA

Fourteen miRNAs were picked out which include miR-15a, miR-16, miR-21, miR-24, miR-26a, miR-27a, miR-27b, miR-126, miR-146a, miR-150, miR-155, miR-221, miR-223, miR-320. Relevant references were presented with PubMed Unique Identifier in Additional file 2: Table S2. The detail information of these miRNAs is shown in Table 1.

General characteristics of the patients with ARDS

A total of 101 patients admitted to the ICU of Zhongda Hospital Affiliated to Southeast University from January 2016 to September 2016; diagnosed ARDS were inspected. Ultimately, 44 patients were excluded (30 malignant tumor patients, six patients administered glucocorticoid in the past 6 months, five patients older than 90 years old and three pregnant women). Fifty-seven were included in the study: 43 cases in ARDSp group and 14 cases in ARDSexp group. Age, BMI, APACHE II score, SOFA score, lactic acid, 28-day mortality rate had no statistical difference ($P > 0.05$) between ARDSp and ARDSexp. General data of the 57 ARDS are listed in Table 2.

Comparison of patient's clinical condition indexes between ARDSp and ARDSexp

Indicators from clinical monitoring and laboratory detection were compared between ARDSp and ARDSexp. Oxygenation index (PO_2/FiO_2) in ARDSp was lower than that in ARDSexp (145 [119–203] vs. 206 [184–253], $P = 0.012$). Murray lung injury score in ARDSp was significantly higher than ARDSexp (2.7 [2–3.3] vs. 1.8 [1.3–2.4], $P = 0.008$). FiO_2 and PEEP had no statistical difference between ARDSp and ARDSexp ($P > 0.05$). The proportion of ECMO, CRRT and invasive mechanical ventilation treatment had no statistical difference between ARDSp and ARDSexp ($P > 0.05$). Indexes related to infection and shock had no statistical difference between two groups ($P > 0.05$) (Table 3).

Comparison of plasma *MSC-VEC*-miRNAs levels between ARDSp and ARDSexp

Plasma miR-221 and miR-27b levels in ARDSexp group exhibited significantly lower than that in ARDSp group

Table 1 Summary of candidate *MSC-VEC*-miRNAs Regulation in vascular endothelial cells

MiRNAs	Function on angiogenic process	Gene targets	Adjusting direction
miR-15a	Inhibits angiogenesis through direct targeting of VEGF and FGF	FGF2, FGFR1, VEGF, VEGFR2	−
miR-16	Inhibits tumor angiogenesis and EC-mediated angiogenesis in vitro and in vivo	FGF2, FGFR1, VEGF, VEGFR2	−
miR-21	Induces tumor angiogenesis in vitro	PTEN	+
miR-24	Decreases endothelial cell proliferation	Sp1	−
miR-26a	Prevents endothelial cell apoptosis	TRPC6	+
miR-27a	Promotes EC angiogenesis in vitro	SEMA6A, Spry2, Dll4	+
miR-27b	Promotes EC angiogenesis in vitro	SEMA6A, Spry2, Dll4	+
miR-126	Promotes EC angiogenesis in vitro and in vivo	Spred-1, PIK3R2, VCAM-1	+
miR-150	Restores vascular barrier function	Ang2	+
miR-146a	Promotes senescence of endothelial cells	NOX4	−
miR-155	Promotes tumor angiogenesis	VHL	+
miR-221	Inhibits EC-mediated angiogenesis in vitro	c-kit, eNOS	−
miR-223	Prevents endothelial cell proliferation	β1 integrin, IGF-1R	−
miR-320	Inhibits diabetic angiogenesis in vitro	IGF-1	−

miR: microRNA, −: Negative regulation, +: Positive adjustment

Table 2 General data comparison between ARDSp and ARDSexp

Variable	Total ($n = 57$)	$ARDS_p$(1) ($n = 43$)	$ARDS_{exp}$(2) ($n = 14$)	*P* value (1) versus (2)
General condition				
Age (years)	59.0 ± 17.5	56.6 ± 20.4	63.7 ± 12.6	0.13
Male *n* (%)	41 (71.9%)	30 (69.8%)	11 (78.6%)	0.52
BMI	23.9 ± 3.6	24.0 ± 3.8	23.6 ± 3.0	0.70
APACHE II score	21.3 ± 8.4	21.8 ± 8.5	20.0 ± 8.4	0.50
SOFA score	10.4 ± 4.9	10.4 ± 4.6	10.3 ± 5.7	0.93
28-day mortality	18 (31.6%)	14 (32.6%)	4 (22.2%)	1.00
Basic diseases				
COPD *n* (%)	1 (1.8%)	0 (0%)	1 (7.1%)	0.25
Hypertension *n* (%)	16 (28.1%)	13 (30.2%)	3 (21.4%)	0.77
CHD *n* (%)	8 (14.0%)	7 (16.3%)	1 (7.1%)	0.68
CVD *n* (%)	8 (14.0%)	8 (18.6%)	0 (0%)	0.19
DM *n* (%)	12 (21.1%)	10 (23.3%)	2 (14.3%)	0.74
HBD *n* (%)	7 (12.3%)	1 (2.3%)	6 (42.9%)	0.001
ISD *n* (%)	0 (%)	0 (%)	0 (%)	1.00
ARDS etiology				
PI *n* (%)	36 (63.2%)	36 (83.7%)	0 (0%)	< 0.001
Inhalation *n* (%)	3 (5.3%)	3 (7.0%)	0 (0%)	0.57
PC *n* (%)	4 (7.0%)	4 (9.5%)	0 (0%)	0.515
Sepsis *n* (%)	3 (5.3%)	0 (0%)	3 (20%)	0.016
Pancreatitis *n* (%)	4 (7.0%)	0 (0%)	4 (26.7%)	0.004
EPT *n* (%)	5 (8.8%)	0 (0%)	5 (33.3%)	0.001
Others *n* (%)	2 (3.5%)	0 (0%)	2 (14.3%)	0.057
Organ dysfunction				
Septic shock *n* (%)	22 (38.6%)	17 (39.5%)	5 (35.7%)	0.23
AKI *n* (%)	14 (24.6%)	10 (23.3%)	4 (28.6%)	0.97

BMI body mass index, *COPD* chronic obstructive pulmonary disease, *ARDS* acute respiratory distress syndrome, *AKI* acute kidney injury, *APACHE* acute physiology and chronic health evaluation, *SOFA* sequential organ failure assessment, *CHD* coronary heart disease, *CVD* cerebrovascular disease, *DM* diabetes mellitus, *HBD* hepatobiliary diseases, *ISD* immune system disease, *PI* pulmonary infection, *PC* pulmonary contusion, *EPT* extrapulmonary trauma

Table 3 Comparison of patient's clinical condition indexes between ARDSp and ARDSexp

Variable	Total ($n = 57$)	$ARDS_p$(1) ($n = 43$)	$ARDS_{exp}$(2) ($n = 14$)	P value (1) versus (2)
Lung injury severity				
PH	7.4 [7.35–7.45]	7.41 [7.36–7.46]	7.37 [7.32–7.43]	0.26
FiO_2	0.5 [0.4–0.6]	0.5 [0.4–0.6]	0.4 [0.4–0.5]	0.06
PEEP(cmH2O)	8 [5–12]	8 [5–12]	5 [5–12]	0.54
PO_2/FiO_2(mmHg)	165 [112–211]	145 [110–203]	206 [184–253]	0.012
Murray score	2.3 [1.7–3.1]	2.7 [2–3.3]	1.8 [1.3–2.4]	0.008
Infection index				
Leukocyte count	10.4 [6–16.7]	10.4 [6.4–14.5]	11.8 [5.5–18.3]	0.81
Platelet count	134 [90–188]	134 [107–195]	128 [49–184]	0.38
CRP	74 [25–128]	74 [31–121]	75 [15–141]	0.87
PCT	1.3 [0.2–12.9]	1. 0 [0.2–13.1]	1.86 [0.7–10.4]	0.60
Shock index				
HR	73 [63–121]	72 [63–120]	76 [63–125]	0.66
NE	5 [0–27.5]	4 [0–20]	5 [0–85]	0.21
Lactic acid	2.1 [1–3.1]	2.0 [0.9–2.9]	2.2[1.2–5.4]	0.11
Organ supporting				
IMV *n* (%)	40 (70.2%)	32 (74.4%)	8 (57.1%)	0.37
ECMO *n* (%)	12 (21.1%)	12 (27.9%)	0 (0%)	0.065
CRRT *n* (%)	10 (17.5%)	7 (16.3%)	3 (21.4%)	0.97

PH arterial blood pH value, PO_2 arterial partial pressure of oxygen, FiO_2 oxygen concentration, *PEEP* positive end expiratory pressure, *Murray score* lung injury score used for ARDS patients, *CRP* C reactive protein, *PCT* procalcitonin, *IMV* invasive mechanical ventilation, *ECMO* extracorporeal membrane oxygenation, *CRRT* continuous renal replacement therapy, *HR* heart rate, *NE* norepinephrine. $P < 0.05$ suggests statistical difference

(0.22 [0.12–0.49] vs. 0.57 [0.22–1.57], $P = 0.008$), (0.34 [0.10–0.46] vs. 0.60 [0.20–1.46], $P = 0.025$). Other 12 kinds of plasma miRNAs levels between two groups showed no statistical difference. Plasma levels of *MSC-VEC*-miRNAs between ARDSp and ARDSexp are shown in Fig. 1.

Comparison of plasma vWF, VCAM-1, IL10, TNFα concentration between ARDSp and ARDSexp

Plasma vWF concentration in ARDSexp group exhibited significantly lower than that in ARDSp group (0.77 [0.29–1.54] vs. 1.80 [0.95–3.51], $P = 0.048$). However, VCAM-1, IL10, TNFα concentration between two groups showed no statistical difference. Plasma concentration of VCAM-1, IL10, TNFα between ARDSp and ARDSexp is shown in Fig. 2.

The correlation of plasma levels between miR-27b/miR-221 and vWF

As plasma miR-27b/miR-221 and vWF levels were significant different between ARDSp and ARDSexp groups, we analyzed the correlation of plasma levels between miR-27b/miR-221 and vWF. We found significant positive correlation between miR-221 and vWF in plasma levels ($r = 0.688$, $P = 0.022$). However, there was no significant correlation between miR-27b and vWF in plasma levels (Fig. 3).

Comparison of plasma patient's clinical illness condition data between survival and non-survival group in ARDSp patients

APACHE II score, SOFA score, P/F, Murray score, CRP, Lactic acid were used as common indicators to evaluate ARDS patients' clinical illness condition. This study showed that APACHE II score, SOFA score and lactic acid in survival group were significantly lower than that in non-survival group (APACHE II score: 18.7 ± 7.6 vs. 28.1 ± 7.6, $P<0.001$; SOFA score: 8.8 ± 4.1 vs. 14.0 ± 3.8, $P<0.001$; lactic acid: 1.7 [0.9–2.2] vs. 2.9 [1.2–3.3], $P = 0.015$) in ARDSp patients. P/F, Murray score and CRP between two groups showed no statistical difference (Table 4).

Comparison of plasma *MSC-VEC*-miRNAs levels between survival and non-survival group in ARDSp patients

In our research, extrapulmonary ARDS was caused by sepsis, pancreatitis, extrapulmonary trauma etc. We just analyzed plasma *MSC-VEC*-miRNAs and vWF, VCAM-1, IL10, TNFα levels between 28 days survival and 28 days non-survival group in ARDSp patients in order to reduce the heterogeneity between patients. Plasma miR-26a and miR-27a levels in non-survival group exhibited significantly lower than that in survival group (miR-26a: 0.17 [0.08–0.20] vs. 0.69 [0.24–2.33] $P = 0.018$; miR-27a: 0.23

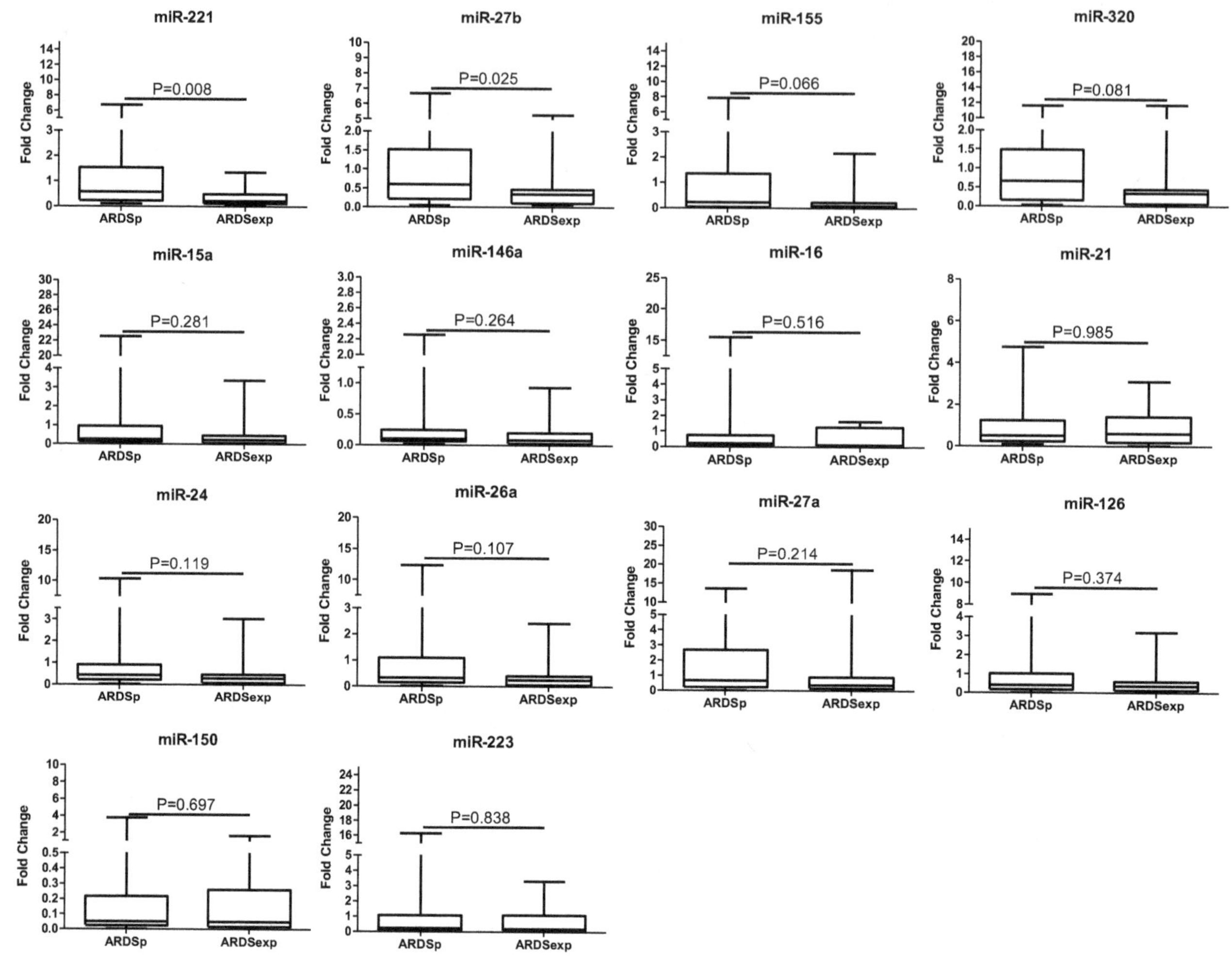

Fig. 1 Comparison of *MSC-VEC*-miRNAs between ARDSp and ARDSexp. Data presented as a relative fold change between ARDSp and ARDSexp for each miRNA. Box plots are displayed where the horizontal bar represents the median, the box represents the IQR, and the whiskers represent the maximum and minimum values. Comparisons made by Mann–Whitney *U* test. *miRNA* microRNA, *IQR* interquartile range

[0.16–0.58] vs. 1.45 [0.38–3.63], $P = 0.021$) in ARDSp patients. Other 12 kinds of miRNAs and vWF, VCAM-1, IL10, TNFα levels in plasma between two groups showed no statistical difference (Figs. 4, 5).

The predictive value of miR-26a and miR-27a for prognosis of ARDSp patients

As APACHE II score, SOFA score, lactic acid, miR-26a and miR-27a were significantly different between non-survival and survival groups in ARDSp patients, ROC curves were drawn and the area under the curve (AUC) values for APACHE II score, SOFA score, lactic acid, miR-26a and miR-27a were, respectively, 0.808 (95%CI: 0.673–0.943), 0.828 (95%CI: 0.693–0.962), 0.782 (95%CI: 0.564–0.897), 0.787 (95%CI: 0.650–0.925), 0.782 (95%CI: 0.650–0.918) (Fig. 6). We also divided the patients into two groups according to median miR-26a or miR-27a value. Survival curve analysis showed that ARDSp patients with lower concentration of miR-26a/miR-27a had higher mortality (Fig. 7). Tables 5 and 6 show the results of the multivariate logistic regression analysis for the death of ARDSp patients. MiR-26a (OR: 1.483, 95% CI: 0.999–2.200, $P = 0.050$), miR-27a (OR: 1.425, 95% CI: 1.008–2.015, $P = 0.045$) were may independently associated with the death of ARDSp patients.

Discussion

The results of this study demonstrate that the expression of plasma miR-221, miR-27b and endothelial markers vWF is significantly different between ARDSp and ARDSexp patients. Plasma miR-26a and miR-27a levels showed significantly different between non-survival group and survival group in ARDSp patients.

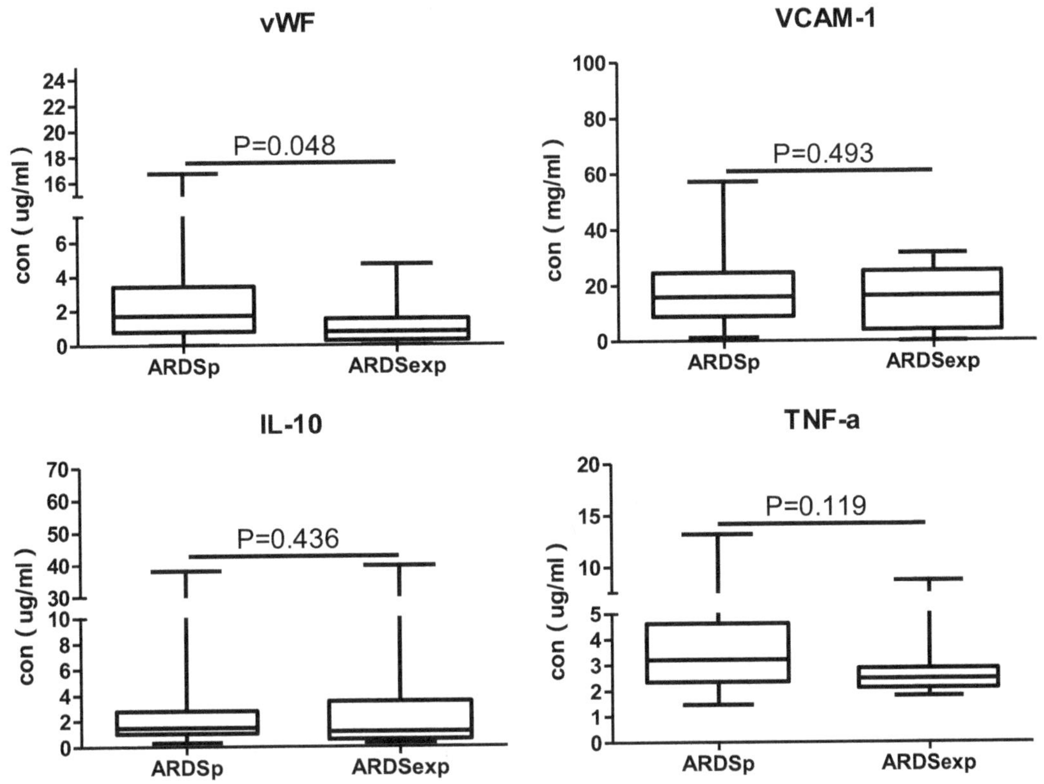

Fig. 2 Comparison of plasma vWF, VCAM-1, IL10, TNFα concentration between ARDSp and ARDSexp. The concentration unit of vWF, IL10, TNFα is ug/ml. The concentration unit of VCAM-1 is mg/ml. Box plots are displayed where the horizontal bar represents the median, the box represents the IQR and the whiskers represent the maximum and minimum values. Comparisons made by Mann–Whitney *U* test

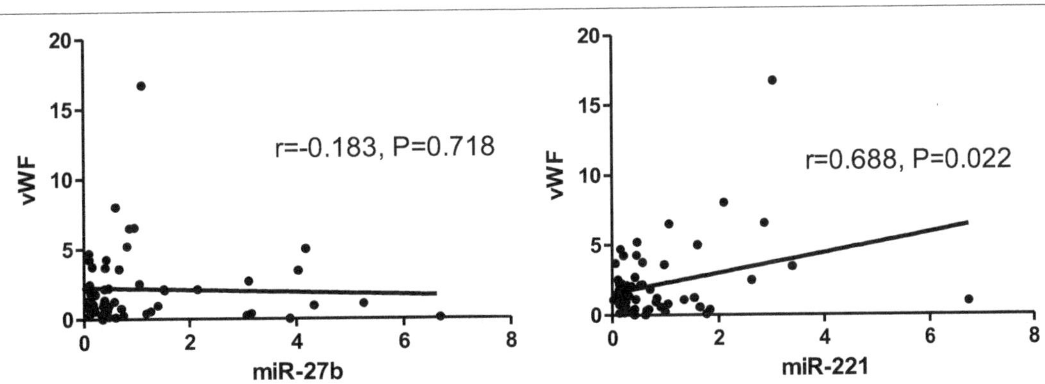

Fig. 3 Correlation between vWF and miR-27b/miR-221

The characteristics of the enrolled patients in this study may impact research results. The ARDSp patients are more serious than the ARDSexp patients in the local lung injury and lung function lesion. The ARDSp patients owned higher Murray lung injury score and lower PO_2/FiO_2 than the ARDSexp patients and included all 12 patients received ECMO treatment. But indicators related to the overall illness condition, such as APACHE II scores, SOFA scores, blood lactate levels, doses of norepinephrine and the proportion of complicating sepsis, septic shock, AKI showed no statistical difference between ARDSp and ARDSexp patients. There was no difference in the 28-day mortality between the two groups, probably because the overall illness condition

Table 4 Comparison of patient's clinical illness condition data in ARDSp patients

Variable	Survival ($n = 29$)	Non-survival ($n = 14$)	*P* value
APACHE II score	18.7 ± 7.6	28.1 ± 7.6	< 0.001
SOFA score	8.8 ± 4.1	14.0 ± 3.8	< 0.001
P/F(mmHg)	150 [113–203]	130 [100–195]	0.39
Murray score	2.6 [2.0–3.0]	3.0 [2.3–3.7]	0.09
CRP	73.7 [31.0–111]	91.3 [33.3–121]	0.76
Lactic acid	1.7 [0.9–2.2]	2.9 [1.2–3.3]	0.015

had no difference between the two groups. Therefore, the survival rate depends on overall illness severity or, say, the systematic condition of the whole organ rather than single organ lesions. We should pay attention to primary disease treatment and, meanwhile, systematic organ maintenance to prevent multiple organ dysfunction on critically ill patients.

In our study, pulmonary vascular endothelium lesion in ARDSp patients may be more serious than that in ARDSexp patients which embody in Murray lung injury score and PO_2/FiO_2. The result is in agreement with the previous research [24–26]. Previous studies show that miR-27b promotes vascular endothelial cell angiogenesis, yet miR-221 inhibits vascular endothelial cell-mediated angiogenesis. So, we deem ARDSp patients will express higher levels of miR-221 and, conversely, express reduced levels of miR-27b than ARDSexp patients. However, our research shows that plasma miR-221 and miR-27b levels

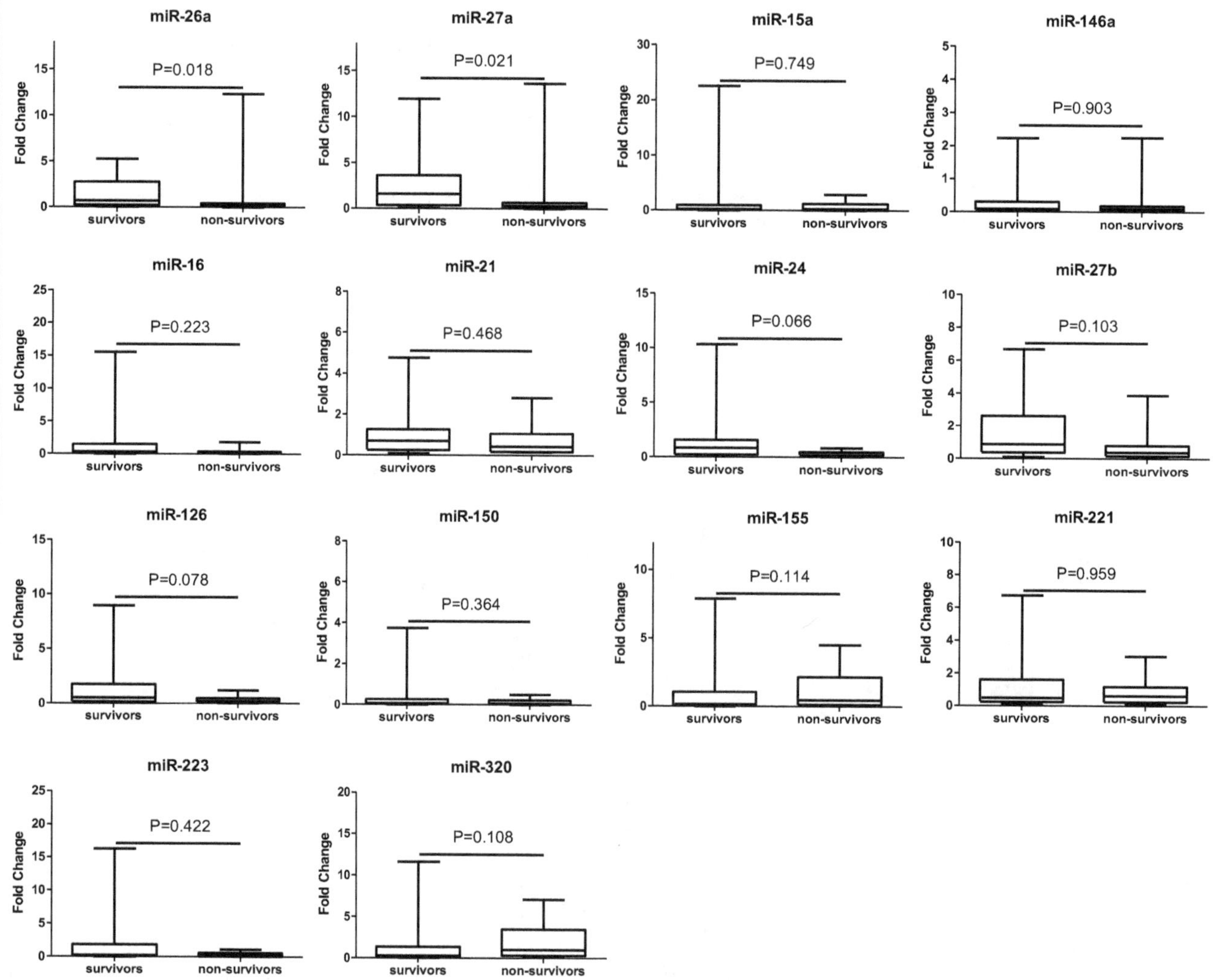

Fig. 4 Comparison of *MSC-VEC*-miRNAs between survival group and death group in ARDSp patients. Data presented as a relative fold change between ARDSp and ARDSexp for each miRNA. Box plots are displayed where the horizontal bar represents the median, the box represents the IQR and the whiskers represent the maximum and minimum values. Comparisons made by Mann–Whitney U test. *miRNA* microRNA, *IQR* interquartile range

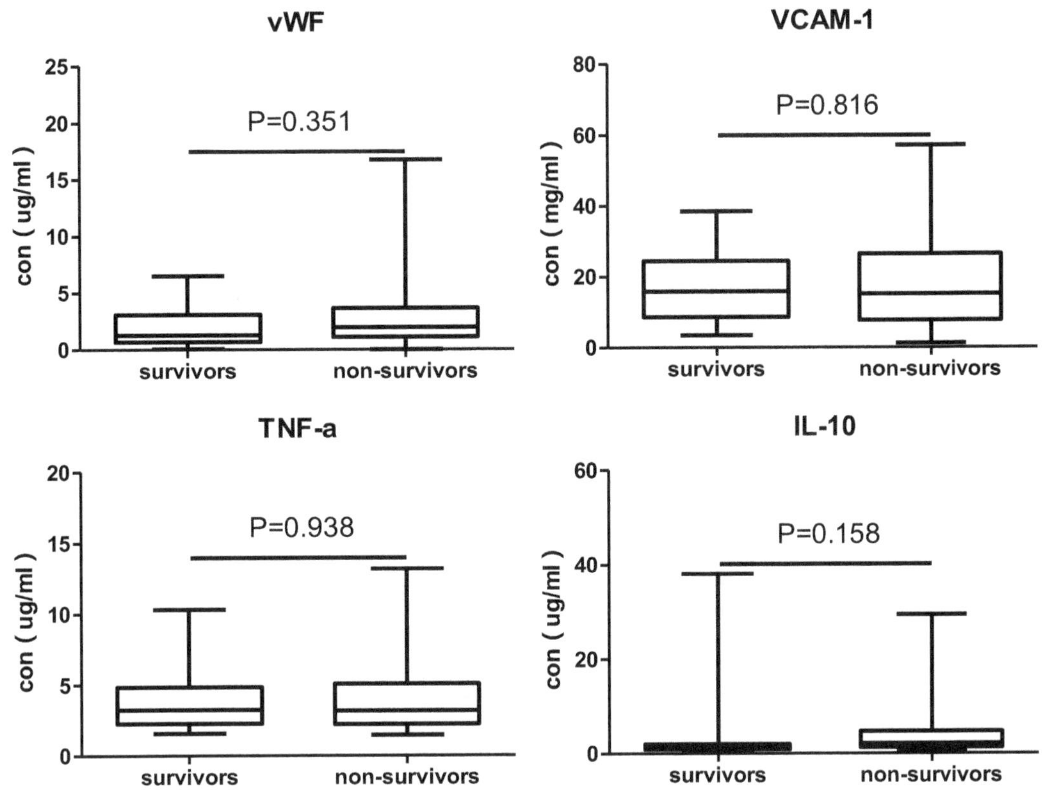

Fig. 5 Comparison of plasma vWF, VCAM-1, IL10, TNFα concentration between survival group and death group in ARDSp patients. The concentration unit of vWF, IL10, TNFα is ug/ml. The concentration unit of VCAM-1 is mg/ml. Box plots are displayed where the horizontal bar represents the median, the box represents the IQR and the whiskers represent the maximum and minimum values. Comparisons made by Mann–Whitney U test

in ARDSexp group exhibited significantly lower than that in ARDSp group which is inconsistent with expected results. We reviewed forepassed clinical researches and acquired contradictory results with each other. Significant increase in miR-27b expression was observed in the serum samples of patients with peripheral artery disease and arteriosclerosis obliterans when compared to the controls [27, 28]. Coskunpinar et al. [29] reported an increased plasma expression level of miR-221 in acute myocardial infarction compared with healthy controls. However, Tsai et al. presented that stroke patients and atherosclerosis subjects had significantly lower miR-221 serum levels than healthy controls [30]. These conclusions give us a hint that the expression of miRNAs is complex in different diseases originating from the similar pathological change.

Meanwhile, this research explored endothelial markers vWF, VCAM-1 and inflammatory cytokines IL10, TNFα. Plasma vWF concentration in ARDSexp group exhibited significantly lower than that in ARDSp group; however, plasma VCAM-1, IL10, TNFα concentration showed no statistical difference between two groups. As far as we know, endothelium can release vWF which forms additional links between the platelets' glycoprotein and the collagen fibrils. To a certain extent, elevated vWF concentration reflected vascular endothelium lesion. But there was much controversy as to whether vWF could serve as a biomarker for ARDS. VWF is considered as in vivo and in vitro marker of endothelial injury in patients with ARDS [31]. It has previously been reported that high plasma level of vWF was associated with a greater risk of developing ARDS in sepsis patients and was associated with higher mortality in patients with established ARDS [31–34]. It also was reported that plasma levels of vWF did not appear to serve as useful markers for predicting ARDS in patients at risk and mortality in ARDS patients [35–37]. The vWF studies in ARDSp and ARDSexp are rare. Calfee et al. [38] reported that plasma vWF levels were significantly lower in ARDSp than that in ARDSexp which was not consistent with our result. It may be because patients in ARDSexp group were severer with higher APACHE III score and mortality in this study which was not consistent with our research, too. Upregulation of VCAM-1 in endothelial cells by cytokines partly occurs as a result of increased gene TNFα transcription. So, in our results,

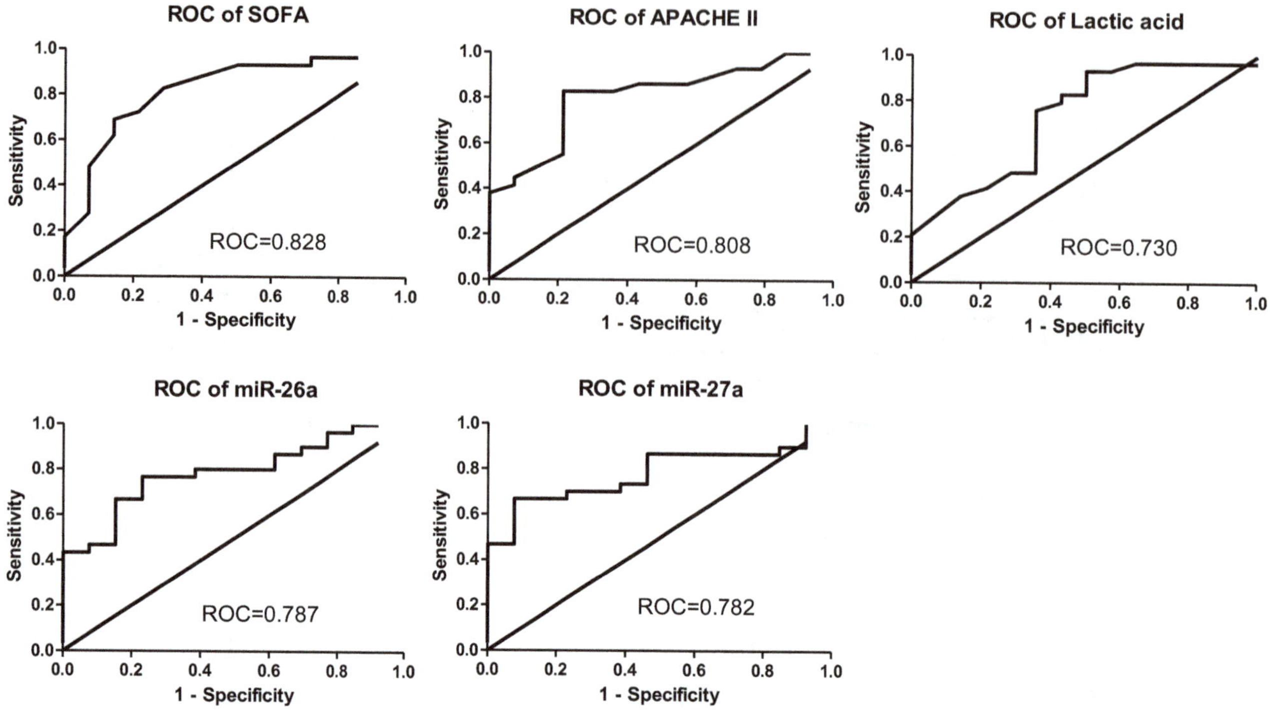

Fig. 6 Receiver operating characteristic curve of SOFA score, APACHE II score, lactic acid value, miR-26a, miR-27a for predicting 28 days mortality in ARDSp patients

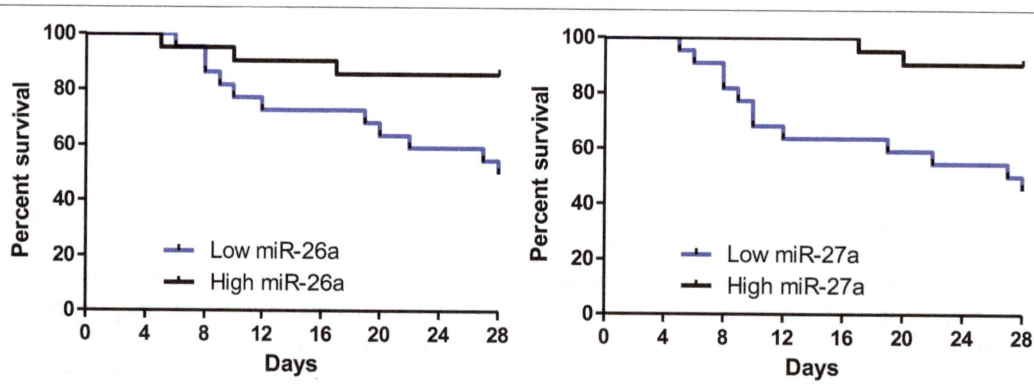

Fig. 7 Probability of survival and subgroup analyses of the risk of death at 28 days

Table 5 Multivariable analysis (miR-26a included) of the death of ARDSp patients

	Odds ratio	95% CI	*P* value
(Intercept)	3931.707	–	0.004
Age	0.959	0.908–1.013	0.133
APACHE II score	0.791	0.679–0.921	0.003
miR-26a	1.483	0.999–2.200	0.050

VCAM-1 and TNFα change in the same direction. In our study, leukocyte count, PCT, CRP showed no statistical difference between two groups, which is consistent with the change direction of IL10, TNFα.

Significant positive correlation between miR-221 and vWF in plasma levels was found in our study. Circulating is mostly released constitutively from endothelial storage organelles, Weibel–Palade bodies (WPBs) [39, 40]. WPBs are released from endothelial cells in response to a large

Table 6 Multivariable analysis (miR-27a included) of the death of ARDSp patients

	Odds ratio	95% CI	*P* value
(Intercept)	1673.348	–	0.007
Age	0.964	0.914–1.017	0.185
APACHE II score	0.803	0.679–0.926	0.002
miR-27a	1.425	1.008–2.015	0.045

number of agonists which include two distinct groups: those that act by elevating intracellular calcium ion (Ca^{2+}) levels and those that act by raising cAMP levels in the cell [41–44]. Xiang et al. [45] identified that miR-24 and miR-335 targeted human vWF 3'UTR. Previous studies with regard to miR-221 regulating vWF production are absent. However, miR-221 increases free Ca^{2+} level of mast cells by PI3 K/Akt/PLCγ/Ca^{2+} signaling pathway [46]. MiR-221 may have the same regulatory role in vascular endothelial cells. The reasons of the positive correlation between miR-221 and vWF in plasma levels need to be studied further.

Because the etiology of extrapulmonary ARDS is diverse, we just analyzed plasma *MSC-VEC*-miRNAs and vWF, VCAM-1, IL10, TNFα levels between 28 days survival and 28 days non-survival group in ARDSp patients in order to reduce the heterogeneity between patients. In ARDSp patients, plasma miR-26a and miR-27a levels in non-survival group exhibited significant statistical differences. Plasma levels of miR-26a and miR-27a were lower in non-survival group, which might be because the two miRNAs were protective factors of vascular endothelial cell. APACHE II score, SOFA score, and lactic acid value showed significant statistical differences between two groups. Receiver operating characteristic curve (ROC curve) showed that SOFA score, APACHE II score, lactic acid value, miR-26a, miR-27a roughly equally predict the prognosis of ARDSp patients. Survival curve intuitively points out that plasma miR-26a and miR-27a levels were associated with mortality in ARDSp patients. So, miR-26a and miR-27a may be potential biomarkers for predicting the prognosis of ARDSp patients, the molecular mechanisms behind this which need to be further studied.

There are limitations in this study. Firstly, as stated above, our candidate miRNAs limited to the *MSC-VEC*-miRNAs, which is associated with MSC, has regulatory effects on VEC and has previously been studied in ARDS. The broader miRNA spectrum needs to be involved in future research. Secondly, this study is a clinical observational study, but not involved the molecular mechanism of miRNA regulation in cell. So, we cannot determine where the differential expression of plasma miR-221 and miR-27b come from and which results the difference contributes to. Thirdly, the sample size is relatively small which may have limited the power of statistical difference in this study.

In conclusion, ARDSp patients have higher Murray lung injury score and worse oxygenation index than ARDSexp patients in our study. Plasma miR-221, miR-27b and vWF levels in ARDSexp patients exhibited significantly lower than that in ARDSp patients. Significant positive correlation was found between miR-221 and vWF in plasma levels. In addition, we found plasma miR-26a and miR-27a levels in non-survival group exhibited significantly lower than that in survival group in ARDSp patients.

Abbreviations

ARDS: acute respiratory distress syndrome; MSC: mesenchymal stem cells; VEC: vascular endothelial cells; ARDSp: pulmonary ARDS; ARDSexp: extrapulmonary ARDS; miRNAs: microRNAs, miR microRNA; ICU: intensive care unit; vWF: von Willebrand factor; APACHE: acute physiology and chronic health evaluation; SOFA: sequential organ failure assessment; KDIGO: kidney disease improving global outcomes; ECMO: extracorporeal membrane oxygenation; CRRT: continuous renal replacement therapy; VCAM-1: vascular cell adhesion molecule 1; IL: interleukin; TNFα: tumor necrosis factor α; CRP: c-Reactive protein; PCT: procalcitonin; ROC: receiver operating characteristic; AUC: area under the curve; AKI: acute kidney injury; IQR: interquartile range.

Authors' contributions

YZH and YZ designed the study. YZ, QS, QL, JFX, and CP conducted experimental operation, performed statistical analyses and interpretation of the data. YZ, SQL collect clinical data and wrote the manuscript. LL, YZH commented on the manuscript. All authors read and approved the final manuscript.

Author details

[1] Department of Critical Care Medicine, Zhongda Hospital, School of Medicine, Southeast University, No. 87, Dingjiaqiao Road, Gulou District, Nanjing 210009, China. [2] Department of Critical Care Medicine, The First Affiliated Hospital of Medical School of Zhejiang University, 79 Qingchun Road, Shangcheng District, Hangzhou 310003, China.

Acknowledgements

The authors thank Hai-bo Qiu, Yi Yang, Ming Xue, Sen Lu, and Rong-rong Huang for their support in the realization of this study.

Competing interests

The authors declare that they have no competing interests

Funding

The study was sponsored by Natural Science Foundation of Jiangsu Province (CN) (BK20141344).

References

1. Bellani G, Laffey JG, Pham T, Fan E, Brochard L, Esteban A, Gattinoni L, van Haren F, Larsson A, McAuley DF, et al. Epidemiology, patterns of care, and mortality for patients with acute respiratory distress syndrome in intensive care units in 50 countries. JAMA. 2016;315(8):788–800.
2. Orfanos SE, Mavrommati I, Korovesi I, Roussos C. Pulmonary endothelium in acute lung injury: from basic science to the critically ill. Intensive Care Med. 2004;30(9):1702–14.
3. Gill SE, Rohan M, Mehta S. Role of pulmonary microvascular endothelial cell apoptosis in murine sepsis-induced lung injury in vivo. Respir Res. 2015;16:109.

4. Gattinoni L, Pelosi P, Suter PM, Pedoto A, Vercesi P, Lissoni A. Acute respiratory distress syndrome caused by pulmonary and extrapulmonary disease. Different syndromes? Am J Respir Crit Care Med. 1998;158(1):3–11.
5. Bernard GR, Artigas A, Brigham KL, Carlet J, Falke K, Hudson L, Lamy M, Legall JR, Morris A, Spragg R. The American–European consensus conference on ARDS. Definitions, mechanisms, relevant outcomes, and clinical trial coordination. Am J Respir Crit Care Med. 1994;149(3 Pt 1):818–24.
6. Rocco PR, Pelosi P. Pulmonary and extrapulmonary acute respiratory distress syndrome: myth or reality? Curr Opin Crit Care. 2008;14(1):50–5.
7. Hoeper MM, Spiekerkoetter E, Westerkamp V, Gatzke R, Fabel H. Intravenous iloprost for treatment failure of aerosolised iloprost in pulmonary arterial hypertension. Eur Respir J. 2002;20(2):339–43.
8. Goodman LR, Fumagalli R, Tagliabue P, Tagliabue M, Ferrario M, Gattinoni L, Pesenti A. Adult respiratory distress syndrome due to pulmonary and extrapulmonary causes: CT, clinical, and functional correlations. Radiology. 1999;213(2):545–52.
9. Rialp G, Betbese AJ, Perez-Marquez M, Mancebo J. Short-term effects of inhaled nitric oxide and prone position in pulmonary and extrapulmonary acute respiratory distress syndrome. Am J Respir Crit Care Med. 2001;164(2):243–9.
10. Lim CM, Kim EK, Lee JS, Shim TS, Lee SD, Koh Y, Kim WS, Kim DS, Kim WD. Comparison of the response to the prone position between pulmonary and extrapulmonary acute respiratory distress syndrome. Intensive Care Med. 2001;27(3):477–85.
11. Riva DR, Oliveira MB, Rzezinski AF, Rangel G, Capelozzi VL, Zin WA, Morales MM, Pelosi P, Rocco PR. Recruitment maneuver in pulmonary and extrapulmonary experimental acute lung injury. Crit Care Med. 2008;36(6):1900–8.
12. Kloot TE, Blanch L, Melynne Youngblood A, Weinert C, Adams AB, Marini JJ, Shapiro RS, Nahum A. Recruitment maneuvers in three experimental models of acute lung injury. Effect on lung volume and gas exchange. Am J Respir Crit Care Med. 2000;161(5):1485–94.
13. Tugrul S, Akinci O, Ozcan PE, Ince S, Esen F, Telci L, Akpir K, Cakar N. Effects of sustained inflation and postinflation positive end-expiratory pressure in acute respiratory distress syndrome: focusing on pulmonary and extrapulmonary forms. Crit Care Med. 2003;31(3):738–44.
14. Pati S, Gerber MH, Menge TD, Wataha KA, Zhao Y, Baumgartner JA, Zhao J, Letourneau PA, Huby MP, Baer LA, et al. Bone marrow derived mesenchymal stem cells inhibit inflammation and preserve vascular endothelial integrity in the lungs after hemorrhagic shock. PLoS ONE. 2011;6(9):e25171.
15. Yang Y, Chen QH, Liu AR, Xu XP, Han JB, Qiu HB. Synergism of MSC-secreted HGF and VEGF in stabilising endothelial barrier function upon lipopolysaccharide stimulation via the Rac1 pathway. Stem Cell Res Ther. 2015;6:250.
16. Hu S, Li J, Xu X, Liu A, He H, Xu J, Chen Q, Liu S, Liu L, Qiu H, et al. The hepatocyte growth factor-expressing character is required for mesenchymal stem cells to protect the lung injured by lipopolysaccharide in vivo. Stem Cell Res Ther. 2016;7(1):66.
17. Wang H, Zheng R, Chen Q, Shao J, Yu J, Hu S. Mesenchymal stem cells microvesicles stabilize endothelial barrier function partly mediated by hepatocyte growth factor (HGF). Stem Cell Res Ther. 2017;8(1):211.
18. Potter DR, Miyazawa BY, Gibb SL, Deng X, Togaratti PP, Croze RH, Srivastava AK, Trivedi A, Matthay M, Holcomb JB, et al. Mesenchymal stem cell derived extracellular vesicles attenuate pulmonary vascular permeability and lung injury induced by hemorrhagic shock and trauma. J Trauma Acute Care Surg. 2017;84(2):245–56.
19. Liu L, He H, Liu A, Xu J, Han J, Chen Q, Hu S, Xu X, Huang Y, Guo F, et al. Therapeutic effects of bone marrow-derived mesenchymal stem cells in models of pulmonary and extrapulmonary acute lung injury. Cell Transplant. 2015;24(12):2629–42.
20. Araujo IM, Abreu SC, Maron-Gutierrez T, Cruz F, Fujisaki L, Carreira H Jr, Ornellas F, Ornellas D, Vieira-de-Abreu A, Castro-Faria-Neto HC, et al. Bone marrow-derived mononuclear cell therapy in experimental pulmonary and extrapulmonary acute lung injury. Crit Care Med. 2010;38(8):1733–41.
21. Zhou Z, You Z. Mesenchymal stem cells alleviate LPS-induced acute lung injury in mice by MiR-142a-5p-controlled pulmonary endothelial cell autophagy. Cell Physiol Biochem. 2016;38(1):258–66.
22. Bao H, Gao F, Xie G, Liu Z. Angiotensin-converting enzyme 2 inhibits apoptosis of pulmonary endothelial cells during acute lung injury through suppressing MiR-4262. Cell Physiol Biochem. 2015;37(2):759–67.
23. Force ADT, Ranieri VM, Rubenfeld GD, Thompson BT, Ferguson ND, Caldwell E, Fan E, Camporota L, Slutsky AS. Acute respiratory distress syndrome: the Berlin definition. JAMA. 2012;307(23):2526–33.
24. Kim SJ, Oh BJ, Lee JS, Lim CM, Shim TS, Lee SD, Kim WS, Kim DS, Kim WD, Koh Y. Recovery from lung injury in survivors of acute respiratory distress syndrome: difference between pulmonary and extrapulmonary subtypes. Intensive Care Med. 2004;30(10):1960–3.
25. Morisawa K, Fujitani S, Taira Y, Kushimoto S, Kitazawa Y, Okuchi K, Ishikura H, Sakamoto T, Tagami T, Yamaguchi J, et al. Difference in pulmonary permeability between indirect and direct acute respiratory distress syndrome assessed by the transpulmonary thermodilution technique: a prospective, observational, multi-institutional study. J Intensive Care. 2014;2(1):24.
26. Luo L, Shaver CM, Zhao Z, Koyama T, Calfee CS, Bastarache JA, Ware LB. Clinical predictors of hospital mortality differ between direct and indirect ARDS. Chest. 2017;151(4):755–63.
27. Signorelli SS, Volsi GL, Pitruzzella A, Fiore V, Mangiafico M, Vanella L, Parenti R, Rizzo M, Volti GL. Circulating miR-130a, miR-27b, and miR-210 in patients with peripheral artery disease and their potential relationship with oxidative stress. Angiology. 2016;67(10):945–50.
28. Li T, Cao H, Zhuang J, Wan J, Guan M, Yu B, Li X, Zhang W. Identification of miR-130a, miR-27b and miR-210 as serum biomarkers for atherosclerosis obliterans. Clin Chim Acta. 2011;412(1–2):66–70.
29. Coskunpinar E, Cakmak HA, Kalkan AK, Tiryakioglu NO, Erturk M, Ongen Z. Circulating miR-221-3p as a novel marker for early prediction of acute myocardial infarction. Gene. 2016;591(1):90–6.
30. Tsai PC, Liao YC, Wang YS, Lin HF, Lin RT, Juo SH. Serum microRNA-21 and microRNA-221 as potential biomarkers for cerebrovascular disease. J Vasc Res. 2013;50(4):346–54.
31. Ware LB, Eisner MD, Thompson BT, Parsons PE, Matthay MA. Significance of von Willebrand factor in septic and nonseptic patients with acute lung injury. Am J Respir Crit Care Med. 2004;170(7):766–72.
32. Rubin DB, Wiener-Kronish JP, Murray JF, Green DR, Turner J, Luce JM, Montgomery AB, Marks JD, Matthay MA. Elevated von Willebrand factor antigen is an early plasma predictor of acute lung injury in nonpulmonary sepsis syndrome. J Clin Invest. 1990;86(2):474–80.
33. Ware LB, Conner ER, Matthay MA. von Willebrand factor antigen is an independent marker of poor outcome in patients with early acute lung injury. Crit Care Med. 2001;29(12):2325–31.
34. Siemiatkowski A, Kloczko J, Galar M, Czaban S. von Willebrand factor antigen as a prognostic marker in posttraumatic acute lung injury. Haemostasis. 2000;30(4):189–95.
35. Bajaj MS, Tricomi SM. Plasma levels of the three endothelial-specific proteins von Willebrand factor, tissue factor pathway inhibitor, and thrombomodulin do not predict the development of acute respiratory distress syndrome. Intensive Care Med. 1999;25(11):1259–66.
36. Moss M, Ackerson L, Gillespie MK, Moore FA, Moore EE, Parsons PE. von Willebrand factor antigen levels are not predictive for the adult respiratory distress syndrome. Am J Respir Crit Care Med. 1995;151(1):15–20.
37. Cartin-Ceba R, Hubmayr RD, Qin R, Peters S, Determann RM, Schultz MJ, Gajic O. Predictive value of plasma biomarkers for mortality and organ failure development in patients with acute respiratory distress syndrome. J Crit Care. 2015;30(1):219.e1–7.
38. Calfee CS, Janz DR, Bernard GR, May AK, Kangelaris KN, Matthay MA, Ware LB. Distinct molecular phenotypes of direct vs indirect ARDS in single-center and multicenter studies. Chest. 2015;147(6):1539–48.
39. Valentijn KM, Eikenboom J. Weibel–Palade bodies: a window to von Willebrand disease. J Thromb Haemost. 2013;11(4):581–92.
40. van den Biggelaar M, Hernandez-Fernaud JR, van den Eshof BL, Neilson LJ, Meijer AB, Mertens K, Zanivan S. Quantitative phosphoproteomics unveils temporal dynamics of thrombin signaling in human endothelial cells. Blood. 2014;123(12):e22–36.
41. Vischer UM, Barth H, Wollheim CB. Regulated von Willebrand factor secretion is associated with agonist-specific patterns of cytoskeletal remodeling in cultured endothelial cells. Arterioscler Thromb Vasc Biol. 2000;20(3):883–91.

42. van den Eijnden-Schrauwen Y, Atsma DE, Lupu F, de Vries RE, Kooistra T, Emeis JJ. Involvement of calcium and G proteins in the acute release of tissue-type plasminogen activator and von Willebrand factor from cultured human endothelial cells. Arterioscler Thromb Vasc Biol. 1997;17(10):2177–87.
43. Vischer UM, Wollheim CB. Epinephrine induces von Willebrand factor release from cultured endothelial cells: involvement of cyclic AMP-dependent signalling in exocytosis. Thromb Haemost. 1997;77(6):1182–8.
44. Kaufmann JE, Oksche A, Wollheim CB, Gunther G, Rosenthal W, Vischer UM. Vasopressin-induced von Willebrand factor secretion from endothelial cells involves V2 receptors and cAMP. J Clin Invest. 2000;106(1):107–16.
45. Xiang Y, Cheng J, Wang D, Hu X, Xie Y, Stitham J, Atteya G, Du J, Tang WH, Lee SH, et al. Hyperglycemia repression of miR-24 coordinately upregulates endothelial cell expression and secretion of von Willebrand factor. Blood. 2015;125(22):3377–87.
46. Xu H, Gu LN, Yang QY, Zhao DY, Liu F. MiR-221 promotes IgE-mediated activation of mast cells degranulation by PI3 K/Akt/PLCgamma/Ca(2+) pathway. J Bioenerg Biomembr. 2016;48(3):293–9.

18

Practice of ultrasound-guided central venous catheter technique by the French intensivists: a survey from the BoReal study group

Julien Maizel[1*], Marie-Anaïs Bastide[1], Jack Richecoeur[2], Eric Frenoy[3], Christian Lemaire[4], Bertrand Sauneuf[5], Hervé Dupont[6], Fabienne Tamion[7], Saad Nseir[8], Damien Du Cheyron[9] and the BoReal Study group

Abstract

Background: The ultrasound (US)-guided technique has been recommended for central venous catheter (CVC) placement in critical care. However, several surveys have shown that the majority of physicians continue to perform landmark procedures. In our region, we have implemented special courses to promote the use of US with formal training and simulators. Ultrasound machines have also been installed in almost every ICU in our area. We designed a survey to investigate whether the training program established for years and the widespread of ultrasound devices in the ICU of our region will be associated with a high rate of physicians performing US procedures.

Methods: A survey comprising 14 questions was designed to elicit information on training in US techniques, the use of US for CVC placement, reasons for nonuse of US and their opinion concerning the need to teach the landmark technique to residents. This survey was electronically sent to every physician of the BoReal study group (32 ICUs located in the North West of France).

Results: We received 190 responses (response rate 66 %) including 34 % of residents. Only 11 % of respondents reported the absence of training in the US technique, and 3 % reported they did not have access to an ultrasound machine. A total of 68 % declared "always" (18 %) or "almost always" (50 %) using US to guide CVC placement. Our results are better than those of previous surveys. The main reasons why physicians did not use the US technique were that they thought that US guidance was unnecessary (36 %) or because the ultrasound machine was not immediately available (33 %). Ninety-one percentages think that the landmark technique should still be taught to the residents. A higher proportion of residents compared to seniors declared that they always or almost always used the US technique.

Conclusion: Training in ultrasound techniques and the widespread availability of ultrasound machines in ICUs seem to improve the rate of US procedures. However, despite strong scientific evidence a proportion of physicians continue to consider the landmark technique as an alternative to US. Training and education are potentially still the best ways to overcome such barriers or conviction.

Keywords: Central venous catheter, Ultrasound, Education

Background

For more than 10 years, the ultrasound (US)-guided technique has been recommended for central venous catheter (CVC) placement in critical care patients [1–5]. The superiority of US over the landmarks technique has been demonstrated in terms of success rate, complications, time and economic burden. However, US-guided procedures are far from being systematic, as several surveys have shown that many physicians continue to perform landmark procedures [6–8]. In a prospective study

*Correspondence: maizel.julien@chu-amiens.fr
[1] Medical ICU and INSERM U1088, University Hospital, Amiens, France
Full list of author information is available at the end of the article

in France, Belgium and Switzerland, only 54 % of central venous lines were placed under ultrasound guidance [9]. More recently, the multicenter randomized controlled trial 3SITES performed in 9 French ICU (4 university hospitals and 5 community hospitals) reported only 67 % of the jugular, 28 % of the femoral and 16 % of the subclavian procedures performed using the ultrasound [10]. The reasons why operators are reluctant to use ultrasound are mainly the absence of training in US techniques, lack of equipment and the belief that US is not necessary [6, 7, 9–12]. The implementation of training session is a key element to increase the rate of US technique. In our region, the US technique has been taught to residents and physicians working in ICU for 10 years. We have implemented special courses to promote the use of US with formal training and simulators. Those training sessions were organized together by the four university hospitals every year in our region. Ultrasound machines have also been installed in almost every ICU in our area. We therefore consider that the great majority of intensivists working in our region are qualified in US procedures and have an ultrasound machine at their disposal, two of the reasons previously reported as obstacles to use the US technique. Consequently, the rate of physicians performing US procedures should be higher in our region than the percentage formerly reported.

We designed a survey to investigate ICU physician CVC placement clinical practices in our region, the reasons why some physicians prefer to use landmarks or US and their opinion concerning the need to continue to teach the landmark technique to residents. The objectives were to observe whether the training program established for years and the widespread availability of ultrasound devices in the ICU of our region will be associated with a high rate of physicians performing US procedures and to list the remaining obstacles persisting against the progression of US technique.

Methods

Survey design

A survey comprising 14 questions was developed. Two physicians that are skilled operators were in charge of elaboration of the questions. The survey was constructed using SurveyMonkey® online software (www.surveymonkey.com) according to guidelines [13]. The 14 questions were presented in a single scrolling page. A group of 5 ICU physicians then tested the questionnaire. A test–retest was performed by the same 5 physicians after an interval of 3 weeks to check reliability, as recommended [13]. Questions were designed to elicit information on physician characteristics, experience in CVC placement, training in US techniques, the use of US for CVC placement, reasons for nonuse of US, reasons for use of US and their opinion concerning the need to teach the landmark technique to residents.

Data collection

The BoReal group is a group of 32 ICUs located in the North West of France (Nord-Pas-de-Calais-Picardie and Normandie regions). This group is composed of 8 university and 24 community ICUs: 5 medical ICUs, 3 surgical ICUs and 24 medical and surgical ICUs. All physicians and residents belonging to the BoReal group provided their e-mail address. Residents had to be currently assigned to the ICU at the time of the survey to be included in the e-mail listing. The survey was sent individually by e-mail to each physician and resident using SurveyMonkey® online software. A cover letter attached to the e-mail briefly explained the study and gave a link to the online survey. Two reminders were sent to nonresponders.

This study was deemed exempt from review by the local ethics committee.

Statistics

Results are expressed as mean ± SD. Descriptive statistics were used to summarize the data. Qualitative items were compared using a Chi-square test. A p value <0.05 was considered to indicate statistically significant differences.

Results

Population

A survey was sent by e-mail to a total of 123 residents and 163 senior physicians, 190 of whom responded (global response rate: 66 %) corresponding to 65 residents (response rate: 53 %) and 125 senior physicians (response rate: 77 %). All surveys were complete. The characteristics of the respondents are presented in Table 1.

Only 11 % of respondents reported the absence of training in the US technique, and 3 % reported they did not have access to an ultrasound machine. A total of 68 % declared "always" (18 %) or "almost always" (50 %) using US to guide CVC placement. About 6 % never and 10 % almost never used the US-guided technique (Fig. 1). The main reasons why physicians did not use the US technique were that they thought that US guidance was unnecessary (36 %) or because the ultrasound machine was not immediately available (33 %) (Table 1). Clotting abnormalities (64 %), obesity (54 %) and anatomic difficulties (52 %) were the main situations that led the physician to use ultrasound for CVC placement.

Fifty-three percent of physicians declared that they had experienced an emergency situation in which they could not wait for the ultrasound machine at least once during the last year, and 91 % considered that the landmark technique should still be taught to residents (Table 1).

Table 1 Results of the survey in the overall population ($n = 190$)

Age (years)	
<30	29 % ($n = 55$)
30–39	37 % ($n = 71$)
40–49	15 % ($n = 29$)
50–60	15 % ($n = 28$)
>60	4 % ($n = 7$)
Main practice (MR)	
ICU only	84 % ($n = 159$)
OR and ICU	15 % ($n = 28$)
ER and ICU	2 % ($n = 3$)
Practice setting (MR)	
Community hospital	47 % ($n = 89$)
University hospital	59 % ($n = 112$)
Experience in CVC placement (years)	
<1	15 % ($n = 28$)
1–5	27 % ($n = 51$)
6–10	22 % ($n = 42$)
>10	36 % ($n = 69$)
Number of CVCs placed during the last 12 months	
<10 (<1/month)	13 % ($n = 25$)
10–24 (1–2/month)	34 % ($n = 65$)
25–50 (1 per week)	33 % ($n = 62$)
>50 (>1/week)	20 % ($n = 38$)
Preferred site of CVC placement	
Jugular > femoral > subclavian	55 % ($n = 105$)
Jugular > subclavian > femoral	15 % ($n = 28$)
Femoral > jugular > subclavian	7 % ($n = 13$)
Femoral > subclavian > jugular	2 % ($n = 4$)
Subclavian > femoral > jugular	6 % ($n = 12$)
Subclavian > jugular > femoral	15 % ($n = 28$)
Technique learned during residency	
Landmark	50 % ($n = 94$)
Ultrasound	9 % ($n = 17$)
Both	41 % ($n = 78$)
Use of ultrasound for CVC placement	
Always	18 % (35)
Almost always	50 % (94)
Half of the time	17 % (32)
Almost never	10 % (18)
Never	6 % (11)
Reasons why you do not use ultrasound (MR)	
You think you do not need it	36 % ($n = 68$)
Not immediately available	33 % ($n = 62$)
No equipment	3 % ($n = 6$)
You think the procedure is longer with ultrasound	19 % ($n = 36$)
Lack of training	11 % ($n = 21$)
Other reasons	17 % ($n = 33$)
Which ultrasound technique do you use?	
Skin mark	8 % ($n = 15$)
Ultrasound guided	71 % ($n = 126$)
Both	21 % ($n = 37$)

Table 1 continued

Which situations would encourage you to use ultrasound? (MR)	
Obesity	54 % ($n = 102$)
Clotting abnormalities	64 % ($n = 122$)
Jugular site	45 % ($n = 85$)
Femoral site	19 % ($n = 37$)
Subclavian site	9 % ($n = 17$)
Anatomic difficulties	52 % ($n = 99$)
Missed landmark procedure	43 % ($n = 81$)
None	3 % ($n = 6$)
How many times have you experienced an emergency situation in which ultrasound was not available sufficiently rapidly enough during the last 12 months?	
0	47 % ($n = 89$)
<2	23 % ($n = 44$)
2–5	24 % ($n = 46$)
6–10	5 % ($n = 9$)
>10	1 % ($n = 2$)
Do you think the landmark procedure should still be taught to residents?	
Yes	91 % ($n = 173$)
No	9 % ($n = 17$)

CVC central venous catheter, *ER* emergency room, *ICU* intensive care unit, *MR* multiple responses, *OR* operating room

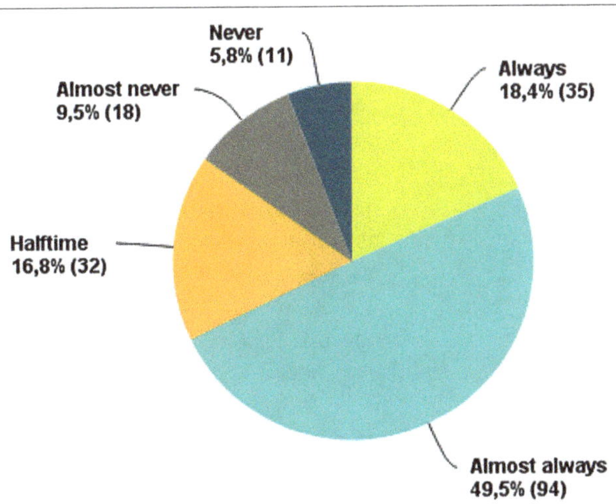

Fig. 1 Use of ultrasound for central venous catheter placement in the overall population ($n = 190$)

Comparisons of residents and seniors

We compared the results of the survey between residents ($n = 65$) and senior physicians ($n = 125$) to determine whether younger physicians behave differently from senior physicians.

The comparison of demographic characteristics between residents and seniors is presented in Table 2. Senior physicians compared to residents preferred more frequently the subclavian site [respectively, 29 % ($n = 36$) vs. 6 % ($n = 4$); $p = 0.01$], while residents tended to prefer the jugular site [61 % ($n = 76$) vs. 88 % ($n = 57$); $p = 0.01$]. The majority of senior physicians only learned the landmark technique (73 %) during their residency training, but this rate dropped to only 5 % for the current residents ($p = 0.001$).

The proportion of physicians who always used US was not different between the residents and seniors [respectively, 23 % ($n = 15$) vs. 16 % ($n = 20$); $p = 0.3$] (Fig. 2; Table 3). However, a higher proportion of residents declared that they "always" or "almost always" used the US technique compared with the seniors [respectively, 89 % ($n = 58$) vs. 57 % ($n = 71$); $p = 0.01$]. Therefore, although residents and seniors both continue to perform landmark procedures, residents more frequently used US guidance than seniors. Unavailability of the ultrasound machine was reported significantly more frequently as a reason for using the landmark procedure by residents than by senior physicians [43 % ($n = 28$) vs. 27 % ($n = 34$); $p = 0.04$]. Subclavian CVC placement was more frequently reported as the reason for using US by residents compared to seniors [respectively, 17 % ($n = 11$) vs. 5 % ($n = 6$); $p = 0.01$]. The very great majority of the two groups reported that the landmark technique should still be taught to residents.

Discussion

All guidelines recommend the use of US for CVC placement because US has been shown to increase successful catheter placement and to reduce complications [1–5]. General barriers to ultrasound-guided CVC include

Table 2 Comparison of the residents and senior physician answers to the first 7 questions of the survey (demographic data)

	Residents $n = 65$	Seniors $n = 125$	*p* value
Age (years)			
<30	82 % ($n = 53$)	2 % ($n = 2$)	0.001
30–39	18 % ($n = 12$)	47 % ($n = 59$)	0.001
40–49	0	23 % ($n = 29$)	–
50–60	0	22 % ($n = 28$)	–
>60	0	6 % ($n = 7$)	–
Main practice			
ICU only	61 % ($n = 40$)	95 % ($n = 119$)	0.001
OR and ICU	37 % ($n = 24$)	3 % ($n = 4$)	0.001
ER and ICU	2 % ($n = 1$)	2 % ($n = 2$)	0.6
Practice setting (MR)			
Community hospital	78 % ($n = 51$)	49 % ($n = 61$)	0.002
University hospital	34 % ($n = 22$)	54 % ($n = 67$)	0.01
Experience in CVC placement (years)			
<1	42 % ($n = 27$)	1 % ($n = 1$)	0.001
1–5	58 % ($n = 38$)	10 % ($n = 13$)	0.001
6–10	0	34 % ($n = 42$)	–
>10	0	55 % ($n = 69$)	–
Number of CVCs placed during the last 12 months			
<10 (<1/month)	8 % ($n = 5$)	16 % ($n = 20$)	0.2
10–24 (1–2/month)	35 % ($n = 23$)	34 % ($n = 42$)	0.9
25–50 (1 per week)	40 % ($n = 26$)	29 % ($n = 36$)	0.2
>50 (>1/week)	17 % ($n = 11$)	22 % ($n = 27$)	0.6
Preferred site of CVC placement			
Jugular > femoral > subclavian	81 % ($n = 53$)	42 % ($n = 52$)	0.001
Jugular > subclavian > femoral	6 % ($n = 4$)	19 % ($n = 24$)	0.03
Femoral > jugular > subclavian	6 % ($n = 4$)	7 % ($n = 9$)	0.9
Femoral > subclavian > jugular	0	3 % ($n = 4$)	–
Subclavian > femoral > jugular	0	10 % ($n = 12$)	–
Subclavian > jugular > femoral	6 % ($n = 4$)	19 % ($n = 24$)	0.03
Technique learned during residency			
Landmark	5 % ($n = 3$)	73 % ($n = 91$)	0.001
Ultrasound	25 % ($n = 16$)	1 % ($n = 1$)	0.001
Both	71 % ($n = 46$)	26 % ($n = 32$)	0.001

CVC central venous catheter, *ER* emergency room, *ICU* intensive care unit, *MR* multiple responses, *OR* operating room

access to equipment and proper training. In our region we have implemented special courses to promote the use of US with formal training and simulators which should be associated with a high rate of US procedures. Our results are encouraging as 68 % of our physicians use "always" or "almost always" the US. In 2007, Bailey et al. [6] reported only 15 % of cardiovascular anesthesiologists in the USA who performed always or almost always US technique. Moreover, the 18 % of our physicians declaring systematically using US is higher than the 5 % reported by Mimoz et al. [14] in a population of French intensivists in 2006. The proportion of physicians who never used US was lower (6 %) in our study compared to previous studies (44 % in the study by Buchanan et al. [12]). Therefore, our results are better than those of previous surveys. We compared residents and senior physicians to identify current trends in the use of US. This comparison confirmed a trend toward increased use of US among younger physicians who also reported less frequently a lack of training to justify the use of landmark technique (Table 3).

The first reason reported by the physicians in our survey for not using US was "they don't need ultrasound"

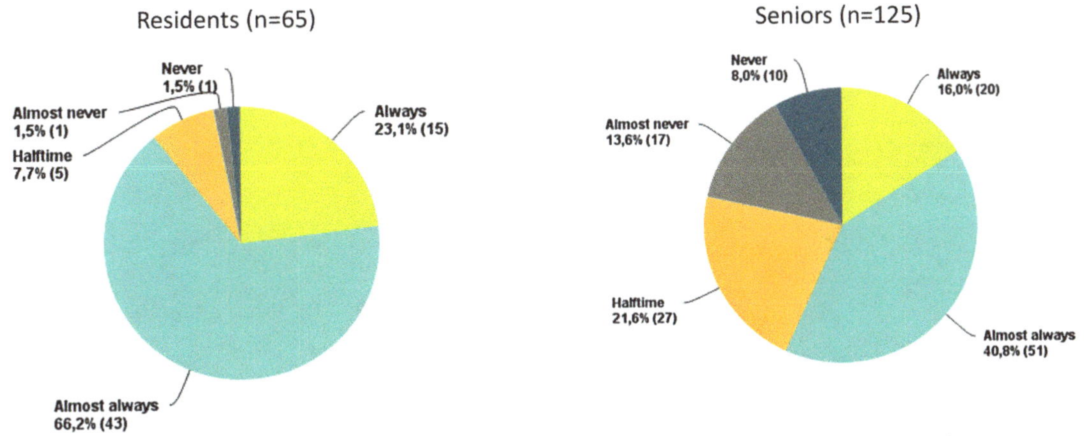

Fig. 2 Use of ultrasound for central venous catheter placement among residents ($n = 65$) and senior physicians ($n = 125$)

(36 %) (Table 1). The same reason of "no apparent need" has already been reported in previous surveys [6, 7]. Despite more than 5 national and international guidelines recommending the use of US, some physicians still consider landmark procedures as a reasonable alternative. More than 40 studies and 7 meta-analyses have shown a clear benefit of using US in terms of success rate and complications. No study has ever demonstrated the superiority of landmark technique over the US-guided technique. However, a proportion of physicians may still consider the benefit of using US to be very minor. It is noteworthy that our survey showed that the subclavian site was the site associated with the lowest rate of US guidance (9 %) compared with the jugular (45 %) and femoral (19 %) sites (Table 1). Although, historically, the jugular vein has been most extensively studied, several studies have now also demonstrated the benefits of US for femoral and subclavian CVC placement, which is why US is now recommended in all sites. For example, in a study based on more than 400 subclavian procedures, Fragou et al. [15] demonstrated the superiority of the US-guided technique over the landmark technique in terms of success rate, number of punctures, complications and procedure time. The recent meta-analysis published by the Cochrane database showed a benefit of US for the jugular site in terms of success rate, complication rate and procedure time [16]. For the subclavian vein, US provides a benefit in terms of arterial puncture and hematoma, but not in terms of success rate and only a benefit in terms of success rate is observed for the femoral site [17]. As stated by the authors of the review, fewer studies have been conducted on the subclavian and femoral veins compared to the jugular vein and the studies included in this meta-analysis were very heterogeneous. More than 5 additional studies on subclavian or femoral vein CVC placement, published since this meta-analysis, have confirmed the superiority of US. Interestingly, our survey shows that residents use more frequently the US for subclavian site than the seniors (Table 3). It is highly possible that in the next years the rate of US subclavian CVC will increase.

In previous surveys, lack of training and absence of an ultrasound machine were cited as the main reasons for not using US [7]. In our region, only 11 % of physicians reported the absence of US training and 3 % reported absence of an ultrasound machine to explain the use of the landmark procedure, which could explain the more frequent use of US procedures in our region compared to previous surveys. However, availability of an ultrasound machine was still a limiting factor for residents, who more frequently reported inaccessibility of the ultrasound machine than seniors to explain use of the landmark technique (Table 3).

Ninety-one percent of physicians recommended teaching the landmark technique, indicating that a large proportion of the physicians who always use US guidance believe that physicians should still be able to perform CVC placement without US. What can justify to perform a landmark procedure if you have an US machine in your setting and you have been trained to US procedures? The only situation remaining is an extreme urgent situation. Fifty-three percent of physicians reported having experienced an emergency situation in which they were unable to wait for the ultrasound machine at least once during the last year. Such situations could justify teaching the landmark technique as a rescue technique, especially as we have demonstrated that residents who have only learned the US-guided technique are unable to perform a landmark procedure [18]. But teaching the landmark procedure during emergency situations where you do not have the time

Table 3 Comparison of the residents and senior physician answers to the last 6 questions of the survey (use of the ultrasound technique)

	Residents $n = 65$	Seniors $n = 125$	p value
Use of ultrasound for CVC placement			
Always	23 % ($n = 15$)	16 % ($n = 20$)	0.3
Almost always	66 % ($n = 43$)	41 % ($n = 51$)	0.001
Half of the time	8 % ($n = 5$)	22 % ($n = 27$)	0.03
Almost never	2 % ($n = 1$)	14 % ($n = 17$)	0.01
Never	2 % ($n = 1$)	8 % ($n = 10$)	0.1
Reasons you do not use ultrasound (MR)			
You think you do not need it	28 % ($n = 18$)	40 % ($n = 50$)	0.1
Not available	43 % ($n = 28$)	27 % ($n = 34$)	0.04
No equipment	9 % ($n = 6$)	0	–
You think the procedure is longer with ultrasound	14 % ($n = 9$)	22 % ($n = 27$)	0.3
Lack of training	5 % ($n = 3$)	14 % ($n = 18$)	0.07
Other reasons	8 % ($n = 5$)	22 % ($n = 28$)	0.02
Which ultrasound technique do you use?			
Skin mark	3 % ($n = 2$)	11 % ($n = 13$)	0.13
Ultrasound guided	81 % ($n = 52$)	65 % ($n = 74$)	0.007
Both	16 % ($n = 10$)	24 % ($n = 27$)	0.4
Which situations would encourage you to use ultrasound? (MR)			
Obesity	57 % ($n = 37$)	52 % ($n = 65$)	0.6
Clotting abnormalities	65 % ($n = 42$)	64 % ($n = 80$))	0.9
Jugular site	51 % ($n = 33$)	42 % ($n = 52$	0.3
Femoral site	12 % ($n = 8$)	23 % ($n = 29$)	0.1
Subclavian site	17 % ($n = 11$)	5 % ($n = 6$)	0.01
Anatomic difficulties	57 % ($n = 37$)	50 % ($n = 62$)	0.4
Missed landmark procedure	37 % ($n = 24$)	46 % ($n = 57$)	0.3
None	0	5 % ($n = 6$)	–
How many times have you experienced an emergency situation in which ultrasound was not available sufficiently rapidly during the last 12 months?			
0	40 % ($n = 26$)	50 % ($n = 63$)	0.2
<2	35 % ($n = 23$)	17 % ($n = 21$)	0.007
2–5	21 % ($n = 14$)	26 % ($n = 32$)	0.6
6–10	3 % ($n = 2$)	6 % ($n = 7$)	0.7
>10	0	2 % ($n = 2$)	–
Do you think the landmark procedure should still be taught to residents?			
Yes	95 % ($n = 62$)	89 % ($n = 111$)	0.4
No	5 % ($n = 3$)	11 % ($n = 14$)	0.2

CVC central venous catheter, *MR* multiple responses

to wait for the US (cardiac arrest for example) is not recommended. The residents will have to perform and learn landmark procedures in nonemergency patients which is associated with a high rate of complications and low success rate during their learning curve. The use of intraosseous catheter could be a good alternative to CVC in case of extreme emergency as previously reported [19, 20].

Our survey presents several limits. The survey responses were self-reported; thus, unknown errors or bias may have resulted from this type of study. In an attempt to keep survey questions brief, questions may have been ambiguous and may have been misinterpreted from their original intent. However, the pilot testing and the test–retest performed by 5 physicians were used to improve the questionnaire as recommended [13]. Our response rate of 66 % may be considered insufficient increasing the risk that our results differ from the non-respondents. But a response rate between 50 and 60 % is usually considered as acceptable, and the mean response rate reported for physicians in published surveys is between 54 and 61 % [13, 21].

In conclusion, training in ultrasound techniques and the widespread availability of ultrasound machines in ICUs seem to improve the rate of US procedures. However, a proportion of physicians still continue to perform landmark techniques and consider this technique as an alternative to US. The translation of evidence to clinical practice regarding the benefits of ultrasound guidance for central venous catheter placement faces many barriers. The belief that they do not need US despite strong scientific evidence and the desire to continue to teach the landmark technique to residents indicate the aspiration of physicians to continue landmark procedures. Training and education are potentially still the best ways to overcome such barriers or conviction.

Abbreviations

CVC: central venous catheter; ER: emergency room; ICU: intensive care unit; OR: operating room; US: ultrasound.

Authors' contributions

JM, MAB designed the study; JM, MAB, JR, EF, CL, BS and HD collected the data; JM did the statistical analysis; and JM, MAB, HD, FT, SN and DDC interpreted the data. All authors read and approved the final manuscript.

Author details

[1] Medical ICU and INSERM U1088, University Hospital, Amiens, France. [2] Medical-Surgical ICU, Medical Center, Beauvais, France. [3] Medical-Surgical ICU, Medical Center, Le Havre, France. [4] Medical-Surgical ICU, Medical Center, Roubaix, France. [5] Medical-Surgical ICU, Medical Center, Cherbourg, France. [6] Department of Anesthesiology and Critical Care and INSERM U1088, University Hospital, Amiens, France. [7] Medical ICU, University Hospital, Rouen, France. [8] Medical ICU, University Hospital, Lille, France. [9] Medical ICU, University Hospital, Caen, France.

Acknowledgements

The authors thank the BoReal study group (by alphabetical order): G Alvado (Bayeux), C Andrejak (Amiens), P Azera (Saint Lô), G Barjon (Compiègne), C Boulle (Douai), O Delastre (Elbeuf), V Delerue (Béthune), M Detave (Montreuil), P Dubosq (Evreux), J Elbaaj (Lisieux), M Fiani (Chateau-thierry), P Jeanjean (Amiens), F Lambiotte (Maubeuge), O Leroy (Tourcoing), M Moubarak (Amiens), R Pordes (Boulogne), E Renaud (Creil), JP Rigaud (Dieppe), A Rivière (Abbeville), R Sahri (Soissons), P Saint Leger (Armentières), D Thevenin (Lens) and T Vanderlinden (Lomme).

Competing interests

The authors declare that they have no competing interests.

References

1. National institute for clinical excellence NICE Technology Appraisal No. 49: guidance on the use of ultrasound locating devices for placing central venous catheters. http://www.nice.org.uk/nicemedia/live/11474/32461/32461.pdf (2002).
2. Troianos CA, Hartman GS, Glas KE, Skubas NJ, Eberhardt RT, Walker JD, et al. Guidelines for performing ultrasound guided vascular cannulation: recommendations of the American Society of Echocardiography and the Society of Cardiovascular Anesthesiologists. J Am Soc Echocardiogr. 2011;24:1291–318.
3. Rupp SM, Apfelbaum JL, Blitt C, Caplan RA, Connis RT, Domino KB, et al. Practice guidelines for central venous access: a report by the American Society of Anesthesiologists Task Force on Central Venous Access. Anesthesiology. 2012;116:539–73.
4. Frykholm P, Pikwer A, Hammarskjöld F, Larsson AT, Lindgren S, Lindwall R, et al. Clinical guidelines on central venous catheterisation. Swedish Society of Anaesthesiology and Intensive Care Medicine. Acta Anaesthesiol Scand. 2014;58:508–24.
5. Lamperti M, Bodenham AR, Pittiruti M, Blaivas M, Augoustides JG, Elbarbary M, et al. International evidence-based recommendations on ultrasound-guided vascular access. Intensive Care Med. 2012;38:1105–17.
6. Bailey PL, Glance LG, Eaton MP, Parshall B, McIntosh S. A survey of the use of ultrasound during central venous catheterization. Anesth Analg. 2007;104:491–7.
7. Matava C, Hayes J. A survey of ultrasound use by academic and community anesthesiologists in Ontario. Can J Anaesth. 2011;58:929–35.
8. Lindgren S, Pikwer A, Ricksten SE, Åkeson J. Survey of central venous catheterisation practice in Sweden. Acta Anaesthesiol Scand. 2013;57:1237–44.
9. Zieleskiewicz L, Muller L, Lakhal K, Meresse Z, Arbelot C, Bertrand PM, et al. Point-of-care ultrasound in intensive care units: assessment of 1073 procedures in a multicentric, prospective, observational study. Intensive Care Med. 2015;41:1638–47.
10. Parienti JJ, Mongardon N, Megarbane B, Mira JP, Kalfon P, Gros A, et al. Intravascular complications of central venous catheterization by insertion site. N Engl J Med. 2015;373:1220–9.
11. Dassinger MS, Renaud EJ, Goldin A, Huang EY, Russell RT, Streck CJ, et al. Use of real-time ultrasound during central venous catheter placement: results of an APSA survey. J Pediatr Surg. 2015;50:1162–7.
12. Buchanan MS, Backlund B, Liao MM, Sun J, Cydulka RK, Smith-Coggins R, et al. Use of ultrasound guidance for central venous catheter placement: survey from the American Board of Emergency Medicine Longitudinal Study of Emergency Physicians. Acad Emerg Med. 2014;21:416–21.
13. Burns KE, Duffett M, Kho ME, Meade MO, Adhikari NK, Sinuff T, et al. A guide for the design and conduct of self-administered surveys of clinicians. CMAJ. 2008;179:245–52.
14. Mimoz O, Moreira R, Frasca D, Boisson M, Dahyot-Fizelier C. Practice assessment of central venous lines care in surgical ICU of French university hospitals. Ann Fr Anesth Reanim. 2010;29:104–12.
15. Fragou M, Gravvanis A, Dimitriou V, Papalois A, Kouraklis G, Karabinis A, et al. Real-time ultrasound-guided subclavian vein cannulation versus the landmark method in critical care patients: a prospective randomized study. Crit Care Med. 2011;39:1607–12.
16. Brass P, Hellmich M, Kolodziej L, Schick G, Smith AF. Ultrasound guidance versus anatomical landmarks for internal jugular vein catheterization. Cochrane Database Syst Rev. 2015;1:CD006962.
17. Brass P, Hellmich M, Kolodziej L, Schick G, Smith AF. Ultrasound guidance versus anatomical landmarks for subclavian or femoral vein catheterization. Cochrane Database Syst Rev. 2015;1:CD011447.
18. Maizel J, Guyomarc'h L, Henon P, Modeliar SS, de Cagny B, Choukroun G, et al. Residents learning ultrasound-guided catheterization are not sufficiently skilled to use landmarks. Crit Care. 2014;18:R36.
19. Lee PM, Lee C, Rattner P, Wu X, Gershengorn H, Acquah S. Intraosseous versus central venous catheter utilization and performance during inpatient medical emergencies. Crit Care Med. 2015;43:1233–8.
20. Leidel BA, Kirchhoff C, Bogner V, Braunstein V, Biberthaler P, Kanz KG. Comparison of intraosseous versus central venous vascular access in adults under resuscitation in the emergency department with inaccessible peripheral veins. Resuscitation. 2012;83:40–5.
21. Asch DA, Jedrzwieski MK, Christakis NA. Response rates to mail surveys published in medical journals. J Clin Epidemiol. 1997;50:1129–36.

Knockout of interleukin-17A protects against sepsis-associated acute kidney injury

Cong-juan Luo[1,2], Feng Luo[1,3], Li Zhang[2*], Yan Xu[1], Guang-yan Cai[2], Bo Fu[2], Zhe Feng[2], Xue-feng Sun[2] and Xiang-mei Chen[2*]

Abstract

Background: Sepsis-associated acute kidney injury (SA-AKI) is an independent risk factor for death in patients with sepsis, but treatment for it is limited. To improve the diagnosis and treatment of SA-AKI, we must first understand its pathogenesis. Recently, interleukin (IL)-17A has been shown to be associated with the pathogenesis of acute kidney injury and sepsis, but its role in SA-AKI remains unclear.

Methods: SA-AKI was induced in male C57BL/6 and IL-17A$^{-/-}$ mice using cecal ligation and puncture (CLP) operations for 24 h.

Results: At 7 days, only seven mice survived in the wild-type septic group, but nine survived in the IL-17A$^{-/-}$ septic group, corresponding to survival rates of 25 % and 45 %, respectively. At 24 h after CLP operations, both wild-type and IL-17A$^{-/-}$ septic mice developed kidney injury. The IL-17A$^{-/-}$ septic mice exhibited decreased serum creatinine and blood urea nitrogen levels and an improved acute tubular necrosis score. The IL-17A$^{-/-}$ septic mice exhibited decreased IL-6, interferon-γ, tumor necrosis factor-α, CXCL1, CXCL2, and CXCL5 expression in kidney tissue, but increased IL-10 expression. In addition, renal neutrophil infiltration was attenuated significantly in the IL-17A$^{-/-}$ septic group. Moreover, IL-17A$^{-/-}$ septic mice showed significantly decreased apoptosis of tubular epithelial cells, including decreased TUNEL-positive tubular cell number and cleaved caspase-3 level, compared with the wild-type CLP group. Their Bax/Bcl-2 expression ratio was also increased.

Conclusions: Our study demonstrates that IL-17A knockout could protect against SA-AKI. We show that IL-17A plays a pathogenic role in SA-AKI by increasing the levels of proinflammatory cytokines and chemokines, and by inducing neutrophil infiltration and apoptosis of tubular epithelial cells. Accordingly, IL-17A may be a novel target in SA-AKI.

Keywords: IL-17A knockout, Sepsis, Sepsis-associated acute kidney injury

Background

Sepsis-associated acute kidney injury (SA-AKI) is an independent risk factor for death in patients with sepsis [1], but its treatment is limited. To improve the diagnosis and treatment of SA-AKI, we must first understand its pathogenesis. In recent years, the majority of studies on this type of injury have focused on hemodynamic factors after bacterial invasion. However, in many patients, SA-AKI occurs without overt signs of global renal hypoperfusion and SA-AKI has been described in the presence of normal or even increased renal blood flow [2]. Therefore, in recent years, apoptosis, neutrophil infiltration, and the production of proinflammatory cytokines have been considered important mechanisms of SA-AKI [3].

Interleukin (IL)-17 is a proinflammatory cytokine secreted mainly by TH17 cells and γδT cells [4]. It constitutes a novel cytokine family that includes six structurally related isoforms, IL-17A to IL-17F [5]. IL-17A, the first identified member of the IL-17 family, now synonymous with IL-17, acts on a variety of cells through its ubiquitous receptors. In addition, it induces the production of other cytokines and chemokines from a variety of cells

*Correspondence: zhangl301@hotmail.com; xmchen301@126.com
[2] State Key Laboratory of Kidney Diseases, Department of Nephrology, Chinese PLA General Hospital and Medical School of Chinese PLA, No.28 Fuxing Road, Beijing 100853, People's Republic of China
Full list of author information is available at the end of the article

and coordinates the recruitment of myeloid cells, such as monocytes and neutrophils, to sites of inflammation [6]. The discovery of the IL-17A cytokine family provided a novel approach to examine the processes underlying inflammatory diseases. It can also help us to identify new therapeutic targets of inflammatory diseases.

Although all clinical research on neutralizing a single mediator of a single target was unsuccessful, the neutralization of IL-17A still showed promise. Studies have reported that IL-17A reached high levels in septic mice after cecal ligation and puncture (CLP) injury, and that the use of antibodies to neutralize IL-17A improved sepsis survival from 10 % to nearly 60 % [7]. Accordingly, targeted IL-17A depletion has been adopted as a therapeutic strategy and is currently undergoing clinical trials for several human autoimmune diseases [8, 9].

Recently, IL-17A has also been shown to be associated with the pathogenesis of kidney and intestine ischemia/reperfusion (I/R) injury [10–12], but its role in SA-AKI remains unclear. Thus, in this study, we used IL-17A$^{-/-}$ mice to evaluate the role of IL-17A in an SA-AKI model induced by CLP injury.

Methods

Animals

Male C57BL/6 mice aged 8–10 weeks were purchased from the animal center at The Chinese People's Liberation Army (PLA) General Hospital (Beijing, China). IL-17A$^{-/-}$ mice in a C57BL/6 background were kindly provided by Professor H. L. Wang (Shanghai Institute of Immunology, Institute of Medical Sciences, Shanghai Jiao Tong University School of Medicine). The mice were maintained on a chow diet in a 12-h light/12-h dark environment at 25 °C at The Chinese PLA General Hospital's Animal Care Facility, in accordance with institutional guidelines. They were acclimated for 1 week prior to the experiments. All animal studies were approved by the Ethics Committee of The Chinese PLA General Hospital.

Mouse model of cecal ligation and puncture

Cecal ligation and puncture-induced sepsis was generated as described previously [13]. Mice were anesthetized with 2 % pentobarbital, and a 1- to 2-cm midline incision was made along the linea alba of the abdominal muscle to isolate and exteriorize the cecum. A total of 75 % of the cecum was ligated with a 4-0 silk suture, and the cecum was punctured twice with a 21-gauge needle. A small amount (droplet) of feces was gently extruded from the holes to ensure patency. The cecum was then returned to the peritoneal cavity and the abdominal incision was closed with 4-0 silk sutures. After the operation, 1 mL of pre-warmed normal saline was administered into the peritoneal cavity. In the sham group, mice underwent the same procedure but were neither ligated nor punctured.

Wild-type and IL-17A$^{-/-}$ mice for blood tests and histological and immunochemical analyses were each divided into two groups: a sham group and a CLP group. Then euthanized 24 h after surgery. Wild-type and IL-17A$^{-/-}$ mice for survival study were also divided into two groups: a sham group and a CLP group. Then euthanized 7d after surgery (Additional file 1).

Survival study

For a survival study, mice in each group were monitored closely for 7 days ($n = 20$/group), after which they were euthanized.

Assessment of kidney function

Kidney injury was assessed based on the levels of serum creatinine and blood urea nitrogen. Mouse serum samples were obtained at 24 h after CLP injury, and the serum was separated by centrifugation at 3000 rpm for 15 min at 4 °C and then stored at −20 °C until use.

Histopathology

For histopathological assessment, kidney tissues were harvested 24 h after CLP. Specimens were fixed in 10 % formaldehyde for at least 24 h. The samples were then embedded in paraffin and sectioned at 4-μm thickness for staining with periodic acid-Schiff. Stained sections were observed using a light microscope (Olympus IX71; Olympus, Tokyo, Japan) at a magnification of 400× and evaluated by three independent pathologists. Histological examinations for acute tubular necrosis were semi-quantified and blinded using the following scoring system, as described previously [14]: 0 = none, 1 = ≤10 %; 2 = 11–25 %, 3 = 26–45 %, 4 = 46–75 %, and 5 = >75 %.

Real-time PCR

Total RNA was extracted from kidney tissue using TRIzol reagent (Invitrogen, Carlsbad, CA, USA) following the manufacturer's instructions. Reverse transcription was performed using the TaqMan Reverse Transcription Kit (Applied Biosystems, Foster City, CA, USA) and a Gene Amp PCR System 9700 (Applied Biosystems) was used to generate cDNA. Real-time quantitative RT-PCR using 2 μL of cDNA from each sample was performed in duplicate with SYBR Mastermix, in accordance with the manufacturer's instructions. All reactions were performed using a 7500 Real-time PCR System (Applied Biosystems). For analysis, glyceraldehyde 3-phosphate dehydrogenase (GAPDH) was used as a normalization control. The relative target mRNA expression normalized to GAPDH expression was analyzed using the $2^{-\Delta\Delta CT}$ method. The primers used are shown in Table 1.

Immunofluorescence studies of kidney samples

Neutrophil granulocyte infiltration into the kidney was evaluated by the detection of Ly6G-positive cells by immunofluorescence; Five-μm-thick kidney sections were cut and incubated overnight with rat anti-Ly6G (1:100; Santa Cruz Biotechnology, Santa Cruz, CA, USA) antibody in a humidified chamber. Secondary antibodies conjugated to CY3 rabbit anti-rat immunoglobulin G (IgG; 1:50; Jackson ImmunoResearch Laboratories, West Grove, PA, USA) were applied for 1 h at room temperature in a darkened humidified chamber. Nuclei were stained with 4′,6-diamidino-2-phenylindole (Zhongshan Goldenbridge Biotechnology, Beijing, China). Each tissue section was observed in a blinded manner under a confocal laser scanning microscope (Olympus FluoView 1000) at a magnification of 600×.

TUNEL staining

For terminal deoxynucleotidyl-transferase-mediated dUTP nick-end labeling (TUNEL) staining, kidneys were fixed in 4 % paraformaldehyde, embedded in paraffin, and cut into 5-μm-thick sections and stained using the DeadEnd Fluorometric TUNEL system (Promega Corporation, Madison, WI, USA), in accordance with the manufacturer's instructions, followed by visualization under an Olympus laser scanning confocal microscope (IX81). Quantitative analysis of TUNEL-positive cells was performed using the Image-Pro software in 20 random fields for each mouse by a technician who was blinded to the treatment groups. The mean of all counts was used for comparisons among the groups.

Western blot analysis

Kidney lysates were prepared by homogenization on ice for 30 min using radioimmunoprecipitation assay buffer [50 mM Tris–Cl (pH 7.6), 150 mM NaCl, 1 % NP-40, 0.1 % sodium dodecyl sulfate, 0.5 % deoxycholic acid, 1 μg/mL leupeptin, 1 μg/mL aprotinin, and 0.5 mM phenylmethylsulfonyl fluoride], and then centrifuged at 12,000 rpm for 30 min at 4 °C, after which supernatants were collected. A total of 100 μg of protein was separated by 15 % sodium dodecyl sulfate–polyacrylamide gel electrophoresis and transferred to a nitrocellulose membrane. Anti-Bax, -Bcl-2, and -cleaved caspase-3 antibodies (Cell Signaling Technology, Danvers, MA, USA) were used as primary antibodies at 4 °C overnight, and horseradish peroxidase-conjugated anti-rabbit/mouse IgG (Santa Cruz Biotechnology) was used as the secondary antibody. Densitometry was performed using Quantity One software (Bio-Rad Laboratories, Hercules, CA, USA).

Table 1 Primers used for real-time PCR

Gene	Forward primers (5′–3′)	Reverse primer (5′–3′)
IL-17	TGGACTCTCCACCGCAATG	TGGGGGTTTCTTAGGGGTCA
IL-6	AGTCAATTCCAGAAACCGCTATG	ACAGGTCTGTTGGGAGTGGT
TNF-α	CTACTGAACTTCGGGGTGAT	CAGGCTTGTCACTCGAATT
IL-10	AGGCAGCCTTGCAGAAAAGA	GCTCCACTGCCTTGCTCTTA
IFN-γ	ATGAACGCTACACACTGCATC	CCATCCTTTTGCCAGTTCCTC
CXCL1	TGGCTGGGATTCACCTCAAGAACA	TGTGGCTATGACTTCG-GTTTGGGT
CXCL2	GAAGTCATAGCCACTCTCAAGG	TTCCGTTGAGGGACAGCA
CXCL5	CGTAACTCCAAAAATTAATCCCAAA	CGAGTGCATTCCGCTTAGCT

Statistics

The survival of mice was estimated by Kaplan–Meier analysis. A log-rank test was used to analyze the survival data. Data are expressed as mean ± standard error. Differences were evaluated using unpaired Student's t tests between two groups and one-way ANOVA for multiple comparisons, followed by a post hoc Student–Newman–Keuls test when necessary. The value of α was corrected by the number of comparisons $[2\alpha/n\ (n-1)]$ to ensure $\alpha = 0.05$ [15]. mRNA levels were calculated using the $2^{-\Delta\Delta CT}$ method. Analyses were performed using SPSS for Windows (version 10.1; SPSS, Chicago, IL, USA). Statistical significance was set at $P < 0.05$.

Results

Effect of IL-17A knockout on the survival of CLP-induced septic mice

In the absence of antibiotic therapy, we investigated whether IL-$17A^{-/-}$ septic mice showed any improvement in terms of survival at 7 days. At 24 h, seven mice had died in the wild-type CLP group, while only five mice had died in the IL-$17A^{-/-}$-CLP group. At 7 days, the survival rate of the wild-type septic group was 25 %, while that of the knockout IL-17A group was 45 % (Fig. 1). IL-17A knockout significantly improved the survival rate at 7 days compared with that in wild-type mice ($P < 0.05$). In addition, no mortality was observed within 7 days in all sham mice (survival rate = 100 %).

Effects of IL-17A knockout on renal function in SA-AKI

Renal injury was assessed by measuring blood urea nitrogen and creatinine levels at 24 h. Baseline levels of these plasma markers of kidney injury did not differ significantly between the wild-type and IL-$17A^{-/-}$ sham groups. Levels of blood urea nitrogen and creatinine were increased in wild-type and IL-$17A^{-/-}$ mice with

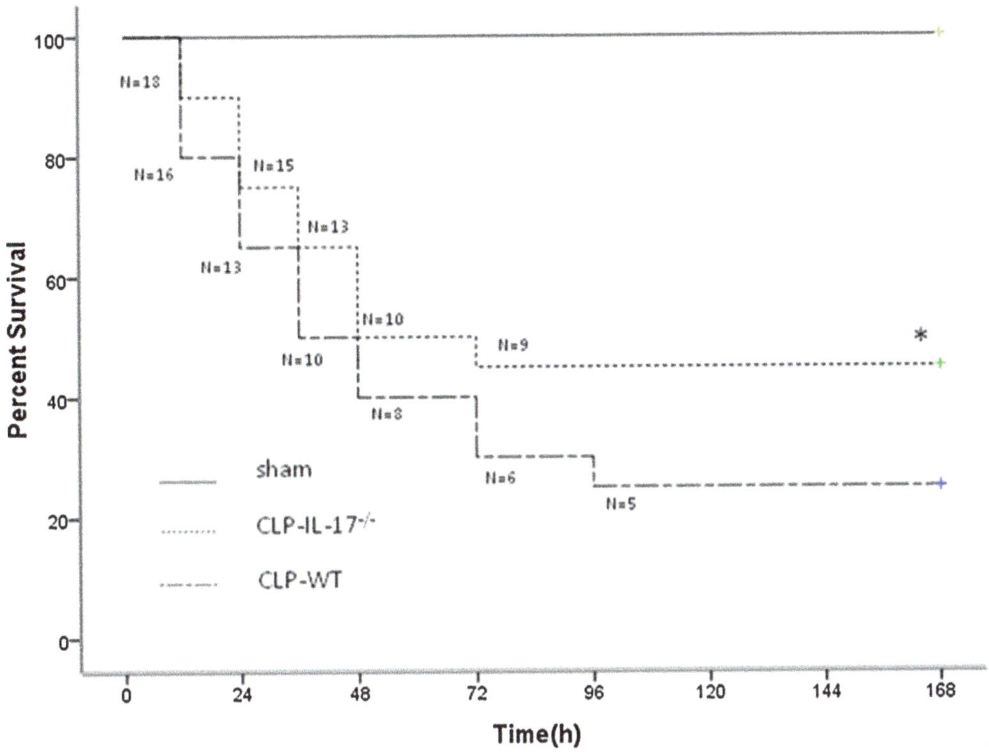

Fig. 1 Survival rate of cecal ligation and puncture (CLP) model mice. Each group consisted of 20 animals. Kaplan–Meier *curves* show the survival rate in each group. The survival rate at 7 days was significantly higher in the interleukin (IL)-17A knockout CLP group than in the wild-type CLP group; *$P < 0.05$

CLP-induced sepsis compared with those in the sham group, indicative of the development of SA-AKI. Compared with wild-type septic mice, IL-17A$^{-/-}$ septic mice showed significantly reduced creatinine and blood urea nitrogen levels ($P < 0.05$; Fig. 2).

Effects of IL-17A knockout on renal histology in SA-AKI

Morphological changes in the sepsis group were scored 24 h after CLP injury based on brush border loss, tubular degeneration, and vacuolization in the proximal tubules. Knockout of IL-17A ameliorated the tissue damage and reduced the tubular injury score ($P < 0.05$; Fig. 3). Taken together, our data show that CLP-induced polymicrobial sepsis resulted in SA-AKI, the severity of which was reduced by IL-17A knockout.

Effect of IL-17A knockout on renal cytokine and chemokine mRNA levels

Previous studies showed that IL-17A in peritoneal fluid plays a critical role during severe polymicrobial sepsis [7]. We hypothesized that IL-17A would play an important role in SA-AKI. To investigate whether IL-17A knockout affected local renal production of inflammatory cytokines and chemokines, we assayed the renal mRNA levels of these cytokines using RT-PCR. The IL-17A, IL-6, interferon (IFN)-γ, tumor necrosis factor (TNF)-α, and IL-10 mRNA levels were increased significantly in both CLP groups at 24 h (Fig. 4). Compared with the wild-type septic group, IL-17A knockout decreased the IL-17A, IL-6, IFN-γ, and TNF-α mRNA levels ($P < 0.05$), but increased the level of IL-10 ($P < 0.05$; Fig. 4).

The chemokines CXCL1, CXCL2, and CXCL5 are not only potent neutrophil chemoattractants but are also encoded by IL-17A target genes. We thus examined the mRNA levels of these chemokine genes related to IL-17A function in the kidney using RT-PCR. The CXCL1, CXCL2, and CXCL5 mRNA levels were increased significantly in the wild-type CLP group and decreased in the IL-17A$^{-/-}$ septic group ($P < 0.05$; Fig. 4). SA-AKI caused a significant increase in the mRNA levels of all five chemokines, consistent with increased neutrophil infiltration. Moreover, IL-17A knockout had the opposite effect on the expression of these chemokines after SA-AKI.

Effect of IL-17A knockout on neutrophil infiltration

Neutrophil infiltration is a hallmark of inflammatory injury after sepsis [16], and one of the main functions of

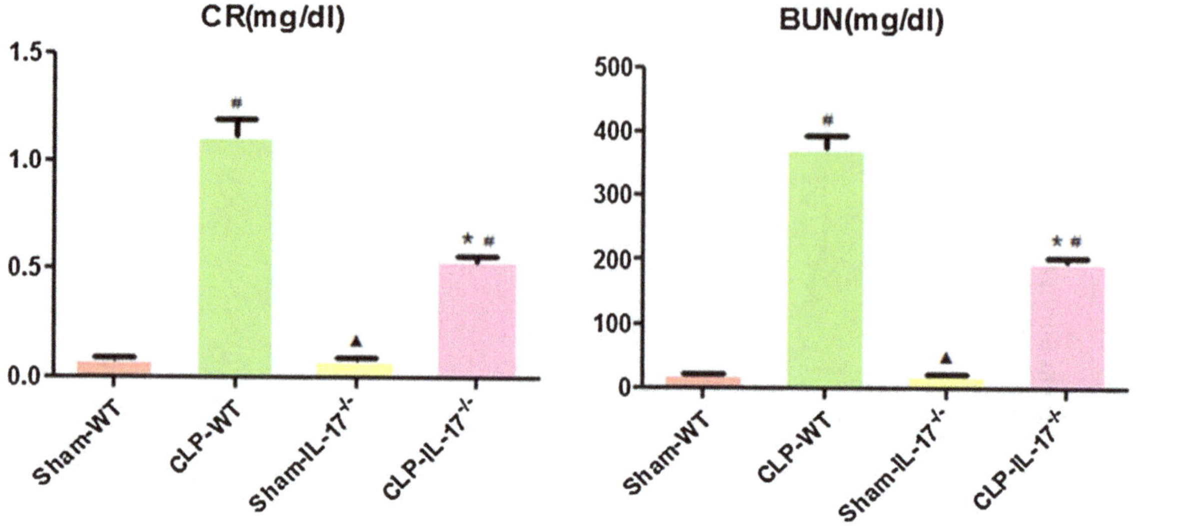

Fig. 2 Changes in creatinine and blood urea nitrogen in the four groups. IL-17 knockout significantly reduced creatinine (Cr) and blood urea nitrogen (BUN) levels 24 h after CLP injury compared with the levels in wild-type CLP mice. $^{\#}P < 0.05$ compared with the sham group. $^{*}P < 0.05$ compared with the wild-type CLP group. Wild-type sham group $n = 20$, IL-17A$^{-/-}$ sham group $n = 20$, wild-type CLP group $n = 1\,2$, and IL-17A$^{-/-}$ septic group $n = 15$

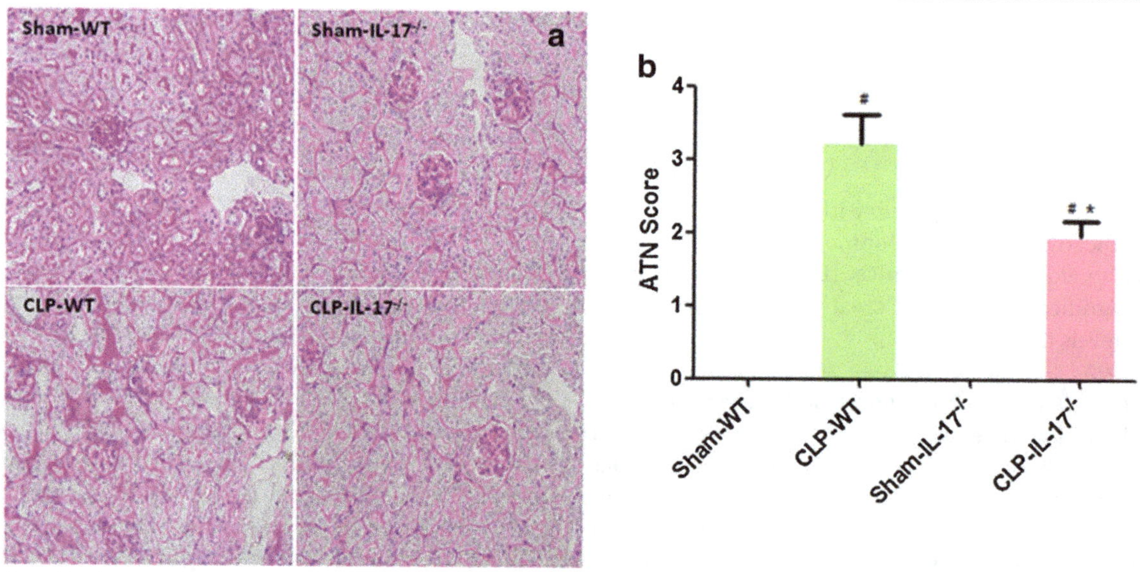

Fig. 3 Renal histology changes in the four groups. **a** Sections were subjected to Periodic acid/Schiff staining to assess kidney morphology. **b** Semi-quantitation of the morphological changes using a histological grading system. The data are presented as mean ± standard deviation (SD). $^{\#}P < 0.05$ compared with the sham group. $^{*}P < 0.05$ compared with the wild-type CLP group. Wild-type sham group $n = 20$, IL-17A$^{-/-}$ sham group $n = 20$, wild-type CLP group $n = 12$, and IL-17A$^{-/-}$ septic group $n = 15$

IL-17A is neutrophil recruitment. To determine whether neutrophil infiltration played a role in our model, we examined the degree of neutrophil infiltration in the kidney using immunofluorescence. No Ly-6G-positive cell infiltration was detected in the sham group of wild-type and IL-17A knockout mice (Fig. 5). In the wild-type septic group, many Ly-6G-positive cells were observed in the renal tissue (Fig. 5), primarily in the renal cortex, including the glomerulus and tubulointerstitium. Compared with the wild-type septic group, the IL-17A$^{-/-}$ septic group exhibited less neutrophil infiltration (Fig. 5).

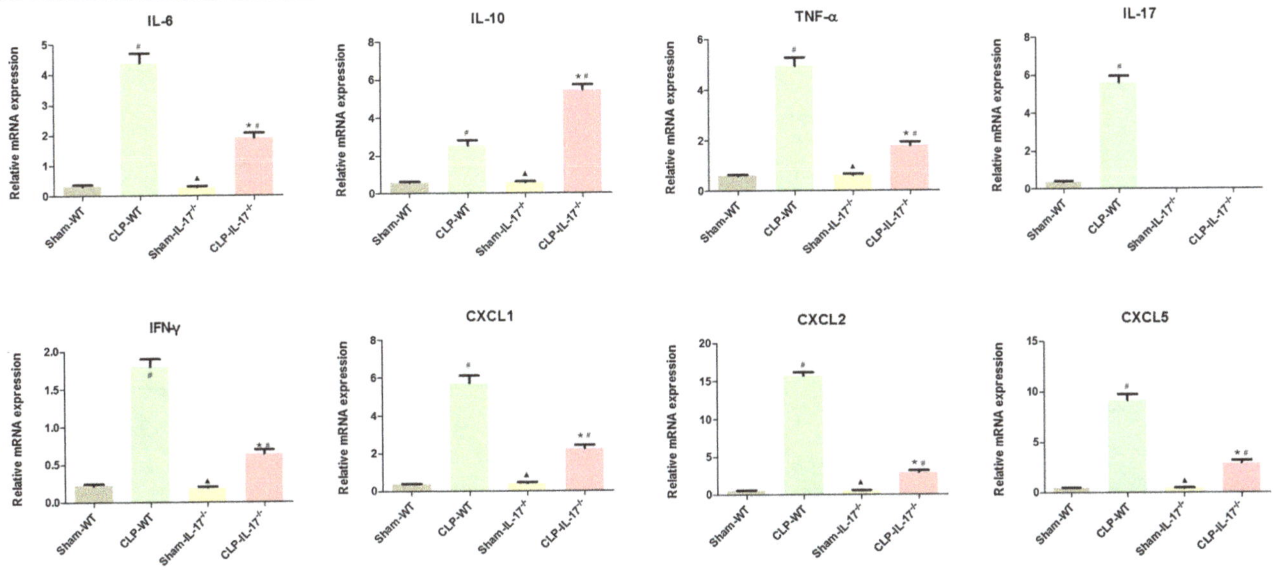

Fig. 4 mRNA levels of inflammatory cytokines and chemokines in the kidneys. The mRNA levels of the inflammatory cytokines IL-10, IL-17, IL-6, interferon-γ, and tumor necrosis factor-α and the chemokines CXCL1, CXCL2, and CXCL5 in kidney tissue 24 h after sham or CLP operation. $^{\#}P < 0.05$ compared with the sham group. $^{*}P < 0.05$ compared with the wild-type CLP group. Wild-type sham group $n = 20$, IL-17A$^{-/-}$ sham group $n = 20$, wild-type CLP group $n = 12$, and IL-17A$^{-/-}$ septic group $n = 15$

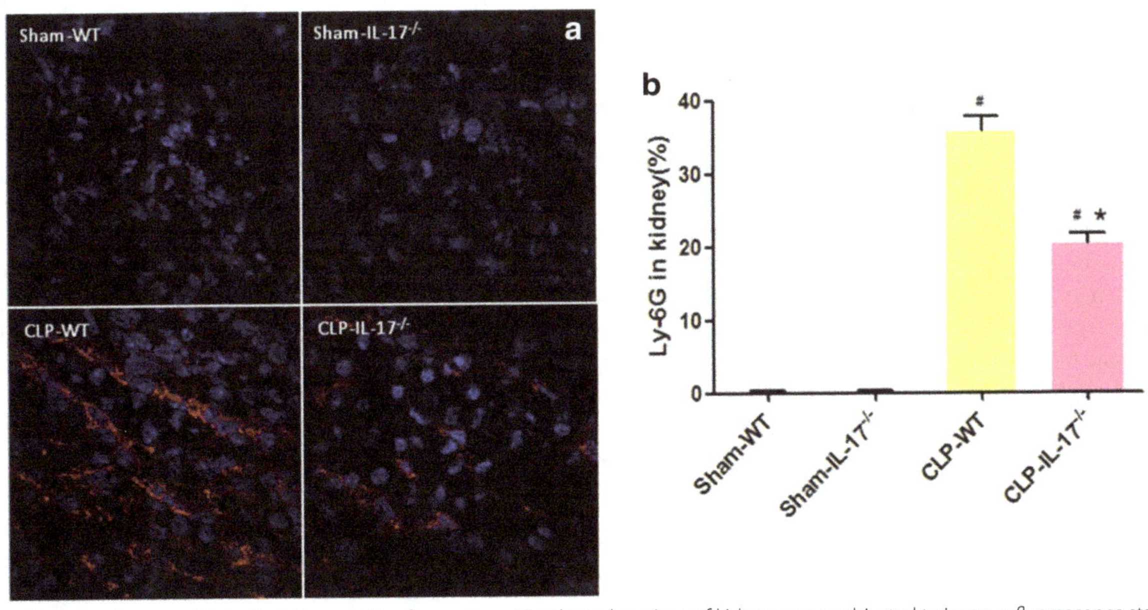

Fig. 5 Infiltration of neutrophils in the kidneys of the four groups. Histological sections of kidneys were subjected to immunofluorescence staining, and the number of positive cells was counted in five high-powered fields per section (original magnification ×400). Values represent mean ± SD. $^{\#}P < 0.05$ compared with the sham group. $^{*}P < 0.05$ compared with the wild-type CLP group. Wild-type sham group $n = 20$, IL-17A$^{-/-}$ sham group $n = 20$, wild-type CLP group $n = 12$, and IL-17A$^{-/-}$ septic group $n = 15$

Anti-apoptotic effects of IL-17A knockout in SA-AKI

Apoptosis contributes significantly to AKI. We hypothesized that the role of IL-17A in SA-AKI is associated with tubular apoptosis. To test this hypothesis, we performed TUNEL assays of renal sections obtained 24 h after CLP injury. As shown in Fig. 6, IL-17A knockout significantly decreased the number of TUNEL-positive tubular cells compared with that in wild-type CLP mice, suggesting

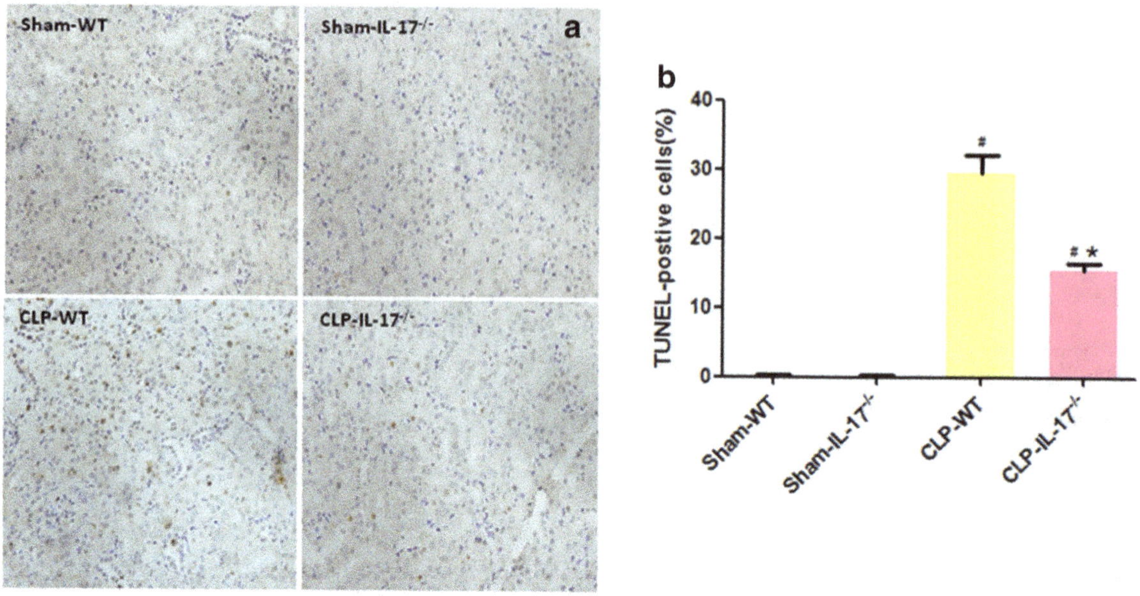

Fig. 6 Numbers of terminal deoxynucleotidyl-transferase-mediated dUTP nick-end labeling (TUNEL)-positive cells in the kidneys. Quantitative analysis of TUNEL-positive cells from 20 random fields per mouse. The data are presented as mean ± SD. $^{\#}P < 0.05$ compared with the sham group. $^{*}P < 0.05$ compared with the wild-type CLP group. Wild-type sham group $n = 20$, IL-17A$^{-/-}$ sham group $n = 20$, wild-type CLP group $n = 12$, and IL-17A$^{-/-}$ septic group $n = 15$

that IL17A knockout reduced the extent of tubular apoptosis.

The expression of cleaved caspase-3, a biomarker of apoptosis, was increased significantly in the wild-type septic group (Fig. 7). The IL-17A$^{-/-}$ septic group also showed an increased cleaved caspase-3 level, albeit significantly less than that in the wild-type septic group (Fig. 7). Furthermore, Bax expression was increased significantly in the wild-type septic group, while there was less expression in the kidney of IL-17A$^{-/-}$ septic mice at the same time (Fig. 7). In addition, Bcl-2 expression decreased slightly in both septic groups. The Bax/Bcl-2 ratio was increased to a greater extent in the wild-type septic group than in the IL-17A$^{-/-}$ septic group. Therefore, IL-17A knockout attenuated the occurrence of kidney cell death induced by CLP injury.

Discussion

In recent years, research has revealed that the main pathogenic factors in SA-AKI are not hemodynamic failure or ischemia, as previously thought, but inflammation and apoptosis [3]. Accordingly, therapies aimed at suppressing apoptosis and inflammation are currently being sought.

In our study, we revealed that IL-17A knockout caused a marked amelioration of SA-AKI, which was associated with a reduction in neutrophil infiltration and tubular cell apoptosis. Moreover, IL-17A enhanced neutrophil infiltration, possibly by inducing CXC chemokine-mediated neutrophil migration. In light of these novel findings, IL-17A may become a new therapeutic target.

Increasing evidence has indicated that both adaptive and innate immunity play a role in the pathogenesis of sepsis [17]. Notably, IL-17A acts as a bridge between adaptive and innate immunity through the inflammatory response [18], and thus occupies a unique position in the pathogenic process of sepsis. A growing body of evidence has also demonstrated that IL-17A is involved in the inflammatory response during kidney injury in acute renal obstruction [19]. However, little was previously known about SA-AKI, although IL-17A is involved in the pathogenesis of sepsis. In this context, we previously reported the important finding that circulating IL-17A levels were elevated in SA-AKI [20]. Therefore, we focused on the effect of IL-17A in SA-AKI using the IL-17A$^{-/-}$ CLP mouse model. Notably, in IL-17A$^{-/-}$ mice, kidney function and morphology were found to be protected after SA-AKI. In this study, genetic deficiency in IL-17A ameliorated SA-AKI markedly, as demonstrated by reduced mortality, improved inflammatory markers, and reduced neutrophil infiltration, which demonstrated a critical role for IL-17A in SA-AKI.

Neutrophil recruitment plays a major role in SA-AKI. Neutrophil chemotaxis and activation may be regulated by CXC chemokines. Interestingly, IL-17A has also been shown to induce the production of CXCL1, CXCL2, and

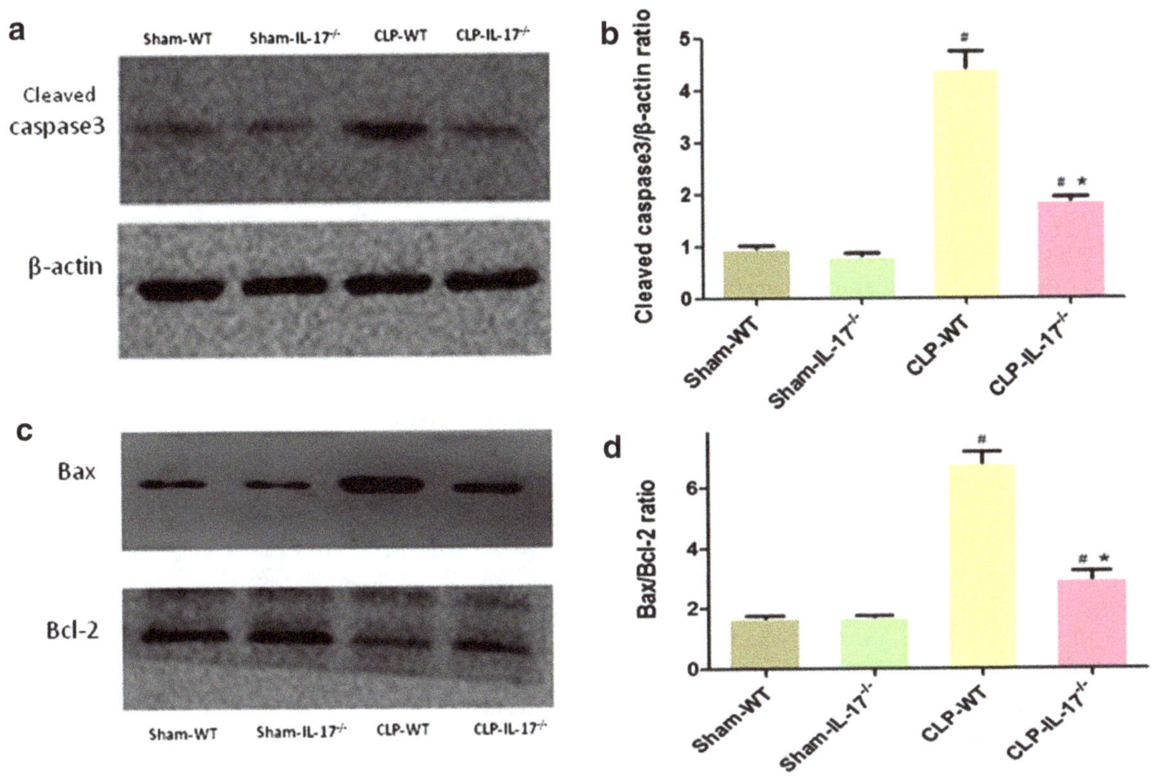

Fig. 7 Expression of Bax, Bcl-2, and cleaved caspase-3 in the kidneys. **a** Western blot results for cleaved caspase-3 protein. **b** Quantitative analysis of cleaved caspase-3. **c** Western blot of Bax and Bcl-2 proteins. **d** Quantitative analysis of Bax and Bcl-2. The protein levels are presented as mean ± SD. $^{\#}P < 0.05$ compared with the sham group. $^{*}P < 0.05$ compared with the wild-type CLP group. Wild-type sham group $n = 20$, IL-17A$^{-/-}$ sham group $n = 20$, wild-type CLP group $n = 12$, and IL-17A$^{-/-}$ septic group $n = 15$

CXCL5 in mouse osteoblastic cells and lung fibroblasts [21, 22]. Moreover, IL-17A has been shown to induce the recruitment of neutrophils into the airways via the production of CXC chemokines [23]. However, the production of IL-17A during infection has not always been correlated with protection. In a murine CLP model of polymicrobial sepsis, IL-17A from γδT cells was detected, but its depletion led to a decrease in bacteremia and reductions in systemic proinflammatory cytokines (TNF-α, IL-1β, and IL-6) and chemokines [24]. In our study, we found that the inhibition of IL-17A markedly decreased renal CXCL1, CXCL2, and CXCL5 expression and neutrophil infiltration. This is consistent with previous reports describing that elevated IL-17A induced neutrophil recruitment and increased inflammation in a more severe CLP model [7]. IL-17A also enhanced cardiomyocyte LIX, KC, and MIP-2 production and neutrophil migration to the supernatant from conditioned cardiomyocytes in vitro [25]. Although we have no further data to validate the pathogenic role of IL-17A in SA-AKI in vitro, which is a limitation of our study, our results still indicate that IL-17A may contribute to SA-AKI, at least in part through the regulation of neutrophil infiltration to the kidney by affecting CXC chemokine expression.

Apoptosis plays an important role in health and disease. It also contributes to kidney dysfunction in I/R or nephrotoxin-induced AKI [26, 27]. However, no consensus has been reached on the role of renal cell apoptosis in the development of SA-AKI. In terms of the histopathological findings from biopsies taken from septic AKI patients, these have been reported to include acute tubular injury or necrosis to varying degrees; leukocyte infiltration into glomeruli, interstitial capillaries, and tubular lumen; and apoptosis in tubular cells and on rare occasions in glomerular cells [28, 29]. In contrast, Langenberg et al. [30] reported a lack of any tubular injury or apoptosis in a sheep SA-AKI model. However, in our study, we observed that a substantial number of tubular cells underwent apoptosis. In addition to increased numbers of TUNEL-positive cells, cleaved caspase-3 activity and Bax were also increased in septic kidneys compared with those in sham kidneys. Meanwhile, the reduced level of the anti-apoptosis protein Bcl-2 also suggested that apoptosis occurred in the kidneys of septic mice after CLP surgery. IL-17A has also been shown to induce apoptosis of vascular smooth muscle cells and airway epithelial cells [31, 32]. However, there are no reports on the role of IL-17A in renal tubular cell apoptosis. Our in vivo study showed that IL-17A knockout reduced tubular cell apoptosis, as confirmed by the decreased number of TUNEL-positive tubular cells, the reduced cleaved caspase-3 activity, and the ratio of pro-apoptotic (Bax) to anti-apoptotic (Bcl-2) proteins. IL-17A may trigger apoptosis directly in tubular cells or indirectly by mediating the production of other factors. However, the regulation of cleaved caspase-3 activity and the Bax/Bcl-2 ratio demonstrated that IL-17A activated intrinsic signaling pathways. These findings indicate that IL-17A plays a pathogenic role in SA-AKI by inducing apoptosis and neutrophil infiltration (Additional file 1).

There are some limitations to this study. A previous study reported that SA-AKI does not result from hypoperfusion alone, but may arise to a large extent from renal inflammation and tubular responses to various sepsis mediators. In many patients, SA-AKI occurs without overt signs of global renal hypoperfusion and SA-AKI has been described in the presence of normal or even increased renal blood flow [33]. Therefore, in our study, we did not perform hemodynamic monitoring, which was one of the limitations. Another previous study also reported that the neutralization of peritoneal IL-17A markedly improves lung injury in severe CLP-induced septic mice [7]. Although we did not prove a beneficial effect of blocking IL-17A in other organ systems in this study, based on the above data, we believe that the beneficial effect of blocking IL-17A could be mediated by other organ systems as well as AKI. Moreover, although we observed decreased levels of IL-17A-related cytokines and chemokines in renal tissues after IL-17A knockout, the mechanism by which IL-17A knockout could protect against SA-AKI remains unclear. It is also needs to be determined whether the improved renal apoptosis is directly related to the knockout of IL-17A.

Conclusions

Overall, our study demonstrated that IL-17A knockout could protect against SA-AKI. We showed that IL-17A may play a pathogenic role in SA-AKI by increasing the levels of proinflammatory cytokines and chemokines, and reducing neutrophil infiltration and apoptosis of tubular epithelial cells. Accordingly, IL-17A may be a novel target in the treatment of SA-AKI.

Abbreviations

AKI: acute kidney injury; IL-17(A): interleukin 17(A); CLP: cecal ligation and puncture; SA-AKI: sepsis-associated acute kidney injury; ANOVA: one-way analysis of variance.

Authors' contributions

LCJ, CXM, and ZL generated the hypothesis; LCJ, CXM, ZL, CGY, and MK participated in study design and coordination; LCJ, FZ, XY, SXF, and FB performed the experiments; LCJ subjected the mice to behavioral tasks during the experimental period; LF and LCJ performed the statistical analysis; LCJ and LF wrote the manuscript; and CXM and ZL made critical revisions to the manuscript. All authors read and approved the final manuscript.

Author details

[1] Department of Nephrology, The Affiliated Hospital of Qingdao University, Shandong 266003, People's Republic of China. [2] State Key Laboratory of Kidney Diseases, Department of Nephrology, Chinese PLA General Hospital and Medical School of Chinese PLA, No.28 Fuxing Road, Beijing 100853, People's Republic of China. [3] Department of Cardiology, Liaocheng People's Hospital, Shandong 252000, People's Republic of China.

Competing interests

The authors declare that they have no competing interests.

Funding

This research was supported by a Grant from the Fund of Chinese PLA 12th Five-Year Plan for Medical Sciences (BWS11J027), National Natural Science Foundation of China (81170643, 81170688, 81470973).

References

1. Coca SG, Yusuf B, Shlipak MG, Garg AX, Parikh CR. Long-term risk of mortality and other adverse outcomes after acute kidney injury: a systematic review and meta-analysis. Am J Kidney Dis. 2009;53:961–73.
2. Langenberg C, Bellomo R, May C, Wan L, Egi M, Morgera S. Renal blood flow in sepsis. Crit Care. 2005;9:R363–74.
3. Wan L, Bagshaw SM, Langenberg C, Langenberg C, Saotome T, May C, Bellomo R. Pathophysiology of septic acute kidney injury: what do we really know? Crit Care Med. 2008;36(Suppl 4):S198–203.
4. Weaver CT, Hatton RD, Mangan PR, Harrington LE. IL-17 family cytokines and the expanding diversity of effector T cell lineages. Annu Rev Immunol. 2007;25:821–52.
5. Chong DL, Ingram RJ, Lowther DE, Muir R, Sriskandan S, Altmann DM. The nature of innate and adaptive interleukin-17A responses in sham or bacterial inoculation. Immunology. 2012;136:325–33.
6. Ley K, Smith E, Stark MA. IL-17A-producing neutrophil-regulatory Tn lymphocytes. Immunol Res. 2006;34:229–42.
7. Li J, Zhang Y, Lou J, Zhu J, He M, Deng X, et al. Neutralisation of peritoneal IL-17A markedly improves the prognosis of severe septic mice by decreasing neutrophil infiltration and proinflammatory cytokines. PLoS One. 2012;7:e46506.
8. Hueber W, Patel DD, Dryja T, Wright AM, Koroleva I, Bruin G, et al. Effects of AIN457, a fully human antibody to interleukin-17A, on psoriasis, rheumatoid arthritis, and uveitis. Sci Transl Med. 2010;2:52–72.
9. Genovese MC, Van den Bosch F, Roberson SA, Bojin S, Biagini IM, Ryan P, et al. LY2439821, a humanized anti-interleukin-17 monoclonal antibody, in the treatment of patients with rheumatoid arthritis: a phase I randomized, double-blind, placebo-controlled, proof-of-concept study. Arthritis Rheum. 2010;62:929–39.
10. Shichita T, Sugiyama Y, Ooboshi H, Sugimori H, Nakagawa R, Takada I, et al. Pivotal role of cerebral interleukin-17-producing gammadeltaT cells in the delayed phase of ischemic brain injury. Nat Med. 2009;15:946–50.
11. Li L, Huang L, Vergis AL, Ye H, Bajwa A, Narayan V, et al. IL-17 produced by neutrophils regulates IFN-gamma-mediated neutrophil migration in mouse kidney ischemia-reperfusion injury. J Clin Invest. 2010;120:331–42.
12. Edgerton C, Crispin JC, Moratz CM, Bettelli E, Oukka M, Simovic M, et al. IL-17 producing CD4 T cells mediate accelerated ischemia/reperfusion-induced injury in autoimmunity-prone mice. Clin Immunol. 2009;130:313–21.

13. Hubbard WJ, Choudhry MA, Schwacha MG, Rue LW 3rd, Bland KI, Chaudry IH, et al. Cecal ligation and puncture. Shock. 2005;24(Suppl 1):52–7.
14. Lien YH, Yong KC, Cho C, Igarashi S, Lai LW. S1P(1)-selective agonist, SEW2871, ameliorates ischemic acute renal failure. Kidney Int. 2006;69:1601–8.
15. Hu J, Zhang L, Wang N, Ding R, Cui S, Zhu F, et al. Mesenchymal stem cells attenuate ischemic acute kidney injury by inducing regulatory T cells through splenocyte interactions. Kidney Int. 2013;84:521–31.
16. Gonçalves GM, Zamboni DS, Câmara NO. The role of innate immunity in septic acute kidney injuries. Shock. 2010;34(Suppl 1):22–6.
17. Stearns-Kurosawa DJ, Osuchowski MF, Valentine C, Kurosawa S, Remick DG. The pathogenesis of sepsis. Annu Rev Pathol. 2011;6:19–48.
18. Ma AI. The ubiquitous nature of IL-17. Nat Immunol. 2012;13:1034–5.
19. Dong X, Bachman LA, Miller MN, Nath KA, Griffin MD. Dendritic cells facilitate accumulation of IL-17 T cells in the kidney following acute renal obstruction. Kidney Int. 2008;74:1294–309.
20. Luo CJ, Zhang FJ, Zhang L, Feng Z, Sun XF, Chen XM, et al. Mesenchymal stem cells ameliorate sepsis-associated acute kidney injury in mice. Shock. 2014;41:123–9.
21. Ruddy MJ, Shen F, Smith JB, Sharma A, Gaffen SL. Interleukin-17 regulates expression of the CXC chemokine LIX/CXCL5 in osteoblasts: implications for inflammation and neutrophil recruitment. J Leukoc Biol. 2004;76:135–44.
22. Zhou X, Chen Q, Moore J, Kolls JK, Halperin S, Wang J. Critical role of the interleukin-17/interleukin-17 receptor axis in regulating host susceptibility to respiratory infection with *Chlamydia* species. Infect Immun. 2009;77:5059–70.
23. Laan M, Cui ZH, Hoshino H, Lotvall J, Sjostrand M, Gruenert DC, Skoogh BE, Linden A. Neutrophil recruitment by human IL-17 via C-X-C chemokine release in the airways. J Immunol. 1999;162:2347.
24. Flierl MA, Rittirsch D, Gao H, et al. Adverse functions of IL-17A in experimental sepsis. FASEB J. 2008;22:2198–205.
25. Liao YH, Xia N, Zhou SF, Tang TT, Yan XX, Lv BJ, et al. Interleukin-17A contributes to myocardial ischemia/reperfusion injury by regulating cardiomyocyte apoptosis and neutrophil Infiltration. J Am Coll Cardiol. 2012;59:420–9.
26. Terada Y, Inoshita S, Kuwana H, Kobayashi T, Okado T, Ichijo H, et al. Important role of apoptosis signal-regulating kinase1 in ischemic acute kidney injury. Biochem Biophys Res Commun. 2007;364:1043–9.
27. Kindt N, Menzebach A, Van de Wouwer M, Betz I, De Vriese A, Conway EM. Protective role of the inhibitor of apoptosis protein, survivin, in toxin-induced acute renal failure. FASEB J. 2008;22:510–21.
28. Hotchkiss RS, Swanson PE, Freeman BD, Tinsley KW, Cobb JP, Matuschak GM. Apoptotic cell death in patients with sepsis, shock and multiple organ dysfunction. Crit Care Med. 1999;27:1230–51.
29. Lerolle N, Nochy D, Guérot E. Histopathology of septic shock induced renal injury: apoptosis and leukocytic infiltration. Intensive Care Med. 2010;36:471–8.
30. Langenberg C, Gobe G, Hood S, May CN, Bellomo R. Renal histopathology during experimental septic acute kidney injury and recovery. Crit Care Med. 2014;42:e58–67.
31. Erbel C, Chen L, Bea F, Wangler S, Celik S, Lasitschka F, et al. Inhibition of IL-17A attenuates atherosclerotic lesion development in apoE-deficient mice. J Immunol. 2009;183:8167–75.
32. Sonnenberg GF, Nair MG, Kirn TJ, Zaph C, Fouser LA, Artis D. Pathological versus protective functions of IL-22 in airway inflammation are regulated by IL-17A. J Exp Med. 2010;207:1293–305.
33. Honore PM, Jacobs R, Hendrickx I, Bagshaw SM, Joannes-Boyau O, Boer W, et al. Prevention and treatment of sepsis-induced acute kidney injury: an update. Ann Intensive Care. 2015;5:51.

20

SAPS 3 score as a predictive factor for postoperative referral to intensive care unit

João M. Silva Jr.[1,2*], Helder Marcus Costa Rocha[1], Henrique Tadashi Katayama[1], Leandro Ferreira Dias[1], Mateus Barros de Paula[1], Leusi Magda Romano Andraus[1], Jose Maria Correa Silva[1] and Luiz Marcelo Sá Malbouisson[1,2]

Abstract

Background: Patients undergoing intermediate-risk surgery are typically taken to the ward postoperatively. However, some may develop complications requiring intensive care later. We aimed to evaluate the characteristics of patients undergoing intermediate-risk surgery who required late postoperative admission to the intensive care unit (ICU) and determine the predictors for this.

Methods: The study included patients undergoing intermediate-risk surgery with preoperative indication for ICU but who were taken to the ward postoperatively, because they appeared to be responding well. However, they required late ICU admission. ICU care and preoperative SAPS 3 score were evaluated. Palliative surgeries and patients readmitted to ICU were excluded.

Results: The study included 100 patients, 27 % of whom had late postoperative admission to the ICU. The preoperative SAPS 3 score was higher (45.4 ± 7.8 vs. 35.9 ± 7.4, $P < 0.001$) in patients who required delayed admission to the ICU postoperatively. Furthermore, they had undergone longer surgery (4.2 ± 1.9 vs. 2.7 ± 1.5 h, $P < 0.001$), and a greater proportion were gastrointestinal surgeries (14.8 vs. 5.5 %, $P = 0.03$) and intraoperative transfusion (18.5 vs. 5.5 % $P = 0.04$). In multivariate analysis, preoperative SAPS 3 and surgery duration independently predicted postoperative ICU admission, respectively (OR 1.25; 95 % CI 1.1–1.4 and OR 3.33; 95 % CI 1.7–6.3).

Conclusion: The identification of high-risk surgical patients is essential for proper treatment; time of surgery and preoperative SAPS 3 seem to provide a useful indication of risk and may help better to characterize patients undergoing intermediate-risk surgery that demand ICU care.

Keywords: Surgical patients, Risk, Intensive care unit, Criteria

Background

A substantial proportion of ICU patients are surgical patients. Nevertheless, high-risk surgical patients are not often identified as such and may experience a more difficult recovery postoperatively [1, 2]. A large observational study has indicated that surgical procedures classified as high risk have a mortality rate as high as 80 % [3]. Although less than 15 % of patients who underwent those procedures were admitted to an intensive care unit (ICU), the individual risk is often underestimated and high-risk patient factors may be overlooked.

As in the rest of the world, the scarcity of ICU beds in Brazil is one of the most important limiting factors for admission to ICU for an eligible patient [2, 4]. Patients with a real chance of recovery are thus prioritized [5, 6]. Surgical patients well illustrate this point, particularly those undergoing elective surgery [2]. The surgical outcome of that population is influenced not only by preoperative physiological status and surgical risk but also by adequate postoperative care [7]. Thus, it is paramount to know the predictors of the risks of increased morbidity and mortality for this group of patients [8].

*Correspondence: joao.s@globo.com
[1] Hospital Servidor Publico Estadual-SP, Rua Pedro de Toledo, 1800/6º A–Vila Clementino, São Paulo, SP 04039-901, Brazil
Full list of author information is available at the end of the article

Aiming for a better use of available resources, the Society of Critical Care Medicine has established criteria for the admission and discharge in ICUs [5, 6] to triage patients who may benefit most from intensive care. The proper use of such criteria is, however, not widespread, particularly in surgical patients.

Several other studies [8–11] have developed prognostic scores for critical patients and even for surgical ones [2, 7, 12, 13]. However, such scores have never been used preoperatively to decide who would or would not require an ICU bed. One of those indices is the SAPS 3 prognostic system [14]. This consists of 20 easily measured parameters [15], and its results, when utilized on high-risk surgical patients, are excellent [16]. Others, such as the ASA physical status index [17], are limited in predicting worse outcomes.

The performance of prognostic models encompasses two objective measures: calibration and discrimination. Calibration refers to how closely the estimated probabilities of mortality correlate with observed mortality over the range of probabilities. Discrimination refers to how well the model discriminates between individuals who will live and those who will die. From the individual patient's point of view, a perfect discrimination would be preferable; however, for clinical trials or comparison of care between ICUs, better calibration is needed. Our intention with this study was to test the discriminatory power of preoperative SAPS 3 scores for ICU indication.

The study objective is thus to evaluate the characteristics and preoperative SAPS 3 scores of surgical patients undergoing intermediate-risk surgery, and who, owing to a decision by the surgical team, were referred to the ward postoperatively, but because of delayed postoperative complications, were admitted to ICU only later. The factors underlying such complications were also investigated.

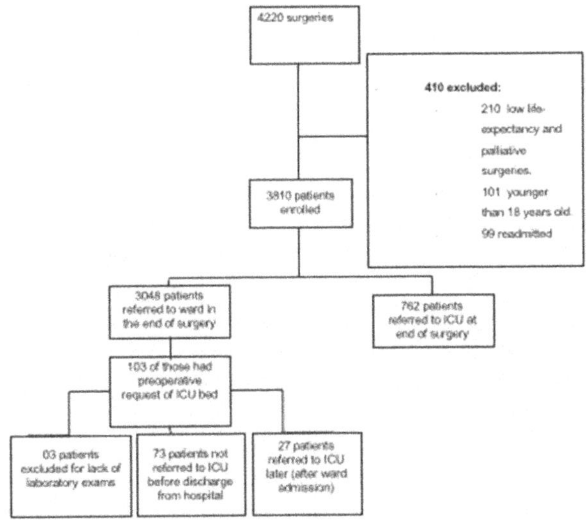

Fig. 1 Flow chart of the number of patients screened

Methods

The study was approved by the Research Ethics Committee and exempted from the signed informed consent form requirement, because it was a case–control medical record review.

The patients included in the study were those undergoing intermediate-risk surgery, defined as those for whom an ICU bed was requested at preoperative assessment for postoperative care but who were not admitted to ICU postoperatively owing to clinical evaluation at the end of the operation. Patients under the age of 18 at the time of hospitalization, patients readmitted to ICU, and those who underwent palliative surgery were excluded from the study (see Fig. 1).

Clinical evaluation performed at the end of surgery included spontaneous breathing, a tidal volume of at least 6–8 ml/kg and respiratory a frequency of less than 25 breaths per minute, as well as peripheral oxygen saturation over 95 % and hemodynamic stability without vasopressor support. These patients needed to be alert and fully oriented, or, in case of preoperative cognitive impairment, the level of consciousness and orientation needed to be the same preoperatively. Other criteria included lack of bleeding, satisfactory control of pain, mobilization (as far as possible), spontaneous micturition, infection parameters within normal range, and non-irritated wound conditions. Patients were evaluated based on these criteria by surgeons and anaesthesiologists who were not involved neither in the study design nor in-group allocation.

Patients who had their medical records reviewed were divided into two groups, those who had an uneventful recovery in the surgical unit and those who, owing to late postoperative complications, had to be admitted to the ICU. The reviewed data allowed the research team to calculate the preoperative SAPS 3 score [14, 18] and the ASA physical status [17] of patients in both groups, as well as to define their demographics, the operative procedure they underwent, operative time, whether intraoperative blood transfusion was required, and hospital mortality. To calculate the SAPS 3 score, physiological data and laboratory analysis were performed on the day before surgery. Records were reviewed from hospitalization to medical discharge or hospital mortality.

At the time of the study, there was no official directive regarding the policy of triage and reservation of ICU beds. Patients were referred to the ICU at the surgical team's discretion based on their experience.

Statistical analysis

According to clinical experience and using the minimal clinically significant difference between groups for calculation, a sample of at least 93 participants would be required to produce a 10 % chance of an alternative hypothesis (late ICU admission) and a 2 % chance of a null hypothesis, accepting a type I error of 0.05 (one-sided) and power of 0.95.

Data were analysed, and the results are expressed as mean ± standard deviation, median (interquartile range), or percentage. For statistical analysis, variables, which followed a Gaussian distribution, were evaluated for significance by using the *t* test. Categorical variables were evaluated by the Chi-square test of contingency.

Binary logistic regression analysis was also performed, applying stepwise selection with backward elimination in order to identify independent risk factors and control confounding effects (variables mutually adjusted). Variables with significant probability (*P* value) of less than 0.05 in univariate analysis were considered candidates and removed in each step in the regression model if they presented a probability (*P* value) higher or equal to 0.10, by likelihood ratio test. Thereafter, selected variables for the regression model were tested to evaluate pairwise interaction possibilities, and those variables with interactions were corrected in the main regression model. If no statistically significant differences were found, variables were excluded. A bootstrap procedure based on 1000 bootstrap samples was applied in the main regression model to investigate the stability of coefficients and predictive ability of the variables included in model. The *P* values presented are from two-tailed tests, and values under 0.05 were considered statistically significant. Odds ratio and 95 % confidence interval (CI) were estimated by logistic regression. A ROC curve was determined for each variable. The cut-off points were estimated by the best sensitivity and specificity for ICU admission.

The Statistical Package for Social Sciences (SPSS-IBM Corp., Armonk, NY, USA) 21.0 was the software used for the statistical analyses.

Results

From June 2013 to December 2013, a total of 4220 patients underwent surgery at the surgical centre of the hospital. Of these patients, 413 were excluded from the study. A total of 100 records were reviewed (see Fig. 1). The mean age of the patients was 66.4 years, with a standard deviation of 14.7 years. Their average SAPS 3 score was 38.5 ± 8.6 and 71 % were classified as ASA physical status 2. In total, 66 % were women. Elective surgery accounted for 84 % of cases, 30 % of patients had undergone gynaecological procedures, 28 % of surgeries were orthopaedic, and 16 % vascular. In the cases reviewed, neuraxial block was the most used type of anaesthesia, 3 % of patients died during hospitalization, and 27 % had a delayed referral to the ICU (see Table 1).

When comparing both groups, SAPS 3 scores were higher among patients admitted to the ICU from the surgical unit (mean 45.4 ± 7.8) than among those who completed their recovery without ICU referral (mean 35.9 ± 7.4, $P < 0.001$). In the group of patients referred to critical care, 40.7 % were considered to be in ASA physical status 3, while only 8.2 % of the patients in the other group fitted that category ($P = 0.001$). In total, 18.5 % of patients in the delayed critical care group had received packed red blood cell transfusion intraoperatively, compared to only 5.5 % of patients who did not need intensive care ($P = 0.004$) (see Table 2).

In the multivariate analysis, the SAPS 3 score was determined as an independent factor for ICU referral (OR 1.25, 95 % CI 1.1–1.4, $P = 0.001$), as well as operative time (OR 3.33, 95 % CI 1.7–6.3, $P < 0.001$) (see Table 3).

The ROC curve area was 0.87 (95 % CI 0.78–0.93) with a 44.2 cut-off point (sensitivity: 63 %; specificity: 87.7 %). For operative time, the ROC curve area was 0.78 (95 % CI

Table 1 Demographics of the patients included in the study

Variable	Value
Age	66.4 ± 14.7
SAPS 3 preoperatively	38.5 ± 8.6
ASA physical status P1 %	12.0
ASA physical status P2 %	71.0
ASA physical status P3 %	17.0
Female gender %	66
Elective surgery %	84.0
Emergency surgery %	16.0
Surgical speciality %	
Gynaecology	30.0
Orthopaedics	28.0
Vascular surgery	16.0
Urological surgery	13.0
Gastrointestinal surgery	8.0
Others	5.0
Postoperative haemoglobin (mg/dL)	12.9 ± 1.5
ICU admission %	27.0
PRBC transfusion %	9.0
Hospital mortality %	3.0
Anaesthesia %	
General anaesthesia	39.0
Neuraxial anaesthesia	49.0
General plus neuraxial anaesthesia	12.0

ICU intensive care unit, *PRBC* packed red blood cell transfusion; all values represent mean ± standard deviation, *Others* neurosurgery, head and neck surgery, thoracic surgery

Table 2 Comparison between patients who had uneventful recoveries in the surgical unit and patients who were referred to the ICU

Variables	ICU delayed (*n* = 27)	Non-ICU (*n* = 73)	*P*
Age (years)	65.7 ± 16.1	66.7 ± 14.3	0.75
Male gender (%)	33.3	34.2	0.93
Female % (%)	66.7	65.8	
SAPS 3	45.45 ± 7.8	35.94 ± 7.4	0.000
ASA (%)			0.002
P1	11.1	12.3	
P2	48.1	79.5	
P3	40.7	8.2	
Surgery (%)			
Elective	81.5	84.9	0.67
Emergence	18.5	15.1	0.29
Type of surgery (%)			
Gynaecology	11.1	37.0	0.02
Orthopaedic	22.2	30.1	0.59
Vascular	22.2	13.7	0.47
Urological	18.5	11.0	0.51
Gastrointestinal	14.8	5.5	0.26
Others	11.1	2.8	0.24
Anaesthesia (%)			0.11
General	55.6	32.9	
Neuroaxis	33.3	54.8	
General + neuroaxis	11.1	12.3	
Surgery time (h)	4.2 ± 1.8	2.7 ± 1.5	0.000
Transfusion requirements intraoperatively (%)	18.5	5.5	0.04
Value of haemoglobin immediately postoperatively(mg/dL)	12.5 ± 1.6	12.9 ± 1.5	0.20
Hospital mortality (%)	11.1	0.0	0.004
Length of hospital stay (days)	23.0 ± 22.2	25.8 ± 31.7	0.410

ICU intensive care unit, *Others* neurosurgery, head and neck surgery, thoracic surgery; all values represent mean ± standard deviation

0.689–0.859), with a 3-h cut-off point (sensitivity: 74.1 %; specificity: 83.6 % (see Fig. 2).

Patients with a preoperative SAPS 3 score exceeding 40 had a higher rate of ICU referral (see Fig. 3).

Discussion

The identification of intermediary-risk surgical patients likely to require ICU care is difficult. To optimize post-surgical care and to prevent under and overuse of ICUs, criteria must be developed. We found that SAPS 3 scores and operative time were significantly higher in patients who eventually require critical care, showing that they could be used to predict early postoperative ICU necessity.

Predicting postoperative ICU need is complex in surgical patients. There are no self-evident criteria because many patient- and procedure-related factors determine ICU need. Because of the lack of objective criteria, many unnecessary admissions occur [11]. In this study, special attention was given to identifying which criteria could be used in practice to triage surgical patients and to determine which population found itself at higher surgical risk.

In multivariate analysis, predictive factors for delayed postoperative ICU admission were SAPS 3 score (OR 1.25 IC 95 % 1.1–1.4) and operative time (3.33 IC 95 % 1.7–6.3). In a recent study, Silva et al. [16] demonstrated the applicability of SAPS-3 in Brazilian hospitals, supporting its validation for surgical patients, consistent with other studies [13]. SAPS 3 is distinct from other prognostic scores because it is simple and does not require the use of sophisticated technological resources or complex data. Operative time is also easily obtained from the anaesthesia record.

Further studies have reached the same conclusion: postoperative risk is easily underestimated in clinical evaluation immediately postoperatively [3, 19]. In our study, 27 % of patients for whom an ICU bed had been

Table 3 Logistic regression for delayed ICU

	P	OR	95 % CI		Bootstrap 95 % CI	
			Lower	Upper	Lower	Upper
SAPS 3 (per unit)	0.001	1.253	1.102	1.425	1.24	1.893
Surgery time (per hour)	0.000	3.327	1.750	6.325	2.235	8.618
ASA physical status (per unit)	0.991	0.991	0.207	4.749	−1.926	6.703
Transfusion requirements	0.593	1.737	0.230	13.145	−1.128	18.526
Gynaecological surgery	0.270	0.199	0.011	3.491	−19.662	4.161

The variables were adjusted in model by ASA, transfusion and surgery. Unless otherwise stated, the bootstrap results are based on 1000 bootstrap samples

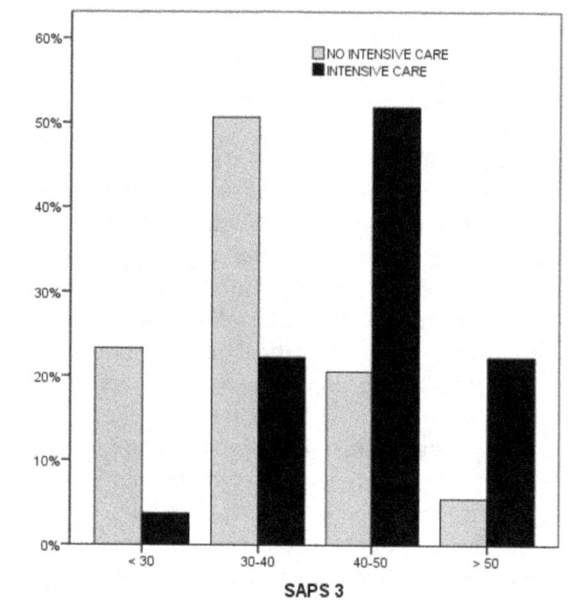

Fig. 2 ROC curves of surgery time and SAPS 3 score for ICU referral

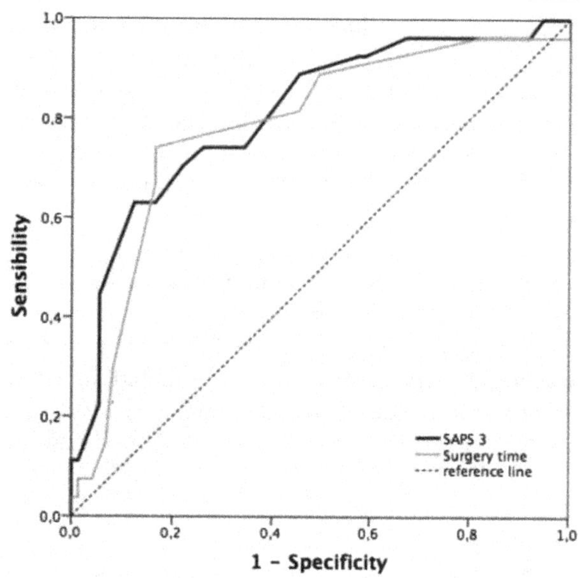

Fig. 3 SAPS 3 score stratification and ICU referral rate

requested but who were not taken to the ICU because they were evaluated as well enough to be cared for in the surgical unit, eventually had to be admitted to the ICU. Their postoperative complications might have been avoided if the request for an ICU bed had been met. This high incidence of late admission to the ICU illustrates the low predictive quality of the criteria used by the surgical team when deciding where the patient should be during the postoperative period, although the rate of refused ICU admissions for surgical patients is lower than that for non-surgical ones [20, 21].

For non-surgical patients, the age, severity of illness, and medical diagnosis are independent factors for ICU admission [22]. For surgical patients, it has been demonstrated that peritonitis, unplanned surgery, age, elevated serum lactate level, and a high central venous pressure on the day of ICU admission were independent predictors of death as a result of multiple organ failure [23]. Most of those factors are measured postoperatively. Identifying early predictors of postoperative complications might assist in the development and implementation of preventive measures.

The importance of preoperative planning is evident in the higher mortality rate of patients with late ICU admission. A late diagnosis and, therefore, a late referral to the ICU severely increase the chance of permanent damage to vital functions [23].

Clinical postoperative evaluation is too imprecise to identify surgical patients with a high risk of complications and may cause costly delays in adequate treatment. For 11 % of late admission patients in our study, this delay proved fatal.

Such complications result in longer hospitalizations, attended by problems such as sepsis, delirium, and organ failure [24]. Therefore, a clear set of objective criteria for ICU admission is important [6].

Findings indicate that subjective, individual analysis of a patient's prognosis as well as isolated clinical parameters may lead to underestimation of the risk of complications and a delay in ICU referral [25].

Nowadays, there are few ICU admission guidelines [2, 4], and they are not widely utilized in clinical practice, particularly in the case of surgical patients.

The prediction of the SAPS 3 model is based exclusively on data evaluated within the first hour, which does not the case with other scores. Besides, the predictive power of the original SAPS 3 score is derived from information evaluated before ICU admission. Prognostic systems that include measurement up the first 24 h of ICU period are unavailable for use in the ICU screening. Furthermore, values above 24 h often capture the standard of care more than the actual clinical state of the patient; in this case, for example, the SOFA or APACHE scores may fall. This is the greatest advantage of SAPS 3, confirming its superiority over other prognostic scores in screening ICU patients. Other scoring systems, such as ASA-PS, do not include variables specific to the surgical procedure and are disadvantageous in their subjectivity.

The current study has some limitations. It is an observational study, which makes renders the potential for error high, even though enough statistical power was achieved. Another limitation is that it was conducted at a single surgical centre and that the sample size is small. Likewise, five variables were included in a logistic regression which evaluates only 27 events, but a bootstrap procedure was made based on 1000 bootstrap samples in order to investigate the stability of coefficients and predictive ability of the variables included in model, and a small amount of variation was found while the number of samples had increased considerably. Additionally, variables might have been overlooked and should constitute the subject of further analysis. For example, all patients requiring ICU care preoperatively could be included; in this way, patients who eventually went to ICU as predicted, those who did not go to ICU but were later admitted and those who never had to go to ICU, might be compared. Although the model applicable to all types of surgery, we have no data on its usefulness and predictability in other groups of patients. Further studies in different patient groups with different models are needed to determine the best predictive model.

Conclusion

Preoperative SAPS 3 scores and surgery time are valuable tools for predicting the severity of illness and the risk of postoperative complications that might require intensive care. They were the most relevant factors analysed in this study.

More studies are required on this subject. The cost-effectiveness of precise indications of postoperative intensive care justifies further research.

Authors' contributions

JMSJ is the guarantor of the integrity of the data and the accuracy of the data analysis. JMSJ, HMCR, and HTK designed the study. LMSM performed the statistical analysis. JMSJ, HMCR, HTK, LFD, MBP, LMRA, JMCS, and LMSM contributed substantially to the collection of data, data analysis, and interpretation and to the writing of the manuscript. All authors read and approved the final manuscript.

Author details

[1] Hospital Servidor Publico Estadual-SP, Rua Pedro de Toledo, 1800/6º A–Vila Clementino, São Paulo, SP 04039-901, Brazil. [2] Anaesthesiology Department, Hospital das Clinicas SP-FMUSP, Av. Dr. Enéas de Carvalho Aguiar, 255 Cerqueira César, São Paulo, SP 05403-000, Brazil.

Competing interests

The authors declare that they have no competing interests.

References

1. Silva JM Jr, Oliveira AM, Segura JL, Ribeiro MH, Sposito CN, Toledo DO, Rezende E, Malbouisson LM. A large venous-arterial PCO(2) is associated with poor outcomes in surgical patients. Anesthesiol Res Pract. 2011;2011:759792.
2. Caldeira VM, Silva Junior JM, Oliveira AM, Rezende S, Araujo LA, Santana MR, Amendola CP, Rezende E. Criteria for patient admission to an intensive care unit and related mortality rates. Rev Assoc Med Bras. 2010;56(5):528–34.
3. Jhanji S, Thomas B, Ely A, Watson D, Hinds CJ, Pearse RM. Mortality and utilisation of critical care resources amongst high-risk surgical patients in a large NHS trust. Anaesthesia. 2008;63(7):695–700.
4. Simchen E, Sprung CL, Galai N, Zitser-Gurevich Y, Bar-Lavi Y, Gurman G, Klein M, Lev A, Levi L, Zveibil F, et al. Survival of critically ill patients hospitalized in and out of intensive care units under paucity of intensive care unit beds. Crit Care Med. 2004;32(8):1654–61.
5. Anonymous. Guidelines for developing admission and discharge policies for the pediatric intensive care unit. Pediatric Section Task Force on Admission and Discharge Criteria, Society of Critical Care Medicine in conjunction with the American College of Critical Care Medicine and the Committee on Hospital Care of the American Academy of Pediatrics. Crit Care Med. 1999;27(4):843–5.
6. Anonymous. Guidelines for intensive care unit admission, discharge, and triage. Task Force of the American College of Critical Care Medicine, Society of Critical Care Medicine. Crit Care Med. 1999;27(3):633–8.
7. Bennett-Guerrero E, Hyam JA, Shaefi S, Prytherch DR, Sutton GL, Weaver PC, Mythen MG, Grocott MP, Parides MK. Comparison of P-POSSUM risk-adjusted mortality rates after surgery between patients in the USA and the UK. Br J Surg. 2003;90(12):1593–8.
8. Marshall JC, Cook DJ, Christou NV, Bernard GR, Sprung CL, Sibbald WJ. Multiple organ dysfunction score: a reliable descriptor of a complex clinical outcome. Crit Care Med. 1995;23(10):1638–52.
9. Le Gall JR, Klar J, Lemeshow S, Saulnier F, Alberti C, Artigas A, Teres D. The Logistic Organ Dysfunction system. A new way to assess organ dysfunction in the intensive care unit. ICU Scoring Group. JAMA. 1996;276(10):802–10.
10. Knaus WA, Draper EA, Wagner DP, Zimmerman JE. APACHE II: a severity of disease classification system. Crit Care Med. 1985;13(10):818–29.
11. Kose I, Zincircioglu C, Cakmak M, Cabbaroglu G, Senoglu N, Gonullu M. Postoperative patients in the intensive care unit: Identifying those who do not really need it. J Crit Care. 2015;30(6):1295–8.
12. Sakr Y, Krauss C, Amaral AC, Rea-Neto A, Specht M, Reinhart K, Marx G. Comparison of the performance of SAPS II, SAPS 3, APACHE II, and their customized prognostic models in a surgical intensive care unit. Br J Anaesth. 2008;101(6):798–803.
13. Nassar APJ, Malbouisson LM, Moreno R. Evaluation of simplified acute physiology score 3 performance: a systematic review of external validation studies. Crit Care. 2014;18(3):R117.
14. Moreno RP, Metnitz PG, Almeida E, Jordan B, Bauer P, Campos RA, Iapichino G, Edbrooke D, Capuzzo M, Le Gall JR. SAPS 3—From evaluation of the patient to evaluation of the intensive care unit. Part 2: Development of a prognostic model for hospital mortality at ICU admission. Intensive Care Med. 2005;31(10):1345–55.
15. Soares M, Salluh JI. Validation of the SAPS 3 admission prognostic model in patients with cancer in need of intensive care. Intensive Care Med. 2006;32(11):1839–44.
16. Silva Junior JM, Malbouisson LM, Nuevo HL, Barbosa LG, Marubayashi LY, Teixeira IC, Nassar Junior AP, Carmona MJ, Silva IF, Auler Junior JO, et al. Applicability of the simplified acute physiology score (SAPS 3) in Brazilian hospitals. Rev Bras Anestesiol. 2010;60(1):20–31.
17. Keats AS. The ASA classification of physical status—a recapitulation. Anesthesiology. 1978;49(4):233–6.
18. Metnitz PG, Moreno RP, Almeida E, Jordan B, Bauer P, Campos RA, Iapichino G, Edbrooke D, Capuzzo M, Le Gall JR. SAPS 3—From evaluation of the patient to evaluation of the intensive care unit. Part 1: Objectives, methods and cohort description. Intensive Care Med. 2005;31(10):1336–44.
19. Lobo SM, Rezende E, Knibel MF, Silva NBd, Páramo JAM, Nácul F, Mendes CL, Assunção M, Costa Filho RC, Grion CC, et al. Epidemiology and outcomes of non-cardiac surgical patients in Brazilian intensive care units. Rev Bras Ter Intensiva. 2008;20(4):376–84.
20. Sprung CL, Danis M, Baily MA, Chalfin DB, Dagi TF, Davila F, De Vita M, Engelhardt TH Jr, Grenvik A, Hofmann PB, Hoyt JW, Kofke WA, Lynn J, Marshall MF, McCartney JJ, Nelson RM, Ninos N, Raphaely RC, Reardon F, Rie MA, Rosenbaum SH, Silverman H, Sottile FD, Spanier A, Steinberg A, Tendier RMD, Teres D, Truog RD, Wallace TE, Wlody G, Yeh TS. Consensus statement on the triage of critically ill patients. Society of Critical Care Medicine Ethics Committee. JAMA 1994;271(15):1200–3.

21. Marshall MF, Schwenzer KJ, Orsina M, Fletcher JC, Durbin CG Jr. Influence of political power, medical provincialism, and economic incentives on the rationing of surgical intensive care unit beds. Crit Care Med. 1992;20(3):387–94.
22. Sinuff T, Kahnamoui K, Cook DJ, Luce JM, Levy MM, Values E. Rationing in critical care task F: rationing critical care beds: a systematic review. Crit Care Med. 2004;32(7):1588–97.
23. Lobo SM, Rezende E, Knibel MF, Silva NB, Paramo JA, Nacul FE, Mendes CL, Assuncao M, Costa RC, Grion CC, et al. Early determinants of death due to multiple organ failure after noncardiac surgery in high-risk patients. Anesth Analg. 2011;112(4):877–83.
24. Higgins TL, McGee WT, Steingrub JS, Rapoport J, Lemeshow S, Teres D. Early indicators of prolonged intensive care unit stay: impact of illness severity, physician staffing, and pre-intensive care unit length of stay. Crit Care Med. 2003;31(1):45–51.
25. Wilkinson D. The self-fulfilling prophecy in intensive care. Theor Med Bioeth. 2009;30(6):401–10.

Outcome of in- and out-of-hospital cardiac arrest survivors with liver cirrhosis

Kevin Roedl[1,3†], Christian Wallmüller[2†], Andreas Drolz[1,3], Thomas Horvatits[1,3], Karoline Rutter[1,3], Alexander Spiel[1,2], Julia Ortbauer[3], Peter Stratil[2], Pia Hubner[2], Christoph Weiser[2], Jasmin Katrin Motaabbed[3], Dominik Jarczak[1], Harald Herkner[2], Fritz Sterz[2] and Valentin Fuhrmann[1,3*]

Abstract

Background: Organ failure increases mortality in patients with liver cirrhosis. Data about resuscitated cardiac arrest patients with liver cirrhosis are missing. This study aims to assess aetiology, survival and functional outcome in patients after successful cardiopulmonary resuscitation (CPR) with and without liver cirrhosis.

Methods: Analysis of prospectively collected cardiac arrest registry data of consecutively hospital-admitted patients following successful CPR was performed. Patient's characteristics, admission diagnosis, severity of disease, course of disease, short- and long-term mortality as well as functional outcome were assessed and compared between patients with and without cirrhosis.

Results: Out of 1068 patients with successful CPR, 47 (4%) had liver cirrhosis. Acute-on-chronic liver failure (ACLF) was present in 33 (70%) of these patients on admission, and four patients developed ACLF during follow-up. Mortality at 1 year was more than threefold increased in patients with liver cirrhosis (OR 3.25; 95% CI 1.33–7.96). Liver cirrhosis was associated with impaired neurological outcome (OR for a favourable cerebral performance category: 0.13; 95% CI 0.04–0.36). None of the patients with Child–Turcotte–Pugh (CTP) C cirrhosis survived 28 days with good neurological outcome. Overall nine (19%) patients with cirrhosis survived 28 days with good neurological outcome. All patients with ACLF grade 3 died within 28 days.

Conclusion: Cardiac arrest survivors with cirrhosis have worse outcome than those without. Although one quarter of patients with liver cirrhosis survived longer than 28 days after successful CPR, patients with CTP C as well as advanced ACLF did not survive 28 days with good neurological outcome.

Keywords: Cardiac arrest, Cirrhosis, Acute-on-chronic liver failure, Multiple organ failure, Intensive care unit

Background

Patients with liver cirrhosis [1] and organ failure admitted to intensive care units (ICU) have high morbidity and mortality [2, 3]. Mortality rates of up to 80% are reported in critically ill cirrhotic patients, progressively increasing with the number of organs failing [4–6]. Recently, chronic liver failure-SOFA (CLIF-SOFA) score [3] was developed as a tool for risk stratification in patients with cirrhosis and acute-on-chronic liver failure (ACLF) [2, 3].

Cardiac arrest (CA) can be the consequence of or lead to multiple organ failure. It is one of the leading causes of death in many parts of the world. Every year estimated 375,000–700,000 citizens are suffering CA in Europe and the USA [7, 8] and receive cardiopulmonary resuscitation (CPR). Patients who achieve return of spontaneous circulation (ROSC) following CA have high morbidity and mortality mainly due to cerebral and cardiac dysfunction that accompany whole-body ischaemia and reperfusion [9]. These disabilities can lead to the post-CA syndrome, which is defined as multiple organ failure after CA. Despite advances in critical and emergency care, survival

*Correspondence: v.fuhrmann@uke.de
†Kevin Roedl and Christian Wallmüller have contributed equally to this work
[1] Department of Intensive Care Medicine, University Medical Center Hamburg-Eppendorf, Martinistraße 52, 20246 Hamburg, Germany
Full list of author information is available at the end of the article

rates after in-hospital cardiac arrest (IHCA) and out-of-hospital cardiac arrest (OHCA) are generally poor and varying greatly for OHCA between 8–16% [10, 11] and for IHCA 14–23% [12–14].

Data on occurrence and outcome of CA in patients with liver cirrhosis are not available. Therefore, the aim of the study was to investigate cause and outcome in patients with liver cirrhosis after CA and ROSC compared to a large cohort of patients with CA and ROSC without liver cirrhosis.

Methods

This study was based on a prospectively maintained registry at the Emergency Department of the Medical University of Vienna. This registry was approved by the ethics committee of the Medical University of Vienna. Due to the observational character of the study, informed consent was waived. The study was performed between January 2005 and January 2012. All consecutive patients admitted to the Emergency Department of the Medical University Vienna after CA and ROSC were included in the analysis. CPR and post-CA care were performed in accordance with the European Resuscitation Council guidelines [15, 16]. The data were collected prospectively according to Utstein-style guidelines [17, 18]. Patients suffering from OHCA were treated by the Viennese two-tier EMS system, featured by an EMS physician and paramedics; the EMS system was described previously in detail [19, 20]. No-flow time was defined as the time period from onset of CA to the start of resuscitation efforts. Low-flow time was defined as the time period from the start of resuscitation efforts until ROSC. Time to ROSC was defined as time from onset of CA until ROSC. CA survivors were followed prospectively for at least 1 year after admission to the emergency department for assessment of survival and neurological outcome. Rates of 28-day mortality, 6-month mortality and 1-year mortality were assessed on site or by contacting the patients or their attending physicians. Cerebral function and overall performance were assessed on admission and after 28 days, 6 months and 1 year, by clinical visits, by physicians on site or contacting the attending physician, the patients or the family of the patient directly by telephone. Cerebral performance categories (CPC) [21] and overall performance categories (OPC) scales were used to assess neurological and overall outcome. A CPC/OPC score of 1–2 was defined as favourable neurological/overall outcome, such as 3–5 as unfavourable. The primary outcome was good neurological survival (CPC 1/2) after 6 months; our secondary outcome was overall mortality after 1 year.

Routine laboratory assessment including coagulation and liver function parameters was performed on daily basis. Furthermore, aetiology of CA (cardiac and non-cardiac origin like pulmonary, traumatic, cerebral, septic, intoxication, drowning, hypothermia, unclear and others) and underlying diseases were assessed and documented.

Severity of illness was evaluated in all patients using Sequential Organ Failure Assessment (SOFA) score [22] and Simplified Acute Physiology Score (SAPS II) [23]. Charlson comorbidity index (CCI) [24] was calculated in all patients. For patients with liver cirrhosis, model of end-stage liver disease score (MELD) [25], Child–Turcotte–Pugh (CTP) score [26] and CLIF-SOFA score [3] were calculated on admission, and CLIF-SOFA was additionally calculated 24 and 48 h after ROSC.

All patients were screened for signs of liver cirrhosis. Presence of liver cirrhosis was defined via histology, if available, otherwise by a combination of clinical characteristics (ascites, spider angiomata, caput medusa), laboratory and radiological findings (typical morphological changes of the liver, sings of portal hypertension, etc. in ultrasonography or computed tomography scanning).

Statistical analysis

Data are presented as count and relative frequency or median and 25–75% interquartile range (IQR). We tabulated clinical variables according to liver cirrhosis status and used Chi-squared, Fisher exact or Mann–Whitney U test for hypothesis testing as appropriate. The prognostic factor of interest was liver cirrhosis, and we used logistic regression to estimate the effect on neurological intact survival. The dependent variable was favourable neurological survival (best CPC 1 or 2; yes vs. no). In a multivariable logistic regression model, we entered liver cirrhosis as main covariable and age, sex, OHCA, witnessed CA, time to ROSC, presence of shockable rhythm, cardiac cause of CA, mechanical ventilation, SOFA on admission, initiation of MTH, CCI and cumulative adrenaline dose as other covariates to the model. To allow for potentially non-random missing data for time to ROSC caused by unwitnessed cardiac arrest, we categorised this variable for 0–4, 5–12, 13–24, 25–44, 45 + minutes as well as 'missing' as the sixth category. We used a similar model to estimate the associations with mortality at one year as the outcome. In all models, we tested for linear effects, first-order interactions and model fit using the likelihood ratio test. Survival function estimates were calculated using Kaplan–Meier method and were compared by the log-rank test. Statistical analysis was conducted using Stata 14 (StataCorp, College Station, TX) and IBM SPSS Statistics version 23.0 (IBM Corp., Armonk, NY). Generally, a p value < 0.05 was considered statistically significant.

Results

Study population

In total, 1068 patients (72% male, median age 61 years) after CA and ROSC were included in this study. Forty-seven (4%) of these patients had liver cirrhosis. Main cause of CA was cardiac in 678 (63%) patients of the total cohort. A total of 798 (75%) patients suffered CA out of hospital. Patients with liver cirrhosis had a significantly higher underlying non-cardiac cause compared to patients without cirrhosis. Median SOFA, SAPS II and CCI on admission were significantly higher in patients with liver cirrhosis. Sex, age, height and weight were distributed equally between both groups. Detailed characteristics of the study population are given in Table 1. Liver function and coagulation parameters were significantly different between patients with and without cirrhosis on hospital admission as illustrated in Additional file 1: Table S1.

Characteristics of patients with liver cirrhosis

Main underlying aetiology of liver cirrhosis was alcoholic liver disease ($n = 35$, 74%) followed by viral hepatitis ($n = 6$, 13%) and others ($n = 6$, 13%). Child–Turcotte–Pugh (CTP) class prior to admission was A in 17 (36%), B in 17 (36%) and C in 13 (28%) patients. Hepatocellular carcinoma (HCC) was present in three patients. Three patients had transjugular intrahepatic portosystemic shunt (TIPS), and one patient was listed for liver transplantation prior to occurrence of CA. No patient had liver transplantation during follow-up. Aetiology of CA was cardiac ($n = 21$, 45%), variceal bleeding ($n = 6$, 13%), sepsis ($n = 5$, 11%), respiratory insufficiency ($n = 5$, 11%), electrolyte disturbances ($n = 4$, 9%) and other causes ($n = 6$, 13%). Detailed data are illustrated in Table 2.

CLIF-SOFA on admission, 24 and 48 h following hospital admission, and MELD, SOFA and SAPS II on admission and CTP score prior to CA were significantly higher in patients with unfavourable neurological outcome or mortality within 28 days.

Thirty-three patients (70%) had ACLF on admission. Four (29%) out of 14 patients without ACLF on admission developed ACLF within 48 h after ROSC. Two (4%) of the patients had ACLF prior to admission. ACLF

Table 1 Patients' characteristics of the study population at admission stratified according to the presence of cirrhosis

Parameters	All patients ($n = 1068$)	Cirrhosis ($n = 47$)	No cirrhosis ($n = 1021$)	*p* value
Age, years *median; IQR*	61 (50–72)	62 (51–67)	61 (50–72)	0.92
Male, *n %*	765 (72)	35 (74)	730 (72)	0.66
Weight, kg *median; IQR*	80 (70–90)	80 (69.5–93)	80 (70–90)	0.72
Height, cm *median; IQR*	175 (168–180)	175 (165–180)	175 (168–180)	0.59
SOFA admission, pts *median; IQR*	9 (6–12)	11 (7.5–13)	9 (6–12)	< 0.05
SAPS II admission, pts *median; IQR*	80 (74–88)	87 (77.5–100)	80 (73–87)	< 0.001
Charlson comorbidity index, pts. *median; IQR*	1 (0–3)	4 (2.5–6)	1 (0–2)	< 0.001
Cause of arrest, *n %*				
Cardiac	678 (63)	21 (45)	657 (64)	< 0.05
Out of hospital, *n %*	798 (75)	31 (66)	767 (75)	0.16
Invasive mechanical ventilation, *n %*	850 (80)	35 (74)	815 (80)	0.37
Before cardiac arrest—normal CPC, *n %*	1043 (98)	45 (96)	998 (98)	0.45
Before cardiac arrest—normal OPC, *n %*	973 (91)	39 (83)	934 (91)	0.09
Ischaemic time, min *median; IQR**				
No flow	0 (0–3)	0 (0–3.5)	0 (0–3)	0.49
Low flow	13 (4–25)	11 (3–23)	13 (4–25)	0.51
Time to ROSC	16 (5–30)	15 (3–27)	16 (5–30)	0.42
Epinephrine cumulative (mg) *median; IQR*	3 (1–4)	3 (1–5.5)	3 (1–4)	< 0.001
Witnessed cardiac arrest, *n %*	921 (86)	42 (89)	879 (86)	0.56
Initial rhythm, *n %*				
VT/VF	550 (51)	10 (21)	540 (53)	< 0.001
PEA/asystole	465 (44)	35 (75)	430 (42)	
Other/unknown	53 (5)	2 (4)	51 (5)	0.82
Defibrillation, *n %*	646 (60)	14 (30)	632 (62)	< 0.001
Therapeutic hypothermia, *n %*	666 (62)	18 (38)	648 (63)	< 0.001

SOFA Sequential Organ Failure Assessment, *SAPS* Simplified Acute Physiology Score, *CPC* cerebral performance categories, *OPC* overall performance categories, *ROSC* return of spontaneous circulation, *VT* ventricular tachycardia, *VF* ventricular fibrillation, *PEA* pulseless electrical activity

* Overall ($n = 926$), cirrhosis ($n = 41$), no cirrhosis ($n = 1021$)

Table 2 Characteristics of patients with cirrhosis stratified according to good 28-day outcome and bad 28-day outcome

Parameters	Overall ($n = 47$)	Good 28-day outcome ($n = 9$)	Bad 28-day outcome ($n = 38$)	*p* value*
Aetiology of cirrhosis, *n* %				0.33
Alcoholic	35 (74)	7 (78)	28 (74)	
Viral	6 (13)	2 (22)	4 (10)	
Other (cryptogenic, cardiac, etc.)	6 (13)	0 (0)	6 (16)	
Hepatocellular carcinoma, *n* %	3 (6)	0 (0)	3 (8)	0.38
Liver TX during follow-up, *n* %	0 (0)	0 (0)	0 (0)	
TIPS, *n* %	3 (6)	0 (0)	3 (8)	0.38
CLIF-SOFA—admission *median; IQR*	10 (6–12.5)	4 (3–4)	11 (9–13)	< 0.001
CLIF-SOFA—24 h *median; IQR*	10 (4.5–14)	4 (2–7)	12 (8.25–15.5)	0.01
CLIF-SOFA—48 h *median; IQR*	7 (2–12.5)	1 (1–7)	11 (6–13.75)	0.01
CTP—before admission, *n* %				0.05
A	17 (36)	6 (67)	11 (29)	
B	17 (36)	3 (33)	14 (37)	
C	13 (28)	0 (0)	13 (34)	
CTP points—before admission *median; IQR*	7 (5.5–10)	6 (5–7)	8 (6–11)	0.03
MELD—admission *median; IQR*	19 (10.5–24)	10 (9–10)	21 (14–24)	< 0.001
SOFA—admission *median; IQR*	11 (7.5–13)	4 (3–7)	12 (10–13.75)	< 0.001
SAPS II—admission *median; IQR*	87 (77.5–100)	66 (66–75)	92 (85–102.75)	< 0.001
Ascites—before admission, *n* %				0.33
None	15 (32)	4 (44)	11 (29)	
Mild	25 (53)	5 (56)	20 (53)	
Severe	7 (15)	0 (0)	7 (18)	
HE—before admission, *n* %				0.22
None	25 (53)	7 (78)	18 (47)	
I–II	17 (36)	2 (22)	15 (40)	
III–IV	5 (11)	0 (0)	5 (13)	
ACLF—on admission, *n* %				< 0.001
Grade 1	11 (23)	1 (11)	10 (26)	
Grade 2	11 (23)	0 (0)	11 (30)	
Grade 3	11 (23)	0 (0)	11 (30)	
No ACLF	14 (30)	8 (89)	6 (16)	
ACLF—during follow-up, *n* %				< 0.001
Grade 1	1 (2)	1 (11)	0 (0)	
Grade 2	3 (6)	1 (11)	2 (5)	
Grade 3	0 (0)	0 (0)	0 (0)	
No ACLF	10 (21)	6 (67)	4 (11)	
Ischaemic time, min *median; IQR*				
No flow	0 (0–3.5)	0 (0–0)	0 (0–5)	< 0.01
Low flow	11 (3–23)	1 (1–3)	16 (8–23.5)	0.06
Time to ROSC	15 (3–27)	1 (1–3)	19.5 (11–28)	< 0.05
Initial rhythm, *n* %				
VT/VF	10 (21)	3 (33)	7 (18)	0.569
PEA/Asystole	35 (75)	4 (45)	31 (82)	< 0.05
Other/unknown	2 (4)	2 (22)	0 (0)	0.305
Witnessed cardiac arrest, *n* %	42 (89)	9 (100)	33 (87)	0.118
Defibrillation, *n* %	14 (30)	3 (33)	11 (29)	0.569
Therapeutic hypothermia, *n* %	18 (38)	1 (11)	17 (45)	< 0.01

CPC cerebral performance categories, *TX* transplantation, *TIPS* transjugular intrahepatic portosystemic shunt, *CLIF-SOFA* chronic liver failure-Sequential Organ Failure Assessment, *CTP* Child–Turcotte–Pugh, *MELD* model for end-stage liver disease, *SOFA* Sequential Organ Failure Assessment, *SAPS* Simplified Acute Physiology Score, *HE* hepatic encephalopathy, *ACLF* acute-on-chronic liver failure

* CPC 1/2 versus CPC 3/4 or mortality

grades 1, 2 and 3 were present in 12 (32%), 14 (38%) and 11 (30%) patients, respectively.

CPR-specific data

The majority of patients of the total cohort (75%) suffered OHCA. This rate did not differ significantly in patients with and without cirrhosis. Cardiac arrest was witnessed in 921 (86%) patients. No-flow time was median 0 (IQR 0–3) minutes, low-flow 13 (IQR 4–25) minutes and time to ROSC 16 (IQR 5–30) minutes, which did not differ significantly between patients with and without cirrhosis. Initial shockable rhythm (VT/VF) was significantly more frequent present in patients without cirrhosis. Accordingly, frequency of defibrillation during CPR was significantly lower in patients with liver cirrhosis. Furthermore, cumulative epinephrine dosage during CPR was significantly higher in patients with cirrhosis. First measured lactate levels were significantly higher in patients with liver cirrhosis. Table 1 and Additional file 1: Table S3 illustrate the detailed CPR data.

Functional outcome and survival after CA

Almost all patients both with and without cirrhosis showed a normal CPC and OPC score prior to occurrence of CA as given in Table 1. Rate of favourable neurological outcome was 19% after 28 days, 6 months and 1 year in patients with cirrhosis, compared to 47% after 28 days and 6 months and 43% after 1 year in patients without cirrhosis, respectively. Rate of favourable neurological outcome in CA survivors after 6 months was significantly lower in patients with liver cirrhosis (19 vs. 47%, crude OR 0.26; 95% CI 0.13–0.53). This association continued to be statistically significant after adjustment for covariables (multivariable-adjusted OR 0.13; 95% CI 0.04–0.36, see Table 3). Mortality in patients with cirrhosis was significantly higher compared to patients without cirrhosis (74, 77 and 79% versus 41, 48 and 50% after 28 days, 6 months and 1 year, respectively; OR for 1-year mortality 3.69; 95% CI 1.82–7.51). Figure 1 demonstrates the survival of patients with and without cirrhosis. Cirrhosis was an independent risk factor for 1-year mortality in multivariate regression analysis (multivariable-adjusted OR 3.25; 95% CI 1.33–7.96, see Table 4).

No patient with liver cirrhosis CTP C as well as no patient with HCC or pre-existing TIPS survived longer than 28 days following ROSC with good neurological outcome. Figure 2 demonstrates the survival of patients with favourable neurological outcome in cirrhosis CTP A + B versus CTP C.

Forty per cent ($n = 4$) of patients with cirrhosis without ACLF died within 28 days following ROSC or had unfavourable neurological outcome compared to 92% ($n = 34$) of patients with ACLF ($p < 0.001$). In detail, 83% ($n = 10$) of patients with ACLF grade 1, 93% ($n = 13$) with ACLF grade 2 and 100% ($n = 11$) with ACLF grade 3 had unfavourable neurological outcome or died within 28 days. Multiple organ failure as cause of death was observed in 30 patients with cirrhosis, one patient had cerebral herniation following hypoxic brain injury, and four patients died with palliative care following irreversible hypoxic brain damage.

Mild therapeutic hypothermia (MTH) was applied in 666 (62%) patients of the total cohort [18 (38%) patients with cirrhosis and 648 (63%) without cirrhosis ($p < 0.001$)]. Furthermore, MTH was significantly

Table 3 Logistic regression model for factors associated with good neurological outcome (CPC 1/2 vs. > 2 or deceased)

Parameter	OR (95% CI)	*p* value
Cirrhosis (yes vs. no)	0.13 (0.04–0.36)	< 0.001
Age (years)	0.96 (0.96–0.98)	< 0.001
Time to ROSC (per category)*	0.56 (0.47–0.67)	< 0.001
Shockable rhythm (yes vs. no)	2.16 (1.45–3.23)	< 0.001
Intubated on admission (yes vs. no)	0.17 (0.09–0.34)	< 0.001
SOFA admission (per category)*	0.73 (0.64–0.82)	< 0.001
Cardiac cause (yes vs. no)	1.73 (1.17–2.58)	0.01
Epinephrine cumulative dose (per mg)	0.91 (0.85–0.98)	0.01
Witnessed cardiac arrest (yes vs. no)	0.62 (0.32–1.23)	0.17
Mild therapeutic hypothermia (yes vs. no)	1.23 (0.80–1.90)	0.36
Out-of-hospital cardiac arrest (yes vs. no)	0.89 (0.58–1.38)	0.61
Male (vs. female)	0.92 (0.65–1.31)	0.65
Charlson comorbidity index (per category)*	0.97 (0.84–1.12)	0.67

OR multivariable-adjusted odds ratio, *CI* confidence interval, *ROSC* return of spontaneous circulation, *SOFA* Sequential Organ Failure Assessment, *mg* milligram

*Time to ROSC categories: 0–4, 5–12, 13–24, 25–44, 45 + min, or missing; SOFA categories (score): 5, 6–8, 9–10, 11–12, 12 +, or missing; Carlson comorbidity categories: 0, 1, 2 + 3, 4 +, or missing

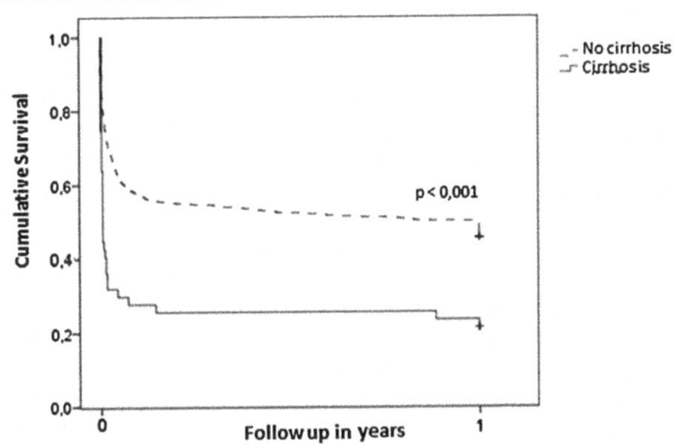

Fig. 1 Survival after ICU admission for cardiac arrest according to the presence and absence of cirrhosis estimated by Kaplan–Meier method

Table 4 Logistic regression model for factors associated with 1-year mortality

1-year mortality	OR	(95% CI)	*p* value
Age	1.05	(1.03–1.06)	< 0.001
Time to ROSC*	1.57	(1.32–1.87)	< 0.001
Shockable rhythm	0.45	(0.31–0.67)	< 0.001
Tube admission	2.33	(1.35–4.03)	< 0.001
SOFA admission*	1.36	(1.20–1.54)	< 0.001
Cirrhosis	3.25	(1.33–7.96)	0.01
Charlson comorbidity index*	1.19	(1.03–1.37)	0.02
Epinephrine cumulative	1.07	(1.01–1.15)	0.03
Male	1.41	(1.00–1.98)	0.05
Cardiac cause of CA	0.68	(0.46–1.00)	0.05
Mild therapeutic hypothermia	0.68	(0.45–1.05)	0.09
OHCA	0.99	(0.66–1.50)	0.98
Witnessed CA	1.00	(0.51–1.94)	0.99

OR multivariable-adjusted odds ratio, *CI* confidence interval, *OHCA* out-of-hospital cardiac arrest, *CA* cardiac arrest, *ROSC* return of spontaneous circulation, *SOFA* Sequential Organ Failure Assessment

* Time to ROSC categories: 0–4, 5–12, 13–24, 25–44, 45 + min, or missing; SOFA categories (score): 5, 6–8, 9–10, 11–12, 12 +, or missing; Charlson comorbidity categories: 0, 1, 2 + 3, 4 +, or missing

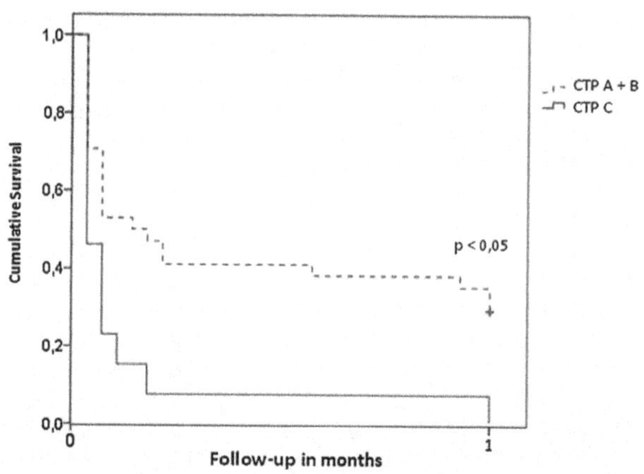

Fig. 2 Probability of having a good neurological outcome after a cardiac arrest among cirrhotic patients according to Child–Turcotte–Pugh score estimated by Kaplan–Meier method

less frequent applied in patients with liver cirrhosis. In the cirrhosis population, patients with MTH were older, had lower SOFA, SAPS II, CLIF-SOFA and MELD score on admission and had significantly longer time to ROSC compared to patients without MTH. We could not observe bleeding or any other complication related to MTH. Twenty-eight-day mortality did not differ significantly between patients with cirrhosis and MTH versus no MTH (78 vs. 72%). Additional file 1: Table S2 illustrates the detailed data on MTH in patients with cirrhosis.

Discussion

In our study, we analysed 1068 critically ill patients following CA and ROSC. Forty-seven of these patients suffered from liver cirrhosis. Presence of cirrhosis was associated with low rates of favourable neurological outcome and increased mortality. Highest rates of unfavourable functional outcome were found in advanced stages of cirrhosis and ACLF.

Cardiac arrest was witnessed in 921 (86%) patients of our cohort, and this is comparable to a previous publication [27]. Seventy-five per cent of the total cohort had OHCA. The first recorded rhythm was shockable in 52% of these patients which is comparable to the reported prevalence of 20–60% in the literature [10, 11, 28]. In contrast, shockable rhythms (35%) were found less frequent in IHCA in accordance with the literature (21–39%) [13, 14, 29]. In the total cohort, 1-year mortality was 50% and favourable functional outcome was observed in 43% of patients following CA. This high rate of favourable outcome may be the consequence of several circumstances. First, we included only patients following ROSC after CA. Accordingly, the rate of good functional outcome was comparable to other studies including only patients with ROSC [27, 30]. Second, we observed in average a short no-flow period in our cohort, which may contribute to the high rate of favourable functional outcome. Third, the vast majority (86%) of CAs was witnessed and we observed a shockable rhythm in about half of the patients.

We identified 47 (4%) patients with cirrhosis in our cohort. This finding is comparable to publications of critical illness, where prevalence of cirrhosis was about 4–7% in the general intensive care setting [31, 32]. These patients had significantly higher SOFA, SAPS II and CCI on hospital admission. Time to ROSC was comparable between patients with and without cirrhosis. However, we observed several significant differences in CA in patients with and without cirrhosis. First, a cardiac aetiology was less frequent and patients with cirrhosis were more likely to have a non-shockable initial ECG rhythm. Second, cumulative epinephrine dosage was higher during CPR and third defibrillations were less frequently performed in patients with cirrhosis. These differences seem to be mainly a consequence of the fact that patients with cirrhosis frequently developed CA following complications of cirrhosis like variceal haemorrhage, severe infection or severe electrolyte disturbances.

Rates of unfavourable functional outcome and mortality were significantly higher in patients with cirrhosis despite no-flow times that were comparable to patients without cirrhosis. This can be explained by the higher comorbidity rate, higher rate of non-cardiac cause and higher rate of non-shockable rhythm in patients with cirrhosis. Furthermore, multivariate regression analysis identified presence of cirrhosis *per se* as an independent predictor of unfavourable outcome.

Overall 38 (81%) patients with cirrhosis had unfavourable neurological outcome or died within 28 days following CA. These patients had a significant higher severity of liver disease and organ failure represented by CTP class, CLIF-SOFA, MELD and ACLF grade as illustrated in Table 2. ACLF was present in 33 (70%) cirrhotic patients at ICU admission following ROSC, and four patients developed ACLF within 48 h after admission. These patients had dramatically worse functional outcome: out of 37 patients with ACLF, 34 (92%) had unfavourable neurology or died within 28 days. Moreover, we observed significant differences in CA characteristics. Patients with cirrhosis and favourable 28-day outcome had a significantly lower no-flow time and time to ROSC and a significantly lower rate of non-shockable rhythm compared to patients with unfavourable neurological outcome or mortality. Furthermore, CA was witnessed in all cases in patients with favourable 28-day outcome. Ischaemic times, especially no flow, seem to be crucial for development of organ failure and unfavourable outcome in patients with cirrhosis. The higher rate of unfavourable 28-day outcome in patients with cirrhosis following CA and ROSC compared to critically ill patients with liver cirrhosis [3, 4, 33] may be explained mainly by the higher severity of illness at baseline in our cohort [4].

The post-CA phase is frequently complicated by the post-CA syndrome, a unique pathophysiological process involving multiple organs [9]. For instance, post-CA brain injury frequently complicates the post-CA phase and accounts for high morbidity and mortality [9, 33]. Factors like hyperglycaemia, impaired cerebral autoregulation as well as pre-existing cerebral impairment in the sense of hepatic encephalopathy could lead to further cerebral injury in patients with cirrhosis. Additionally, post-CA myocardial dysfunction and systemic ischaemia and reperfusion response are frequent findings and account for high morbidity and mortality after CA [15]. The severity of the post-CA syndrome varies according to duration and cause of CA [15]. In our cohort of patients with cirrhosis, death was mainly related to multiple organ failure (86%). Post-anoxic encephalopathy as solitaire cause of death was observed in a minority of patients with cirrhosis, only. Patients with cirrhosis seem to be more prone to organ impairment following CA. This seems to be a consequence of a higher vulnerability for new onset of organ failure and higher severity of illness during CA as discussed previously.

Mild therapeutic hypothermia, i.e. targeted temperature 32–36 °C for 24 h [15], is frequently used despite recent controversial findings as standardised post-CA care [27, 30, 34]. MTH was performed in 666 (62%) patients of our total cohort and in 18 (38%) patients with cirrhosis. Main reason for withholding MTH in cirrhosis was severely abnormal coagulation. A recent study of patients with cirrhosis demonstrated that abnormal coagulation parameters, especially fibrinogen and platelet counts, predict new onset of major bleeding in patients with cirrhosis at the ICU [33]. Data on bleeding complications due to MTH in patients with liver diseases are scarce. Two small case series [35, 36], a randomised controlled trial [37] and a retrospective study [38] of MTH in patients with acute liver failure did not observe an association of MTH and increased rate of bleeding complications. We could not observe new onset of bleeding or any other complication related to MTH in our cohort of critically ill patients with cirrhosis. Twenty-eight-day mortality did not differ significantly in patients with cirrhosis and MTH compared to patients with cirrhosis without MTH. This may be a consequence of the rather small number of patients with cirrhosis, the higher rate of OHCA and a significantly longer time to ROSC in the MTH group. In addition, this study was not powered to analyse the effect of MTH on prognosis in cirrhotic patients. Additional file 1: Table S2 illustrates the detailed data.

Multiple organ failure is associated with high mortality in patients with liver cirrhosis. ACLF is a dynamic condition, which can improve or worsen in a short period of time [39]. Early and repeated risk stratification may help and guide clinical decision making in this extremely sick population [40, 41]. Although our study is able to identify the population that is at highest risk of worst outcome (patients with advanced stages of ACLF and patients with cirrhosis CTP C), we do not believe that current knowledge is already sufficient to provide (i.e. score-based) cut-offs in regard to the decision whether to continue or to stop treatment due to futility. Rather, we are convinced that further therapeutic decisions, especially for withdrawal of care, must take individual patient based factors (i.e. severity of acute and chronic illness, patient's wishes, etc.) into account. Furthermore, remaining treatment options (e.g. liver transplantation), course of the disease and severity of acute illness should be taken into account for further decisions by the attending physician. Future studies are warranted for end-of-life decisions in critically ill patients with cirrhosis [41, 42].

Our study has some limitations. The number of patients with cirrhosis is rather small. However, this is the first study investigating CA in patients with cirrhosis. Furthermore, this study was conducted in a medical intensive care setting. Thus, our data may not be transferable to surgical ICUs. Residual confounding arising from unmeasured covariates cannot be entirely excluded.

In conclusion, CA survivors with cirrhosis have worse outcome than those without pre-existent chronic liver disease. Although one quarter of patients with liver cirrhosis survived longer than 28 days after successful CPR, patients with CTP C as well as advanced ACLF did not survive 28 days with good neurological outcome.

Abbreviations

CA: cardiac arrest; ROSC: return of spontaneous circulation; ICU: intensive care unit; OHCA: out-of-hospital cardiac arrest; IHCA: in-hospital cardiac arrest; MTH: mild therapeutic hypothermia; CPC: cerebral performance categories; OPC: overall performance categories; SOFA: Sequential Organ Failure Assessment; SAPS: Simplified Acute Physiology Score; CCI: Charlson comorbidity index; MELD: model of end-stage liver disease; CTP: Child–Turcotte–Pugh; TIPS: transjugular intrahepatic portosystemic shunt; HCC: hepatocellular carcinoma; PCI: percutaneous coronary intervention.

Authors' contributions

KRo, CWa, FS and VF participated in study conception and design. AD, TH, KRu, AS, JO, PH, CWe, JKM, DJ, CWa, VF and KRo were involved in acquisition of data. KRo, VF, FS, CWa and HH contributed to analysis and interpretation of data. KRo and CWa drafted the manuscript. VF, FS and HH were involved in critical revision of the manuscript for important intellectual content. VF and FS participated in supervision. All authors read and approved the final manuscript.

Author details

[1] Department of Intensive Care Medicine, University Medical Center Hamburg-Eppendorf, Martinistraße 52, 20246 Hamburg, Germany. [2] Department of Emergency Medicine, Medical University of Vienna, Vienna, Austria. [3] Division of Gastroenterology and Hepatology, Department of Internal Medicine 3, Medical University of Vienna, Vienna, Austria.

Acknowledgements

The authors would like to thank the staff of the Emergency Department and ICUs of the Medical University of Vienna and appreciate their work.

Competing interests

The authors declare that they have no competing interests.

Funding

No financial support has been received conducting this study.

References

1. Shellman RG, Fulkerson WJ, DeLong E, Piantadosi CA. Prognosis of patients with cirrhosis and chronic liver disease admitted to the medical intensive care unit. Crit Care Med. 1988;16:671–8.
2. Jalan R, Gines P, Olson JC, Mookerjee RP, Moreau R, Garcia-Tsao G, et al. Acute-on chronic liver failure. J Hepatol. 2012;57:1336–48.
3. Moreau R, Jalan R, Gines P, Pavesi M, Angeli P, Cordoba J, et al. Acute-on-chronic liver failure is a distinct syndrome that develops in patients with acute decompensation of cirrhosis. Gastroenterology. 2013;144:1426–37 **(1437.e1421–1429)**.
4. McPhail MJW, Shawcross DL, Abeles RD, Chang A, Patel V, Lee G-H, et al. Increased survival for patients with cirrhosis and organ failure in liver intensive care and validation of the chronic liver failure-sequential organ failure scoring system. Clin Gastroenterol Hepatol. 2015;13(1353–1360):e1358.
5. Arabi Y, Ahmed QA, Haddad S, Aljumah A, Al-Shimemeri A. Outcome predictors of cirrhosis patients admitted to the intensive care unit. Eur J Gastroenterol Hepatol. 2004;16:333–9.
6. Cholongitas E, Senzolo M, Patch D, Kwong K, Nikolopoulou V, Leandro G, et al. Risk factors, sequential organ failure assessment and model for end-stage liver disease scores for predicting short term mortality in cirrhotic patients admitted to intensive care unit. Aliment Pharmacol Ther. 2006;23:883–93.
7. Berdowski J, Berg RA, Tijssen JGP, Koster RW. Global incidences of out-of-hospital cardiac arrest and survival rates: systematic review of 67 prospective studies. Resuscitation. 2010;81:1479–87.
8. Mozaffarian D, Benjamin EJ, Go AS, Arnett DK, Blaha MJ, Cushman M, et al. Heart disease and stroke statistics-2016 update: a report from the American Heart Association. Circ. 2016;133(4):e38–360.
9. Neumar RW, Nolan JP, Adrie C, Aibiki M, Berg RA, Böttiger BW, et al. Post-cardiac arrest syndrome: epidemiology, pathophysiology, treatment, and prognostication. A consensus statement from the International Liaison Committee on Resuscitation (American Heart Association, Australian and New Zealand Council on Resuscitation, European Resuscitation Council, Heart and Stroke Foundation of Canada, InterAmerican Heart Foundation, Resuscitation Council of Asia, and the Resuscitation Council of Southern Africa); the American Heart Association Emergency Cardiovascular Care Committee; the Council on Cardiovascular Surgery and Anesthesia; the Council on Cardiopulmonary, Perioperative, and Critical Care; the Council on Clinical Cardiology; and the Stroke Council. Circulation. 2008;118:2452–83.
10. Atwood C, Eisenberg MS, Herlitz J, Rea TD. Incidence of EMS-treated out-of-hospital cardiac arrest in Europe. Resuscitation. 2005;67:75–80.
11. Nichol G, Thomas E, Callaway CW, Hedges J, Powell JL, Aufderheide TP, et al. Regional variation in out-of-hospital cardiac arrest incidence and outcome. JAMA. 2008;300:1423–31.
12. Peberdy MA, Kaye W, Ornato JP, Larkin GL, Nadkarni V, Mancini ME, et al. Cardiopulmonary resuscitation of adults in the hospital: a report of 14720 cardiac arrests from the National Registry of Cardiopulmonary Resuscitation. Resuscitation. 2003;58:297–308.
13. Meaney PA, Nadkarni VM, Kern KB, Indik JH, Halperin HR, Berg RA. Rhythms and outcomes of adult in-hospital cardiac arrest. Crit Care Med. 2010;38:101–8.
14. Girotra S, Nallamothu BK, Spertus JA, Li Y, Krumholz HM, Chan PS. Trends in survival after in-hospital cardiac arrest. N Engl J Med. 2012;367:1912–20.
15. Nolan JP, Soar J, Cariou A, Cronberg T, Moulaert VRM, Deakin CD, et al. European Resuscitation Council and European Society of Intensive Care Medicine Guidelines for Post-resuscitation Care 2015: Section 5 of the European Resuscitation Council Guidelines for Resuscitation 2015. Resuscitation. 2015;95:202-22.
16. Soar J, Nolan JP, Böttiger BW, Perkins GD, Lott C, Carli P, et al. Section 3. Adult advanced life support: European Resuscitation Council guidelines for resuscitation 2015. Resuscitation. 2015;95:100-47.
17. Cummins RO, Chamberlain D, Hazinski MF, Nadkarni V, Kloeck W, Kramer E, et al. Recommended guidelines for reviewing, reporting, and conducting research on in-hospital resuscitation: the in-hospital 'Utstein style'. A statement for healthcare professionals from the American Heart Association, the European Resuscitation Council, the Heart and Stroke Foundation of Canada, the Australian Resuscitation Council, and the Resuscitation Councils of Southern Africa. Resuscitation. 1997;34:151–83.
18. Cummins RO, Chamberlain DA, Abramson NS, Allen M, Baskett PJ, Becker L, et al. Recommended guidelines for uniform reporting of data from out-of-hospital cardiac arrest: the Utstein Style. A statement for health professionals from a task force of the American Heart Association, the European Resuscitation Council, the Heart and Stroke Foundation of Canada, and the Australian Resuscitation Council. Circulation. 1991;84:960–75.
19. Schober A, Sterz F, Laggner AN, Poppe M, Sulzgruber P, Lobmeyr E, et al. Admission of out-of-hospital cardiac arrest victims to a high volume cardiac arrest center is linked to improved outcome. Resuscitation. 2016;106:42–8.
20. Nurnberger A, Sterz F, Malzer R, Warenits A, Girsa M, Stockl M, et al. Out of hospital cardiac arrest in Vienna: incidence and outcome. Resuscitation. 2013;84:42–7.
21. Jennett B, Bond M. Assessment of outcome after severe brain damage. Lancet. 1975;1:480–4.
22. Vincent JL, Moreno R, Takala J, Willatts S, De Mendonça A, Bruining

H, et al. The SOFA (Sepsis-related Organ Failure Assessment) score to describe organ dysfunction/failure. On behalf of the Working Group on Sepsis-Related Problems of the European Society of Intensive Care Medicine. Intensive Care Med. 1996;22:707–10.

23. Le Gall JR, Lemeshow S, Saulnier F. A new Simplified Acute Physiology Score (SAPS II) based on a European/North American multicenter study. JAMA. 1993;270:2957–63.
24. Charlson ME, Pompei P, Ales KL, MacKenzie CR. A new method of classifying prognostic comorbidity in longitudinal studies: development and validation. J Chronic Dis. 1987;40:373–83.
25. Kamath PS, Wiesner RH, Malinchoc M, Kremers W, Therneau TM, Kosberg CL, et al. A model to predict survival in patients with end-stage liver disease. Hepatology. 2001;33:464–70.
26. Cholongitas E, Papatheodoridis GV, Vangeli M, Terreni N, Patch D, Burroughs AK. Systematic review: the model for end-stage liver disease—should it replace Child-Pugh's classification for assessing prognosis in cirrhosis? Aliment Pharmacol Ther. 2005;22:1079–89.
27. Nielsen N, Wetterslev J, Cronberg T, Erlinge D, Gasche Y, Hassager C, et al. Targeted temperature management at 33 °C versus 36 °C after cardiac arrest. N Engl J Med. 2013;369:2197–206.
28. Schober A, Sterz F, Herkner H, Locker GJ, Heinz G, Fuhrmann V, et al. Post-resuscitation care at the emergency department with critical care facilities—a length-of-stay analysis. Resuscitation. 2011;82:853–8.
29. Wallmuller C, Meron G, Kurkciyan I, Schober A, Stratil P, Sterz F. Causes of in-hospital cardiac arrest and influence on outcome. Resuscitation. 2012;83:1206–11.
30. Group HaCAS. Mild therapeutic hypothermia to improve the neurologic outcome after cardiac arrest. N Engl J Med. 2002;346:549–56.
31. Piton G, Chaignat C, Giabicani M, Cervoni JP, Tamion F, Weiss E, et al. Prognosis of cirrhotic patients admitted to the general ICU. Ann Intensive Care. 2016;6:94.
32. Fuhrmann V, Kneidinger N, Herkner H, Heinz G, Nikfardjam M, Bojic A, et al. Impact of hypoxic hepatitis on mortality in the intensive care unit. Intensive Care Med. 2011;37:1302–10.
33. Drolz A, Horvatits T, Roedl K, Rutter K, Staufer K, Kneidinger N, et al. Coagulation parameters and major bleeding in critically ill patients with cirrhosis. Hepatology. 2016;64:556–68.
34. Bernard SA, Gray TW, Buist MD, Jones BM, Silvester W, Gutteridge G, et al. Treatment of comatose survivors of out-of-hospital cardiac arrest with induced hypothermia. N Engl J Med. 2002;346:557–63.
35. Jalan R, Olde Damink SWM, Deutz NEP, Hayes PC, Lee A. Moderate hypothermia in patients with acute liver failure and uncontrolled intracranial hypertension. Gastroenterology. 2004;127:1338–46.
36. Jalan R, ODamink SW, Deutz NE, Lee A, Hayes PC. Moderate hypothermia for uncontrolled intracranial hypertension in acute liver failure. Lancet. 1999;354:1164–8.
37. Bernal W, Murphy N, Brown S, Whitehouse T, Bjerring PN, Hauerberg J, et al. A multicentre randomized controlled trial of moderate hypothermia to prevent intracranial hypertension in acute liver failure. J Hepatol 2016;65(2):273-9.
38. Karvellas CJ, Todd Stravitz R, Battenhouse H, Lee WM, Schilsky ML, Group UALFS. Therapeutic hypothermia in acute liver failure: a multicenter retrospective cohort analysis. Liver Transpl. 2015;21:4–12.
39. Arroyo V, Moreau R, Jalan R, Gines P. Acute-on-chronic liver failure: a new syndrome that will re-classify cirrhosis. J Hepatol. 2015;62:S131–43.
40. Saliba F, Ichai P, Levesque E, Samuel D. Cirrhotic patients in the ICU: prognostic markers and outcome. Curr Opin Crit Care. 2013;19:154–60.
41. Gustot T, Fernandez J, Garcia E, Morando F, Caraceni P, Alessandria C, et al. Clinical course of acute-on-chronic liver failure syndrome and effects on prognosis. Hepatology. 2015;62:243–52.
42. McPhail MJ, Auzinger G, Bernal W, Wendon JA. Decisions on futility in patients with cirrhosis and organ failure. Hepatology. 2016;64:986.

22

Carotid and femoral Doppler do not allow the assessment of passive leg raising effects

Valentina Girotto[1*], Jean-Louis Teboul[1], Alexandra Beurton[1], Laura Galarza[1], Thierry Guedj[2], Christian Richard[1] and Xavier Monnet[1]

Abstract

Background: The hemodynamic effects of the passive leg raising (PLR) test must be assessed through a direct measurement of cardiac index (CI). We tested whether changes in Doppler common carotid blood flow (CBF) and common femoral artery blood flow (FBF) could detect a positive PLR test (increase in CI ≥ 10%). We also tested whether CBF and FBF changes could track simultaneous changes in CI during PLR and volume expansion. In 51 cases, we measured CI (PiCCO2), CBF and FBF before and during a PLR test (one performed for CBF and another for FBF measurements) and before and after volume expansion, which was performed if PLR was positive.

Results: Due to poor echogenicity or insufficient Doppler signal quality, CBF could be measured in 39 cases and FBF in only 14 cases. A positive PLR response could not be detected by changes in CBF, FBF, carotid nor by femoral peak systolic velocities (areas under the receiver operating characteristic curves: 0.58 ± 0.10, 0.57 ± 0.16, 0.56 ± 0.09 and 0.64 ± 10, respectively, all not different from 0.50). The correlations between simultaneous changes in CI and CBF and in CI and FBF during PLR and volume expansion were not significant ($p = 0.41$ and $p = 0.27$, respectively).

Conclusion: Doppler measurements of CBF and of FBF, as well as measurements of their peak velocities, are not reliable to assess cardiac output and its changes.

Keywords: Volume expansion, Fluid responsiveness, Hemodynamic monitoring, Cardiac output

Background

Since it has been demonstrated that fluid overload can be deleterious in patients with acute respiratory distress syndrome [1] and severe sepsis [2], it is of paramount importance to avoid excessive fluid administration in such cases. The decision to give fluids must be guided by a reliable prediction of fluid responsiveness as only 50% of patients respond to fluid administration by increasing cardiac output [3]. In order to predict the response of cardiac output to fluid infusion, the passive leg raising (PLR) test has been validated. It consists in lifting the legs passively at 45° and moving the trunk down horizontally, starting from a semi-recumbent position. By transferring a consistent amount of venous blood from the legs and the splanchnic compartment toward the intrathoracic compartment, it increases the mean systemic pressure [4], the cardiac preload and consequently cardiac output in the case of preload responsiveness of both ventricles [5]. However, it must be coupled with a direct and real-time measurement of cardiac output, which is often invasive [6–8].

The Doppler measurement of blood flow and its velocity in the carotid as well as in the femoral arteries may be interesting for estimating the changes in cardiac output during a PLR test, since changes in arterial blood flow and in cardiac output might be proportional. Nevertheless, contradictory results have been published regarding this issue [9–14].

*Correspondence: girotto.valentina@gmail.com
[1] Service de Réanimation Médicale, Hôpital de Bicêtre, Hôpitaux Universitaires Paris-Sud, Insert UMR_999, Université Paris-Sud, Assistance Publique – Hôpitaux de Paris, Le Kremlin-Bicêtre, France
Full list of author information is available at the end of the article

Our study had two aims. The first was to test whether changes in carotid and femoral Doppler measurements were able to detect a positive PLR test. The second was to investigate the ability of carotid and femoral Doppler measurements to track the changes in cardiac index, during PLR and fluid administration.

Methods

Patients

Before starting the study, we obtained the agreement of our institutional review board (*Comité pour la protection des personnes Ile-de-*France VI, ref # 2016-A00959-42). All patients or their relatives accepted to participate in the study. It took place at a 25-bed medical intensive care unit of a university hospital between June and November 2016.

Patients were included in the study if they met the following criteria:

- Age ≥ 18 years.
- A PiCCO2 device (Pulsion Medical Systems, Feldkirchen, Germany) already in place for clinical purposes.
- Decision to perform a PLR test made by the attending physicians.

Patients were excluded if the PLR maneuver was contraindicated (intracranial hypertension), if PLR was supposed to be unreliable (venous compression stocking and intraabdominal hypertension) or if it was impossible to perform vascular Doppler measurements.

Hemodynamic measurements

All patients were equipped with a jugular or subclavian venous catheter and a thermistor-tipped femoral arterial catheter (PV2024, Pulsion Medical Systems). Hemodynamic variables were recorded continuously by using a data acquisition software (HEM 4.2, Notocord, Croissy-sur-Seine, France). Cardiac Index was recorded by the PiCCO Win 4.0 software (Pulsion Medical Systems). For all thermodilution measurements, the results obtained from three consecutive saline boluses were averaged [15, 16].

Doppler measurements

One investigator (VG) performed all ultrasound measurements. Images were analyzed and measurements were performed offline by two investigators (VG and TG). Ultrasound examination was performed with a CX50 (Philips Healthcare, Eindhoven, The Netherlands) by using a 12–5 MHz flat linear probe.

At each step of the protocol, we obtained images of the common carotid artery. First, a long-axis view of the carotid artery was obtained approximately 1–2 cm before its bifurcation. We assessed pulsed wave Doppler, the sampling volume being positioned in the middle of the lumen with caliper parallel to blood flow (Fig. 1). Time average mean velocity (TAMEAN) and peak systolic velocity (PSV) were automatically estimated by the echograph software. Velocity-time integral (VTI) was measured by manually tracing the flow envelope for each image (Fig. 1). We kept an insonation angle of 60° between Doppler beam and sample. In longitudinal view, the maximal diameter was measured from intima to intima with an angle of 90° to the vessel.

To determine carotid blood flow, we used two different methods, one based on VTI (cm) and the other on TAMEAN (cm/s):

- Carotid blood flow (mL/min) = TAMEAN $\times \pi r^2 \times 60$.
- Carotid blood flow (mL/min) = VTI $\times \pi r^2 \times$ Heart rate (beats/min).

where "*r*" (in cm) represents the radius of the vessel that was assumed to be circular.

In addition, we measured TAMEAN with both narrow and large sampling windows within the arterial lumen, in order to compare two different ways of calculating carotid blood flow.

Measurements were also performed at the level of the common femoral artery before the bifurcation into superficial femoral artery and deep femoral artery. Blood flow, peak systolic velocity and diameter were measured with the same method and formulas as described before. Nevertheless, at this level, the only method that was used to measure femoral blood flow was the one based on VTI. Indeed, the contour of the femoral velocity that was automatically traced by the device for measuring time average mean velocity included both positive and negative values of femoral velocities, eventually providing very low values of TAMEAN. We decided to trace the contour manually, including only the positive values in the measurement of VTI.

Study design

At baseline, a first set of transpulmonary thermodilution and Doppler measurements were recorded (Additional file 1: Figure S1). Two PLR tests ("PLR1" and "PLR2") were then consecutively performed because it was not feasible to simultaneously record carotid and femoral Doppler indices during the same PLR test. The PLR position was maintained until the maximal value of pulse contour analysis-derived cardiac index was reached, what always occurs within 1 min [5]. Between the two PLR tests, we waited for approximately 5 min to obtain

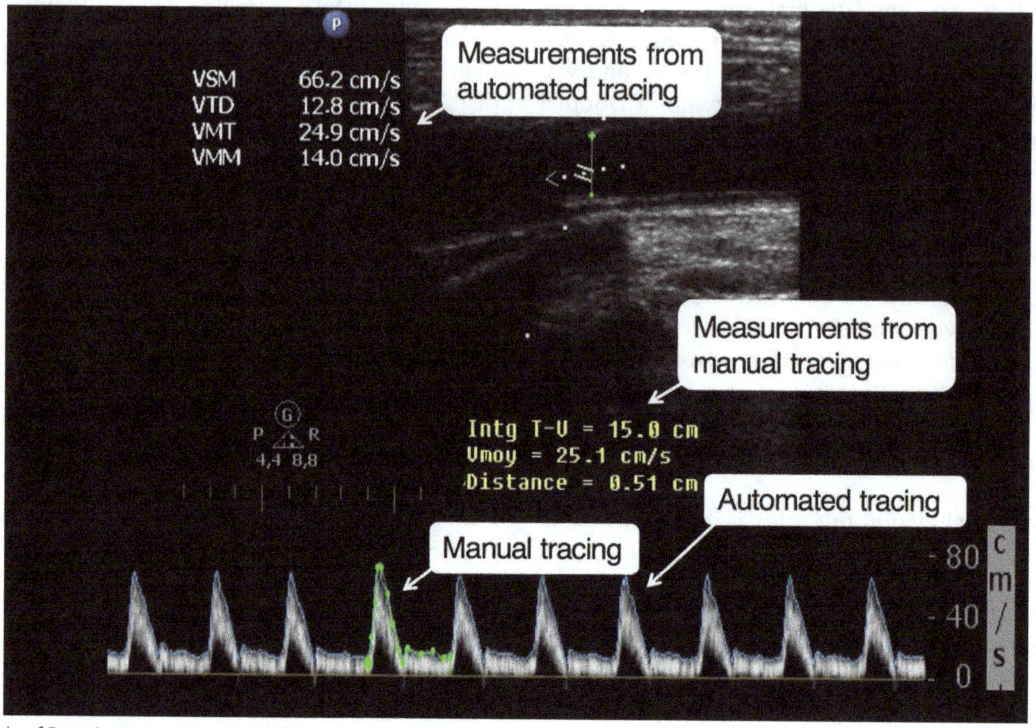

Fig. 1 Example of Doppler measurements performed in a patient

stable hemodynamic baseline values. Each PLR test was performed as previously described [6]. At its maximum effect, a second set of hemodynamic and Doppler measurements was performed (Additional file 1: Figure S1). The effects of PLR on cardiac output were measured by pulse contour analysis and not by transpulmonary thermodilution because these effects must be assessed by a real-time monitoring technique [6]. In practice, we observed the continuously changing value of pulse contour analysis-derived cardiac index while performing the Doppler measurements. As soon as the cardiac index value started to decrease, we considered that it had reached its maximum. At this precise time, we froze the image of the echograph and performed the Doppler measurements on the values displayed during the previous seconds. If pulse contour analysis-derived cardiac index increased ≥ 10% during the PLR tests, compared to the baseline value, the patient was regarded as responder to the tests [8]. In total, the two PLR tests were performed within 15 min.

After the second PLR, another transpulmonary thermodilution was performed. Then, according to the decision of the clinicians in charge, only responders to the first PLR test were given 500 mL of normal saline over 10 min. All echographic and hemodynamic variables were then recorded at the end of fluid infusion, including transpulmonary thermodilution (Additional file 1: Figure S1). Catecholamines dosages and ventilation settings were kept constant during the study period.

Data analysis

All data were normally distributed (Kolmogorov–Smirnov test for normality). Date are expressed as mean ± standard deviation (SD) or number and frequency (*n*, %). Comparison between time points of the study was performed using paired Student's t tests. Comparison between PLR responders and non-responders was performed using two-tailed Student's *t* tests. Pearson correlation coefficient was calculated to compare carotid/femoral blood flow and cardiac index as well as their relative changes following PLR and fluid infusion. A receiving operating characteristics (ROC) curve was constructed to evaluate the ability of the PLR-induced changes in carotid and femoral blood flows and velocities to detect responsiveness to PLR. The inter- and intraindividual variability of carotid Doppler measurements were also calculated. Considering a α-risk of 20% and a β-risk of 10%, to evidence an increase in 20% of carotid and femoral blood flows during PLR [9, 10], we planned to include 50 cases in the study. Statistical significance was defined by a p value < 0.05. The statistical analysis was performed using MedCalc 11.6.0 software (MedCalc, Mariakerke, Belgium).

Results

Patient characteristics

Thirty-three patients were included in the study. Patients could be included more than once at different days, so that we collected 51 cases in total, which were considered as individual cases (Fig. 2). Their characteristics are summarized in Table 1.

At the time of inclusion, in 48 (94%) cases, patients were intubated and ventilated in the volume-controlled mode. Patients received catecholamines in 46 (90%) cases (norepinephrine alone in 41 cases, dobutamine and norepinephrine in three cases, dobutamine alone in two cases).

Feasibility of carotid and femoral Doppler examination

Among all carotid Doppler measurements, two cases were excluded because of carotid stenosis and 10 because of poor image quality that prevented to reliably trace the contour of the signal (Fig. 2). Among the remaining 39 cases, in one case we could not assess carotid blood flow by TAMEAN (Fig. 2).

Among all cases, two were excluded because the femoral site was not accessible for performing Doppler measurement (obesity), 16 cases were excluded because of a poor 2D echogenicity that prevented to precisely define the intima edge of the femoral artery and 19 cases because of poor quality of the Doppler signal (Fig. 2).

Table 1 Baseline patient characteristics

Gender (male)	22 (67%)
Age (years)	67 ± 14
Weight (kg)	68 ± 12
Height (cm)	165 ± 9
SAPS II	62 ± 19
Diagnostic	
Septic shock	16 (49%)
Cardiogenic shock	7 (21%)
ARDS	6 (18%)
Coma	2 (6%)
Pancreatitis	1 (3%)
Acute renal failure	1 (3%)
LVEF < 50%	8 (24%)

N = 33

Data are presented as mean ± standard deviation or number (percentage)

SAPS II simplified acute physiology score, *ARDS* acute respiratory distress syndrome, *LVEF* left ventricular ejection fraction

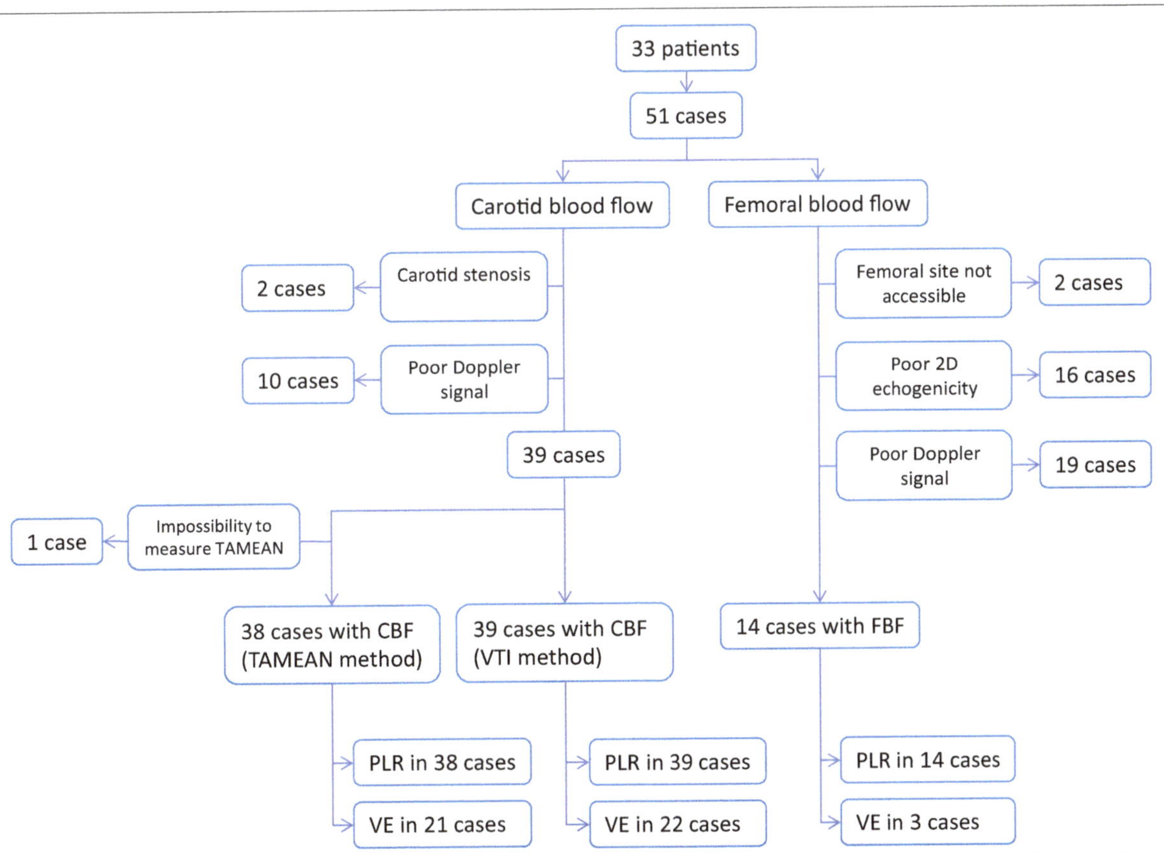

Fig. 2 Flowchart. *CBF* carotid blood flow, *PLR* passive leg raising, *TAMEAN* time average mean velocity, *VE* volume expansion, *VTI* velocity time integral

An increase in cardiac index ≥ 10% during the first PLR predicted fluid responsiveness with a positive predictive value of 93%. The specificity, sensitivity and negative predictive of PLR as a predictor of the response to fluid infusion value could not be calculated since we performed fluid infusion only in patients with a positive PLR test. An increase in cardiac index ≥ 10% during the second PLR predicted fluid responsiveness with the same positive predictive value because both PLR tests exerted similar effects on cardiac index.

The results of ROC curves analysis are presented in Additional file 1: Table S1 and Fig. 3. Neither the changes in carotid blood flow measured with the VTI method nor the carotid blood flow measured the TAMEAN method or the carotid PSV could detect a positive response to the PLR1 test. Neither the changes in femoral blood flow measured with the VTI method nor the femoral PSV could detect a positive response to the PLR2 test (Additional file 1: Table S1, Fig. 3). Results were not different when the analysis was performed with only the first case measured in each of the patients who had been included several times in the study (data not shown).

Relationship between cardiac index and carotid Doppler measurements in absolute values and relative changes

Absolute values of carotid blood flow and of PSV as well as the ratio of carotid blood flow over cardiac index during each study step are reported in Table 2.

For TAMEAN, the inter-individual variability was 8.9 ± 8.7% and the intraindividual variability was 12.7 ± 12.2%. For PSV, the inter-individual variability was 5.0 ± 4.1% and the intraindividual variability was 2.2 ± 1.7%. No difference was found between values of carotid blood flow calculated from TAMEAN sampled in large and narrow sampling windows ($p = 0.28$).

Considering all measurements at different study steps (Fig. 2), only weak correlations were found between absolute values of cardiac index and absolutes values of carotid blood flow calculated from TAMEAN ($n = 135$; $r = 0.54$, $p < 0.01$) (Additional file 1: Figure S2) and absolutes values of carotid PSV ($n = 139$; $r = 0.26$, $p < 0.01$). Absolute values of carotid blood flow calculated with TAMEAN were almost systematically lower than the corresponding values calculated with VTI (data not shown).

Considering all changes observed during the first PLR test ($n = 38$) and fluid infusion ($n = 21$) (Fig. 2), we found no correlation between changes in cardiac index and changes in carotid blood flow calculated from TAMEAN ($n = 59$; $r = 0.07$, $p = 0.61$) and between changes in cardiac index and changes in carotid blood flow calculated from VTI ($n = 61$; $r = 0.11$, $p = 0.41$). The ability of changes in carotid blood flow calculated from VTI and TAMEAN to detect changes in cardiac index are illustrated by 4-box tables in Additional file 1: Table S2. Results were not different when the analysis was performed with only the first case measured in each of the patients who had been included several times in the study (data not shown).

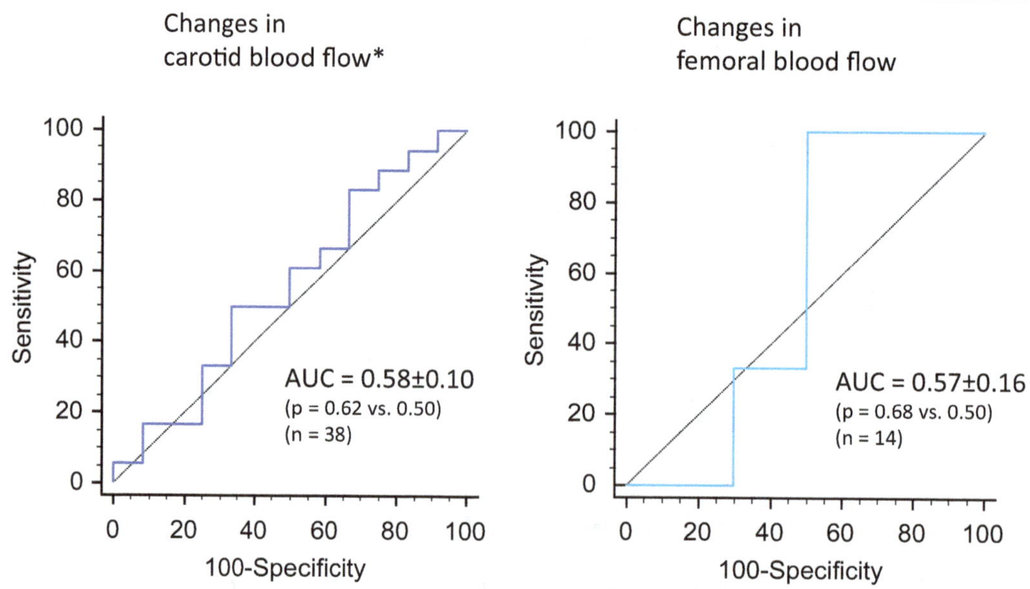

Fig. 3 Receiver operating characteristic curves describing the ability of changes in carotid femoral blood flows to detect a positive response of cardiac index to a passive leg raising test (increase ≥ 10%). *AUC* area under the curve. Asterisks results are provided for carotid blood flow measured by the velocity time integral method

Table 2 Hemodynamic and Doppler measurements

	Baseline 1	PLR1	Baseline 2	PLR2	Baseline 3	After fluid infusion
Heart rate (beats/min)						
PLR responders ($n=27$)	91 ± 19	92 ± 22	89 ± 17	93 ± 17	92 ± 15	93 ± 15
PLR non-responders ($n=24$)	91 ± 18	91 ± 17	87 ± 14	92 ± 14	89 ± 19	–
Systolic arterial pressure (mmHg)						
PLR responders ($n=27$)	117 ± 26	129 ± 32*	115 ± 25	130 ± 34#	115 ± 32	129 ± 33$
PLR non-responders ($n=24$)	125 ± 21	130 ± 24*	122 ± 18	127 ± 20#	125 ± 20	–
Diastolic arterial pressure (mmHg)						
PLR responders ($n=27$)	57 ± 13	62 ± 11*	52 ± 16	62 ± 11#	57 ± 14	63 ± 18$
PLR non-responders ($n=24$)	61 ± 9	64 ± 11*	60 ± 7	64 ± 9#	61 ± 10	–
Central venous pressure (mmHg)						
PLR responders ($n=27$)	11 ± 4	14 ± 5*	9 ± 4	15 ± 5#	11 ± 4	12 ± 4$
PLR non-responders ($n=24$)	10 ± 6	14 ± 6*	10 ± 6	13 ± 7#	10 ± 6	–
Cardiac index (L/min/m^2)						
PLR responders ($n=27$)	3.11 ± 1.21	3.62 ± 1.29*	2.98 ± 1.15	3.63 ± 1.27#	2.91 ± 0.91	3.53 ± 1.16$
PLR non-responders ($n=24$)	3.16 ± 1.07	3.23 ± 1.12	3.14 ± 1.10	3.23 ± 1.24#	3.17 ± 1.13	–
Carotid artery flow (TAMEAN) (mL/min)						
PLR responders ($n=21$)	371 ± 138	407 ± 144	–	–	335 ± 118	390 ± 141$
PLR non-responders ($n=17$)	293 ± 128	344 ± 159	–	–	321 ± 130	–
Carotid artery flow (VTI) (mL/min)						
PLR responders ($n=21$)	615 ± 194	674 ± 202	–	–	601 ± 214	690 ± 221$
PLR non-responders ($n=17$)	593 ± 225	617 ± 218	–	–	577 ± 227	–
Carotid PSV (cm/s)						
PLR responders ($n=22$)	88 ± 23	82 ± 21	–	–	81 ± 22	88 ± 22
PLR non-responders ($n=17$)	83 ± 30	77 ± 28	–	–	82 ± 23	–
Cardiac index to common carotid artery (TAMEAN) (%)						
PLR responders ($n=21$)	13 ± 5	12 ± 4	–	–	12 ± 3	13 ± 5
PLR non-responders ($n=17$)	9 ± 2	10 ± 3	–	–	10 ± 3	–
Femoral artery flow (VTI) (mL/min)						
PLR responders ($n=3$)	–	–	408 ± 331	404 ± 319	433 ± 400	733 ± 800
PLR non-responders ($n=11$)	–	–	368 ± 126	386 ± 127	382 ± 78	–
PSV femoral (cm/s)						
PLR responders ($n=17$)	–	–	84 ± 28	111 ± 45#	77 ± 28	86 ± 31$
PLR non-responders ($n=18$)	–	–	78 ± 17	89 ± 17	78 ± 20	–

Data are presented as mean ± standard deviation. PLR responders: cases with increase in pulse contour analysis-derived cardiac index ≥ 10% during passive leg raising, PLR non-responders: cases with increase in pulse contour analysis-derived cardiac index < 10% during passive leg raising

TAMEAN time average mean velocity, *PSV* peak systolic velocity

* $p<0.05$ versus Baseline 1; # $p<0.05$ versus Baseline 2; $ $p<0.05$ versus Baseline 3

Relationship between cardiac index and femoral Doppler measurements in absolute values and relative changes

Considering all measurements at different study steps ($n=45$, Fig. 2), a weak correlation was found between absolute values of femoral blood flow and cardiac index ($r=0.21$, $p=0.17$). Still considering all measurements performed at the femoral level at different study steps ($n=118$, Fig. 2), a weak correlation was found between absolute values of PSV and cardiac index ($r=0.32$, $p<0.01$) (Additional file 1: Figure S3).

Considering all changes observed during the second PLR test and during fluid infusion ($n=17$, Fig. 2), the correlation coefficient between changes in femoral blood flow and changes in cardiac index was $r=0.28$ ($p=0.27$). The ability of changes in carotid blood flow calculated from VTI and TAMEAN to detect changes in cardiac index are illustrated by 4-box tables in Additional file 1: Table S2. Results were not different when the analysis was performed with only the first case measured in each of the patients who had been included several times in the study (data not shown).

Discussion

The main finding of our study is that carotid and femoral blood flow and their peak velocities did not allow the detection of a positive PLR test and that their changes were not correlated with the simultaneous changes in cardiac index.

The previous results regarding the ability of Doppler measurements of peripheral arteries to estimate cardiac output and its changes are very controversial. Marik et al. [9] have demonstrated an excellent ability of changes in carotid blood flow to detect the PLR effects. Nevertheless, the authors used bioreactance as the reference for measuring cardiac output, while the accuracy of this technique has been seriously questioned [17, 18]. In a study by Préau et al. [10], the variation in femoral artery peak systolic velocity during PLR could reliably predict fluid responsiveness in critically ill patients. Nevertheless, in this study, the carotid blood flow was not investigated and, on the femoral site, only the peak systolic velocity was investigated [10]. Moreover, in this study, the diagnostic threshold that they measured for PLR-induced increases in femoral peak velocity was 8%, while the inter-observer variability of this variable was as large as 8.4 ± 9.2%.

In contrast with these results, other studies in cardiac surgery patients [11, 12] and healthy volunteers [13, 14] showed that the correlation between changes in cardiac output and in common carotid blood flow either was weak or had wide limits of agreement. Our results corroborate these negative studies. Rohering et al. [12] found a strong correlation between absolute values and changes of carotid blood flow and cardiac index. However, limits of agreement in the Bland–Altman analysis (± 20%) were so wide that they concluded that carotid Doppler should not replace direct cardiac output monitoring, especially for performing the PLR test [12]. In the study by Peatchy et al. [13], changes in carotid diameter were not measured during PLR. We measured this diameter in our study, but this did not improve the reliability of the estimation of cardiac index by carotid blood flow.

Several reasons may explain these findings. First, regarding the carotid Doppler signal, from a physiological point of view, the proportion of cardiac output that is directed toward the carotid artery may vary depending on cerebral blood flow regulation, impairing the correlation between carotid blood flow and cardiac output and controversial results have been reported regarding this point [19–24]. Second, another explanation may be the lack of reliability of the carotid and femoral Doppler measurements themselves. In the literature, we could not find a gold standard to calculate femoral and carotid blood flows. Many different methods exist [25], and they provide discordant results [26] with numerous sources of error [27]. In our study, absolute values of carotid blood flow measured by TAMEAN were in accordance with values shown in literature [22], but they were almost systematically half of the values obtained from VTI. Even in patients that had not been excluded from the study, the echogenicity and the quality of the Doppler signal prevented to obtain precise measurements in many cases, especially at the femoral level. This likely led to errors in the measurement of the vessel diameter and hence to even larger miscalculations of blood flow values, as the squared value of arterial diameter is taken into account for measuring them. The measurement of femoral blood flow was impeded by the fact that, at this level, the anatomical landmarks tended to change with PLR. This likely explained the large intra- and inter-variability, indicating that these techniques are not suitable for the precise measurement of changes of small amplitude. Finally, access to the femoral site was difficult in obese patients, such that two of such patients were excluded. Eventually, we obtained a limited number of Doppler measurements for femoral artery. This fact may be enough to conclude that the method is not adapted to current practice in the ICU setting.

Limitations

First of all, we obtained only a limited number of measurements of Doppler variables, what has reduced the power of our analysis. Nevertheless, given the poor results we observed, it is unlikely that including more patients would have led to better results. Regarding femoral measurements, the fact that it was impossible to acquire them in a so large proportion of patients itself indicates that the technique is not appropriate. Second, some patients have been included several times in the study. Nevertheless, the analysis performed with only the first measurement performed in these patients did not show different results from the main analysis. Third, Doppler measurements were performed on one side only, while the opposite one may have provided better results. Fourth, although we took the precaution to exclude it, it is still possible that a mild degree of arterial stenosis may have influenced the relationship between cardiac output and arterial flow. Fifth, Doppler examinations were performed at the bedside in the ICU, while measurements performed in an echographic laboratory could provide more reliable measurements. Nevertheless, our methodology reflects the real-life practice. Finally, fluid infusion was not performed in non-responders, so that we could not assess the specificity and sensitivity of PLR-induced changes in arterial blood flows or velocity to assess fluid responsiveness. Nevertheless, given the poor reliability of Doppler measurements obtained in PLR responders, it is very likely that they did not perform better in PLR non-responders.

Conclusions

Carotid and femoral blood flows and peak systolic velocities were not reliable to assess the effects of a PLR test. These methods were not reliable to estimate cardiac output and its variations in intensive care patients. Many technical and physiological reasons may explain this lack of reliability.

Abbreviations

AUROC: area under the receiver operating characteristics curve; PLR: passive leg raising; PSV: peak systolic velocity; ROC: receiving operating characteristics; SD: standard deviation; TAMEAN: time average mean velocity; VTI: velocity–time integral.

Authors' contributions

VG collected the data, performed data analysis and drafted the manuscript and approved its final version. J-LT conceived the study, participated to analyzing the data and to writing the manuscript and approved its final version. LG and AB contributed to data recording and approved its final version. TG contributed to data analysis and approved its final version. CR supervised the study and approved its final version. XM conceived the study, supervised data analysis and manuscript writing and coordinated the study. All authors read and approved the final manuscript.

Author details

[1] Service de Réanimation Médicale, Hôpital de Bicêtre, Hôpitaux Universitaires Paris-Sud, Insert UMR_999, Université Paris-Sud, Assistance Publique – Hôpitaux de Paris, Le Kremlin-Bicêtre, France. [2] Service de Radiologie, Hôpital de Bicêtre, Hôpitaux Universitaires Paris-Sud, Assistance Publique – Hôpitaux de Paris, Le Kremlin-Bicêtre, France.

Acknowledgements

None.

Competing interests

Profs. Jean-Louis Teboul and Xavier Monnet are members of the Medical Advisory Board of Pulsion Medical Systems. The other authors declare that they have no competing interests.

Funding

No funding.

References

1. Wiedemann HP, Wheeler AP, Bernard GR, et al. Comparison of two fluid-management strategies in acute lung injury. N Engl J Med. 2006;354:2564–75.
2. Vincent JL, Sakr Y, Sprung CL, et al. Sepsis in European intensive care units: results of the SOAP study. Crit Care Med. 2006;34:344–53.
3. Monnet X, Marik PE, Teboul JL. Prediction of fluid responsiveness: an update. Ann Intensive Care. 2016;6:111.
4. Guérin L, Teboul JL, Persichini R, et al. Effects of passive leg raising and volume expansion on mean systemic pressure and venous return in shock in humans. Crete Care. 2015;19:411.
5. Monnet X, Rienzo M, Osman D, et al. Passive leg raising predicts fluid responsiveness in the critically ill. Crit Care Med. 2006;34:1402–7.
6. Monnet X, Teboul JL. Passive leg raising: five rules, not a drop of fluid! Crit Care. 2015;19:18.
7. Monnet X, Marik P, Teboul JL. Passive leg raising for predicting fluid responsiveness: a systematic review and meta-analysis. Intensive Care Med. 2016;42:1935–47.
8. Teboul JL, Saugel B, Cecconi M, et al. Less invasive hemodynamic monitoring in critically ill patients. Intensive Care Med. 2016;42:1350–9.
9. Marik PE, Levitov A, Young A, et al. The use of bioreactance and carotid Doppler to determine volume responsiveness and blood flow redistribution following passive leg raising in hemodynamically unstable patients. Chest. 2013;143:364–70.
10. Préau S, Saulnier F, Dewavrin F, et al. Passive leg raising is predictive of fluid responsiveness in spontaneously breathing patients with severe sepsis or acute pancreatitis. Crit Care Med. 2010;38:819–25.
11. Weber U, Glassford NJ, Eastwood GM, et al. A pilot assessment of carotid and brachial artery blood flow estimation using ultrasound Doppler in cardiac surgery patients. J Cardiothorac Vasc Anesth. 2016;30:141–8.
12. Roehrig C, Govier M, Robinson J, et al. A carotid Doppler flowmetry correlates poorly with thermodilution cardiac output following cardiac surgery. Acta Anaesthesiol Scand. 2017;61:31–8.
13. Peachey T, Tang A, Baker EC, et al. The assessment of circulating volume using inferior vena cava collapse index and carotid Doppler velocity time integral in healthy volunteers: a pilot study. Scand J Trauma Resusc Emerg Med. 2016;24:108.
14. Weber U, Glassford NJ, Eastwood GM, et al. A pilot study of the relationship between Doppler-estimated carotid and brachial artery flow and cardiac index. Anaesthesia. 2015;70:1140–7.
15. Monnet X, Teboul JL. Cardiac output monitoring: throw it out... or keep it? Crit Care. 2018;22:35.
16. Monnet X, Persichini R, Ktari M, Jozwiak M, Richard C, Teboul JL. Precision of the transpulmonary thermodilution measurements. Crit Care. 2011;27:15.
17. Kupersztych-Hagege E, Teboul JL, Artigas A, et al. Bioreactance is not reliable for estimating cardiac output and the effects of passive leg raising in critically ill patients. Br J Anaesth. 2013;111:961–6.
18. Fagnoul D, Vincent JL, De Backer D. Cardiac output measurements using the bioreactance technique in critically ill patients. Crit Care. 2012;16:460.
19. Eicke BM, von Schlichting J, Mohr-Ahaly S, et al. Lack of association between carotid artery volume blood flow and cardiac output. J Ultrasound Med. 2001;20:1293–8.
20. Gassner M, Killu K, Bauman Z, et al. Feasibility of common carotid artery point of care ultrasound in cardiac output measurements compared to invasive methods. J Ultrasound. 2014;18:127–33.
21. Tranmer BI, Keller TS, Kindt GW, et al. Loss of cerebral regulation during cardiac output variations in focal cerebral ischemia. J Neurosurg. 1992;77:253–9.
22. Yazici B, Erdoğmuş B, Tugay A. Cerebral blood flow measurements of the extracranial carotid and vertebral arteries with Doppler ultrasonography in healthy adults. Diagn Interv Radiol. 2005;11:195–8.
23. Sato K, Ogoh S, Hirasawa A, et al. The distribution of blood flow in the carotid and vertebral arteries during dynamic exercise in humans. J Physiol. 2015;589:2847–56.
24. Meng L, Hou W, Chui J, et al. Cardiac output and cerebral blood flow: the integrated regulation of brain perfusion in adult humans. Anesthesiology. 2015;123:1198–208.
25. Blanco P. Volumetric blood flow measurement using Doppler ultrasound: concerns about the technique. J Ultrasound. 2015;18:201–4.

23

Fluoroscopy-guided simultaneous distal perfusion as a preventive strategy of limb ischemia in patients undergoing extracorporeal membrane oxygenation

Woo Jin Jang[1], Yang Hyun Cho[2], Taek Kyu Park[3], Young Bin Song[3], Jin-Oh Choi[3], Joo-Yong Hahn[3], Seung-Hyuk Choi[3], Hyeon-Cheol Gwon[3], Eun-Seok Jeon[3], Woo Jung Chun[1], Ju Hyeon Oh[1] and Jeong Hoon Yang[3*]

Abstract

Background: Limited data are available regarding prevention of limb ischemia in femorally cannulated patients on venoarterial extracorporeal membrane oxygenation (VA-ECMO). We investigated the association between strategy of distal perfusion catheter (DPC) insertion and vascular complications like limb ischemia in patients undergoing VA-ECMO.

Methods: We evaluated 230 patients from two tertiary hospitals who received VA-ECMO via femoral cannulation between August 2014 and July 2017. The patients were divided into two groups according to DPC insertion strategy: patients who underwent DPC insertion at the time of primary cannulation (DPC group, $n = 96$) and patients who were provisionally treated with DPC (No-DPC group, $n = 134$). The primary outcome was limb ischemia.

Results: Of the 96 patients in the DPC group, 61 (63.5%) underwent insertion under fluoroscopic guidance. The DPC group had a significantly lower incidence of limb ischemia (2.1% vs. 8.2%, $p = 0.047$) and a lower tendency of in-hospital mortality (38.5% vs. 50.7%, $p = 0.067$) than the No-DPC group. In the multivariable analysis, fluoroscopy-guided simultaneous insertion of the DPC (odds ratio 0.11; 95% confidence interval 0.01–0.98; $p = 0.048$) was a significant predictor of reduction of limb ischemia.

Conclusions: Simultaneous insertion of a DPC, particularly under fluoroscopy guidance, can be considered as a preventive strategy for limb ischemia in femorally cannulated patients on VA-ECMO.

Keywords: Distal perfusion catheter, Limb ischemia, Extracorporeal membrane oxygenation

Background

Venoarterial extracorporeal membrane oxygenation (VA-ECMO) has been widely used as a salvage therapy in critically ill patients with refractory cardiogenic shock [1]. The femoral vessel approach for VA-ECMO insertion is regarded as the default route because the equipment can be placed rapidly and easily [2]. In patients undergoing VA-ECMO using transfemoral cannulation, limb ischemia is a lethal complication that can be influenced by vessel size, increased vascular tone due to hemodynamic instability, size of the indwelling arterial cannula, and use of vasopressors [3–6]. To prevent limb ischemia after cannulation, the guidance of an antegrade distal perfusion catheter (DPC) into the proximal superficial femoral artery (SFA) has been assisted by various techniques such as ultrasound and fluoroscopy

*Correspondence: jhysmc@gmail.com
[3] Division of Cardiology, Department of Critical Care Medicine and Medicine, Heart Vascular Stroke Institute, Samsung Medical Center, Sungkyunkwan University School of Medicine, 81, Irwon-dong, Gangnam-gu, Seoul 135-710, Republic of Korea
Full list of author information is available at the end of the article

[2, 7]. However, the optimal timing of and strategy for DPC insertion have not been fully elucidated for patients undergoing VA-ECMO via femoral cannulation. Therefore, we investigated whether simultaneous insertion of a DPC, particularly fluoroscopy-guided DPC insertion, at the time of primary ECMO cannulation can reduce critical limb ischemia compared with a provisional approach.

Methods

Study population

We investigated 257 consecutive patients who underwent VA-ECMO from a retrospective multicenter registry at Samsung Medical Center, Seoul, South Korea, and Samsung Changwon Hospital, Gyeongnam, South Korea, from August 2014 through July 2017. Of these, we included only patients who were placed on peripheral VA-ECMO via femoral cannulation and excluded patients who were under 18 years of age or who underwent ECMO using central aortic or axilla-arterial cannulation. Ultimately, 230 patients were enrolled in this study and were divided into two groups according to timing of DPC insertion: patients who underwent DPC insertion at the time of the primary cannulation (DPC group) and patients who did not undergo DPC insertion at the primary femoral cannulation including provisional DPC insertion after the onset of distal limb ischemia (No-DPC group) (Fig. 1). The local institutional review board of each participating hospital approved this study and waived the requirement for informed consent.

Extracorporeal membrane oxygenation implantation and management

The decision to implant ECMO was made by an experienced team, and the ECMO was placed by either cardiovascular surgeons or interventional cardiologists. The Capiox Emergency Bypass System (Capiox EBS™; Terumo, Inc., Tokyo, Japan) and Permanent Life Support (PLS) System (MAQUET, Rastatt, Germany) were used. Heparin was intravenously administered as a bolus of 5000 units, followed by continuous intravenous infusion to maintain an activated clotting time between 150 and 180 s. After initiation of ECMO, the pump blood flow rate was initially set above 2.2 L/min/body surface area (m^2) and subsequently adjusted to maintain a mean arterial pressure above 65 mmHg. Blood pressure was continuously monitored through an arterial catheter, and arterial blood gas analysis was performed in the artery of the right arm to estimate cerebral oxygenation. Additional fluids, blood transfusion, and/or catecholamines (i.e., norepinephrine, epinephrine, or dobutamine) were supplied to maintain intravascular volume and/or to achieve a mean arterial pressure above 65 mmHg if necessary [8].

Cannulation of extracorporeal membrane oxygenation and distal perfusion catheter

Percutaneous cannulation of the femoral artery and vein was mainly performed by the attending staff interventional cardiologist or cardiovascular surgeon using the Seldinger technique. The femoral vessels (either unilateral, one-side arterial, or one-side venous) were accessed

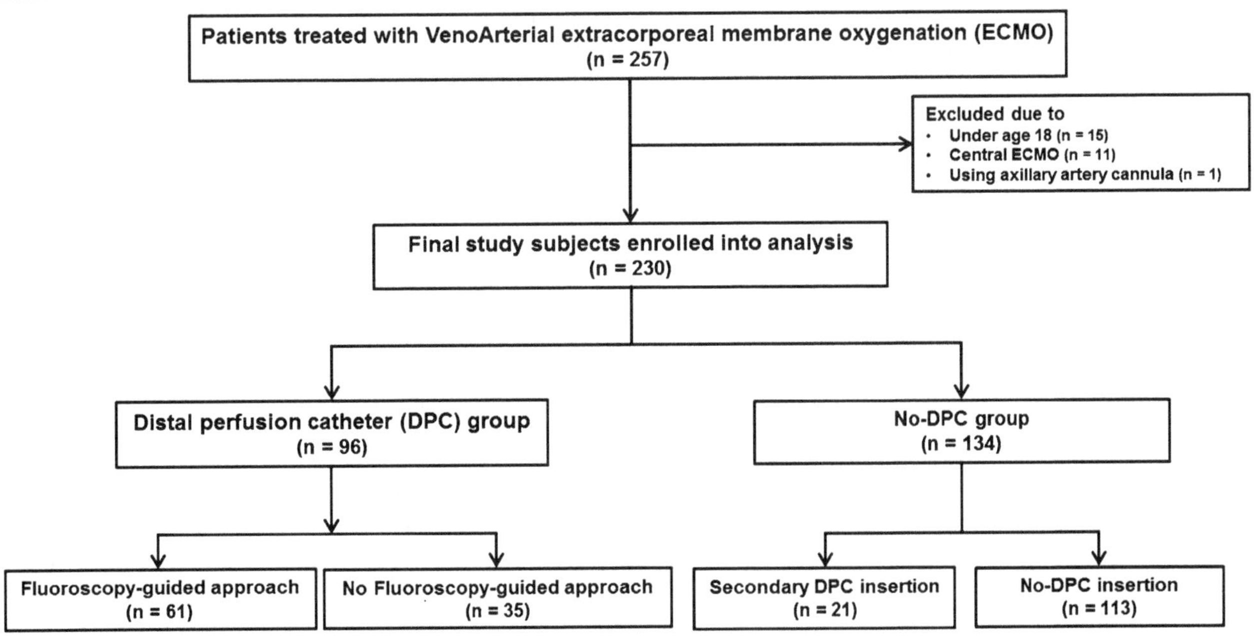

Fig. 1 Schematic illustration of study cohort selection

retrograde using an angiogram needle. The venous cannula was either 55 or 68 cm in length and from 21 to 28 Fr.; the arterial cannula was 24 cm and from 14 to 21 Fr. The final selection of cannula was based on manufacturer pressure–flow curves for each cannula size and patient size. Femoral cut-down procedures were performed when it was difficult to puncture the femoral artery percutaneously, for example, in patients with peripheral artery disease or severe obesity. At bedside, the DPC placement site was accessed antegrade using a micropuncture needle followed by a 0.018-inch nitinol wire (Cook Medical Inc, Bloomington, IN, USA) at the proximal SFA ipsilateral to the arterial cannula. A 6- or 7-Fr. sheath was then advanced into the mid-SFA. In the catheterization laboratory, we first inserted another sheath at the common femoral artery (CFA) contralateral to the arterial ECMO cannula and advanced a hydrophilic wire from the CFA sheath (through the aortic bifurcation and the ipsilateral common iliac artery, then between the arterial ECMO cannula and the vessel wall of the ipsilateral common iliac artery) to the distal portion of the ipsilateral SFA. The DPC was then safely inserted into the distal portion of the arterial cannula (ipsilateral to the SFA) using a micropuncture needle as the reference point of the previously placed hydrophilic wire. The catheter was attached to the side port of the arterial cannula using 6-inch extension tubing with an intervening three-way stopcock (Fig. 2).

Data collection, definitions, and study outcomes

Baseline characteristics, procedural characteristics, laboratory data, and clinical outcome data were obtained by reviewing medical records or by telephone contact, if necessary. Laboratory findings, including creatinine and lactate, were collected just before VA-ECMO insertion. The primary outcome was limb ischemia, which was defined as cases requiring surgical management or involving neurologic sequelae. In-hospital mortality, successful weaning rate of ECMO, thrombotic events, major bleeding, and catheter-related complications (defined as a composite of limb ischemia, major bleeding, and thrombotic events) were assessed in addition to the primary outcome. Major bleeding was defined as cases involving hemodynamic instability or those that occurred in a critical area or organ such as intracranial, retroperitoneal, pericardial, or intramuscular with compartment syndrome.

Statistical analysis

Continuous variables were compared using Student's *t* test or the Wilcoxon rank-sum test. The results were presented as mean $\pm$ standard deviation or median with interquartile range. Categorical data were tested using Fisher's exact test or the Chi-square test. Multivariable logistic regression analysis was performed via a stepwise backward selection process to determine the independent predictors of limb ischemia. Clinical variables (i.e., fluoroscopy-guided simultaneous DPC, age ≥ 65 years, gender, duration of ECMO > 5 days, and large arterial cannula) were included in the regression models. All variables associated with limb ischemia were analyzed using univariate analysis. Factors with $p < 0.2$ and those that were clinically relevant were included in the multivariable analysis. All tests were two-tailed, and p value < 0.05 was considered statistically significant. Statistical analyses were performed using SPSS software, version 23 (IBM, Armonk, New York, USA).

Results

Baseline, procedural, and laboratory characteristics

The baseline and procedural characteristics of the study population are shown in Table 1. There were no significant differences between the DPC group and the No-DPC group except body mass index (BMI) in baseline characteristics. Of the 134 patients in the No-DPC group, 21 (15.7%) underwent secondary DPC insertion. ECMO was mainly inserted in either catheterization laboratory room, intensive care unit, or emergency room. Extracorporeal cardiopulmonary resuscitation (ECPR) was more frequently performed in the No-DPC group than in the DPC group ($p = 0.003$). The size of femoral arterial cannula was similar between the DPC group and the No-DPC group ($p = 0.080$), but venous cannular size was larger in the DPC group than in the No-DPC group ($p = 0.019$). Anticoagulation therapy ($p = 0.004$) and left ventricular venting during ECMO support ($p = 0.029$) were more frequently performed in the DPC group than in the No-DPC group, and large arterial cannula ($p = 0.066$) tended to be used less frequently in the DPC group compared to the No-DPC group. The median duration of ECMO support was 3 days [interquartile range (IQR) 1–7 days]. The median total length of stay in the intensive care unit was 6 days (IQR 1–16 days), and the median total length of stay in the hospital was 20 days (IQR 6–45 days).

Limb ischemia and other catheter-related complications in VA-ECMO patients

Thirty-four cases of ischemic complication (13 limb ischemia, 18 thrombotic events, and 3 ischemic strokes) occurred. Of the 13 patients with distal limb ischemia, 3 were recovered through medical treatment, while 3

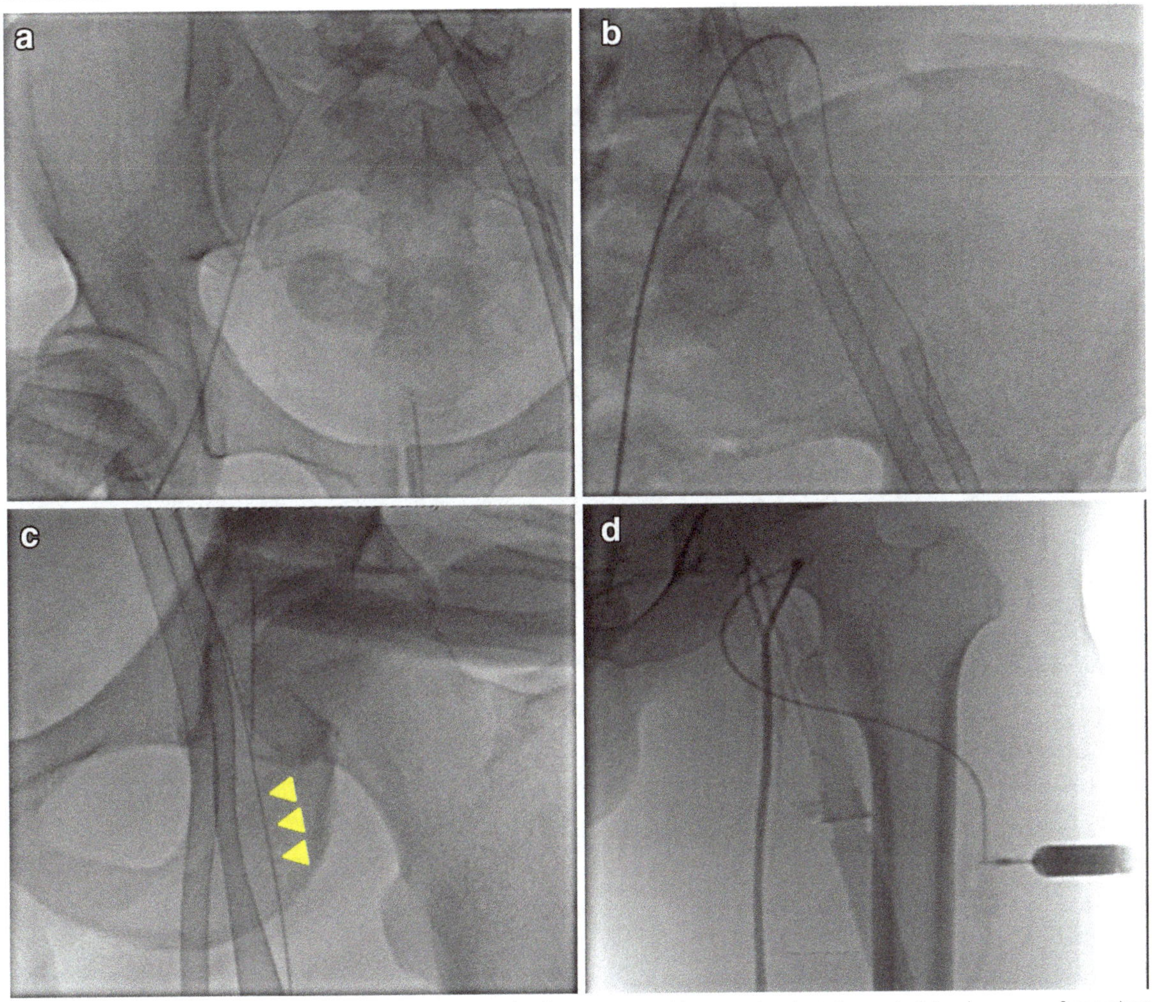

Fig. 2 Percutaneous insertion of a distal perfusion catheter. **a** Under fluoroscopy guidance, a sheath at the contralateral common femoral artery (CFA) was inserted using a micropuncture needle followed by a 0.018-inch nitinol wire. **b** A hydrophilic wire was advanced from the sheath of the contralateral CFA (through the aortic bifurcation and the ipsilateral common iliac artery, between the arterial ECMO cannula and the vessel wall of the ipsilateral common iliac artery) to the distal portion of the ipsilateral superficial femoral artery (SFA). **c** The proximal SFA ipsilateral to the arterial cannula was punctured using a micropuncture needle followed by a 0.018-inch nitinol wire as the reference point of the previously placed wire (yellow arrow heads). A distal perfusion catheter (6- or 7-Fr. sheath) was inserted antegrade and advanced safely into the mid-SFA. **d** The distal perfusion catheter was attached to the side port of the arterial cannula using 6-inch extension tubing with an intervening three-way stopcock

underwent fasciotomy, 3 received surgical thrombectomy, and 4 underwent surgical amputation of the distal lower limb implanted with ECMO. Limb ischemia was less frequent in the DPC group than in the No-DPC group (2.1% vs. 8.2%; $p=0.047$). The incidences of major bleeding (8.3% vs. 4.5%; $p=0.228$), thrombotic events (5.2% vs. 9.7%; $p=0.211$), and catheter-related complications (24.0% vs. 19.4%; $p=0.405$) were not different between the two groups. The rate of successful ECMO weaning was greater in the DPC group than in the No-DPC group (79.2% vs. 61.9%; $p=0.005$), and the DPC group had a lower tendency of in-hospital mortality than the No-DPC group (38.5% vs. 50.7%; $p=0.067$) (Table 2).

Fluoroscopy-guided distal perfusion and predictors on lower limb ischemia

Of the 96 patients in the DPC group, 61 (63.5%) underwent DPC insertion under fluoroscopic guidance (Table 1). Fluoroscopy-guided DPC group had a numerically low incidence of catheter-related complication including limb ischemia, cannular site bleeding, and thrombotic event compared to no fluoroscopy-guided DPC group (Table 2). Furthermore, the incidence of limb ischemia tended to be lower in the fluoroscopy-guided DPC group than in the No-DPC group ($p=0.057$). We performed multivariable logistic regression analysis to identify predictors of limb ischemia in patients

Table 1 Baseline and procedural characteristics

	DPC group ($n=96$)			No-DPC group ($n=134$)	p value DPC versus No-DPC
	Fluoroscopy-guided ($n=61$)	No fluoroscopy-guided ($n=35$)	p value		
Age (years)	55.2±16.7	55.7±16.2	0.143	58.5±13.7	0.106
Gender (male)	39 (63.9)	20 (57.1)	0.735	89 (66.4)	0.439
Body mass index (kg/m²)	23.0±3.1	25.0±3.9	<0.001	25.6±3.9	<0.001
Diabetes mellitus	16 (26.2)	10 (28.6)	0.260	46 (34.3)	0.243
Hypertension	22 (36.1)	10 (28.6)	0.790	51 (38.1)	0.462
Dyslipidemia	11 (18.0)	2 (5.7)	0.016	9 (6.7)	0.083
Current smoker	13 (21.3)	12 (34.3)	0.959	29 (21.6)	0.438
Chronic kidney disease	4 (6.6)	2 (5.7)	0.688	11 (8.2)	0.576
Peripheral vascular disease	2 (3.3)	0 (0)	0.670	3 (2.2)	0.936
Previous MI	10 (16.4)	7 (20.0)	0.396	29 (21.6)	0.462
Previous PCI	9 (14.8)	7 (20.0)	0.217	30 (22.4)	0.285
Previous CABG	1 (1.6)	1 (2.9)	0.136	9 (6.7)	0.104
Previous CVA	5 (8.5)	2 (5.7)	0.858	10 (7.5)	0.961
Clinical presentation			0.002		0.061
Ischemic cardiomyopathy	32 (52.5)	10 (28.6)		58 (43.3)	
Non-ischemic cardiomyopathy	13 (21.3)	5 (14.3)		21 (15.7)	
Septic shock	0 (0)	6 (17.1)		4 (3.0)	
Refractory arrhythmia	8 (13.1)	1 (2.9)		4 (3.0)	
Other causes	8 (13.1)	13 (37.1)		47 (35.1)	
Purpose of ECMO implantation			0.035		0.121
Bridge to recovery	49 (80.3)	32 (91.4)		122 (91.0)	
Bridge to transplantation	12 (19.7)	3 (8.6)		12 (9.0)	
ECPR	24 (39.3)	17 (48.6)	0.002	84 (62.7)	0.003
Initial ECMO pump flow (L/min)	3.0±0.8	3.3±0.5	0.722	3.1±1.1	0.729
Operating site of ECMO			<0.001		<0.001
Intensive care unit	0 (0)	21 (60.0)		31 (23.1)	
Catheterization laboratory room	56 (91.8)	0 (0)		33 (24.6)	
Emergency room	4 (6.6)	7 (20.0)		27 (20.1)	
Operating room	0 (0)	4 (11.4)		17 (12.7)	
Others	1 (1.6)	3 (8.6)		26 (19.4)	
Arterial catheter size (Fr.)	15.3±0.7	15.4±0.9	0.061	15.3±0.8	0.080
Venous catheter sized (Fr.)	22.4±1.5	21.9±0.7	0.010	21.5±2.4	0.019
Large arterial cannula[a]	10 (16.4)	9 (25.7)	0.055	41 (30.6)	0.066
During ECMO support					
Anticoagulation therapy	52 (85.2)	25 (71.4)	0.001	84 (62.7)	0.004
Left ventricular venting	16 (26.2)	3 (8.6)	0.003	13 (9.7)	0.029
Distal perfusion	61 (100.0)	35 (100.0)	<0.001	21 (15.7)	<0.001
Continuous renal replacement therapy	18 (29.5)	16 (45.7)	0.177	53 (39.6)	0.524
Intra-aortic balloon pump	2 (3.3)	1 (2.9)	0.696	6 (4.5)	0.602
Mechanical ventilation	47 (77.0)	27 (77.1)	0.318	94 (70.1)	0.243
Laboratory findings					
Creatinine (mg/dL) (just before ECMO insertion)	1.4 (1.0–1.54)	1.2 (0.8–1.4)	0.391	1.3 (0.9–1.9)	0.779
Lactate (mmol/L) (just before ECMO insertion)	4.9 (2.8–9.2)	5.7 (2.0–10.4)	0.051	5.3 (2.1–10.1)	0.683
Lactate (mmol/L) (24 h after ECMO insertion)	1.9 (1.4–3.1)	2.2 (1.1–4.9)	0.300	2.1 (0.0–3.9)	0.700
Duration of ECMO support (day)	3.4 (2.1–7.5)	4.0 (2.0–6.3)	0.013	2.0 (1.0–5.0)	0.052
Length of ICU stay (day)	10.0 (3.5–19.0)	6.0 (1.0–15.5)	0.518	5.0 (1.0–10.0)	0.012
Length of hospital stay (day)	27.0 (14.0–73.0)	24.0 (7.5–49.8)	0.271	14.0 (5.0–34.0)	0.030

Values are mean ± standard deviation, median (interquartile range), or n (%)

CABG coronary artery bypass grafting, *CVA* cerebrovascular accident, *DPC* distal perfusion catheter, *ECPR* extracorporeal cardiopulmonary resuscitation, *ICU* intensive care unit, *MI* myocardial infarction, *PCI* percutaneous coronary intervention, *ECMO* extracorporeal membrane oxygenation

[a] We considered patient used 16–21-Fr. catheter as patient used large arterial catheter

Table 2 Clinical outcomes and complications

	DPC group ($n=96$)			No-DPC group ($n=134$)	p value DPC versus No-DPC
	Fluoroscopy-guided ($n=61$)	No fluoroscopy-guided ($n=35$)	p value		
Limb ischemia	1 (1.6)	1 (2.9)	0.688	11 (8.2)	0.047
Major bleeding	5 (8.2)	3 (8.6)	0.949	6 (4.5)	0.228
Thrombotic event	2 (3.3)	3 (8.6)	0.261	13 (9.7)	0.211
Catheter-related complication[a]	12 (19.7)	11 (31.4)	0.194	26 (19.4)	0.405
Successful weaning from ECMO	49 (80.3)	27 (77.1)	0.711	83 (61.9)	0.005
In-hospital mortality	22 (36.1)	15 (42.9)	0.510	68 (50.7)	0.067

Values are n (%)

DPC distal perfusion catheter, *ECMO* extracorporeal membrane oxygenation

[a] Catheter-related complication was defined as a composite of limb ischemia, cannular site bleeding, and thrombotic event

undergoing VA-ECMO. Simultaneous DPC insertion (OR 0.13, 95% CI 0.03–0.68, $p=0.016$) and ICU stay ≥ 11 days (OR 4.34, 95% CI 1.26–14.97, $p=0.020$) on model I, and fluoroscopy-guided simultaneous DPC insertion (OR 0.11, 95% CI 0.01–0.98, $p=0.048$) and ICU stay ≥ 11 days (OR 3.71, 95% CI 1.12–12.32, $p=0.032$) on model II were significant prognostic factors for lower limb ischemia (Table 3).

Table 3 Predictors of lower limb ischemia

	Odds ratio	95% CI	p value
Model I			
Simultaneous DPC insertion	0.13	0.03–0.68	0.016
Age ≥ 65 years	0.27	0.06–1.35	0.111
Male	1.37	0.40–4.76	0.618
BMI ≥ 25 kg/m^2	0.46	0.13–1.66	0.235
Diabetes mellitus	0.91	0.25–3.35	0.891
Clinical presentation	0.77	0.52–1.14	0.189
ICU stay ≥ 11 days	4.34	1.26–14.97	0.020
Model II			
Fluoroscopy-guided DPC insertion	0.11	0.01–0.98	0.048
Age ≥ 65 years	0.28	0.06–1.36	0.114
Male	1.46	0.42–5.10	0.554
BMI ≥ 25 kg/m^2	0.48	0.14–1.70	0.255
Diabetes mellitus	0.93	0.25–3.45	0.910
Clinical presentation	0.73	0.49–1.10	0.131
ICU stay ≥ 11 days	3.71	1.12–12.32	0.032

Model I: adjusted with simultaneous DPC insertion, age ≥ 65 years, male, BMI ≥ 25 kg/m^2, diabetes mellitus, clinical presentation, and ICU stay ≥ 11 days

Model II: adjusted with fluoroscopy-guided simultaneous DPC insertion, age ≥ 65 years, male, BMI ≥ 25 kg/m^2, diabetes mellitus, clinical presentation, and ICU stay ≥ 11 days

BMI body mass index, *CI* confidence interval, *DPC* distal perfusion catheter, *ICU* intensive care unit

Discussion

We investigated the association between the method and timing of distal perfusion and vascular complications, including limb ischemia, major bleeding, and thrombotic events, in patients undergoing VA-ECMO. Our main finding is that simultaneous DPC insertion at the time of primary ECMO cannulation reduced the incidence of lower limb ischemia. In the multivariable analysis, fluoroscopy-guided simultaneous insertion of DPC, duration of ECMO implantation > 5 days, and use of a large arterial cannula (over 16 Fr.) were significant predictors of limb ischemia. In general, our findings correspond well with earlier studies that established an association between distal perfusion and adverse clinical outcomes [2, 9]. The present study showed for the first time that fluoroscopy-guided DPC insertion via a contralateral approach might be a safe and effective strategy to prevent limb ischemia in femorally cannulated patients on VA-ECMO.

VA-ECMO implantation for patients with refractory cardiopulmonary failure is quick and convenient when using a percutaneous femoral approach, but limb ischemia and other catheter-related complications frequently develop due to partial luminal obstruction or injury to the common femoral artery or vein. Muehrcke et al. [10] reported an ischemia rate of 70% in an ECMO population of 24 patients without DPC placement at the time of cannulation. Their cannulation protocol was modified to include simultaneous DPC placement, with noted improvement in limb salvage. Foley et al. [5] reported an ischemia rate of 21% in 58 patients without DPCs, although they found no difference in limb ischemia or mortality between prophylactic and expectant placement of a DPC. These findings strongly suggest that limb ischemia can be avoided in a large number of patients undergoing ECMO if the physician can safely insert a DPC. Additionally, Lamb et al. [2] reported that placement of a DPC at the time of cannulation and intensive monitoring of limb perfusion may decrease the incidence of ischemic complication. Ranney et al. [9] investigated the indication and timing of DPC placement and reported that DPC placement at the time of primary cannulation may lower the incidence of limb ischemia. However, both studies had a limited number of patients and focused only on the occurrence of complicated limb ischemia in ECMO patients; therefore, no definite conclusion can be drawn from these studies. The strength of our study is in the comparison of overall clinical outcomes and ECMO-related vascular complications, as well as limb ischemia, between two timings of DPC insertion using a large, dedicated ECMO registry.

In the real-world practice, additional procedures, like DPC insertion, could be harmful in critically ill patients who are vulnerable to bleeding or who had received anticoagulation therapy while on ECMO. Therefore, finding a method to insert the DPC that avoids bleeding complications caused by multiple needle thrusts would make it possible to avoid fatal complications in the lower limb. In the present study, DPCs were preferentially inserted in all VA-ECMO patients unless limited by technical considerations, typically an inability to cannulate the SFA, and no procedural-related limb complication occurred in patients treated with fluoroscopy-guided DPC insertion. Our findings suggest that simultaneous DPC insertion at the time of primary ECMO cannulation should be considered to prevent limb ischemia, and image-guided insertion methods, such as fluoroscopy, are more effective and safe.

Study limitations

This study has several limitations. First, its design was non-randomized, retrospective, and observational, which may have affected the results due to confounding factors. Second, the selection of treatment strategy for the cannulated limb was at the discretion of the operator and could have influenced the results by introducing bias. Third, the impact of limb ischemia on long-term outcomes and the influence of eventual distal perfusion in the No-DPC group were not assessed in this study. Fourth, patients undergoing simultaneous DPC insertion may be comparatively more stable to those who do not undergo the procedure. The DPC and No-DPC groups were different in baseline BMI, rate of ECPR, and operating site of ECMO in the present study. This might have influenced study outcomes and produced a higher rate of ECMO weaning in patients undergoing simultaneous DPC insertion. Finally, we did not compare our fluoroscopy-guided contralateral DPC strategy with previous methods such as ultrasound-guided DPC insertion or ipsilateral DPC insertion. Therefore, this method cannot be chosen with certainty as the best method of DPC insertion.

Conclusion

Simultaneous insertion of DPC at the time of primary ECMO cannulation using a femoral approach could prevent advanced limb ischemia. In particular, fluoroscopy-guided DPC insertion via a contralateral approach can be considered as a new strategy for prevention of disastrous vascular complications.

Abbreviations

DPC: distal perfusion catheter; SFA: superficial femoral artery; VA-ECMO: venoarterial extracorporeal membrane oxygenation.

Authors' contributions

WJJ and JHY had full access to all of the data and take responsibility for the integrity of the data and the accuracy of the data analysis. WJJ, YHC, and JHY contributed to the study concept and design. All authors contributed to the acquisition, analysis, or interpretation of data. WJJ and JHY drafted the manuscript. WJJ, YHC, and JHY contributed to critical revision of the manuscript for important intellectual content. WJJ and JHY performed statistical analysis. SHC and JHY were responsible for study supervision. All authors gave final approval of the version to be published and agreed to be accountable for all aspects of the work, thereby ensuring that questions related to the accuracy or integrity of any part of the work are appropriately investigated and resolved. All authors read and approved the final manuscript.

Author details

[1] Division of Cardiology, Department of Internal Medicine, Samsung Changwon Hospital, Sungkyunkwan University School of Medicine, Changwon, Republic of Korea. [2] Department of Thoracic and Cardiovascular Surgery, Samsung Medical Center, Sungkyunkwan University School of Medicine, Seoul, Republic of Korea. [3] Division of Cardiology, Department of Critical Care Medicine and Medicine, Heart Vascular Stroke Institute, Samsung Medical Center, Sungkyunkwan University School of Medicine, 81, Irwon-dong, Gangnam-gu, Seoul 135-710, Republic of Korea.

Acknowledgements

None.

Competing interests

The authors declare that they have no competing interests.

Funding

None.

References

1. Kar B, Gregoric ID, Basra SS, Idelchik GM, Loyalka P. The percutaneous ventricular assist device in severe refractory cardiogenic shock. J Am Coll Cardiol. 2011;57:688–96.
2. Lamb KM, DiMuzio PJ, Johnson A, Batista P, Moudgill N, McCullough M, et al. Arterial protocol including prophylactic distal perfusion catheter decreases limb ischemia complications in patients undergoing extracorporeal membrane oxygenation. J Vasc Surg. 2017;65:1074–9.
3. Bisdas T, Beutel G, Warnecke G, Hoeper MM, Kuehn C, Haverich A, et al. Vascular complications in patients undergoing femoral cannulation for extracorporeal membrane oxygenation support. Ann Thorac Surg. 2011;92:626–31.
4. Huang SC, Yu HY, Ko WJ, Chen YS. Pressure criterion for placement of distal perfusion catheter to prevent limb ischemia during adult extracorporeal life support. J Thorac Cardiovasc Surg. 2004;128:776–7.
5. Foley PJ, Morris RJ, Woo EY, Acker MA, Wang GJ, Fairman RM, et al. Limb ischemia during femoral cannulation for cardiopulmonary support. J Vasc Surg. 2010;52:850–3.

6. Aziz F, Brehm CE, El-Banyosy A, Han DC, Atnip RG, Reed AB. Arterial complications in patients undergoing extracorporeal membrane oxygenation via femoral cannulation. Ann Vasc Surg. 2014;28:178–83.
7. Zimpfer D, Heinisch B, Czerny M, Hoelzenbein T, Taghavi S, Wolner E, et al. Late vascular complications after extracorporeal membrane oxygenation support. Ann Thorac Surg. 2006;81:892–5.
8. Park TK, Yang JH, Jeon K, Choi SH, Choi JH, Gwon HC, et al. Extracorporeal membrane oxygenation for refractory septic shock in adults. Eur J Cardiothorac Surg. 2015;47:e68–74.
9. Ranney DN, Benrashid E, Meza JM, Keenan JE, Bonadonna D, Mureebe L, et al. Vascular complications and use of a distal perfusion cannula in femorally cannulated patients on extracorporeal membrane oxygenation. ASAIO J. 2018;64:328–33.
10. Muehrcke DD, McCarthy PM, Stewart RW, Seshagiri S, Ogella DA, Foster RC, et al. Complications of extracorporeal life support systems using heparin-bound surfaces. The risk of intracardiac clot formation. J Thorac Cardiovasc Surg. 1995;110:843–51.

Permissions

All chapters in this book were first published in AIC, by Springer; hereby published with permission under the Creative Commons Attribution License or equivalent. Every chapter published in this book has been scrutinized by our experts. Their significance has been extensively debated. The topics covered herein carry significant findings which will fuel the growth of the discipline. They may even be implemented as practical applications or may be referred to as a beginning point for another development.

The contributors of this book come from diverse backgrounds, making this book a truly international effort. This book will bring forth new frontiers with its revolutionizing research information and detailed analysis of the nascent developments around the world.

We would like to thank all the contributing authors for lending their expertise to make the book truly unique. They have played a crucial role in the development of this book. Without their invaluable contributions this book wouldn't have been possible. They have made vital efforts to compile up to date information on the varied aspects of this subject to make this book a valuable addition to the collection of many professionals and students.

This book was conceptualized with the vision of imparting up-to-date information and advanced data in this field. To ensure the same, a matchless editorial board was set up. Every individual on the board went through rigorous rounds of assessment to prove their worth. After which they invested a large part of their time researching and compiling the most relevant data for our readers.

The editorial board has been involved in producing this book since its inception. They have spent rigorous hours researching and exploring the diverse topics which have resulted in the successful publishing of this book. They have passed on their knowledge of decades through this book. To expedite this challenging task, the publisher supported the team at every step. A small team of assistant editors was also appointed to further simplify the editing procedure and attain best results for the readers.

Apart from the editorial board, the designing team has also invested a significant amount of their time in understanding the subject and creating the most relevant covers. They scrutinized every image to scout for the most suitable representation of the subject and create an appropriate cover for the book.

The publishing team has been an ardent support to the editorial, designing and production team. Their endless efforts to recruit the best for this project, has resulted in the accomplishment of this book. They are a veteran in the field of academics and their pool of knowledge is as vast as their experience in printing. Their expertise and guidance has proved useful at every step. Their uncompromising quality standards have made this book an exceptional effort. Their encouragement from time to time has been an inspiration for everyone.

The publisher and the editorial board hope that this book will prove to be a valuable piece of knowledge for researchers, students, practitioners and scholars across the globe.

List of Contributors

Oliver Karam
Pediatric Intensive Care Unit, Geneva University Hospital, Geneva, Switzerland
Univ. Lille, EA 2694 - Santé Publique: épidémiologie et qualité des soins, 59000 Lille, France

Pierre Demaret
Univ. Lille, EA 2694 - Santé Publique: épidémiologie et qualité des soins, 59000 Lille, France
Pediatric Intensive Care Unit, CHC Liège, Liège, Belgium

Alain Duhamel
Univ. Lille, EA 2694 - Santé Publique: épidémiologie et qualité des soins, 59000 Lille, France
Department of Biostatistics, CHU Lille, 59000 Lille, France

Alison Shefler
Pediatric Intensive Care Unit, Oxford University Hospitals, Oxford, UK

Philip C. Spinella
Division of Critical Care, Department of Pediatrics, Washington University in St. Louis, St. Louis, MO, USA

Simon J. Stanworth
NHS Blood and Transplant, John Radcliffe Hospital, Oxford, UK

Marisa Tucci
Pediatric Intensive Care Unit, CHU Sainte-Justine, Montreal, Canada

Stéphane Leteurtre
Univ. Lille, EA 2694 - Santé Publique: épidémiologie et qualité des soins, 59000 Lille, France
Pediatric Intensive Care Unit, CHU Lille, 59000 Lille, France

Cécile Aubron
The Australian and New Zealand Intensive Care Research Centre, Department of Epidemiology and Preventive Medicine, Monash University, Melbourne, Australia
The Transfusion Research Unit, Department of Epidemiology and Preventive Medicine, Monash University, Melbourne, Australia
Medical Intensive Care Unit, Centre Hospitalier Régional et Universitaire de Brest, site La Cavale Blanche, Bvd Tanguy Prigent, 29609 Brest Cedex, France
LUBEM, EA 3882 - Université de Bretagne Occidentale, 29 200 Brest, France

Joris DePuydt
The Intensive Care Unit, The Alfred Hospital, Melbourne, Australia
University Hospital of Antwerp, 2000 Antwerp, Belgium

Carlos Scheinkestel, Vincent Pellegrino and Deirdre Murphy
The Intensive Care Unit, The Alfred Hospital, Melbourne, Australia
School of Public Health and Preventive Medicine, Monash University, Melbourne, Australia

Matthieu Schmidt
The Australian and New Zealand Intensive Care Research Centre, Department of Epidemiology and Preventive Medicine, Monash University, Melbourne, Australia
Medical Intensive Care Unit, iCAN, Institute of Cardiometabolism and Nutrition, Hôpital de la Pitié–Salpetrière, Assistance Publique–Hôpitaux de Paris, Paris, France

Marie-Alix Espinasse, Armelle Biola-Vidamment, Benoît Noël and Marc Pallardy
INSERM UMR-996 - Inflammation, Chemokines and Immunopathology, Univ Paris-Sud, Faculté de pharmacie, Université Paris-Saclay, 5 rue JB Clément, 92296 Châtenay-Malabry Cedex, France

Vanessa Granger, Luc de Chaisemartin and Sylvie Chollet-Martin
INSERM UMR-996 - Inflammation, Chemokines and Immunopathology, Univ Paris-Sud, Faculté de pharmacie, Université Paris-Saclay, 5 rue JB Clément, 92296 Châtenay-Malabry Cedex, France
Laboratoire d'immunologie, «Autoimmunité et hypersensibilités», Hôpital Bichat-Claude Bernard, AP-HP, Paris, France

Philippe Montravers, Pascale Piednoir and Guillaume Dufour
Département d'Anesthésie-Réanimation, Hôpital Bichat-Claude Bernard, AP-HP, Paris, France
Université Paris Diderot, Sorbonne Paris Cité, Paris, France

David Hajage and Florence Tubach
Département d'Epidémiologie et Recherche Clinique, Assistance Publique-Hôpitaux de Paris Hôpital Bichat, INSERM, CIE 801, Université Paris Diderot, Sorbonne Paris Cité, Paris, France

Konstantin A Popugaev, Ivan A Savin, Andrew U Lubnin, Alexander S Goriachev, Boris A Kadashev, Pavel L Kalinin, Andrew V Oshorov, Alexander A Polupan, Ekaterina U Sokolova, Maxim A Kutin and Valeriy I Lukianov
Department of Neurological Intensive Care Unit (NICU), Burdenko Neurosurgical Research Institute, 16 4th Tverskaya-Yamskaya, Moscow, 125047, Russia

Michael Bailey
The Australian and New Zealand Intensive Care Research Centre, Department of Epidemiology and Preventive Medicine, Monash University, Melbourne, Australia

Zoe McQuilten
The Australian and New Zealand Intensive Care Research Centre, Department of Epidemiology and Preventive Medicine, Monash University, Melbourne, Australia
The Transfusion Research Unit, Department of Epidemiology and Preventive Medicine, Monash University, Melbourne, Australia

D Jamie Cooper and David Pilcher
The Australian and New Zealand Intensive Care Research Centre, Department of Epidemiology and Preventive Medicine, Monash University, Melbourne, Australia
The Intensive Care Unit, The Alfred Hospital, Melbourne, Australia

Jayne Sheldrake
The Intensive Care Unit, The Alfred Hospital, Melbourne, Australia

Gilles Capellier and François Belon
The Intensive Care Unit, Jean Minjoz Hospital, 25030 Besançon, France

Pedro Vitale Mendes, Eduardo Leite Vieira Costa and Luciano Cesar Pontes Azevedo
Intensive Care Unit, Hospital das Clinicas, University of São Paulo School of Medicine, Rua Dr. Enéas Carvalho de Aguiar, 255, Sala 5023, São Paulo, SP 05403000, Brazil
Research and Education Institute, Hospital Sírio-Libanês, São Paulo, Brazil

Cesar de Albuquerque Gallo, Bruno Adler Maccagnan Pinheiro Besen, Adriana Sayuri Hirota, Raquel de Oliveira Nardi, Edzangela Vasconcelos dos Santos, Ho Yeh Li, Daniel Joelsons, Flavia Krepel Foronda and Marcelo Park
Research and Education Institute, Hospital Sírio-Libanês, São Paulo, Brazil

Jinfeng Luo, Jing Xue, Jin Liu, Bin Liu, Li Liu and Guo Chen
Department of Anesthesiology and Translational Neuroscience Center, West China Hospital, Sichuan University, No. 37 Guoxue Xiang, Wuhou District, Chengdu 610041, Sichuan, People's Republic of China

Sergi Vaquer, Candelaria de Haro, Paula Peruga and Antonio Artigas
Critical Care Center, CIBER de Enfermedades Respiratorias, Corporació Sanitària Universitària Parc Taulí, Autonomous University of Barcelona, Parc Taulí 1, 08208 Sabadell, Spain

Joan Carles Oliva
Fundació Parc Taulí, Parc Taulí University Institute, Parc Taulí 1, 08208 Sabadell, Spain

Lise Piquilloud and Alain Mercat
CHU d'Angers, 4 rue Larrey, 49000 Angers, France
Medical Intensive Care Department, University Hospital, Angers, France

Pierre-Yves Olivier, François Beloncle, Nicolas Lerolle and Pierre Asfar
CHU d'Angers, 4 rue Larrey, 49000 Angers, France
Medical Intensive Care Department, University Hospital, Angers, France
BNMI Laboratory, CNRS UMR 6214—INSERM U1083, Angers University, Angers, France

Valérie Seegers
CHU d'Angers, 4 rue Larrey, 49000 Angers, France
Statistical Department, University Hospital, Angers, France

Paul Cales
CHU d'Angers, 4 rue Larrey, 49000 Angers, France
HIFIH, UPRE-EA 3859, SFR 4208, LUNAM University, Angers, France

Maher Tabka, Mathilde Renou de La Bourdonnaye and Daniel Henrion
BNMI Laboratory, CNRS UMR 6214—INSERM U1083, Angers University, Angers, France
Faculté de medicine d'Angers, 4 rue haute de reculée, 49000 Angers, France

Peter Radermacher
Universitätsklinikum, Ulm Helmholtzstr. 8/1, 89081 Ulm, Germany
Institut für Anästhesiologische Pathophysiologie und Verfahrensentwicklung, Universitätsklinikum, Ulm, Germany

Xuefeng Xu
National Clinical Research Centre for Respiratory Diseases, Beijing Hospital, Beijing 100730, China
Department of Surgical Intensive Care Medicine, Beijing An Zhen Hospital, Capital Medical University, No. 2 Anzhen Rd., Chao-Yang District, Beijing 100029, China

Chen Wang
National Clinical Research Centre for Respiratory Diseases, Beijing Hospital, Beijing 100730, China
Department of Pulmonary and Critical Care Medicine, China-Japan Friendship Hospital, 2 Yinghua Dongjie, Beijing 100029, China

Yanming Li
National Clinical Research Centre for Respiratory Diseases, Beijing Hospital, Beijing 100730, China
Department of Pulmonary and Critical Care Medicine, Beijing Hospital, Beijing 100730, China

Fei Xiao
National Clinical Research Centre for Respiratory Diseases, Beijing Hospital, Beijing 100730, China
Key Laboratory of Geriatrics, Beijing Hospital and Beijing Institute of Geriatrics, Ministry of Health, Beijing, China

Chune Jia, Sa Luo and Huaping Dai
Department of Pulmonary and Critical Care Medicine, China-Japan Friendship Hospital, 2 Yinghua Dongjie, Beijing 100029, China

Dominik Jarczak
Department of Intensive Care Medicine, University Medical Center Hamburg- Eppendorf, Martinistraße 52, 20246 Hamburg, Germany

Alexander Spiel
Department of Intensive Care Medicine, University Medical Center Hamburg- Eppendorf, Martinistraße 52, 20246 Hamburg, Germany
Department of Emergency Medicine, Medical University of Vienna, Vienna, Austria

Christian Wallmüller, Peter Stratil, Pia Hubner, Christoph Weiser, Harald Herkner and Fritz Sterz
Department of Emergency Medicine, Medical University of Vienna, Vienna, Austria

Kevin Roedl, Andreas Drolz, Thomas Horvatits, Karoline Rutter and Valentin Fuhrmann
Department of Intensive Care Medicine, University Medical Center Hamburg- Eppendorf, Martinistraße 52, 20246 Hamburg, Germany
Division of Gastroenterology and Hepatology, Department of Internal Medicine 3, Medical University of Vienna, Vienna, Austria

Julia Ortbauer and Jasmin Katrin Motaabbed
Division of Gastroenterology and Hepatology, Department of Internal Medicine 3, Medical University of Vienna, Vienna, Austria

Guillemette Thomas, Christophe Guervilly, Mélanie Adda and Stéphanie Dizier
Hôpital Nord, Réanimation des Détresses Respiratoires et des Infections Sévères, Assistance Publique–Hôpitaux de Marseille, 13015 Marseille, France

Sami Hraiech, Samuel Lehingue, Romain Rambaud, Fanny Klasen, Laurent Papazian and Jean-Marie Forel
Hôpital Nord, Réanimation des Détresses Respiratoires et des Infections Sévères, Assistance Publique–Hôpitaux de Marseille, 13015 Marseille, France
URMITE, UMR CNRS 7278, Faculté de Médecine, Aix-Marseille Université, 13005 Marseille, France

Antoine Roch
URMITE, UMR CNRS 7278, Faculté de Médecine, Aix-Marseille Université, 13005 Marseille, France
Hôpital Nord, Service des Urgences, Assistance Publique–Hôpitaux de Marseille, 13015 Marseille, France

Nadim Cassir
URMITE, UMR CNRS 7278, Faculté de Médecine, Aix-Marseille Université, 13005 Marseille, France

Sandrine Wiramus
Hôpital de la Conception, Réanimation des brulés Assistance Publique–Hôpitaux de Marseille, 13005 Marseille, France

Song-qiao Liu, Qin Sun, Jian-feng Xie, Jing-yuan Xu, Qing Li, Chun Pan, Ling Liu and Ying-zi Huang
Department of Critical Care Medicine, Zhongda Hospital, School of Medicine, Southeast University, No. 87, Dingjiaqiao Road, Gulou District, Nanjing 210009, China

Yi Zheng
Department of Critical Care Medicine, Zhongda Hospital, School of Medicine, Southeast University, No. 87, Dingjiaqiao Road, Gulou District, Nanjing 210009, China
Department of Critical Care Medicine, The First Affiliated Hospital of Medical School of Zhejiang University, 79 Qingchun Road, Shangcheng District, Hangzhou 310003, China

Izumi Nakayama
Intensive Care Unit, Department of Internal Medicine, Okinawa Chubu Hospital, 281 Miyazato, Uruma, Okinawa 904-2293, Japan

Junichi Izawa
Intensive Care Unit, Department of Anesthesiology, The Jikei University School of Medicine, 3-19-18 Nishi-Shinbashi, Minato-ku, Tokyo 105-8471, Japan
The Center for Critical Care Nephrology, Clinical Research, Investigation, and Systems Modeling of Acute Illness Center, Department of Critical Care Medicine, University of Pittsburgh School of Medicine, Pittsburgh, PA 15213, USA

Hideyuki Mouri and Junji Shiotsuka
Department of Anesthesiology and Critical Care, Jichi Medical University, Saitama Medical Center, 1-847 Amanuma, Oomiya-ku, Saitama, Saitama 330-8503, Japan

Tetsuhisa Kitamura
Division of Environmental Medicine and Population Sciences, Department of Social and Environmental Medicine, Graduate School of Medicine, Osaka University, 1-1 Yamada-oka, Suita, Osaka 565-0871, Japan

Valentina Girotto, Jean-Louis Teboul, Alexandra Beurton, Laura Galarza, Christian Richard and Xavier Monnet
Service de Réanimation Médicale, Hôpital de Bicêtre, Hôpitaux Universitaires Paris-Sud, Insert UMR_999, Université Paris-Sud, Assistance Publique - Hôpitaux de Paris, Le Kremlin-Bicêtre, France

Thierry Guedj
Service de Radiologie, Hôpital de Bicêtre, Hôpitaux Universitaires Paris-Sud, Assistance Publique - Hôpitaux de Paris, Le Kremlin-Bicêtre, France

Constance Vuillard, Olivier Pajot, Hervé Mentec, Gaëtan Plantefève and Damien Contou
Service de Réanimation Polyvalente, Centre Hospitalier Victor Dupouy, 69 rue du Lieutenant Colonel Prudhon, 95100 Argenteuil, France

Marc Pineton de Chambrun and Matthieu Schmidt
Service de Réanimation Médicale, Centre Hospitalier Universitaire Pitié-Salpétrière - Assistance Publique Hôpitaux de Paris, 47-83 boulevard de l'Hôpital, 75013 Paris, France

Nicolas de Prost
Service de Réanimation Médicale, Centre Hospitalier Universitaire Henri Mondor - Assistance Publique Hôpitaux de Paris, 51 avenue du Maréchal de Lattre de Tassigny, 94010 Créteil, France

Claude Guérin
Service de Réanimation Médicale, Hôpital de la Croix-Rousse, 103 Grande rue de la Croix-Rousse, 69004 Lyon, France
INSERM 955, Créteil, France

Auguste Dargent and Jean-Pierre Quenot
Service de Médecine Intensive Réanimation, Centre Hospitalier Universitaire François Mitterrand de Dijon, 14 rue Paul Gaffarel, 21000 Dijon, France

Sébastien Préau and Geoffrey Ledoux
Service de Réanimation, Centre Hospitalier Régional Universitaire de Lille, 2 avenue Oscar Lambret, 59000 Lille, France

Mathilde Neuville
Service de Réanimation Médicale, Centre Hospitalier Universitaire Bichat Claude-Bernard - Assistance Publique Hôpitaux de Paris, 46 rue Henri Huchard, 75877 Paris, France

Guillaume Voiriot and Muriel Fartoukh
Service de Réanimation médico-chirurgicale, Centre Hospitalier Universitaire Tenon - Assistance Publique Hôpitaux de Paris, 5 rue de la Chine, 75020 Paris, France

Rémi Coudroy
Service de Réanimation médicale, Centre hospitalier universitaire de Poitiers, 2 rue de la Milétrie, 86021 Poitiers, France

Guillaume Dumas and Eric Maury
Service de Réanimation médicale, Centre Hospitalier Universitaire Saint-Antoine - Assistance Publique Hôpitaux de Paris, 184 rue du Faubourg Saint-Antoine, 75012 Paris, France

Nicolas Terzi
Service de Réanimation, Centre Hospitalier Universitaire de Grenoble Alpes, avenue Maquis du Grésivaudan, 38700 La Tronche, France

Yacine Tandjaoui-Lambiotte
Service de Réanimation médico-chirurgicale, Centre Hospitalier Universitaire Avicennes - Assistance Publique Hôpitaux de Paris, 125 rue de Stalingrad, 93000 Bobigny, France

Francis Schneider
Service de Réanimation, Centre Hospitalier Universitaire de Strasbourg, 1 avenue Molière, 67200 Strasbourg, France

Maximilien Grall
Service de Réanimation Médicale, Centre Hospitalier Universitaire de Rouen, 1 rue de Germont, 76000 Rouen, France

Emmanuel Guérot
Service de Réanimation Médicale, Centre Hospitalier Universitaire Hôpital Européen Georges-Pompidou - Assistance Publique Hôpitaux de Paris, 20 rue Leblanc, 75015 Paris, France

Romaric Larcher
Service de Réanimation Médicale, Centre Hospitalier Universitaire de Montpellier, 191 avenue du Doyen Gaston Giraud, 34000 Montpellier, France

Sylvie Ricome
Service de Réanimation Polyvalente, Centre Hospitalier Robert-Ballanger, Boulevard Robert Ballanger, 93600 Aulnay-sous-Bois, France

Raphaël Le Mao
Service de Réanimation médicale, Centre Hospitalier Régional Universistaire de Brest, Site La Cavale Blanche, Boulevard Tanguy Prigent, 29200 Brest, France

Gwenhaël Colin
Service de réanimation médico-chirurgicale, Centre Hospitalier Départemental de Vendée, Les Oudairies, 85925 La Roche sur Yon Cedex 9, France

Christophe Guitton
Service de Réanimation médico-chirurgicale, Centre Hospitalier du Mans, 194 avenue Rubillard, 72037 Le Mans, France

Lara Zafrani
Service de Réanimation médicale, Hôpital Saint-Louis, Assistance Publique Hôpitaux de Paris, 1 avenue Claude Vellefaux, 75010 Paris, France

Elise Morawiec
Unité de Réanimation et de Surveillance continue, Service de Pneumologie et Réanimation médicale, Groupe hospitalier Pitié-Salpêtrière, 47-83 bd de l'hôpital, 75651 Paris, France

Marie Dubert
Service d'Immunologie Clinique, Hôpital Saint-Louis, Assistance Publique Hôpitaux de Paris, 1 avenue Claude Vellefaux, 75010 Paris, France

Christian Lemaire
Medical-Surgical ICU, Medical Center, Roubaix, France

Bertrand Sauneuf
Medical-Surgical ICU, Medical Center, Cherbourg, France

Hervé Dupont
Department of Anesthesiology and Critical Care and INSERM U1088, University Hospital, Amiens, France

Fabienne Tamion
Medical ICU, University Hospital, Rouen, France

Saad Nseir
Medical ICU, University Hospital, Lille, France

Damien Du Cheyron
Medical ICU, University Hospital, Caen, France

F. Sanfilippo
Department of Anesthesia and Intensive Care, IRCCS-ISMETT (Istituto Mediterraneo per i Trapianti e Terapie ad alta specializzazione), Palermo, Italy

S. Scolletta
Unit of Intensive Care Medicine, Department of Medical Biotechnologies, University of Siena, Siena, Italy

A. Morelli
Department of Anaesthesiology and Intensive Care, University of Rome, "La Sapienza", Rome, Italy

A. Vieillard-Baron
Hospital Ambroise Paré, Assistance Publique-Hôpitaux de Paris, Boulogne, France

Nicolas S. Marjanovic
Emergency Department and Prehospital Care, University Hospital of Poitiers, 86000 Poitiers, France
CIC1402 U5 ALIVE - University Hospital of Poitiers, 86000 Poitiers, France
ABS-Lab - Laboratory of Anatomy, Biomechanics and Simulation, Poitiers University, School of Medicine, 86000 Poitiers, France

Christelle Teiten
Emergency Department, University Hospital of Brest - La Cavale Blanche, 29609 Brest Cedex, France

Nicola Pallamin
B-com, Institute of Research and Technology, Brest University, 29609 Brest Cedex, France

Erwan L'Her
Department of Intensive Care Medicine, University Hospital of Brest - La Cavale Blanche, Boulevard Tanguy Prigent, 29609 Brest Cedex, France
CeSIM/LaTIM UMR 1101, Western Brittany University - School of Medicine, Rue Camille Desmoulins, 29200 Brest, France

Pierre-Louis Declercq, Stéphanie Gelinotte, Kévin Guernon, Jean-Baptiste Michot, Vincent Royon, Dorothée Carpentier and Fabienne Tamion
Department of Medical Intensive Care, Rouen University Hospital, Rouen Cedex, France

Michael Bubenheim
Department of Clinical Research Support, Biostatistics Unit, Rouen University Hospital, Rouen Cedex, France

Gaëtan Béduneau
Department of Medical Intensive Care, Rouen University Hospital, Rouen Cedex, France
UPRES EA 3830-IRIB, Institute for Biomedical Research, Rouen University, Rouen Cedex, France

Christophe Girault
Department of Medical Intensive Care, Rouen University Hospital, Rouen Cedex, France
UPRES EA 3830-IRIB, Institute for Biomedical Research, Rouen University, Rouen Cedex, France
Service de Réanimation Médicale, Hôpital Charles Nicolle, Centre Hospitalier Universitaire-Hôpitaux de Rouen, 1, Rue de Germont, 76031 Rouen Cedex, France

Julien Maizel and Marie-Anaïs Bastide
Medical ICU and INSERM U1088, University Hospital, Amiens, France

Jack Richecoeur
Medical-Surgical ICU, Medical Center, Beauvais, France

Eric Frenoy
Medical-Surgical ICU, Medical Center, Le Havre, France

Yan Xu
Department of Nephrology, The Affiliated Hospital of Qingdao University, Shandong 266003, People's Republic of China

Cong-juan Luo
Department of Nephrology, The Affiliated Hospital of Qingdao University, Shandong 266003, People's Republic of China
State Key Laboratory of Kidney Diseases, Department of Nephrology, Chinese PLA General Hospital and Medical School of Chinese PLA, No.28 Fuxing Road, Beijing 100853, People's Republic of China

Feng Luo
Department of Nephrology, The Affiliated Hospital of Qingdao University, Shandong 266003, People's Republic of China
Department of Cardiology, Liaocheng People's Hospital, Shandong 252000, People's Republic of China

Li Zhang, Guang-yan Cai, Bo Fu, Zhe Feng, Xue-feng Sun and Xiang-mei Chen
Department of Cardiology, Liaocheng People's Hospital, Shandong 252000, People's Republic of China

Helder Marcus Costa Rocha, Henrique Tadashi Katayama, Leandro Ferreira Dias, Mateus Barros de Paula, Leusi Magda Romano Andraus and Jose Maria Correa Silva
Hospital Servidor Publico Estadual-SP, Rua Pedro de Toledo, 1800/6º A–Vila Clementino, São Paulo, SP 04039-901, Brazil

João M. Silva Jr. and Luiz Marcelo Sá Malbouisson
Hospital Servidor Publico Estadual-SP, Rua Pedro de Toledo, 1800/6º A–Vila Clementino, São Paulo, SP 04039-901, Brazil
Anaesthesiology Department, Hospital das Clinicas SP-FMUSP, Av. Dr. Enéas de Carvalho Aguiar, 255 Cerqueira César, São Paulo, SP 05403-000, Brazil

Woo Jin Jang, Woo Jung Chun and Ju Hyeon Oh
Division of Cardiology, Department of Internal Medicine, Samsung Changwon Hospital, Sungkyunkwan University School of Medicine, Changwon, Republic of Korea

Yang Hyun Cho
Department of Thoracic and Cardiovascular Surgery, Samsung Medical Center, Sungkyunkwan University School of Medicine, Seoul, Republic of Korea

Taek Kyu Park, Young Bin Song, Jin-Oh Choi, Joo-Yong Hahn, Seung-Hyuk Choi, Hyeon-Cheol Gwon, Eun-Seok Jeon and Jeong Hoon Yang
Division of Cardiology, Department of Critical Care Medicine and Medicine, Heart Vascular Stroke Institute, Samsung Medical Center, Sungkyunkwan University School of Medicine, 81, Irwon-dong, Gangnam-gu, Seoul 135-710, Republic of Korea

Index

A

Abdominal Compartment Syndrome, 37, 42-44

Acetaminophen, 77, 86

Acute Tubular Necrosis, 188-189

Airway Scope, 154-155, 160-166

Anti-synthetase, 122-123, 125-132

Autoimmune Inflammatory Myopathies, 122-123, 130

B

Bacteremia, 72, 80, 88-95, 195

Bloodstream Infection, 26, 68, 70-73, 88-89, 91-94

C

Cardiac Arrest, 48, 89-90, 146, 186, 205-210, 212-213

Cardiopulmonary Resuscitation, 47, 205, 212, 224, 226

Cardiovascular Anesthesiologists, 184, 187

Carotid Blood Flow, 100, 103, 214-215, 217-220

Cecal Ligation And Puncture, 99, 188-189, 191, 196-197

Central Venous Catheter, 49, 68, 73-75, 180, 183-187

Charlson Comorbidity Index, 206-207, 209-210, 212

Conservative Therapy, 37, 41-42

Crystalloid Solution, 8-10, 104

Cytokine Storm, 105-107, 114, 116, 119, 121

Cytoplasmic Protein, 77

D

Device-related Infections, 67, 72

Diastolic Function, 134-135, 137-138, 140-145

Diencephalon Dysfunction, 37-38, 41-43

Distal Perfusion Catheter, 222-223, 225-228

E

End-stage Liver Disease, 79, 81, 86, 206, 208, 212-213

Endotracheal Intubation, 146-147, 152-154, 160-165

Epithelial Cells, 62, 188, 196

Extracorporeal Life Support, 2-4, 6-7, 16, 18, 22, 24-25, 31-32, 35-36, 45, 47, 51, 53-54, 67, 74-76, 228-229

Extracorporeal Membrane Oxygenation, 7, 15-17, 20-25, 35-36, 45-46, 49, 53-54, 56, 59, 62, 65-67, 70-71, 74-75, 167, 171, 177, 222-223, 226-229

F

Fatty Acid-binding Proteins, 78, 86

Femoral Artery Blood Flow, 214

Femorally Cannulated Patients, 222, 227, 229

G

Gastrointestinal Dysmotility, 37-38

Gene Expression, 55, 57-59, 62, 168

Glucocorticoid-induced Leucine Zipper, 55-56, 60-61, 65-66

Goal-directed Fluid Therapy, 8, 12, 14

H

Haemorrhage, 31, 33, 35, 45-46, 49, 52, 210

Hepatic Encephalopathy, 77, 81, 86, 208, 211

Hypotension, 8-9, 21, 44, 97, 99-100, 103

I

Inflammatory Myositis, 122, 124, 126, 129

Intensive Care Units, 25, 35, 98, 132, 177, 187, 203, 205, 221

Interstitial Lung Disease, 122-123, 130, 132-133

Intra-abdominal Hypertension, 37, 40, 42-44

L

Limb Ischemia, 222-225, 227-228

Liver Cirrhosis, 205-207, 209-212

Low Cardiac Index, 8, 10

M

Mechanical Ventilation, 3-4, 10, 15-20, 24-25, 32, 35-36, 40-41, 43, 47, 49, 56, 61-62, 66-69, 74, 80-86, 123, 127, 135, 137, 139-141, 144, 167, 169, 171, 206-207, 226

Membrane Oxygenator, 22, 68, 72

Mesenchymal Stem Cells, 167-168, 177-178, 197

Metabolic Acidosis, 97-98, 103-104

Multiple Organ Dysfunction, 1, 6, 37, 40, 43, 174, 197, 203

N

Neutrophil Infiltration, 188, 191-192, 194-197

Neutrophils, 55-63, 65-66, 116, 120, 124, 126, 128, 189, 193, 195-196

O

Oxygen Saturation, 147, 155, 199

P

Passive Leg Raising, 144, 214, 217-219, 221

Pediatric Intensive Care Unit, 1, 6, 203

Plasma Exchange, 122-123, 127-128, 130

Plasma Transfusion, 1-3, 5-7, 69, 71

Porcine Model, 66, 105-107, 118, 121

Proinflammatory Cytokines, 66, 114, 188, 195-196

Pulmonary Edema, 10, 12, 106-107, 114, 120-121, 123, 134, 140-143, 167

Q

Quick Sequential Organ Failure Assessment, 88, 90-95

R

Randomized Controlled Trials, 2, 14-15, 25, 34, 144

Renal Hemodynamics, 97, 101-103

S

Sellar Region Tumors, 37, 43

Sepsis, 2, 7, 12, 35, 37-38, 40-44, 58-59, 61-62, 65-66, 69, 75, 88-99, 101-104, 106-107, 114, 118, 120-121, 123, 125, 130, 132, 173, 175, 177-178, 188-189, 213-214, 221

Septic Shock, 2, 6-7, 13, 17, 56, 58-59, 65-66, 69, 89, 94-98, 103-104, 106, 121, 135, 140-142, 144-145, 170, 173, 197, 217, 226, 229

Sinus Rhythm, 140, 147

Sodium Chloride, 97, 104

Superficial Femoral Artery, 215, 222, 225, 228

Systemic Inflammatory Response Syndrome, 46, 89, 94-96

Systolic Velocities, 214, 221

T

Thoracic Epidural Anesthesia, 37-38, 44

Thromboembolic Events, 45, 47

Tissue Doppler Imaging, 134-135, 138, 143

Transesophageal Echocardiography, 135, 143

Tumor Necrosis Factor, 121, 177, 188, 191, 193

V

Vascular Endothelial Cells, 167-168, 170, 177

Ventilator-induced Lung Injury, 25, 144

Video-laryngoscopes, 154-155, 165

W

Weaning Failure, 134, 141, 144

www.ingramcontent.com/pod-product-compliance
Lightning Source LLC
LaVergne TN
LVHW080915210926
848485LV00004B/655